Applied Pathophysiology for Occupational Therapy

A Guide for Clinical Decision Making

Applied Pathophysiology for Occupational Therapy

A Guide for Clinical Decision Making

Natalie Norman Michaels, PT, EdD, GCS Emeritus

Professor, School of Occupational Therapy
College of Pharmacy and Health Sciences
Belmont University
Nashville, Tennessee
United States

Sandy Stevens, PhD, OTR/L

Assistant Professor, School of Occupational Therapy
College of Pharmacy and Health Sciences
Belmont University
Nashville, Tennessee
United States

Roya Rezadoost, OTD, OTR/L

Occupational Therapist
Pediatric Therapist, Early Childhood
School-Based Intervention
Belmont University
United States

Ashley Rabuck, OTD, OTR/L, CSRS

Occupational Therapist
Certified Stroke Rehab Specialist
Inpatient Rehabilitation
Neonatal Occupational Therapy Services
Belmont University
United States

ELSEVIER

Elsevier
3251 Riverport Lane
St. Louis, Missouri 63043

APPLIED PATHOPHYSIOLOGY FOR OCCUPATIONAL THERAPY: A GUIDE FOR CLINICAL DECISION MAKING

ISBN: 978-0-443-12078-7

Content Strategist: Laura Klein
Senior Content Development Specialist: Shilpa Kumar/Priyadarshini Pandey
Publishing Services Manager: Deepthi Unni
Senior Project Manager: Beula Christopher
Senior Book Designer: Brian Salisbury

Printed in India

Last digit is the print number: 9 8 7 6 5 4 3 2 1

This book is dedicated to the memories of those who have been inspirational individuals in our lives in days past and to those still living who continue to inspire us each and every day.
Dedicated to the memory of Pauline Norman, Rudy Norman, Lillian Michaels, Charles Michaels, Donald Potter, Roycana Potter, Mahmoud Rezadoost, and Malihe Sayahi.

Those inspirational to **Dr. Natalie Norman Michaels***:*
I wish to dedicate this book to my caring, loving, and handsome husband, Richard Michaels; my fun and extremely supportive kids, Heather Marie Slaughter, Thomas Mark Housel, Tiffany Rae Housel, Austin Michaels, and Alexandra Michaels, COTA; my inspiration, Catherine C. Goodman; my patient co-authors, Roya Rezadoost and Ashley Rabuck; and my co-author, forever friend, and intellectual confidant, Sandy Stevens.

Those inspirational to **Dr. Sandy Stevens***:*
I wish to dedicate this book to my supportive friends and family and celebrate a friendship with Natalie Michaels who keeps both of us grounded, productive, and excited in the quest to educate others about the power of health care and occupational therapy.

Those inspirational to **Dr. Roya Rezadoost***:*
I wish to dedicate this book to my beautiful and loving partner, Audrey, thank you for your unwavering support, encouragement, and love. To my parents, Debbie and Mir, thank you for instilling in me the values of hard work, perseverance, passion, kindness, and respect, and for always cheering me on. To my brothers, Jonathan and Justin, and sisters-in-law, Olivia and Megan, thank you for seeing the importance of this profession and always supporting me in my career and life. To Amy Neal, who introduced me to occupational therapy, thank you for seeing something special in me and encouraging me to pursue this beautiful profession. To my best friends, both near and far, thank you for your companionship, laughter, and steadfast belief in my dreams. To current and future occupational therapists, may your passion for this world continue to burn bright.

Those inspirational to **Dr. Ashley Rabuck***:*
I wish to dedicate this book to my grandparents, Leo and Stephanie Gordon, my very best friends, for their insurmountable love, support, encouragement, guidance, confidence, and dedication to friendly competition over nail-biting card games; to all other family members, close friends, patients, and colleagues, both near and far, past and present, thank you for molding me into the human, friend, and clinician I am today; and to the cuddliest honorable mention, my fur baby Jasper, thank you for your energetic, playful, and comforting spirit.

List of Contributors

Katy Schmidt, OTD, OTR/L

Assistant Professor, School of Occupational Therapy
College of Pharmacy and Health Sciences
Belmont University
Nashville, Tennessee

About the Authors

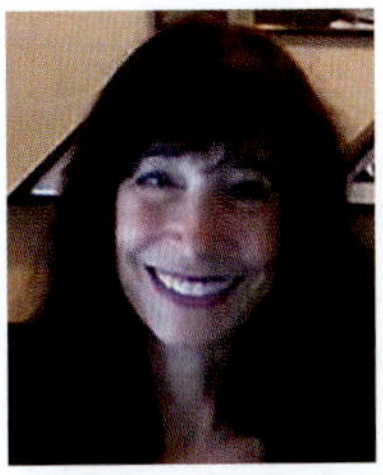

Natalie Norman Michaels, PT, EdD, GCS Emeritus, is a physical therapist and professor in the School of Occupational Therapy at Belmont University in Nashville, Tennessee. Dr. Michaels received her bachelor's degree in physical therapy from Ithaca College, her master's degree in applied psychology from Fairfield University, and her doctorate in curriculum and instruction from the University of Central Florida. She has taught pathophysiology to physical therapy and occupational therapy students for over 20 years. She created one of the first online differential diagnosis courses that met the direct access requirements in Tennessee for physical therapists. Dr. Michaels is a certified Geriatric Clinical Specialist Emeritus with the American Board of Physical Therapy Specialties. She serves as a reviewer for multiple journals, has published over 50 peer-reviewed papers, and is a co-editor for the *Journal of Aquatic Physical Therapy*.

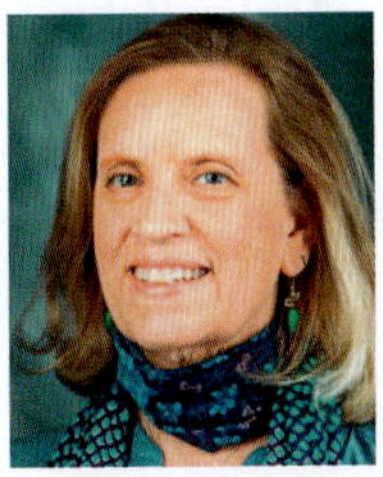

Sandy Stevens is an associate professor in the Department of Occupational Therapy at Belmont University. In addition to teaching neurophysiology, pathophysiology, and research classes, she is coordinating a community wellness program. Her research focuses on physical activity interventions to improve health and function in individuals with chronic disabilities. She is an avid researcher with interests in physical activity, health and well-being, and aquatic therapy.

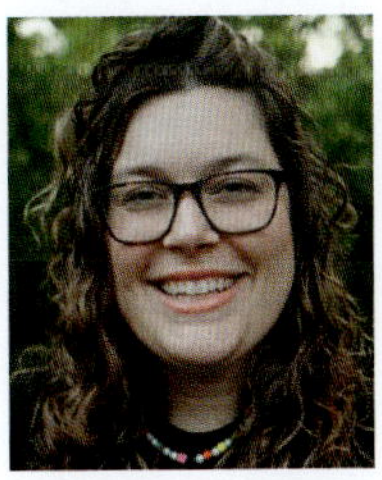

Roya Rezadoost is an occupational therapist specializing in early childhood education within the public school system. She graduated in 2020 with a doctorate in occupational therapy from Belmont University in Nashville, Tennessee. She has since gained 5 years of experience working passionately to support the developmental needs of young children, helping to facilitate their individual success in the classroom and beyond. Roya cherishes the relationships she creates with each of her students. Roya enjoys finding that just-right challenge for her students, while meeting them where they are developmentally. She is passionate about facilitating their transition into a school setting, providing environmental adaptations, and individualized plans to facilitate their success. Roya combines evidence-based practices with a compassionate approach to address the unique challenges faced by our youngest learners. Roya is passionate about sensory integration, child and adolescent mental health, trauma-informed practices, and advocating for diversity, equity, and inclusion within all aspects of the field. Roya is a member of local professional organizations, presents at colleges and educational conferences, and continually strives to enhance the quality of early childhood occupational therapy in schools.

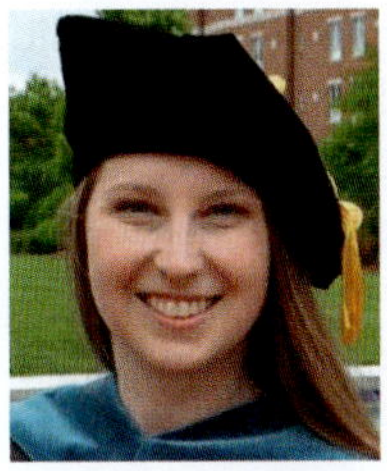

Ashley Rabuck is a licensed and registered occupational therapist who earned her doctoral degree from Belmont University in May 2022. During her graduate-level capstone project, Dr. Rabuck proposed enhancement and reorganization of the pathophysiology course to encompass greater clinical application and whose research helped justify the need for this occupational therapy-centric pathophysiology textbook. Following her passion for pediatrics after graduation, Dr. Rabuck worked at an outpatient pediatric clinic in Tennessee before accepting an acute care position at a local Level II trauma hospital in Virginia. Within her first year of employment, Dr. Rabuck became the hospital's first neonatal occupational therapist for their Level II NICU. Dr. Rabuck also transitioned to, and currently spends most of her clinical time in, the Inpatient Rehab setting, treating adults with various neurological, orthopedic, and cardiopulmonary conditions. Outside of work, Dr. Rabuck enjoys cooking, playing pickleball, and spending time with family and friends.

Foreword

Applied Pathophysiology for Occupational Therapy: A Guide for Clinical Decision Making has been written by an experienced and talented team of educators with backgrounds in physical therapy and occupational therapy to address a gap in texts directly addressing foundational knowledge in pathophysiology applied to occupational therapy practice. True to the roots of occupational therapy, the text not only addresses the expected foci on the physical conditions commonly addressed by occupational therapy practitioners (OTPs) but also intentionally includes a focus on mental health conditions, conveying the distinct value of occupational therapy as a profession working with people in an integrated manner across biopsychosocial factors impacting participation in everyday life, and resultant quality of life, health, and wellbeing.

I appreciated the text's organization looking across the lifespan, at the systems level, and then directly addressing mental health conditions that can be primary or comorbid to the challenges faced by the person seeking occupational therapy services. The text includes important case exemplars that help the readers (OT students and practitioners) to recognize the complex challenges that are faced by OTPs every day and to make a tremendous difference in the outcomes associated with occupational therapy as a part of the health care team.

Dr. Ginny Stoffel, PhD, OT, FAOTA
Associate Professor Emeritus, University of Wisconsin-Milwaukee and Past President, American Occupational Therapy Association, 2013–16

Virginia ("Ginny") C. Stoffel, PhD, OT, FAOTA is well known in the field of occupational therapy for her work in mental health. Her research has focused on the lived experience of disability for individuals with mental illness and substance use disorders, and she is co-author of *Occupational Therapy in Mental Health: A Vision for Participation*. Dr. Stoffel served as the 29th president of the American Occupational Therapy Association, during which time she gave a powerful presidential address focusing on building capacity through attitude, authenticity, and action. She has been inspirational to many, including these authors, through her patience, kindness, advice, and wisdom. The following quote, one of many, is a demonstration of Dr. Stoffel's faith in the field and in the compassionate care provided by OTP's.

"OT practitioners do not ask, 'What's the matter with you?' Instead they ask 'What matters to you?'"

Natalie Norman Michaels
Sandy Stevens
Roya Rezadoost
Ashley Rabuck

A Note From Catherine C. Goodman

A note from Catherine C. Goodman, PT, MBA, author of *Differential Diagnosis for the Physical Therapist* (seventh edition) and *Pathology: Implications for the Physical Therapist* (fifth edition) [Elsevier Publisher].

Natalie Michaels, PT, EdD, GCS Emeritus, ATRIC, her co-authors, and her team of contributors have brought full circle the concept of recognizing cautionary/red flags and screening for medical referral for the occupational therapy practitioner (OTP). They have brilliantly incorporated a systematic and structured approach to pathophysiology and medical screening.

The material in this text goes beyond basic pathophysiology. The authors show the "whys" and "hows" for everyday utilization of pathophysiology and screening specifically applicable to the OTP.

Anyone practicing in the rehabilitation arm of health care, whether via Zoom triage or with a more direct hands-on approach, must have this information and clinical knowledge to evaluate, treat, and/or refer and to do so in the fastest and safest manner possible.

Dr. Michaels must be commended for bringing this information to our partners in the field of occupational therapy for the first time, thereby advancing the occupational therapy curriculum and thus the entire profession.

Catherine C. Goodman, PT, MBA

Preface

The mission statement of the American Occupational Therapy Association (AOTA) is to advance the practice and research of occupational therapy and to advocate "on behalf of its members, the profession, and the public."[1] The AOTA *Vision 2025* further defines occupational therapy as an inclusive profession that, "...maximizes health, wellbeing, and quality of life for all people, populations, and communities through effective solutions that facilitate participation in everyday living."[1,2] Occupational therapists (OTRs) and occupational therapy assistants (COTAs), known collectively in this book as occupational therapy practitioners (OTPs), do this throughout their day, especially during their client care from the initial evaluation to discharge. The AOTA position statement, *Occupational Therapy Scope of Practice,* defines the process of occupational therapy as "the delivery of services," including evaluation, intervention, and determination of outcomes.[3] The *Scope of Practice* further explains that the process of evaluation is focused on discerning "what the client wants and needs to do; determining what the client can do and has done; and identifying supports and barriers to health, well-being, and participation."[4] Understanding the symptomatology of a specific disorder is essential to accurately assess what a client can and should be able to do, as well as to identify potential barriers to health, well-being, and participation. This rationale inspired the development of this textbook. Although there were other pathology textbooks on the market for occupational therapy students, none followed both a developmental and systemic approach, with inclusion of mental health, and application to the field of occupational therapy. The writers of this textbook hope to fill that gap.

This textbook seeks to inform occupational therapy students about the signs and symptoms typically expected for their client's condition, as well as those that may be present but fall outside the norm for the diagnosis. Although OTPs have a strong scope of practice, this does not include making a definitive medical diagnosis. This would be in the jurisdiction of the client's physician. Yet, it is imperative that OTPs are able to identify signs and symptoms outside of the cluster of those expected and clearly articulate this information to a client's physician so that appropriate testing can be completed. OTPs need to stay within their scope of practice, and although they must work inside the box, they still need to think outside the box. OTPs are an important part of client care, often noticing symptoms outside the box before other practitioners.

It is a pleasure to present the first edition of this textbook, *Applied Pathophysiology for Occupational Therapy: A Guide for Clinical Decision Making*. This book is the first of its kind, not only addressing normal human physiology along the developmental progression, but also the physical and mental health conditions most likely encountered by OTPs. This book first focuses on pathophysiology throughout the lifespan and then migrates to a systems approach, including multiple case studies for application. Elements of cognitive pathophysiology are added as well as mental health conditions. This book concludes with a glossary of some of the pathophysiological conditions most frequently encountered by OTPs.

Section I addresses the *Client Interview* and screening procedures for the appropriate OT treatment intervention and then moves along the stages of development depicting normal physiology and some of the pathological conditions encountered at each stage: *Pediatric, Adolescent, Adult, and Older Adult*. Section II takes on a systems approach, first explaining pathophysiology on a cellular level, and then covering the conditions mostly like seen in ten of the physiological systems such as hematological, cardiovascular, and pulmonary. Section III focuses on pathophysiology and cognition by first reviewing the theoretical constructs of cognition and then focusing on cognitive pathophysiology. Section IV covers pathophysiology and mental health. These seven chapters cover disorders often seen by OTPs such as mood disorders, anxiety disorders, and personality disorders. Section V sums it all up by depicting pathology and the OTP and how their scope of practice fits into the bigger picture as a client advocate. Beginning with the definitions of domain and process from the fourth edition of the *Occupational Therapy Practice Framework*: Domain and Practice (OTPF-4),[5] and applying them to the World Health Organization's International Classification of Functioning, Disability, and Health,[6] this section, consisting of one chapter, pulls together the content of this textbook, the unique skill set of OTPs, and their knowledge of pathophysiology to the meaningful participation of OT clients. This is all followed by a quick-reference Glossary of some of the medical conditions most likely to be encountered by OTPs.

We are thrilled to be collaborating with an amazing scholar and author, Dr. Catherine C. Goodman who has graciously allowed us to use some of the content of her book, *Differential Diagnosis for Physical Therapists*[7] to embellish the richness of this text, while maintaining the focus on occupational therapy and the conditions most likely encountered and treated by OTPs. We are also very fortunate to have had Charlene Marshall, author of *Pathology for the Physical Therapist Assistant*, serve as executive reviewer for Section II, and Dr. Katy Schmidt, Assistant Professor in the School of OT at Belmont University and alumna of the Johns Hopkins Mental Health Occupational Therapy Fellowship, serve as our primary author for the mental health chapters in Section IV.

We hope that this text will be a valuable asset in the occupational therapy classroom and an important text when studying for the board examination. We also see this text as a possible quick reference providing valuable information for the OTP in the clinical setting. It is our intention to provide the future OTP with the needed tools for critical thinking and decision-making when dealing with both expected and unexpected client signs and symptoms. We also hope that this text will help the future OTP provide "effective solutions"[6] and to serve as strong client advocates, helping the profession to move one step closer to the realization of *Vision 2025*.

Natalie Norman Michaels
Sandy Stevens
Roya Rezadoost
Ashley Rabuck

References

1. American Occupational Therapy Association *About AOTA. Mission and Vision. The American Occupational Therapy Association*. AOTA Mission & Vision | AOTA; 2024. https://www.aota.org/about/mission-vision.
2. American Occupational Therapy Association Vision 2025. *Am J Occup Ther*. 2017;71(3): https://doi.org/10.5014/ajot.2017.713002. 7103420010p1.
3. *Am J Occup Ther*. 2020;74(suppl2):7412410010p1–7412410010p87. https://doi.org/10.5014/ajot.2020.74S2001.
4. American Occupational Therapy Association Occupational therapy scope of practice. *Am J Occup Ther*. 2021;75(suppl 3): 7513410030. https://doi.org/10.5014/ajot.2021.75S3005.
5. American Occupational Therapy Association The occupational therapy practice framework: domain and practice: 4th ed. *Am J Occup Ther*. 2020;74(suppl 2). https://www.cdc.gov/nchs/icd/icf/index.html.
6. CDC. International Classification of Functioning, Disability and Health. World Health Organization. Centers for Disease Control and Prevention, 2024. https://www.cdc.gov/nchs/icd/icf/index.html.
7. Heick J, Lazaro RT. *Goodman and Snyder's Differential Diagnosis for Physical Therapists: Screening for Referral*. 7th ed. Elsevier; 2023.

Contents

SECTION I

Pathophysiology Through the Lifespan

Introduction to Section I

In the intricate world of health care, occupational therapists and occupational therapy assistants, collectively referred to in this book as occupational therapy practitioners (OTPs), play a unique and pivotal role in enhancing the quality of life for individuals through engagement in meaningful and purposeful activities. Occupational therapy is deeply rooted in understanding the human body's functions and the various factors that can interfere with them. As an OTP, a thorough grasp of pathophysiology is essential. Pathophysiology is defined as the functional changes that occur with disease and the scientific research related to these changes with respect to the body's normal functions and processes.[1] This knowledge not only informs clinical reasoning but also guides the development of effective, evidence-based intervention strategies tailored to each client's unique needs.

In Section I of this textbook, the reader will learn crucial concepts essential for occupational therapy practice across different stages of life. It will lay the groundwork for understanding how pathophysiological processes impact human development and health, guiding OTPs in providing effective, personalized care to their clients.

There are nine chapters in this section. Chapter 1 focuses on the pivotal role of the client interview in occupational therapy. Chapter 2 examines critical red flags within the occupational therapy scope, guiding ethical decision-making and timely intervention for urgent medical conditions. Chapter 3 explores the impact of prenatal and genetic factors on health and development. Chapter 4 addresses developmental milestones and common pathophysiological conditions in infants. Chapter 5 analyzes developmental stages in early and middle childhood, focusing on pathophysiological conditions seen during this stage of life. Chapter 6 investigates health challenges specific to female adolescents, including hormonal changes and psychosocial influences. Chapter 7 explores unique health issues and pathophysiological considerations during male adolescence. Chapter 8 examines prevalent pathophysiological conditions in early and middle adulthood. Finally, Chapter 9 focuses on health issues and pathophysiological changes in late adulthood and age-related conditions.

Occupational therapy promotes health and well-being through meaningful occupations utilizing a client-centered approach.[2] Section I will help provide OTPs with the foundational knowledge necessary to integrate pathophysiological insights into client-centered care across the lifespan. By understanding developmental milestones, common health challenges, and specific age-related pathologies, OTPs are better equipped to identify when a symptom may need further intervention. Recognizing red flags and knowing when to take immediate action will be critical skills emphasized throughout this section.

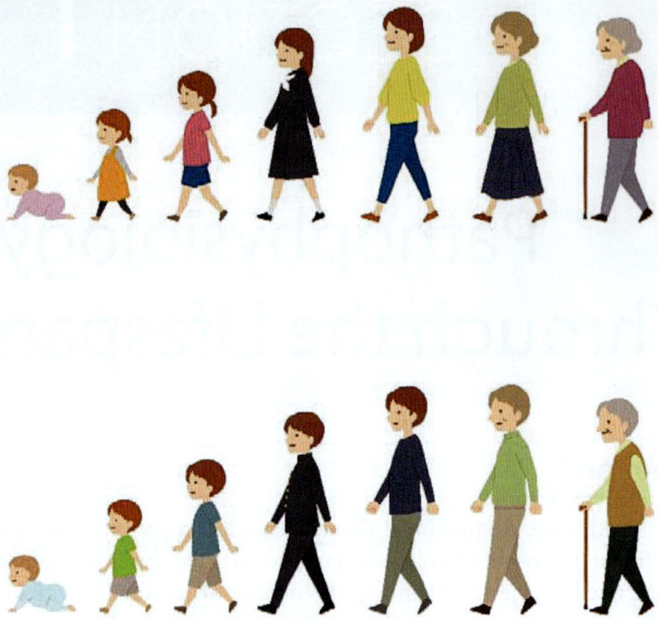

(From www.istockphoto.com/perisuta.)

References

1. Medical Dictionary. Pathophysiology. In: *The Free Dictionary by Farlex: Medical Dictionary*; N.D. Pathophysiology | definition of pathophysiology by Medical dictionary (thefreedictionary.com)
2. WFOT. *About Occupational Therapy*. World Federation of Occupational Therapy; 2024.

1 Screening for Occupational Therapy

OBJECTIVES

By the end of this chapter, the reader should be able to:

- Differentiate the roles of the occupational therapist and the roles of the occupational therapy assistant with respect to pathophysiology.
- Briefly summarize the occupational therapy screening process.
- Differentiate between a red flag, a yellow flag, and a green flag.
- List ways to properly interview a client.
- Explain the importance of HIPAA guidelines.
- Define the occupational therapy scope of practice.

Pathophysiology and the Occupational Therapy Practitioner

The term occupational therapy practitioner, also known as *OTP*, will be used throughout this chapter to represent registered occupational therapists (OTRs) and certified occupational therapy assistants (COTAs).[1] Although OTRs and COTAs have distinct scopes of practice, there is a significant overlap in their responsibilities related to pathophysiology.

All OTPs are responsible for using evidence-based practice, staying updated on medical and therapeutic advances, maintaining knowledge of signs and symptoms of pathophysiological conditions, taking vitals, using clinical reasoning skills, and communicating with the medical team regarding changes in medical status or unusual signs and symptoms.[2,3] OTPs are responsible for understanding how pathophysiological conditions impact occupational performance, body structures and functions, movement quality, overall wellbeing, and mental health.[2,3] OTPs must recognize the impact of pathophysiology on a client's functional abilities and apply this knowledge when choosing and implementing interventions to promote their recovery. Finally, OTPs should always advocate for the client and work together for the purpose of the client's functional progress.[2,3]

The OTR will perform a client's initial evaluation and create a treatment plan with therapeutic short-term and long-term goals.[2,3] This process will be further outlined in Chapter 30. A solid understanding of pathophysiology is imperative to recognize signs and symptoms that may fall outside what is expected for a given diagnosis. The COTA is responsible for communication with their supervising OTR when an individual presents differently than what was documented during their initial evaluation or last treatment session.[3] The COTA will also report relevant clinical observations of the client's response to a specific intervention. The COTA must be familiar with the physiology associated with a given condition, recognize symptoms of concern, and report these promptly to the OTR. The OTR can then adjust the therapeutic plan of care and communicate further with the referring physician as needed.[3] Collaboration between the OTR and COTA in interpreting subjective and objective pathophysiological information gathered during client interactions is essential for identifying appropriate yellow and red flags.

Introduction to the Occupational Therapy Screening Process

As the field of health care changes, OTPs must be even more cognizant of the increased need to screen their clients for appropriateness of occupational therapy intervention. According to the fourth edition of the *Occupational Therapy Practice Framework* (OTPF-4), *occupational therapy (OT)* is

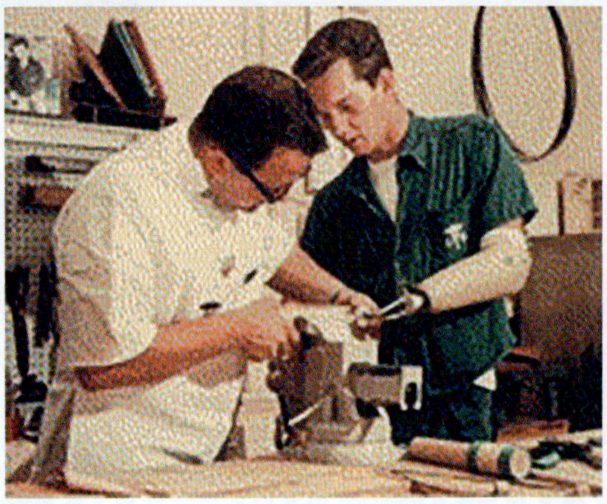

• Yakobina SC, Yakobina SR, Harrison-Weaver S. War, what is it good for? Historical contribution of the military and war to occupational therapy and hand therapy. *J Hand Ther*. 2008; 111. Article #083.

defined as the enhancement of participation through the therapeutic use of everyday occupations with individuals, groups, or populations.[4] The term *client* refers to the recipient of OT intervention and can include the families of the recipient, groups, and/or populations served. In this text, these terms are used in accordance with the OTPF-4 definitions. The focus of this book, *Applied Pathophysiology for Occupational Therapy: A Guide for Clinical Decision Making*, is to help enable the OTP to recognize signs and symptoms of disorders and diseases and to make a decision whether or not to treat a client, staying within the OT scope of practice. This text is not to teach OTPs to be medical diagnosticians. However, OTPs can utilize critical thinking strategies to differentiate the occupational implications of a client's condition as it impacts their everyday life. Although OTPs must work inside the box pertaining to the allowed scope of service, they must also be able to think outside the box (Fig. 1.1).

The OT scope of practice, such as the scope of practice of other professions, varies state by state. This variation is not dramatic, but it is there, and practicing OTPs must remember to check with their state guidelines. What remains unchanged are the set cornerstones of OT practice stated in the OTPF-4. These cornerstones include, but are not limited to, values and beliefs that are rooted in occupation and the therapeutic use of self.[4] There are also included contributors that influence the cornerstones, and they include client-centered practice, clinical and professional reasoning, and evidence-informed practice. These elements of client care are mandatory but cannot be performed well without a good knowledge base.

The Screening Process

The OTPF-4 defines *screening* as a consultation process that helps produce an occupational profile and possible recommendations for OT evaluation and possible intervention. The occupational profile is a summary of the client's experiences and interests. This is a very important part of the process to understand the client's perspective and background, but the need to set realistic goals must always be in the back of the therapist's mind. Understanding the underlying pathophysiology is imperative. According to Heick and Lazaro, a healthcare provider must be able to recognize the signs and symptoms of possible disorders that can mimic musculoskeletal or neuromuscular dysfunction.[5] OT screening differs from OT evaluation. The screening provides information about whether or not to proceed to a more thorough evaluation. The OTPF-4 outlines *evaluation* as the utilization of multiple methods to assess the client, the contexts, the occupations, and the occupational performance.[4] This helps to establish client goals and OT intervention needed to get there.

Clinical Presentation: Yellow and Red Flags

According to Catherine C. Kellogg (formerly Catherine C. Goodman), an important part of the screening process is the ability to identify yellow flags (those signifying caution) and red flags (those signifying warning).[5] To do this, the signs and symptoms are placed into identifiable clusters that could signify a possible disorder. Remember, as OTPs, we do NOT provide a medical diagnosis, but we do need to be able to identify unexpected signs and symptoms and refer the client back to the physician when warranted. It is also important to know how to communicate this to the physician so that the appropriate tests can be ordered to rule out the possibilities that might make OT contraindicated.

Yellow flags signal caution to the OTP. This means to slow down and take a second look at relevant questions regarding the suspicious symptom or symptoms. A useful tool to help determine yellow flags is the Optimal Screening for Prediction of Referral and Outcome for Yellow Flags (OSPRO-YF).[2,3] This tool uses a questionnaire to look at the client's negative coping, negative moods, and positive affective/coping domains. An additional tool to help determine yellow flags is the Optimal Screening for Prediction of Referral and Outcome—Review of Symptoms (OSPRO-ROS).[2,3] This tool uses a questionnaire to look at symptoms that should be addressed by the client's physician or another healthcare provider before OT intervention is even considered. A yellow flag presents no immediate danger, but the potential for a health problem if it is not addressed. When a yellow flag presents itself, it is best to inform the physician.

Red flags are those features of the client's medical history and/or clinical presentation that signify a high risk for serious illness. Where a yellow flag might mean "Slow down," a red flag is a warning to "Stop." Although red flags could be a sign of a serious condition, they are rarely cause for immediate medical intervention. Each symptom must be viewed within the context of the entire person. For example, seeing clonus in a person after a stroke does not require immediate medical attention because it is expected in this population; however, chest pain in a client with obesity and diabetes, who does not typically have episodes of angina, could constitute a medical emergency.

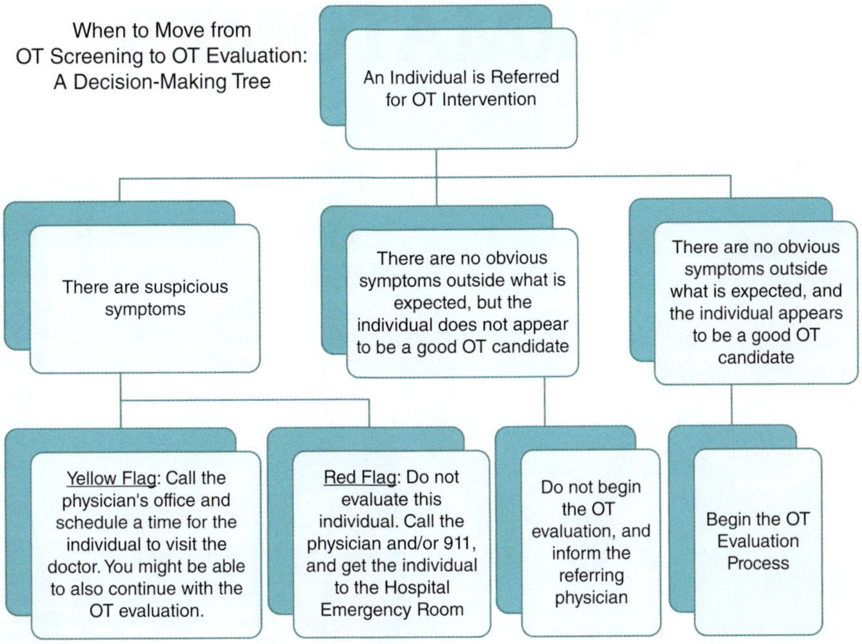

• **Fig. 1.1** Simplified version of the occupational therapist decision-making process. *ER*, Emergency room; *OT*, occupational therapy.

Pain Patterns

The word "pain" is defined in the OTPF-4 on page 53 as an "unpleasant feeling indicating potential or actual damage to some body structure."[4] The National Institutes of Health's (NIH) National Institute of Neurologic Disorders and Stroke defines acute pain *as a normal sensation triggered in the nervous system to alert you to possible injury and the need to take care of yourself,* and chronic pain as persistent pain with signals *firing in the nervous system for weeks, months, or even years.*[7] The NIH's National Center for Complimentary and Integrative Health reports that pain is the most common reason for seeking medical care,[8] and it is often the reason for seeking occupational therapy intervention, as pain can limit function and, therefore, participation; these pain patterns can often be the key to understanding underlying disease processes.[5]

Because each organ system in the body is supplied by the nervous system via cranial nerves and/or nerve roots from various levels of the spinal cord, problems in these systems can sometimes mimic musculoskeletal difficulties in corresponding areas. Each chapter of Section II of this text, "Pathophysiology by System" includes a discussion about the symptoms that can sometimes mimic musculoskeletal conditions: the yellow flags and the red flags.

Sensory innervation of the human body via nerve roots is indicative of a central nervous system phenomenon and is shown in dermatome charts. A quick review of the dermatomes of the human body can be seen in Fig. 1.2.

Sensory innervation of the human body via nerves is indicative of a peripheral nervous system phenomenon. A comparison in the human body can be seen in Fig. 1.3.

Common sites of referred pain from abdominal viscera can be seen in Fig. 1.4.

The Interview as a Screening Tool

Although medical questionnaires completed in the waiting room can provide good information about the reason for the visit and past medical history, nothing compares to the conversation you have with the client.

Asking the Right Questions

The initial discussion you have with the OT client can serve as a good screening interview, but knowing how to ask the right questions is paramount. Yet this is a skill set that is developed gradually over time and can always be improved, even in the most seasoned clinicians.[5] Using a compassionate, caring, and professional attitude can help gain the client's trust.

A good way to start is with an open-ended question, such as "Can you tell me the reason for your visit today?" This enables the client to embellish a bit and tell you a few sentences to give you a better understanding of the reason for their visit. The interview can then slowly move toward more closed-ended questions for clarification such as "So, you are saying that the pain is worse when you lie down to rest?" This provides a simple yes or no answer, but wait for the client to talk more if they feel the need for further clarification. This helps to prevent miscommunication. As the therapist you need to show empathy and compassion, but be sure to maintain control of the interview.

Also maintain an awareness of nonverbal cues. This can be even more important than the verbal interview.[5] Body language, such as wincing with movement or leaning to one side, can provide relevant clues to the client's condition. This can be especially important when English is a second language or when using an interpreter.

DERMATOMES

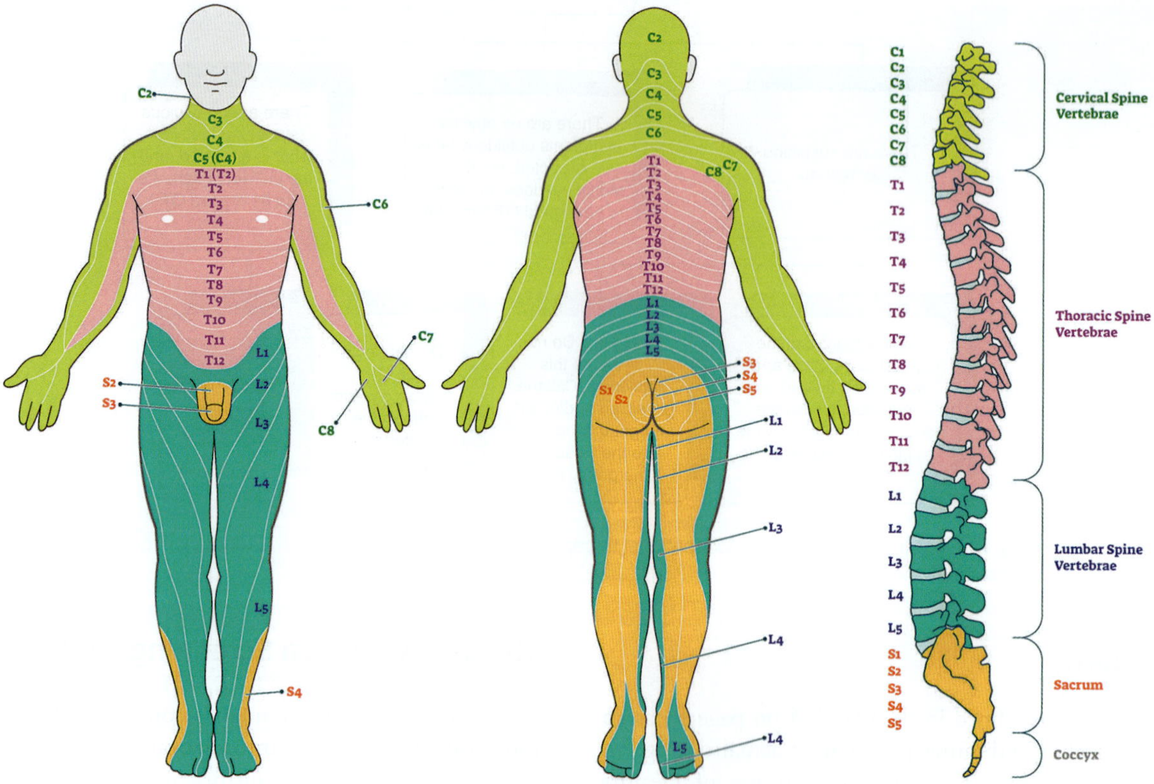

• **Fig. 1.2** Dermatomes of the human body. (From iStock.com/VectorMine.)

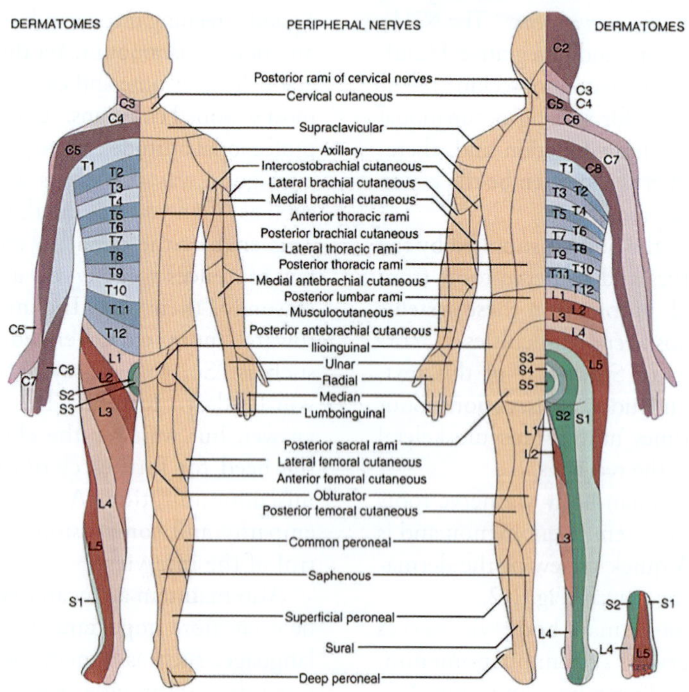

• **Fig. 1.3** Cutaneous innervation via peripheral nerves of the human body. (From Lundy-Ekman L. *Neuroscience: Fundamentals for Rehabilitation.* 3rd ed. Saunders; 2007.)

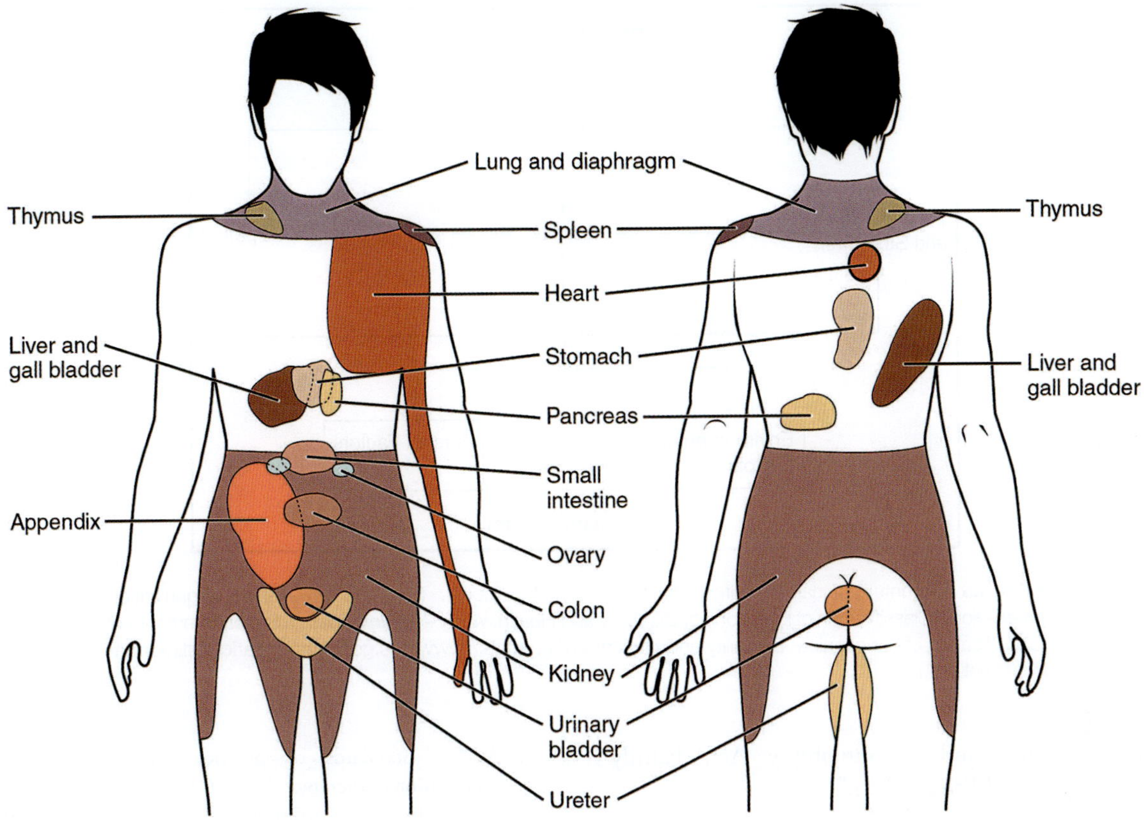

• **Fig. 1.4** Common sites of referred pain from abdominal viscera. (From https://commons.wikimedia.org/wiki/File:1506_Referred_Pain_Chart.jpg.)

What to Report to the Physician

In each section of this textbook, there is information regarding the yellow and red flags to consider. As you progress through each chapter, it is our hope that you will have a better understanding of what to document for the healthcare team, when to report findings immediately to the physician, and when immediate intervention is needed that may require emergency room or intervention. Again, it is not the goal of this book to teach you to diagnose. That is outside the scope of OT intervention. What this book hopes to achieve is a good working knowledge to help with the clinical decision-making when choosing whether to treat a client, to refer them back to their physician, or both.

Maintaining HIPAA Guidelines

Throughout the screening, evaluation, decision-making, and intervention process, the OT must remain cognizant of the Health Insurance Portability and Accountability Act (HIPAA) of 1996. This is a set of national standards created to maintain the privacy of health information.[9] This act was originally created to improve the portability of health insurance coverage for people who were between jobs.[10] To streamline health care, the Administrative Simplification Rule was added. This rule made recommendations for health information privacy and security.[10] In 2003, the US Department of Health and Human Services (HHS) issued the Privacy Rule to implement the requirements of HIPAA. This Privacy Rule focuses on the use and disclosure of protected health information. Although these rules were written in a firm language, there was no way to ensure compliance, so in 2006, the Enforcement Rule was added, giving the HHS authority to enforce compliance with HIPAA guidelines.[10] With the increased utilization of electronic health records (EHRs), the HITECH Act was added in 2009, providing guidelines for these records and encouraging providers to use EHRs through the use of financial incentives. The most recent addition to the HIPAA guidelines since the writing of this chapter was the Omnibus Final Rule, defining terms, addressing gaps, and adding clarity to the original legislation.[10]

For the OTP, these laws help provide rules and guidelines regarding the most private way to document medical information and to share it with the physician. Information in the medical record can only be shared with the consent of the client and never in a way where it could fall into the wrong hands. Page 8 of the 2020 American Occupational Therapy Association (AOTA) Code of Ethics states that the OTP must "Maintain the confidentiality of all verbal, written, electronic, augmentative, and nonverbal communications in compliance with applicable laws, including all aspects of privacy laws and exceptions thereto (e.g., Health

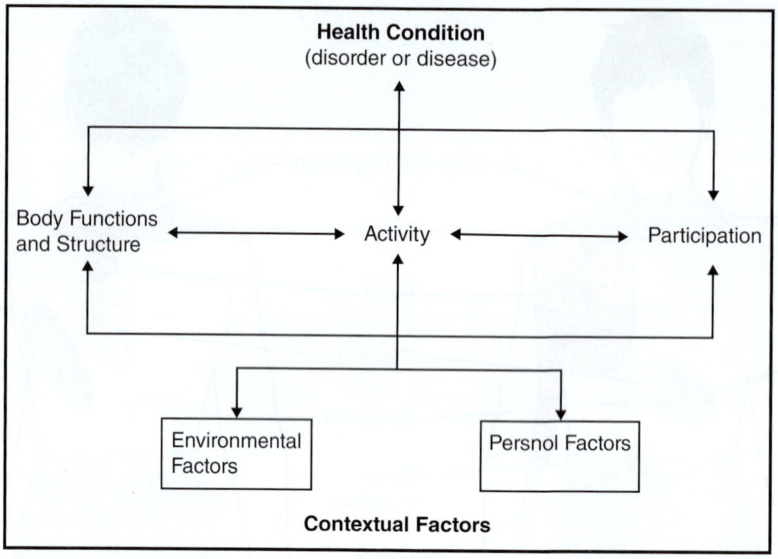

• **Fig. 1.5** The International Classification of Functioning model. (From World Health Organization International Classification of Functioning, Disability and Health. *WHO – FIC Information Sheet*. International Classification of Functioning, Disability and Health; 2012. https://www.cdc.gov/nchs/data/icd/icfinformationsheet.pdf.)

Insurance Portability and Accountability Act, Family Educational Rights and Privacy Act)."[11]

Staying Within the Scope of OT

The AOTA reports that the scope of practice for OT is continuously evolving.[12] The *Scope of Occupational Therapy Practice* includes the focus of OT or the *domain*, and the delivery of OT or the *process*. This document clarifies the roles as well as the relationship between the occupational therapists and the occupational therapy assistants. The World Health Organization (WHO) created a framework called the International Classification of Functioning (ICF) model to provide healthcare practitioners with a common language for measuring health and disability (Fig. 1.5).[13]

In the document published by the AOTA, *Scope of Occupational Therapy Practice*, WHO is quoted as stating that the field of OT incorporates basic constructs of the ICF model, such as context, body structures, and activities to enable full participation. Although the OT curriculum will inform you of most of the possibilities that the field of OT has to offer, you must always stay within the guidelines of your state regulations, the AOTA Scope of Practice, HIPAA, and the rules of your clinical setting.

References

1. AOTA. *About the Profession*. American Occupational Therapy Association; 2025. Available from: https://www.aota.org/career/become-an-ot-ota/about-the-profession.
2. AOTA. Occupational therapy scope of practice. *Am J Occup Ther*. 2021;75(suppl 3):7513410020. https://doi.org/10.5014/ajot.2021.75S3005.
3. AOTA. Standards of practice for occupational therapy. Occupational therapy. *Am J Occup Ther*. 2021;75(suppl 3): 7513410030. https://doi.org/10.5014/ajot.2021.75S3004.
4. American Occupational Therapy Association. The occupational therapy practice framework: domain and practice: 4th ed. *Am J Occup´ Ther*. 2020;74(suppl 2):1–87. doi: 10.5014/ajot.2020.74S2001.
5. Heick J, Lazaro RT. *Goodman and Snyder's Differential Diagnosis for Physical Therapists: Screening for Referral*. 7th ed. 2023, Elsevier.
6. George SZ, Benecuik JM, Lentz TA, et al. Optimal Screening for Prediction of Referral and Outcome for Yellow Flags (OSPRO) for musculoskeletal pain conditions: results from the validation cohort. *J Orthop Sports Phys Ther*. 2018;48(6):460–475.
7. NINDS. *Chronic Pain*. The National Institute of Neurologic Disorders and Stroke; 2023. https://www.ninds.nih.gov/health-information/disorders/chronic-pain.
8. NCCIH. *Pain*. The National Center for Complementary and Integrative Health; 2023. https://www.nccih.nih.gov/health/pain.
9. HHS. *Summary of the HIPAA Privacy Rule*. The United States Department of Health & Human Services; 2023. https://www.hhs.gov/hipaa/for-professionals/privacy/laws-regulations/index.html.
10. HIPAA Guide. *History of HIPAA*. The HIPAA Guide; 2023. https://www.hipaaguide.net/history-of-hipaa/.
11. The American Occupational Therapy Association. The AOTA Occupational Therapy Code of Ethics. *Am J Occup Ther*. 2023;74(suppl 3):1–13. https://research.aota.org/ajot/article/74/Supplement_3/7413410005p1/6691/AOTA-2020-Occupational-Therapy-Code-of-Ethics.
12. AOTA Scope. *Occupational Therapy Scope of Practice*. American Occupational Therapy Association; 2023. https://www.aota.org/practice/practice-essentials/scope-of-practice.
13. CDC. *The ICF: An Overview*. Centers for Disease Control and Prevention; 2010. https://www.cdc.gov/nchs/data/icd/icfoverview_finalforwho10sept.pdf.

2

Red Flags and the Occupational Therapy Scope of Practice

OBJECTIVES

By the end of this chapter, the reader should be able to:

- Explain the importance of a client's family history as well as their past medical history.
- Look for symptoms that could be outside what is expected for an individual's condition.
- Define the therapeutic use of self and the importance of client confidence in their therapist.
- List the recommended ten steps for occupational therapy decision-making.
- Assess the occupational therapist's decision-making process in a case example.
- Differentiate between the basic roles of the occupational therapist and the occupational therapy assistant with respect to pathophysiology as well as the importance of the interaction and communication with all occupational therapy practitioners (OTPs).
- Recognize some of the major pathophysiological symptoms that would require immediate medical attention.

The Screening Process in More Detail

As already mentioned in Chapter 1, an important part of the screening process is the ability to identify yellow flags (those signifying caution) and red flags (those signifying warning).[1] The occupational therapist is responsible for the initial evaluation of the client, but both the therapist and the occupational therapy assistant should be aware of symptoms that could signify potential yellow or red flags. Although yellow flags rarely present a reason for immediate concern, there is no question that during an OTP's time working in a clinical setting, the practitioner will encounter one or more red flag episodes that require immediate intervention. The alert OTP will often notice signs and symptoms that are a concern and should not be ignored. It is better to contact the doctor with a concern that ends up being insignificant than to not contact the doctor when the situation really did constitute an emergency. It is always best to err on the side of caution.

Occupational therapy practitioners (OTPRs) are in an excellent position to be advocates for their clients. The well-seasoned OTP will typically begin the screening interview with open-ended questions and then focus on specifics with more closed-ended questions. These questions can paint a more complete picture of the client's current condition. Because it is the occupational therapist who performs the evaluation and much of the screening, a good portion of this chapter centers around the occupational therapist. It is the occupational therapy assistant, however, who follows through, communicating new findings and changes in a client's medical condition to the therapist so decisions can be made accordingly.

Family History

Family history is sometimes overlooked in the clinical setting, with the current symptoms taking center stage. Yet, this information can be vital when understanding the possible conditions that this client might be experiencing. Open-ended questions/requests can provide more information than simple yes/no questions. See Fig. 2.1 for some ideas. When asking open-ended questions, let the client talk and really listen. The occupational therapist can then zoom into more focused, closed-ended questions to gain more insight, letting the conversation lead the way.

Past Medical History

You cannot know where a hurricane is going unless you know where it has been and the path it has been following. The same is true of a client's medical history. A clinician who treats a client knowing only about the here-and-now will miss valuable information about the path the client's health has taken to get to this point. This past information will help to better understand the client's current condition, which will not only help to achieve their OT goals but could even save a life. Fig. 2.2 provides some questions to help gain insight into the client's past medical history.

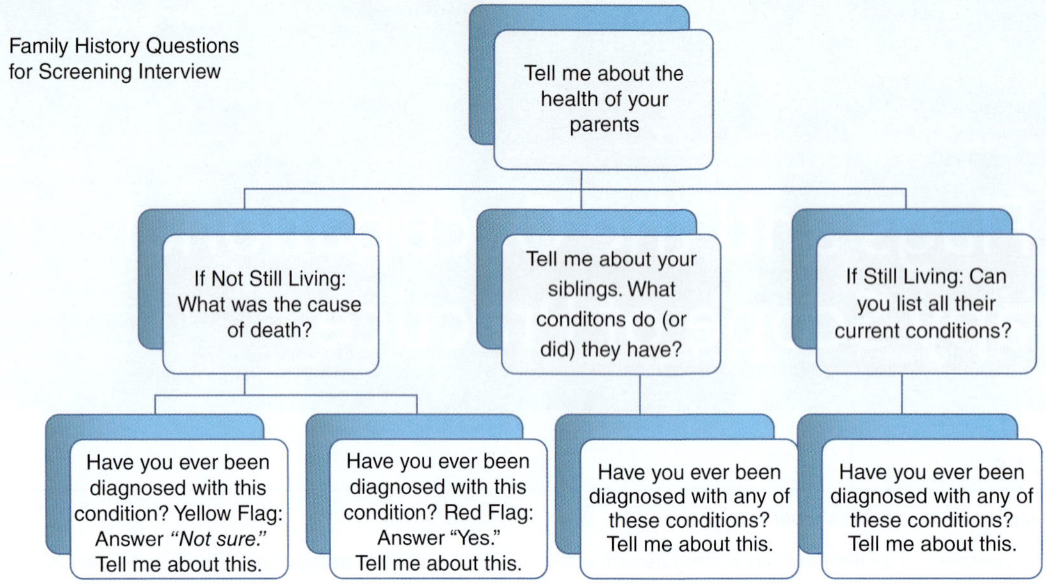

• **Fig. 2.1** Simplified version of the occupational therapy open-ended interview for family history.

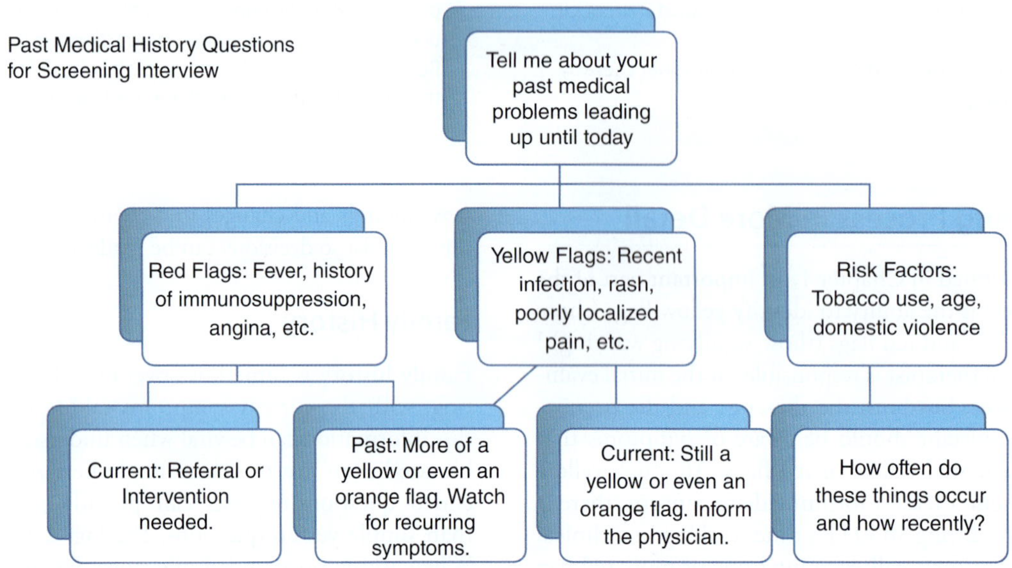

• **Fig. 2.2** Simplified version of the occupational therapy open-ended interview for past medical history.

Clinical Presentation

Interview questions regarding clinical presentation might seem straightforward with easy interview questions that do not need embellishment, but unfortunately that is not the case. Often, valuable information is lost as the clinician focuses on the body part or specific function that led to the physician's order for OT. One of the most valuable questions is simply, "What other symptoms have you been experiencing?" Specific questions like "Are you having any bowel or bladder problems?" can be asked as the interview moves from the open-ended questions to the more closed-ended questions, depending on the answers given by the client. Although the interview should be controlled by the therapist, the answers given by the client should determine the direction of the interview. Fig. 2.3 provides some questions to help gain insight regarding the client's clinical presentation.

Vital Signs and Warnings

Screenings will sometimes include vital signs. According to Heick and Lazaro, vital signs, along with the reported symptomatology and observation, are among the best screening tools available to the therapist.[1] Primary vital signs are pulse rate, blood pressure, respiratory rate, and body temperature.[1] Additional signs include oxygen saturation, pain level, and sensation. Normal values for vital signs, according to Johns Hopkins Medicine and the Mayo Clinic, can be found in Table 2.1.

The Client's Confidence in the Therapist

The *Occupational Therapy Practice Framework* (OTPF) discusses the therapeutic use of self, where OTPs not only develop but also manage their relationship with their

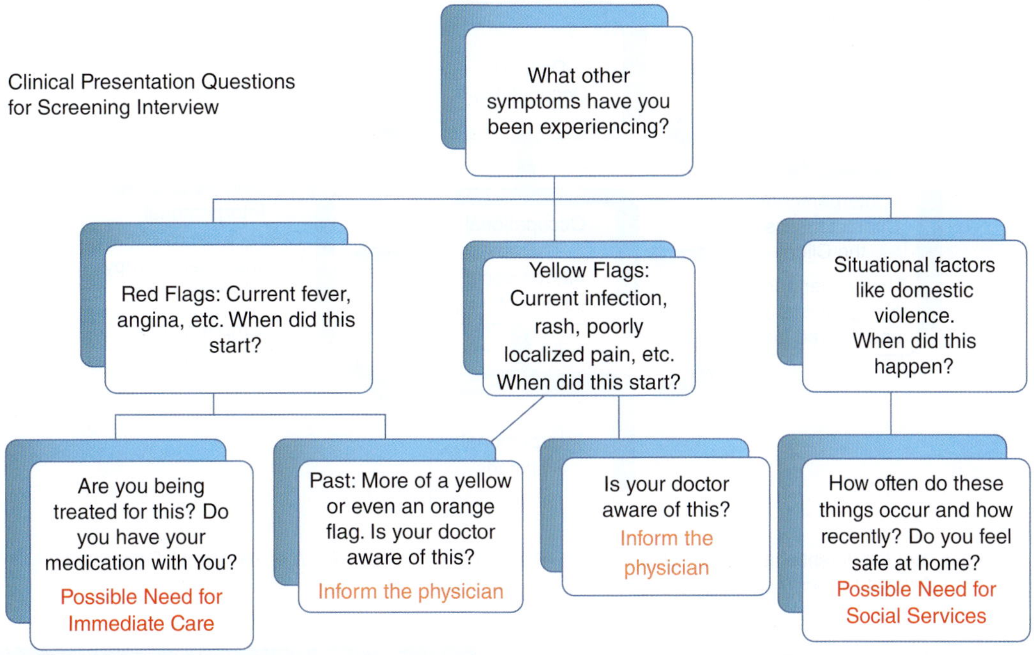

• **Fig. 2.3** Simplified version of the occupational therapy open-ended interview for clinical presentation.

TABLE 2.1 Normal Vital Sign Values

Vital Sign	Normal Value
Pulse Rate[2]	Normal: 60 but can vary between 60 and 100 bpm based on exercise and relaxation
Blood Pressure[2]	Normal: 120/80 Elevated: 120–129/less than 80 Stage 1 HBP: 130–139/ 80–89 Stage 2 HBP: 140 or higher/90 or higher
Respiratory Rate[2]	Normal: 12–16 breaths per minute; this might increase with fever or illness
Body Temperature[2]	Normal: 98.6°F Fever: high temperature, typically above 99°F Hypothermia: low temperature, typically below 95°F
Pulse Oximeter Readings[3]	Normal: 95%–100% Low: under 90%[3]

bpm, Beats per minute; *HBP*, high blood pressure.
Adapted in part from the Johns Hopkins Medicine[2] and Mayo Clinic.[3]

clients using professional reasoning and empathy for a more client-centered approach.[4] This close working relationship can sometimes create a level of trust on the part of the client, leading to more open and honest communication. The occupational therapist must, therefore, be on the lookout for new signs and symptoms disclosed to the them but not to other practitioners, who see the client less frequently and work with the client less closely. According to Pelloquin, this strong therapist interaction can help the occupational therapist recommit to having the client act as a vital partner in a more collaborative relationship.[5]

In the book *The Intentional Relationship: Occupational Therapy and the Use of Self*, Taylor expounds on the importance of a positive relationship with the client and discusses the use of the Intentional Relationship Model.[6] This model is described by Bonsaksen et al. as redirecting attention to the more interpersonal aspects of OT.[7] Taylor et al. first introduced this model in 2008 as a depiction of the relationship between a therapist and a client and to express the need for the client to first participate in the therapy process as a precursor to participation in life's desired occupations (Fig. 2.4).

OTPs are in a unique position to gain the client's participation and trust. This trusting relationship is essential if a client is to disclose important information during a screening interview, examination, or intervention.[1] The OTP might be the first, and possibly the only person, to whom a client discloses personal information about important signs and symptoms. The focus of this textbook will hopefully help the reader to gain a better understanding of what these signs and symptoms could potentially mean.

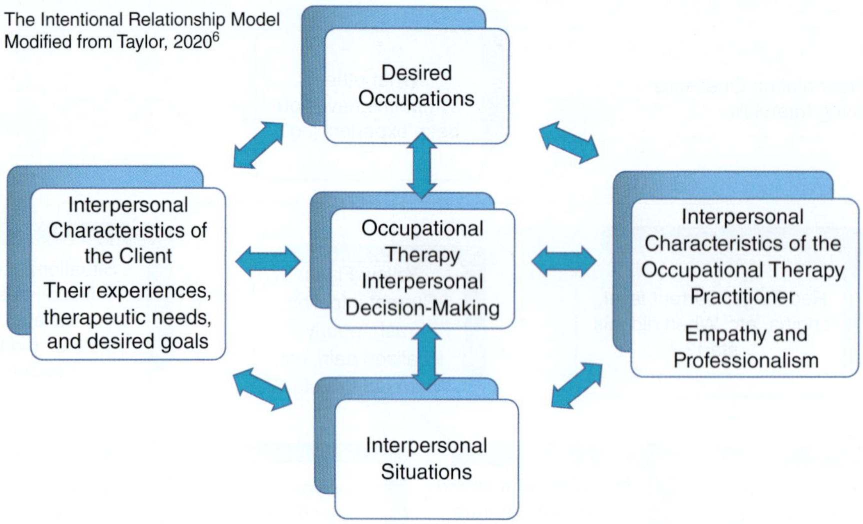

• **Fig. 2.4** The Intentional Relationship Model.[6] (Revised from Taylor RR. *The Intentional Relationship: Occupational Therapy and the Use of Self*. FA Davis; 2020.)

The Decision-Making Process

OTPs must always treat within the scope of their practice guidelines as determined by the government, the state, the American Occupational Therapy Association (AOTA), and their clinical settings. They must work inside the box but always be thinking outside the box. OTPs cannot diagnose, but they can make a determination regarding whether or not a client is a good candidate for OT intervention, whether or not their symptoms require contacting the physician, and whether or not the symptoms constitute an emergency situation.

To Treat or to Refer Back to the Physician

Yellow flags signify caution. They are symptoms to take note of and possibly keep an eye on to see if they change. They need to be included in the documentation, regardless of whether or not they pertain to the reason for the OT visit. Keeping a watch on yellow flags is important because they can become red flags in time. Red flags signify a warning and could mean immediate intervention is warranted. A good rule of thumb for decision-making is to follow these 10 steps:

1. Screen
2. Take a Closer Look at Anything Suspicious
3. Determine Flag Status (Yellow or Red and whether to notify the physician)
4. Take Action if Needed
5. Document the Findings
6. Take a Second Look
7. Determine Flag Status (Yellow or Red and whether to notify the physician)
8. Take Action if Needed
9. Document the Findings
10. Repeat steps 6 through 9 as often as needed, always looking for new signs or symptoms

An example of this can be found in Case Study 2.1.

CASE EXAMPLE 2.1

A 75-year-old male presented in the occupational therapy department with left carpal tunnel syndrome.

1. **Screen:** The therapist interviewed and screened the client.
2. **Take a Closer Look:** On examination, the occupational therapist discovered a suspicious mole on the individual's back over the right scapula.
3. **Determine Flag Status:** The mole was smaller than the ¼-inch size that might signal a warning (see Chapter 12), so the occupational therapist decided that, for now, it was a yellow flag.
4. **Take Action if Needed:** The client was treated for the carpal tunnel syndrome.
5. **Document the Findings:** The occupational therapist described it in her documentation and, with the client's consent, added a picture of this mole with a ruler next to it for size and included this picture in the medical record.
6. **Take a Second Look:** After 4 weeks of therapy for carpal tunnel, the occupational therapist again measured the suspicious mole. It was now slightly larger than the ¼ inch and darker in color. She again took a picture of the mole with a ruler next to it to show the change in size.
7. **Determine the Flag Status:** Because of the change in mole appearance in such a short time and because it was now larger than ¼ inch in size, the occupational therapist considered it a red flag.
8. **Take Action if Needed:** The doctor was informed that same day. The physician made an appointment for the next morning.
9. **Document the Findings:** The OTR again documented her findings and her phone call to the doctor for the medical record.
10. **Repeat steps 6 through 9 as often as needed.**

This is a true case. The client had skin cancer called *malignant melanoma*. The area of skin was excised (removed) by the physician, and the client did well. Thanks to the OTR, this was caught early.

TABLE 2.2 Guidelines for Physician Referral

Medical Category	Warning Flags or Conditions
General Systemic	• Pain or limitation is due to an unknown cause • Not the typical NMS signs and symptoms • Lack of progress with OT intervention • Development of constitutional signs and symptoms (fever, fatigue, etc.) anytime during the weeks of therapy • New findings related to PMH, unknown to referring physician • Changes in health status that persist a week or longer • Untreated or undiagnosed jaundice
For Females	• Low back, pelvic, groin, or sacroiliac (SI) symptoms without known cause and with constitutional signs and symptoms • Symptoms that happen along with menses • Spontaneous bleeding after menopause • Vaginal bleeding, elevated blood pressure, or Braxton-Hicks contraction during exercise in a pregnant female
Vital Signs	• A continuous rise or fall in BP • Increased BP in a female on birth control pills • Pulse amplitude that increases with expiration and decreases with inspiration • Increase pulse over 120 bpm lasting more than 3 minutes after rest • Difference of more than 40 mm Hg between systolic BP and diastolic BP • Persistent low-grade (or high) fever along with sweats and other constitutional signs • Any fever that is unexplained
Cardiac	• More than the prescribed amount (typically three) sublingual nitroglycerine tabs needed for the relief of angina • Continued increase in angina even after the stimulus like exercise or cold has been eliminated • Changes in the pattern of angina • Abnormally severe chest pain • Angina pain that radiates to the jaw or to the left arm • The upper part of the back feels unusually cool, sweaty, or moist to the touch • Client expresses doubts about their condition • Palpitations especially if frequent (6 or more in a minute) or accompanied with pain • New arrhythmias in a neurologically unstable client • Unable to climb a flight of stairs without feeling winded • Awakened at night with shortness of breath when lying down • Dyspnea that worsens in a client with known cardiac involvement • Syncope (fainting) without warning
Cancer	• Skin lesions that flag signs mentioned in the CAUTION pneumonic listed in Chapter 12 • Any female with chest, axillary, breast, or shoulder pain, especially with a family history of cancer • Any male with SI, pelvic, groin, or low back pain, especially with a family history of prostate cancer • New episode of acute back pain in anyone with a previous history of cancer • Bone pain especially on weight bearing that lasts more than a week and is worse at night • Any bleeding from any area that is unexpected
Pulmonary	• Shoulder pain that is aggravated by respiratory movements that can be reduced by holding one's breath • Shoulder pain that is worse when lying down but increases when sitting up and leaning forward • Shoulder or chest pain that feels better with autosplinting (lying on the affected side or supporting it firmly with a pillow) • For individuals with asthma, signs of asthma when exercising • A weak and rapid pulse with a fall in BP • Presence of persistent cough or constitutional signs and symptoms
Genitourinary	• Change in the color, clarity, amount, and/or odor of the urine • Any indication of blood in the urine • Cervical spine pain along with urinary incontinence
Gastrointestinal	• Back pain and abdominal pain located at the same level with constitutional signs and symptoms • Back pain of unknown cause in a person who has a history of cancer • Back pain and shoulder pain in an individual taking NSAIDs, especially when there is also GI upset or blood in the stools • Back or shoulder pain that comes and goes with meals or is relieved after a bowel movement

(Continued)

TABLE 2.2 **Guidelines for Physician Referral—cont'd**

Medical Category	Warning Flags or Conditions
Musculoskeletal	• Symptoms that seem to not be proportionate to the injury or persist longer than expected • Severe increase in back pain along with constitutional signs and symptoms, especially fever • New joint pain without injury, especially following surgery, with signs of inflammation (red, warm, swelling, and pain)
Precautions/ Contraindications to Therapy	• Uncontrolled pulmonary edema or chronic heart failure • Active myocarditis • Resting heart rate of 120 bpm or higher • Resting systolic BP of 180 mm Hg or higher • Resting diastolic BP of 105 mm Hg or higher • Unexplained dizziness or near syncope • Dyspnea • Increased fatigue • Unsteadiness • Irregular heart rate with signs of dizziness, nausea, or lack of a palpable pulse • Posterior calf pain post-surgically • Individuals with diabetes who have chronically unstable blood sugar levels

BP, Blood pressure; *bpm*, beats per minute; *NMS*, neuromusculoskeletal; *NSAIDs*, nonsteroidal anti-inflammatory drugs; *OT*, occupational therapy; *PMH*, past medical history.
Adapted from Heick J, Lazaro RT. *Goodman and Snyder's Differential Diagnosis for Physical Therapists: Screening for Referrals. 7th ed.* Elsevier. 2023:25–26.

Flag Status

As you progress through this text, you will become better able to determine red and yellow flags and those who fall within the orange area between the two. For now, we are including the following information from Goodman and Snyder's *Differential Diagnosis for Physical Therapists: Screening for Referral.*[1]

Guidelines for Immediate Medical Attention

Although these guidelines will be available following each of Chapters 10 through 20, having a list here might help to align your thinking in the decision-making process. The ability to identify red flags can be very important, especially when new symptoms develop that were not present at an individual's last physician visit, but the OTP must take into account as much information from the individual as possible before assuming that immediate medical attention is warranted. However, it is the opinion of these authors that it is always better to err on the side of caution. It is a better choice to inform the doctor and risk appearing incompetent than to assume that "it is likely nothing" and risk missing signs of a serious condition. So, although the big picture is important, the following symptoms are considered by Heick and Lazaro to be the major red flags that would require immediate medical attention[1]:

- Angina or chest pain not relieved after 20 minutes of rest or after administration of medication (nitroglycerin)
- Angina at rest
- Angina accompanied by sweating or nausea
- Bowel or bladder incontinence with saddle anesthesia from cauda equine syndrome or bladder incontinence with cervical spine pain
- Anaphylactic shock (see Chapter 18)
- Compromised ventilation with increased levels of CO_2 (see Chapter 14)
- If the client with diabetes becomes confused or lethargic, finger stick glucose test will help here if possible
- Rebound tenderness or positive McBurney's point (see Chapter 15)
- Sudden worsening of intermittent claudication (could be due to a thromboembolism)
- Throbbing pain in the chest, back, or abdomen with exertion with pulsation when recumbent and a pulsing, palpable mass
- Changes in size, tenderness, or shape of lymph nodes with a fixed or irregular mass in the breast or axilla, especially when there is a history of cancer

See Table 2.2 for more guidelines on physician referral.

The Evolving Occupational Therapy Scope of Practice

The American Medical Association defines *Scope of Practice* as the activities that licensed healthcare professionals are allowed to perform, as determined by statutes enacted by their state legislatures and the rules that are adopted by their licensing entity.[8] This is important because of the high-stakes nature of the field of medicine, and it is done to ensure that each professional is acting within the education and experience required by their specific field of care. It is the OTP's responsibility to visit the licensing entity for their specific state to see their state guidelines and to abide by them. For more on the OT scope of practice, see Chapter 1.

Use the American Occupational Therapy Association as a Guide

One of the best resources available regarding the scope of practice for OTPs is the AOTA website.[9] According to the AOTA, the scope of practice of OT is evolving. This requires all OTPs, new and seasoned, to stay on top of changes that may be occurring within their state. The AOTA website can direct you to the appropriate state for more information.[10]

References

1. Heick J, Lazaro RT. *Goodman and Snyder's Differential Diagnosis for Physical Therapists: Screening for Referral.* 7th ed. Elsevier. 2023.
2. Johns Hopkins Medicine. *Vital Signs (Body Temperature, Pulse Rate, Respiration Rate, Blood Pressure).* John Hopkins Medicine. https://www.hopkinsmedicine.org/health/conditions-and-diseases/vital-signs-body-temperature-pulse-rate-respiration-rate-blood-pressure.
3. Mayo Clinic. *Mayo Clinic Symptoms: Hypoxemia.* https://www.mayoclinic.org/symptoms/hypoxemia/basics/definition/sym-20050930.
4. The occupational therapy practice framework: domain and practice: 4th ed. *Am J Occup Ther.* 2020;74(suppl 2). https://doi.org/10.5014/ajot.2020.74S2001.
5. Peloquin SM. The patient-therapist relationship in occupational therapy: understanding visions and images. *Am J Occup Ther.* 1990;44(1):13–21. https://doi.org/10.5014/ajot.44.1.13.
6. Taylor RR. *The Intentional Relationship: Occupational Therapy and the Use of Self.* FA Davis; 2020.
7. Bonsaken T, Vollestad K, Taylor RR. The Intentional Relationship Model: use of the therapeutic relationship in Occupational therapy practice. *Ergoterapeuten.* 2013;05:26–31.
8. AMA. *What Is Scope of Practice?* American Medical Association. https://www.ama-assn.org/practice-management/scope-practice/what-scope-practice.
9. AOTA. *Occupational Therapy Scope of Practice.* American Occupational Therapy Association. https://www.aota.org/practice/practice-essentials/scope-of-practice.
10. AOTA. *Licensure.* American Occupational Therapy Association. https://www.aota.org/career/state-licensure.

3 Prenatal and Genetic Pathophysiology

OBJECTIVES

By the end of this chapter, the reader should be able to:

- Demonstrate a basic understanding of the DNA molecule.
- Differentiate mutations from genetic inheritance.
- Provide a basic understanding of prenatal development.
- List various pathologies related to genetic inheritance.
- Interpret the possible genotype behind congenital conditions.
- Provide a basic understanding of teratogens that can lead to congenital anomalies.

Conception and Genetics

Science and the understanding of human development have come a long way since the 17th and 18th centuries. During this time period, there was a debate between the Animalculists (who believed all the information needed to produce a person was in the head of the sperm) and the Ovists (who believed all the information was stored in the ovum).[1] It was not until the late 18th century when Kasper Frederich Wolff contended that both parents contribute equally to the development of a new baby.[1] Since then, science has moved quickly toward a better understanding of human genetics. In 1990, an international group of scholars launched the Human Genome Project in an effort to study the sequence of human DNA (deoxyribonucleic acid) that constitutes our genetic makeup.[2] By the year 2003, about 90% of the human blueprint had been sequenced. This information about the human blueprint has helped to better understand genetic inheritance and mutations.[2]

The Study of Genetics

Fertilization or conception occurs when the sperm and the ovum meet, creating a zygote. When there are two ova at the time of conception and both are fertilized, this results in fraternal (dizygotic) twins, and when there is one ovum that splits, producing two babies, this results in identical (monozygotic) twins (Fig. 3.1).

Each of our cells contains 46 (23 pairs of) chromosomes, except for the gametes (the ovum and the sperm), which contain only 23 chromosomes. The chromosomes are made up of strands of DNA[1] (Fig. 3.2). DNA is a complex molecule shaped like a twisted ladder (called a double helix), and the rungs of this ladder consist of pairs of nucleotide bases (adenine, thymine, cytosine, and guanine). There are 3 billion base pairs in human DNA that are distributed across 23 chromosomes,[3] which carry 50 million to about 300 million base pairs each. Of the 23 pairs of chromosomes, 22 pairs are autosomes (unrelated to sexual expression), along with 1 pair of sex chromosomes (XX = female and XY = male).[1]

Segments of the DNA that contain the recipe for making a protein are called genes. Proteins are the basic building blocks for our cells and tissues.[4] There are about 20,000 protein-coding genes in the human genome.[4] These genes are the basic units of our inheritance. Pairs of genes that affect a trait are called alleles. If two alleles are the same, they are called homozygous; if they are different, they are called heterozygous.[1]

Some alleles are dominant, and some are recessive. A dominant gene is more likely to be expressed if partnered with a recessive gene. For example, when considering eye color, brown (B) is dominant over blue (b), which is recessive. If a brown and a blue allele occur together, the person will typically have brown eyes (Fig. 3.3). The pair of alleles (Bb) for a specific trait is called the genotype, and the expressed trait itself (brown eyes) is known as the phenotype.[5] For a recessive trait to show as a phenotype, the person must have a homozygous genotype of recessive alleles. If a recessive trait is not expressed because of the presence of a dominant allele, the person could still be a carrier and pass the recessive trait on to their children.

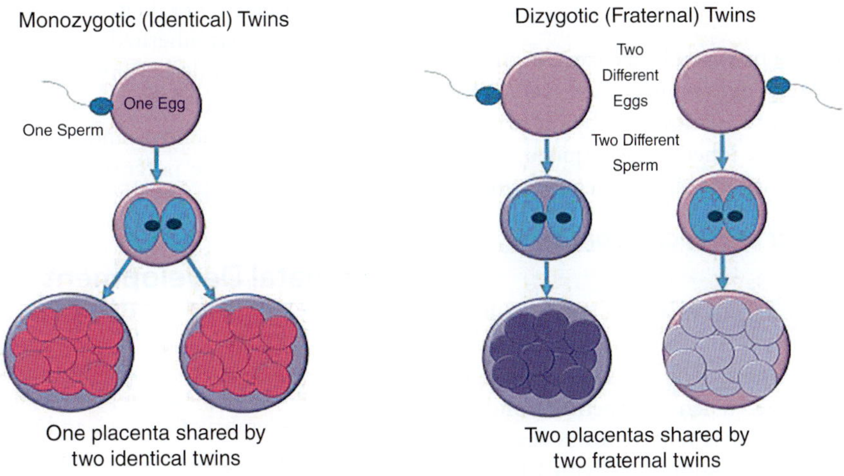

• **Fig. 3.1** Monozygotic and dizygotic twins.

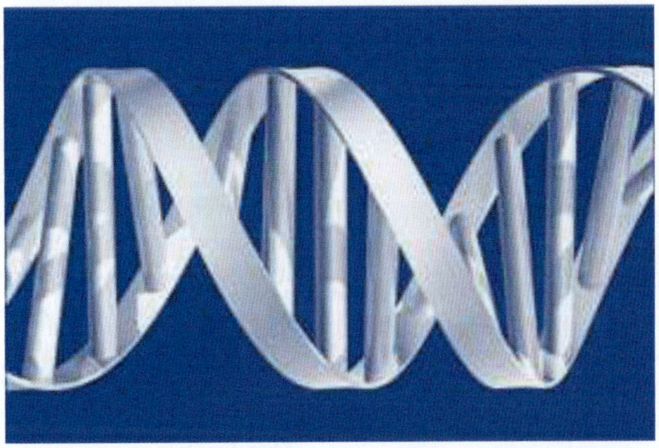

• **Fig. 3.2** The double helix of DNA. (From Matloff ET, Brierley KL. The double-helix derailed: the story of the BRCA patent. *Lancet*. 2010;376(9738):314–315.)

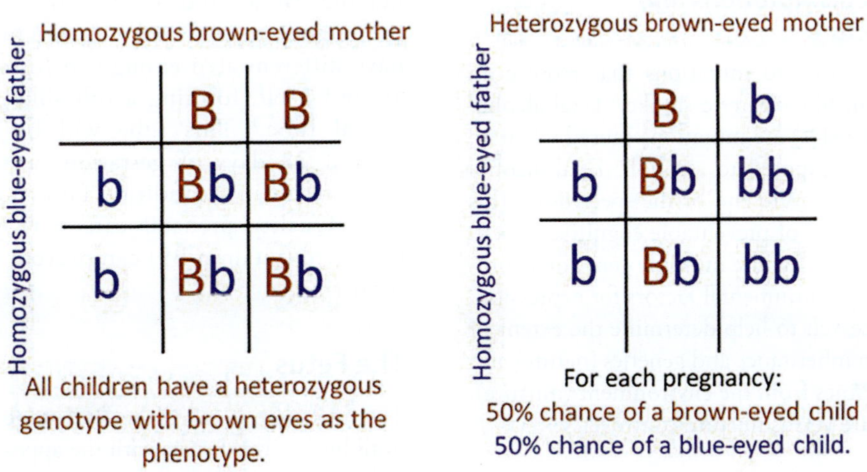

• **Fig. 3.3** Depiction of dominant and recessive inheritance.

Genetic Disorders

Genetic disorders are caused primarily by a change in the normal DNA sequence.[6] These disorders can be caused by a change in the number or structure of chromosomes, by mutations in one or more genes that can be inherited or acquired, or by a combination of gene mutations and environmental factors.

Changes in the Number or Structure of the Chromosomes

Some conditions in this category include Down syndrome (trisomy 21), which occurs when there is an extra 21st chromosome, and Turner syndrome, which occurs when a girl is missing an X chromosome. When an inherited condition affects the sex chromosomes, it is referred to as sex-linked. There can be an extra X chromosome (like with Klinefelter syndrome), or there can be a missing X chromosome (like with Turner syndrome). Fragile X is a condition caused by an incomplete X chromosome. It is one of the most common inherited causes of intellectual disability.[7] Because males have only one X chromosome, the symptoms are more pronounced in males (XY) than in females (XX) who, if their second X is healthy, may have no symptoms and simply be carriers.

Mutations (Inherited or Acquired)

An inherited predisposition is when an allele is inherited that produces the possibility of getting a trait or phenotype (like heart disease or obesity) but can be delayed or even prevented with a change in lifestyle. Phenylketonuria is a genetic predisposition for symptoms which can be prevented with a special milk-free diet. Late-appearing symptoms are not visible at birth but occur months to years down the road. Conditions in which this is the case include cystic fibrosis and Tay-Sachs disease. You can also inherit a certain type of Alzheimer's disease or heart disease, which will not show until you are older. Some diseases are carried via recessive genes, like sickle cell and Tay-Sachs.[1] In contrast, some mutations are acquired and not inherited, like progeria.

Combination of Gene Mutations and Environmental Factors

Some cancers develop due to mutations that require an environmental element like cigarette smoke.[6] Fetal alcohol spectrum disorders (FASDs) are mutations caused when an individual is prenatally exposed to alcohol.[8] Fetal alcohol syndrome is at the most severe end of the spectrum.[9] This is the most common cause of preventable cognitive deficit. Because many of our traits require multiple genes or a combination of genes and environmental factors for expression, there is a need for research to help determine the extent of effect that comes from inheritance and genetics (nature) and extent of effect that comes from the environment (nurture). This is called the nature versus nurture controversy.

Genetic Counseling

Genetic counseling can help prospective parents learn the odds of passing a trait on to their children. This counseling can also help to evaluate people for genetic predisposition (e.g., if one has inherited the gene for breast cancer). Lastly, counseling can determine the reaction range of a trait (the potential for variability in a heritable trait based on environmental influences) and the canalization of a trait (the limitation of the potential for variance in expression of a heritable trait).

Prenatal Development

The Zygote

There are three stages of prenatal development: the germinal stage, the embryonic stage, and the fetal stage. As previously mentioned, conception occurs when the sperm enters the ovum, producing a zygote. This is the start of the **germinal stage of development** (lasting about 2 weeks), during which the cells immediately begin to divide. Within the first 3 or 4 days, the zygote makes its way down the fallopian tube to the uterus, and its cells form a fluid-filled sphere called a blastocyst.[1] This will float freely for a day or 2 before embedding itself into the uterine wall. The cells continue to divide until two layers are formed: the outer ectoderm (which will later become the skin, nails, hair, teeth, and nervous system) and the inner endoderm (which will become the digestive system, liver, pancreas, salivary glands, and respiratory system). Soon after, a middle layer will form between the two. This layer is called the mesoderm (which will later develop into the inner layer of skin, muscles, skeleton, excretory, and circulatory systems). This ball created from the blastocyst, with the above three layers of cells, is called a gastrula (Fig. 3.4).

The Embryo

The next stage, the **embryonic stage** (from about 2 to 8 weeks) is characterized by rapid cellular division and differentiation as major body organs begin to form. This is a critical stage when the embryo is most vulnerable. By around 21 days of gestation, the cells in the mesoderm that make up the brain and spinal cord have differentiated enough to form a sheet that wraps around itself, forming a tube-like structure called the neural tube.[1] This tube will be completely formed around 28 days of gestation; an incomplete closure could result in a condition known as spina bifida (Fig. 3.5). Quality prenatal care with adequate intake of folic acid (vitamin B9) can prevent this condition from occurring.

The Fetus

The final stage is called the **fetal stage** (from about 8 weeks until birth). This begins with the appearance of the first bone cells. The fetus will grow rapidly during this stage, to about 20 times its previous length. The fetus will typically not be passive in the womb and will kick, tumble, swallow, make fists, hiccup, and suck their thumbs.[1]

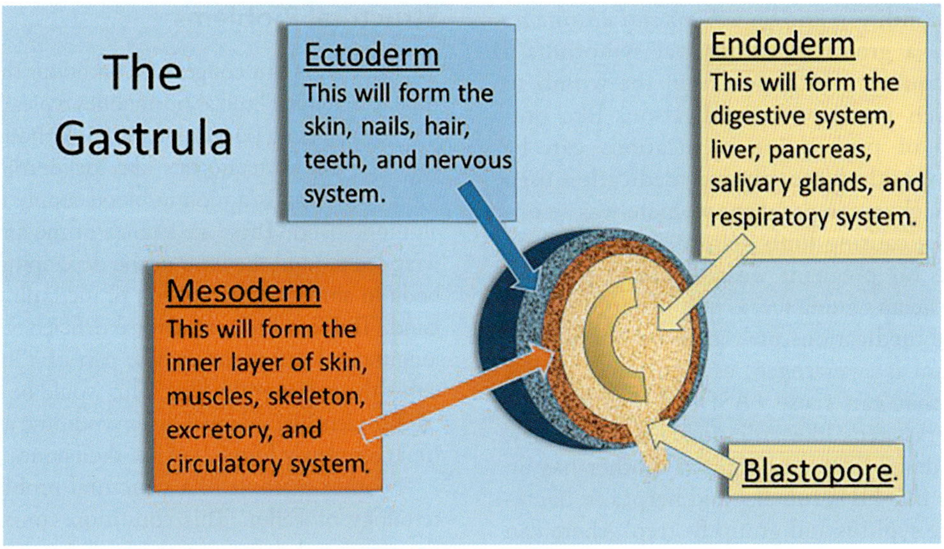

• **Fig. 3.4** The layers of the gastrula.

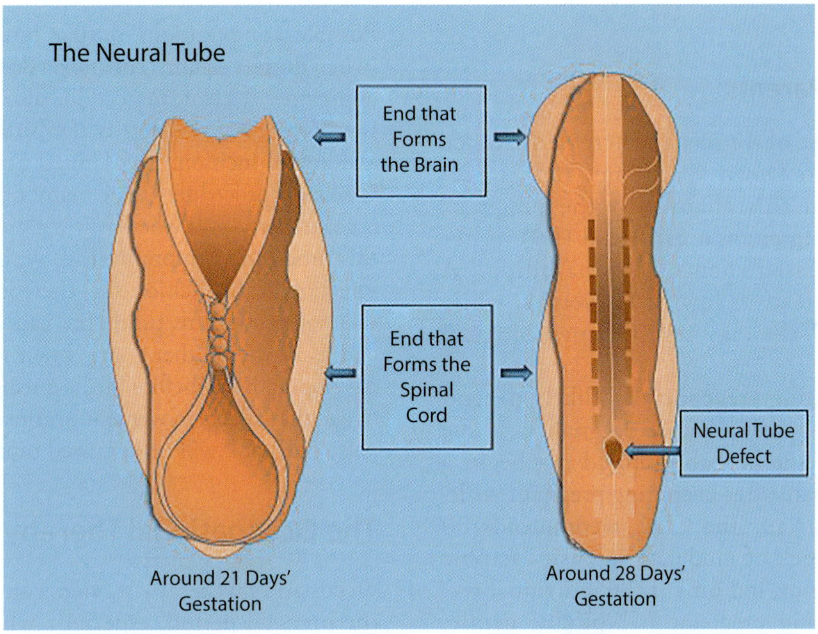

• **Fig. 3.5** The neural tube showing a defect that would result in spina bifida.

Congenital Anomalies

There are many congenital anomalies that can occur, affecting various systems in the human body. Some will be mentioned here, but most of the more common congenital anomalies seen by occupational therapy practitioners (OTPs) will be covered in this text for each system at the end of Chapters 10 through 20.

Teratogens

The word *teratogen* is from the Greek word for "monster" and refers to any environmental agent that can cause a congenital disorder by interfering with normal embryologic or fetal development.[10] Illegal drugs can act as teratogens. Babies can actually be born with crack-cocaine addiction, and substances like cocaine, heroin, and even marijuana can lead to low birth weight, heart problems, and a condition known as *neonatal abstinence syndrome*. This is a group of withdrawal symptoms a newborn baby acquires after exposure in the womb to certain drugs, even prescription medications like opioids.[10] A variety of prescription medications can be teratogens. Thalidomide, a prescription medication used to treat morning sickness in pregnant women, was a concern in the 1960s, causing limb deformities, and is no longer prescribed for pregnant women. Good prenatal care, under a physician's guidance, is important to ensure females only take medications proven to be safe during pregnancy. Alcohol is a teratogen, as mentioned earlier in this chapter, that can cause FASDs. There are also environmental teratogens like radiation, lead, mercury, and some pesticides.[10] When a pregnant mother has an infection (viruses like HIV, rubella, and herpes or bacterial infections like syphilis and group B strep), there can be detrimental problems in the developing fetus. The fetus can acquire the infection from the mother through the placenta. A newborn baby can also get the infection through vaginal fluid when passing through the birth canal or when breastfeeding from an infected mother.[1] This is another reason that thorough prenatal care is paramount.

The Health of the Parents

A mother over the age of 40 has an increased chance of having a baby with Down syndrome, and as previously mentioned in this chapter, if the pregnant woman is not receiving enough folic acid (B9) in her diet, there is an increased chance of spina bifida.[1] A diet low in zinc can lead to low birth weight, while insufficient iodine intake may result in neurological abnormalities.

Physical activity during pregnancy will likely depend on the activity of the mother before pregnancy. If she was not active before, she probably should not begin a vigorous exercise program after becoming pregnant without consulting a physician. The CDC recommends 30 minutes, 5 days per week of moderate-intensity aerobic exercise during pregnancy, but only if the individual was healthy before becoming pregnant.[11] Typically, gentle, low-impact exercises are reserved for the last 3 months of pregnancy.

The father's health is also very important. If he is exposed to large amounts of alcohol, radiation, or certain pesticides, it may result in abnormal sperm. Males who smoke are at an increased risk of impotence or of transmitting genetic abnormalities.[1] A pregnant woman's exposure to secondhand smoke has been linked to low-birth-weight infants and cancer in childhood. Low vitamin C (for either parent) increases the risk of birth defects, and a man of advanced age (over the age of 60) might have an increased chance of fathering a child with Down syndrome, dwarfism, or Marfan syndrome (with head and limb deformities).[1]

Structural Problems

There are also some congenital conditions that are simply structural. Congenital limb abnormalities typically involve a missing limb or a missing portion of a limb. Although these can sometimes be due to teratogens like thalidomide, the most common cause is a disruption in blood supply to a limb due to an amniotic band. These are strands of the amnion that become wrapped around the limb of the developing fetus, causing the body to amputate the portion of the limb that is distal to the band. This is called a transverse deficiency. There can also be longitudinal deficiencies where part of a limb is missing, like either the radius or the ulna. This would be caused by congenital disorders like Adams-Oliver syndrome and includes aplasia (not completely formed) of the skull bones.

Another example of a structural problem in utero is the tetralogy of Fallot. This condition consists of four different structural defects in the fetal heart, causing the blood to carry very little oxygen to the rest of the body. The only treatment for this is surgery. Tetralogy of Fallot will be discussed more in Chapter 13.

Mishaps During Birth

Possible complications during birth include breech birth (when the feet exit first) or anoxia (lack of oxygen to the baby). Sometimes a cesarean section, also known as a C-section, is required. A C-section is the birth of a baby through an abdominal incision. The United States has a higher rate of C-section procedures than many other countries, and there is controversy over whether it is always indicated.[12] Although this procedure is more invasive with an increased chance of infection at the incision site, there is some evidence to show that sometimes this procedure can save the life of the fetus and assist the mother.[13] Any brain injury that occurs to the developing brain before birth, during birth, or up to 2 years of age that affects movement or muscle tone is called cerebral palsy (CP). CP will be discussed more in Chapter 4.

The Occupational Therapy Scope of Practice

Occupational therapy services can be beneficial as early as the prenatal period, especially when working with pregnant women. Pregnant women will sometimes visit OTPs for discomfort in their back or inguinal area. Positioning instructions, posture exercises, gentle soft tissue stretching, and client/family education might be ordered by the physician (see Table 3.1).

Early intervention is extremely important for newborns who are born prematurely or with congenital anomalies. OTPs are also often seen in neonatal intensive care neonatal intensive care units (NICUs), providing this early care. NICUs serve newborn infants who have congenital conditions or respiratory/cardiac complications at birth that require continuous monitoring by nursing staff. OTPs perform gentle sensory integration techniques, range of motion, positioning, and parent education for these infants.

TABLE 3.1 Some Prenatal Conditions Seen by Occupational Therapy Practitioners

Pathologies Related to Genetic Inheritance	Genetic Anomaly	Symptoms
Cystic fibrosis	A progressive, degenerative disorder related to a gene found on chromosome 7, with an inherited autosomal recessive cause. The production of thick secretions leads to blockages in multiple bodily systems.[14]	• Difficulty breathing • Intestinal blockage/abdominal distension • Gastrointestinal complications (pain, diarrhea, constipation, greasy or foul-smelling stools) • Blocked biliary or pancreatic ducts • Trouble absorbing nutrients • Jaundice • Low body mass index • Muscle and joint pain • Clubbed feet or hands • Delayed growth or puberty[14]
Fragile X syndrome	An X-linked dominant inheritance caused by changes in the FRM1 gene.[15]	• Intellectual disability • Learning disorders • Speech impairment • Craniofacial deformities • Facial features: elongated face, prominent jaw and forehead, large ears • High-arched palate • Flat feet • Joint laxity/hypermobility • Hypotonia • Seizures • Social and behavioral concerns • ADHD[15]
Pathologies Related to Genetic Anomalies and Mutations (Not Inherited)	**Genetic Anomaly**	**Symptoms**
Trisomy 21—Down syndrome	Caused by an extra copy of chromosome 21.[16]	Distinct facial features/physical characteristics: • Short stature • Low-set ears • Thick, protruding tongue with high-arched palate • Epicanthal folds in eyes • Shorter extremities • Broad, short fingers and toes • Smaller hands with a single palmar crease (lacks palmar arches) Common comorbidities: • Vision problems (i.e., strabismus, nystagmus) • Hearing loss • Sleep disturbances (i.e., sleep apnea) • Heart defects, cardiovascular anomalies • Low muscle tone (i.e., difficulties with swallowing and sucking, weaker cervical spine) • AAI • More likely to develop infections • Developmental delays • Cognitive deficits[16]
Progeria	A rare genetic condition caused by a mutation of the LMNA gene with a life expectancy of about 14.5 years old.[17]	• Advanced aging in children • Cardiovascular complications • Hair loss • Wrinkled skin • Prominent eyes • Beaked nose • Scleroderma[17]

(Continued)

TABLE 3.1 Some Prenatal Conditions Seen by Occupational Therapy Practitioners—cont'd

Turner syndrome	Females born with only one X chromosome (XO).[18]	• Webbed neck • Skeletal abnormalities • Congenital swelling of extremities, hands, feet • Kidney problems • Congenital heart defect • Hormone imbalances • May lack secondary sex characteristics • Cognitive deficits[18]
Klinefelter syndrome	Males born with an extra X chromosome (XXY).[19]	• Learning disabilities • Behavioral and emotional problems • Abnormal body proportions (including small genitalia) and tall stature • Increased risk for cancer and autoimmune disorders • Infertility[19]
XYY syndrome	Males born with an extra Y chromosome.[20]	• Increased height • Mild developmental delays • Behavioral concerns • Increased incidence of dyslexia[20]
Pathologies Related to Teratogens	**Cause**	**Symptoms**
FASDs	A group of conditions caused by maternal exposure to alcohol in utero during pregnancy, with physical, pathological, cognitive, and behavioral effects.[21]	• Abnormal physical development (affects weight, height) • Facial anomalies with wider spaced eyes and a flat philtrum • CNS problems • Sleep and sucking problems as an infant • Vision or hearing problems • Cognitive deficit (attention, memory, etc.) • Learning disabilities • Developmental delays • Hyperactivity • Difficulty forming friendships[21]
Pathologies Related to Health of the Parents	**Cause**	**Symptoms**
Spina bifida	Can be caused by a lack of folic acid (vitamin B9) in the maternal diet, causing a defect in the developing neural tube.[22]	An opening in the developing spinal cord that can be very mild and hidden (occulta) • A small tuft of hair over the area To very severe (myelomeningocele) • Protrusion of neural tissue • Infections • Possible paralysis[22]
Childhood cancer	Childhood cancer can be caused by a number of variables, but one of them is paternal smoking.[23,24]	Paternal cigarette smoking and maternal exposure to secondhand smoke have been found to be related to a significantly elevated risk of childhood cancers, especially acute leukemia and lymphoma.[23,24]
Structural Problems	**Cause**	**Symptoms**
Caudal regression syndrome (sacral agenesis)	A rare congenital condition resulting in the underdevelopment of the sacrum in utero (can impact the lumbar spine as well).[25]	• A possible fluid-filled sac near the spinal cord • Difficulty urinating and having bowel movements • Underdeveloped lower extremities • May be unable to walk • Might have lower extremity and/or low back paralysis[25]
Torticollis	Shortening of one of the neck muscles (the sternocleidomastoid) with possible causes including abnormal development of muscle or abnormal positioning in the womb.[26]	Thickened or shortened neck muscles, impacting range of motion and motor development. • Neck pain • Headaches • Very tight sternocleidomastoid on one side of the child's neck • Head is laterally flexed and slightly extended toward one side, and rotated toward the opposite side[26]

TABLE 3.1 Some Prenatal Conditions Seen by Occupational Therapy Practitioners—cont'd

Mishaps During Birth or In Utero	Cause	Symptoms
CP	This is a group of disorders caused by damage to the movement centers of the brain, typically occurring before birth, but this can happen during birth or during the first 2 years of life.[27]	These disorders affect movement, posture, and muscle tone. There are many variations of symptoms in individuals with CP. Some possible symptoms are listed below: • Spasticity • Fluctuations in muscle tone • Ataxia (loss of balance and ambulatory coordination) • Delayed speech development • Problems swallowing • Cognitive deficits and learning difficulties are sometimes present[27]
DDH or congenital hip dislocation	This is a malformation of the infant's hip, typically with the acetabulum too shallow to accommodate the femoral head. It is more common in females, first-born babies, or babies born breech.[28]	• Positive Barlow test. Confirmed with "clunking" sound. See Fig. 3.6 • Positive Ortolani maneuver. See Fig. 3.7 • Leg length discrepancy • Abnormal gait pattern • Typically presents bilaterally, with genetic causes (hereditary laxity, hormonal secretions in utero) and environmental causes (increased uterine pressure, positions in utero) • Developmental delays and Trendelenburg sign, if not treated early

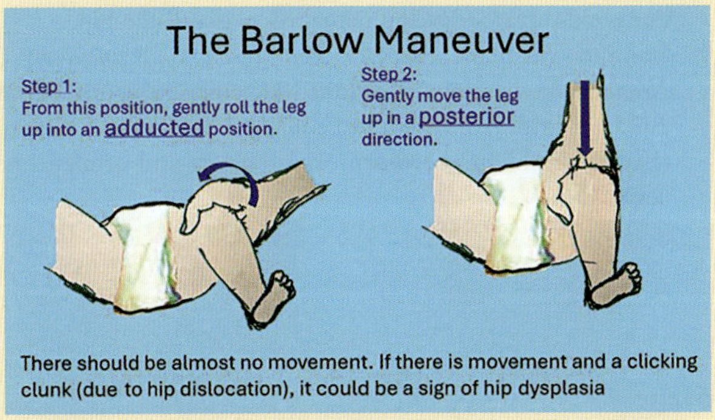

• **Fig. 3.6** The Barlow maneuver: The infant's thigh in the above position is gently moved posteriorly. There should be little to no movement, but if there is mobility in this direction and a "clunk" as the head femoral pops out of joint, it could possibly be hip dysplasia.[29] Courtesy *Natalie Norman Michaels*.

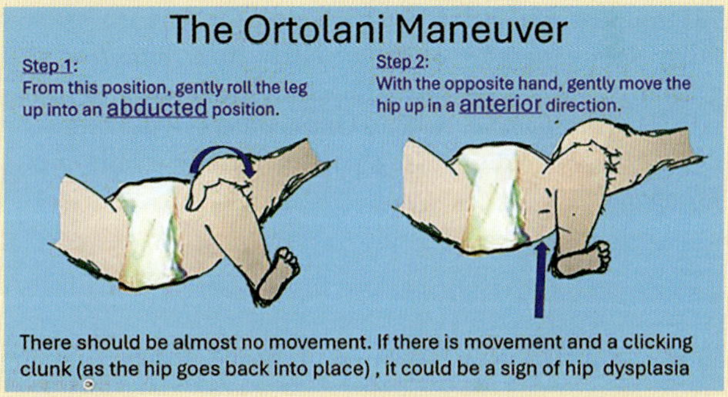

• **Fig. 3.7** The Ortolani maneuver: The infant's thigh in the above position is gently abducted, and pressure is applied to the posterior thigh in an anterior direction. There should be little to no movement, but if there is mobility in this direction, and a "clunk" as the femoral head pops back into place, it could possibly be hip dysplasia.[29] Courtesy *Natalie Norman Michaels*.

AAI, Atlantoaxial insecurity; *ADHD*, attention deficit hyperactivity disorder; *CP*, cerebral palsy; *DDH*, developmental dysplasia of the hip; *FASDs*, fetal alcohol syndrome disorders.

References

1. Papalia DE, Martorell G. *Experience Human Development*. 14th ed. McGraw Hill; 2021.
2. NIH. *The Human Genome Project*. The National Human Genome Research Institute; 2022. https://www.genome.gov/human-genome-project.
3. NIH. *Base Pair*. The National Human Genome Research Institute; 2022. https://www.genome.gov/genetics-glossary/Base-Pair.
4. NIH. *Gene*. The National Human Genome Research Institute; 2022. https://www.genome.gov/genetics-glossary/Gene.
5. National Geographic Society. *Genotypes*. The National Geographic Society. https://education.nationalgeographic.org/resource/genotypes.
6. NIH. *Genetic Disorders*. The National Human Genome Research Institute; 2018. https://www.genome.gov/For-Patients-and-Families/Genetic-Disorders.
7. CDC. *Fragile X Syndrome (FXS)*. Centers for Disease Control and Prevention; 2024. https://www.cdc.gov/fragile-x-syndrome/?CDC_AAref_Val=https://www.cdc.gov/ncbddd/fxs/index.html.
8. FASD United. *FASD*. FASD United: The National Voice on Fetal Alcohol Spectrum Disorders. https://fasdunited.org/fasd/.
9. CDC. *Fetal Alcohol Spectrum Disorders*. Centers for Disease Control and Prevention. https://www.cdc.gov/

physical-activity-basics/guidelines/healthypregnant-or-postpartum-women.html.
10. Cleveland Clinic. *Teratogens*. Cleveland Clinic; 2023. https://my.cleve-landclinic.org/health/articles/24325-teratogens.
11. CDC. *Physical Activity Recommendation for Pregnant and Postpartum Women*. Centers for Disease Control; 2023. https://www.cdc.gov/physicalactivity/basics/pregnant-and-postpartum-women.html.
12. WHO. *Cesarean Section Rates Continue to Rise, Amid Growing Inequalities in Access*. World Health Organization. https://www.who.int/news/item/16-06-2021-caesarean-section-rates-continue-to-rise-amid-growing-inequalities-in-access.
13. Mayo Clinic. *C-Section*. Mayo Clinic. https://www.mayoclinic.org/tests-procedures/c-section/about/pac-20393655.
14. NIH. *Cystic Fibrosis Symptoms*. NIH; 2022. https://www.nhlbi.nih.gov/health/cystic-fibrosis/symptoms.
15. GARD. *Fragile X Syndrome*. Genetic and Rare Diseases Information Center. NIH; 2023. https://rarediseases.info.nih.gov/diseases/6464/fragile-x-syndrome/living.
16. NIH. *What Conditions or Disorders Are Commonly Associated With Down Syndrome?* NIH; 2017. https://www.nichd.nih.gov/health/topics/down/conditioninfo/associated.
17. Cleveland Clinic. *Progeria*. Cleveland Clinic; 2022. https://my.clevelandclinic.org/health/diseases/17850-progeria.
18. GARD. *Turner Syndrome*. Genetic and Rare Diseases Information Center. NIH; 2023. https://rarediseases.info.nih.gov/diseases/7831/turner-syndrome.
19. NIH. *About Klinefelter Syndrome*. NIH; 2023. https://www.genome.gov/Genetic-Disorders/Klinefelter-Syndrome.
20. NORD. *XYY-Syndrome*. National Organization of Rare Diseases; 2023. https://rarediseases.org/rare-diseases/xyy-syndrome/#symptoms.
21. CDC. *Basics About FASDs*. Centers for Disease Control and Prevention; 2022. https://www.cdc.gov/ncbddd/fasd/facts.html.
22. Mayo Clinic. *Spina Bifida*. Mayo Clinic; 2022. https://www.mayoclinic.org/diseases-conditions/spina-bifida/symptoms-causes/syc-20377860.
23. Ji BT, Shu XO, Linet MS, et al. Paternal cigarette smoking and the risk of childhood cancer among offspring of nonsmoking mothers. *J Natl Cancer Inst*. 1997;89(3):238–244. https://doi.org/10.1093/jnci/89.3.238.
24. Chunxia D, Meifang W, Jianhua Z, et al. Tobacco smoke exposure and the risk of childhood acute lymphoblastic leukemia and acute myeloid leukemia: a meta-analysis. *Medicine (Baltimore)*. 2019(28):e16454. https://doi.org/10.1097/MD.0000000000016454.
25. Cleveland Clinic. *Caudal Regression Syndrome*. Cleveland Clinic; 2022. https://my.clevelandclinic.org/health/diseases/23425-caudal-regression-syndrome.
26. Cleveland Clinic. *Torticollis*. Cleveland Clinic; 2022. https://my.clevelandclinic.org/health/diseases/22430-torticollis.
27. Mayo Clinic. *Cerebral Palsy*. Mayo Clinic; 2021. https://www.mayoclinic.org/diseases-conditions/cerebral-palsy/symptoms-causes/syc-20353999.
28. John Hopkins. *Developmental Dysplasia of the Hip*. John Hopkins. Health; 2023. https://www.hopkinsmedicine.org/health/conditions-and-diseases/developmental-dysplasia-of-the-hip.
29. Stanford Medicine. *Barlow and Ortolani Maneuvers: The Newborn Examination*. Stanford Medicine. Newborn Nursery; 2023. https://med.stanford.edu/newborns/clinical-rotations/residents/residents-newborn-exam/barlow-and-ortalani-maneuvers.html.

4

Typical Development and Pathophysiology During Infancy

OBJECTIVES

By the end of this chapter, the reader should be able to:

- Explain the importance of understanding typical development before attempting to understand what is atypical.
- Demonstrate a basic understanding of the typical stages of childbirth.
- Provide a basic understanding of the APGAR scale.
- Differentiate between typical child birth and atypical child birth.
- Differentiate between typical infant development and atypical infant development.
- List various pathophysiological conditions related to atypical infant development.
- List various pathophysiological conditions related to atypical infant brain development.
- Differentiate between conditions caused by infection and congenital anomalies.

The term "infancy" typically refers to the period from birth until about 12 months of age. This chapter will give a short overview of the typical development from newborn until 1 year of age and then review some of the more common pathological conditions typically seen by occupational therapy practitioners.

Parturition

Parturition is the process of giving birth. When childbirth goes smoothly, it follows the typical path explained below. This chapter will briefly summarize the events that take place during a typical birth, followed by those of an atypical birth.

Typical Birth

Childbirth or parturition occurs in three stages: dilation, expulsion, and placental stage.[1,2] Dilation, also called early labor, is when the cervix first begins to dilate and continues until the cervix is completely dilated. There are two phases of dilation. The latent phase (typically lasting 5–6 hours, although it can be longer for a first-time birth) is when the cervix moves from 0 to about 4 cm of dilation. The active phase (typically lasting 3–6 hours) is dilation from 4 to 10 cm.[1] As the cervix dilates, the uterus contracts. At the beginning of the stage of dilation, the contractions occur every 20 to 30 minutes, but as labor progresses, the contractions increase in frequency and intensity. By the end of this stage, the contractions are more intense and about 3 minutes apart.[2]

The second stage of parturition is expulsion. This stage begins from complete dilation until after the birth of the baby. This stage has two phases: active and passive. The passive phase is when the baby's head is moving down through the vaginal canal, and the active phase is when the mother feels the urge to push or bear down, along with the uterine contractions.[1] The back of the baby's head is typically the first to present through the birth canal.

The third stage of parturition is the placental stage. This starts right after birth and ends with uterine contractions causing separation and release of the placenta from the vaginal canal.[1] In some cases, however, this separation can lead to bleeding, and the placenta sometimes needs to be surgically removed[2] (Fig. 4.1).

Within 5 minutes after birth, doctors will typically assess the health of a baby using the APGAR scale.[3] This is a scoring system that looks at five dimensions: appearance, pulse, grimace, activity, and respiration. The highest score on each of the five dimensions is a 2, so the highest total score is 10 (Table 4.1). A score of 7 or above means the baby is in good health. A lower score means that immediate medical care is needed, such as suctioning, to clear the airways. A score of less than 7 is common during the 60-second period immediately after birth for babies born after complicated pregnancies or cesarean sections. Typically, this improves within minutes. If the APGAR score is still low 5 minutes after suctioning, then something else may be wrong that requires more intensive intervention.[3]

The Neonatal Behavioral Assessment Scale developed by Dr. Berry Brazelton is another measurement tool that is typically completed within 24 to 36 hours after birth, in which 28 behavioral items and 20 neurological items are used to

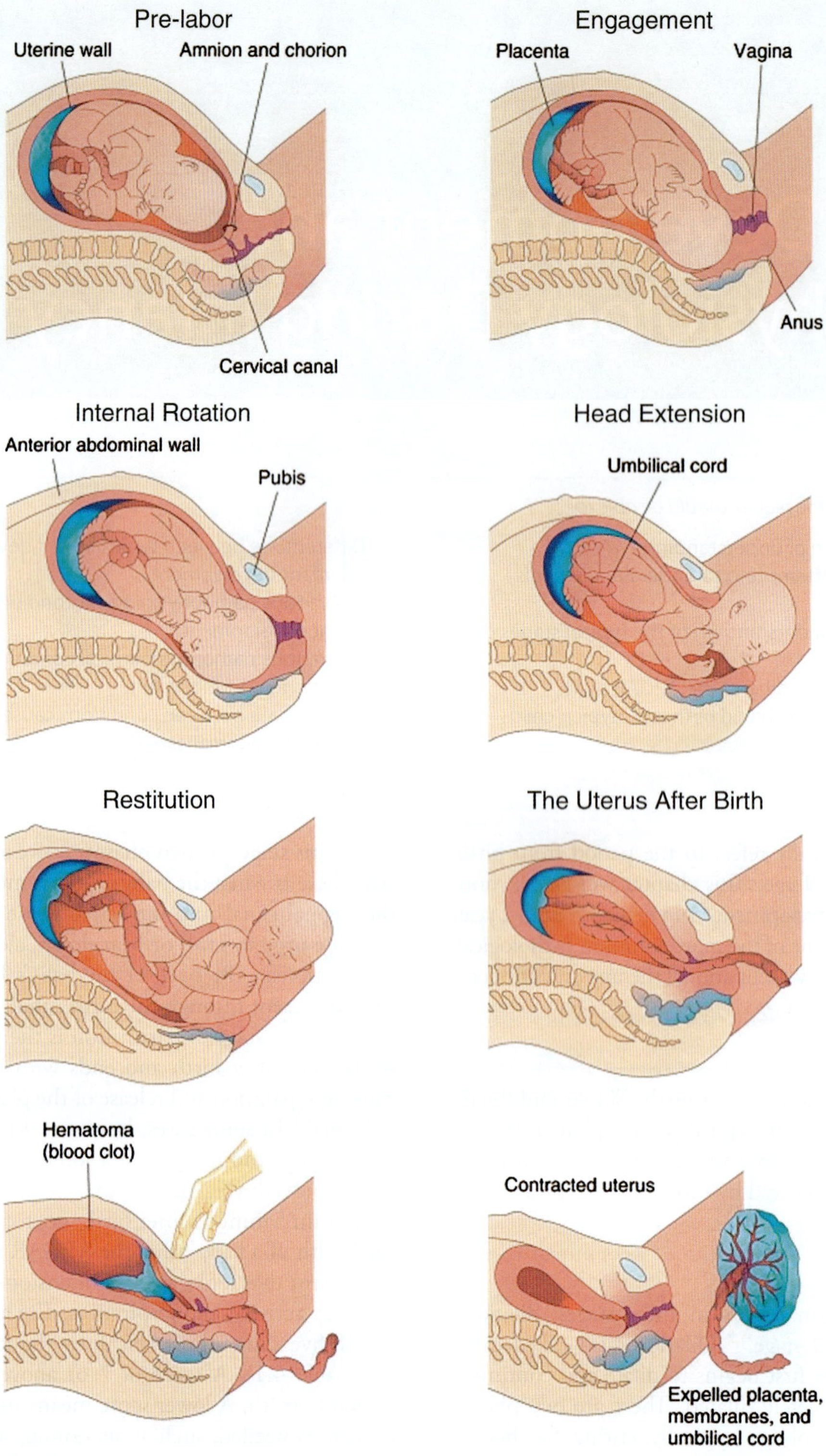

• **Fig. 4.1** Normal birth. (Used with permission from Clinical Overview. Normal Labor. Elsevier Point of Care. ClinicalKey. https://www.clinicalkey.com/#!/content/clinical_overview/67-s2.0-ba02ba6f-f40e-480b-81ac-787414c07c1b?scrollTo=%2367-s2.0-ba02ba6f-f40e-480b-81ac-787414c07c1b-77633564-f268-4d80-a1ba-b699183428c3-annotated.)

examine infants and newborns up to 2 months of age. It helps to describe a newborn's response to the world outside the womb and to see how certain behaviors are integrated into the child's development.[4,5] There are many other scales used as well.

Atypical Birth

Maternal Complications

During birth, there is the potential for some maternal complications, such as uterine rupture, hemorrhage, or

TABLE 4.1 The APGAR Scale[3]

APGAR Sign	2	1	0
Appearance (skin coloration)	Normal color all over (hands and feet are pink)	Normal color (but hands and feet are bluish)	Bluish-gray or pale all over
Pulse (heart rate)	Normal (above 100 beats per minute)	Below 100 beats per minute	Absent (no pulse)
Grimace (responsiveness or "reflex irritability")	Pulls away, sneezes, or coughs with stimulation	Facial movement only (grimace) with stimulation	Absent (no response to stimulation)
Activity (muscle tone)	Active, spontaneous movement	Arms and legs flexed with little movement	No movement, "floppy" tone
Respiration (rate and effort)	Normal rate and effort, nice loud cry	Slow or irregular breathing	Absent (no breathing)

From *What Is the Apgar Score?* Johns Hopkins All Children's Hospital; 2023. https://www.hopkinsallchildrens.org/Patients-Families/Health-Library/HealthDocNew/What-Is-the-Apgar-Score.

infection. Other maternal comorbidities such as diabetes or obesity can put the mother at higher risk.[6] Obesity during pregnancy not only puts females at a higher risk for eventual cardiometabolic disorders but can restrict the growth of a normal term baby or lead to a preterm delivery.[7]

The Position of the Baby

There can be variations in the position of the fetus at birth. A face presentation occurs when the baby's chin leads the way, a breech presentation is when the baby's feet lead the way, and transverse position is when the baby is lying horizontally. These variations will either require rotation for better positioning or what is known as a cesarean section birth (the surgical removal of the fetus through an abdominal incision).[2]

Problems During Expulsion

As already mentioned, possible complications during birth include breech birth (when the feet exit first) or anoxia (lack of oxygen to the baby), which may require a cesarean section (birth of the baby through an abdominal incision). The United States has a higher rate of cesarean section procedures than any other country, and there is controversy over whether this is always indicated. Although this procedure is more invasive with an increased chance of infection at the incision site, there is some evidence to show that sometimes this procedure can save the life of the fetus and assist the mother.[8]

Preterm and Low Birth Weight

Although a "normal" pregnancy lasts 37 to 42 weeks, some infants are born prematurely (shorter than 37 weeks gestation) and some are born small-for-date (weighing less than expected for the number of weeks gestation).[9] The term low birth weight applies to any baby weighing less than 5.5 pounds (2500 g) at birth.[10] Factors that can lead to a low birth weight baby include poor nutrition for the pregnant mother, teratogens like alcohol (that can lead to Fetal Alcohol Spectrum Disorders or FASD, see Chapters 3 and 19), multiple births,[8] or the age of the mother (younger than age 15).[11] Pregnancy during adolescence was also associated with higher rates of preeclampsia and threatened abortion.[12]

Length of gestation and birth weight are important predictors of infant survival.[9] Low birth weight has been found to be a risk factor for Sudden Infant Death Syndrome (SIDS). SIDS is the death of an apparently healthy infant prior to 12 months of age and is the third leading cause of death in infants.[12] Although the 2020 National Vital Statistics Report from the CDC listed congenital malformations as the first leading cause of infant death, the second leading cause of death was short gestation and low birth weight.[13] Infant death rate varies in the United States by race, with the highest mortality rate of infants born from non-Hispanic Black females (10.38 deaths per 1000), followed by non-Hispanic American Indians and Alaska Natives (7.68), Hispanic (4.69), White (4.40), and Asian (3.14).[14]

Postmaturity

A baby can also be born later than expected, and like prematurity, this can lead to problems. Postmaturity is when a baby is born at a gestation greater than 42 weeks. Because of an inadequate blood supply, these babies tend to be long and thin and can increase the need for a cesarean section delivery.[9]

Other Atypical Conditions Sometimes Seen at Birth

There are other possible conditions that are typically diagnosed at the time of birth that will be discussed in subsequent chapters. Cardiac anomalies like Tetralogy of Fallot will be covered in Chapter 13, gastrointestinal disorders like tracheoesophageal fistula will be discussed in Chapter 15, metabolic disorders like phenylketonuria and jaundice will be discussed in Chapter 18, and orthopedic and structural anomalies like congenital transverse limb deficiency will be covered in Chapter 20.

Typical Development During Infancy

The term neonate typically refers to a newborn who is less than 4 weeks of age.[14]

According to the CDC growth charts, the weight range (at the 50th female baby percentile to the 75th male baby percentile) of the typical newborn in the United States in 2021 was around 7.5 to 8.5 pounds,[15] and the length was around 19.4 to 20.4 inches.[16]

Infant Physical Development

Infant development for healthy, full-term infants continues the way it did in utero, in a cephalocaudal (from head to foot) and proximodistal (from trunk to fingers and toes) pattern.[9] This growth is very fast during the first 3 years of life, with the highest rate of growth during the first 2 months.[9] In 2021, the typical child increased in size (at the 50th female baby percentile to the 75th male baby percentile) from around 11.5 to 13.5 pounds at 2.5 months to around 30.6 to 34.1 pounds at 3 years.[15] As the baby grows, primitive reflexes emerge. There are estimated to be around 27 of these reflexes that emerge right at birth or soon after and disappear (or are integrated) by 6–12 months of age (Table 4.2).[9]

Typical development can also be monitored by looking closely at a child's developmental milestones. These consist of the typical gross motor milestones, like rolling over and crawling (Fig. 4.2) and the typical fine motor milestones, like reaching and grasping (Table 4.3).

TABLE 4.2 Primitive Reflexes

Primitive Reflex	Purpose of the Reflex	What Is the Movement?	When It Appears	When It Becomes Integrated
Moro reflex	Survival—an arousal response	This is an arching of the trunk and abduction of the arms in response to a sudden startle stimulus.	Birth	2–4 months
Rooting reflex	Survival—for feeding	Babies will automatically turn their head toward a touch sensation on the cheek.	Birth	3–4 months
Palmer or grasp reflex	To assist the baby with grasp development	The baby's hand will close when you touch the palm.	Birth	5–6 months
ATNR	To help the baby pass through the canal during a vaginal delivery cross pattern movements	When you turn the baby's head to one side, the extremities on that side extend at the elbow and knee and abduct at the shoulder and hip. The two extremities on the opposite side will flex. This is also called the fencer's pose.	Birth	6 months
Spinal Galant reflex	Assists with crawling and creeping	When the baby is held in prone suspension, stroking the lateral side of the spine will make the trunk laterally flex in that direction.	Birth	3–9 months
STNR	To prepare the baby to move from prone to quadruped for crawling	When in quadruped, and the neck flexes for the baby to look down, the arms will flex and the legs will extend, and when the neck extends, the arms extend and the legs flex.	6–9 months	9–11 months
Landau reflex	To assist with posture	When the baby is held in the air in prone with hands supporting the stomach, the baby will look up, arch the back, and extend the extremities.	4–5 months	1 year
Babinski reflex	This can test the CST	When you stroke the bottom of the foot, the ankle will dorsiflex and toes with fan out.*	Birth	At around 24 months
TLR		When the baby's neck is flexed in prone, the arms, legs, and trunk flex, and when the neck extends in supine, the arms and legs extend.	In utero	3½ years

*Information on the Babinski sign is from Acharya AB, Jamil RT, Dewey JJ. Babinski reflex. In: *StatPearls*. StatPearls Publishing; 2022. https://www.ncbi.nlm.nih.gov/books/NBK519009/.

ATNR, Asymmetric tonic neck reflex; *CST*, corticospinal tract; *STNR*, symmetric tonic neck reflex; *TLR*, tonic labyrinthine reflex.

Adapted in part from https://www.sprockettherapy.com/primitive-reflexes.html.

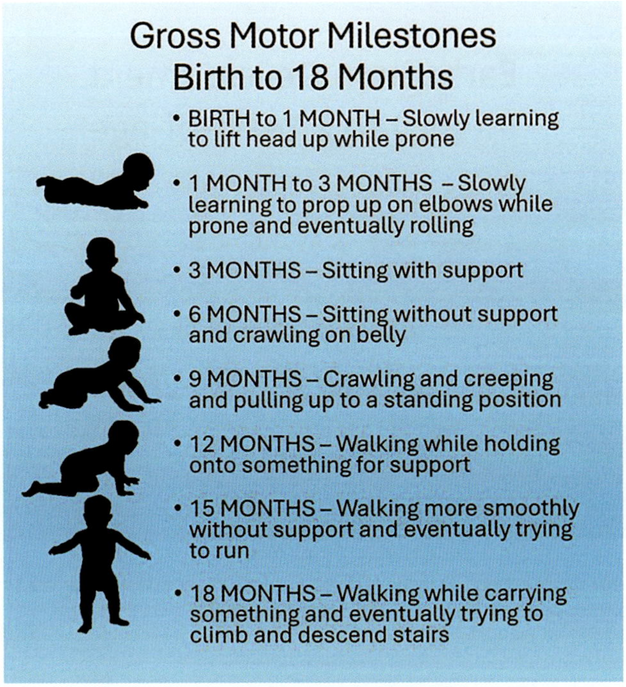
Gross Motor Milestones
Birth to 18 Months
• BIRTH to 1 MONTH – Slowly learning to lift head up while prone
• 1 MONTH to 3 MONTHS – Slowly learning to prop up on elbows while prone and eventually rolling
• 3 MONTHS – Sitting with support
• 6 MONTHS – Sitting without support and crawling on belly
• 9 MONTHS – Crawling and creeping and pulling up to a standing position
• 12 MONTHS – Walking while holding onto something for support
• 15 MONTHS – Walking more smoothly without support and eventually trying to run
• 18 MONTHS – Walking while carrying something and eventually trying to climb and descend stairs

• **Fig. 4.2** Gross motor developmental milestones. (Image modified from Etsy/Happysept; data from https://www.cdc.gov/ncbddd/actearly/milestones/milestones-2yr.html.)

TABLE 4.3 Fine Motor Developmental Milestones

Approximate Age (months)	Fine Motor Skill
1	Will tightly grasp objects placed in their hand. This is the grasp reflex.
2	Will begin to notice and play with their own hands. Can briefly hold a toy.
3	Able to bring hands to mouth and begins to develop voluntary grasp. The child will look at an object and reach for it (visually directed reaching).
4–6	Can reach for toys while prone and can transfer toys from one hand to the other when supine. Can bang an object on a table and can shake a rattle.
7–9	Can reach for toys while seated and grasp smaller objects with fingers. Can use thumb and index finger opposition.
10–12	Can clasp hands and can drop and pick up objects upon request.
13–15	Can scribble, begins to stack blocks to make towers, and tries to place pegs into board. Can place objects into medium or large containers.

Adapted from https://www.choc.org/userfiles/file/Rehab-Developmental%20Milestones%20final.pdf.

Infant Brain Development

The human brain weighs 25% of its adult weight (of 3.5 pounds) at birth but grows to 70% by 1 year of age and to 80% by 2 years of age (Fig. 4.3).[9] Some of this increase in brain weight is due to myelination. Myelin is a fatty substance found in glial cells that insulate the axons of the neurons.[9] When these cells are found in the central nervous system (the brain and the spinal cord), they are called oligodendrocytes, and when found in the

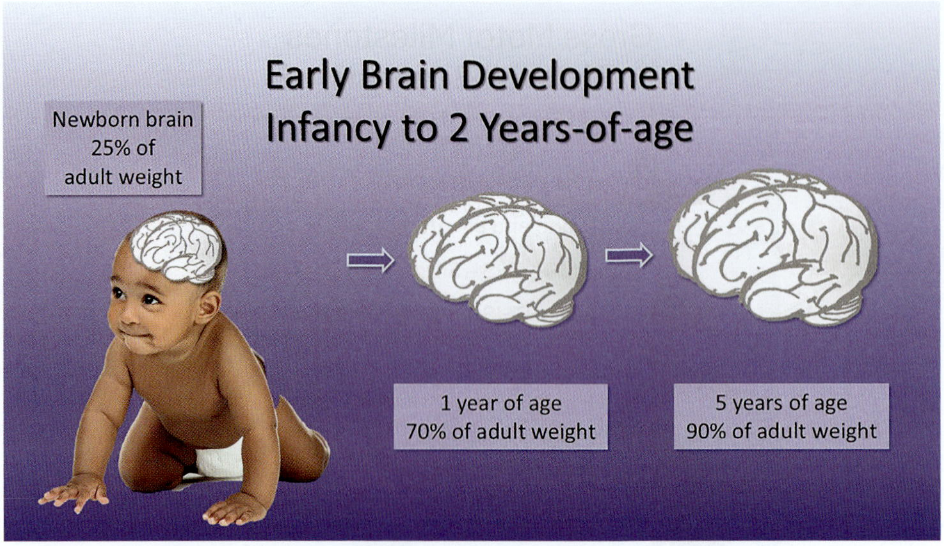

• **Fig. 4.3** Infant brain development. (Image modified from iStock.com/5second; data from https://www.cdc.gov/ncbddd/childdevelopment/earlybrain-development.html.)

extremities, they are called Schwann cells. These cells are responsible for the provision of nutrients to the nearby neurons and for the insulation needed for efficient transfer of neural information. Myelination begins to form in utero at around 20 weeks of gestation and continues to form throughout infancy, accelerating from 12 months of age until around age 2, but the process begins to slow down and continues until around age 5.[18]

During the first year of life, the cerebellum (for balance and coordination) grows rapidly, almost tripling in size.[19] Areas of the cerebral cortex responsible for vision and hearing are mature by about 6 to 12 months of age, but areas of the frontal lobe used for reasoning and cognition are not fully developed for several years. Early in life, there is an overproduction of neuronal synapses, with up to twice as many synapses as in adulthood.[19] This period is followed by a pruning or elimination of unused synapses that gradually reduces the number closer to what is seen in adults.[20]

The sense of touch and pain is believed to be fairly well developed in newborns as well as smell and taste. Hearing is also well developed, and newborn babies tend to prefer a higher pitched voice (female) to a lower pitched voice (male).[21] Visual acuity is the last to develop. According to the American Academy of Ophthalmology, a newborn's vision is estimated to be about 20/400.[22] By 6 months of age, vision has improved to about 20/120 and continues to improve until age 2 when it reaches 20/20.

The CDC recommends the following for healthy brain development: good nutrition, protection from exposure to toxins and infections, and healthy experiences with other people and the world.[23] It is very important that infants receive adequate nutrition because inadequate nutrition can result in a decline in motor and cognitive development. Breast milk is believed to be the ideal food for infants because it is easiest to digest and because it contains a proper balance of nutrients as well as immunoglobulins to help the baby fight infection.[24] Bottle-feeding with a well-balanced formula can also have benefits. Others can feed the baby if a bottle is used, and the amount consumed can be controlled. It is important for the parents to take the child to a qualified pediatrician or a lactation consultant and to ask questions.

Atypical Development During Infancy

Atypical Physical Development

There are many conditions that can result in atypical physical development during infancy. These conditions can cause minor to severe developmental delays. The three discussed here are failure to thrive (FTT), large intestinal atresia/stenosis, and osteogenesis imperfecta. Some of the conditions affecting physical development in this age group that are commonly seen by occupational therapy practitioners (OTPs) in the clinical setting can be found in Table 4.4.

Failure to Thrive

The term *FTT* in infancy refers to an inability to gain weight at the typical rate.[25] These children are typically at the third to fifth percentile of the pediatric growth charts.[26] The problem can be organic or nonorganic.[25,26] If the baby has an organic cause, it means that a physiologic reason has been determined, such as vomiting, diarrhea, or some other medical disorder. When a child has FTT with no

TABLE 4.4 Conditions Affecting Physical Development Commonly Seen by OTPs

Condition	Symptoms	Implications for Occupational Therapy Treatment
Spina bifida[34]	A type of neural tube defect. The symptoms vary depending on the type and severity of the condition. *Spina Bifida Occulta* • Mild or "hidden" • No involvement of spinal cord or nerves • One or two affected vertebrae leaving a gap but no neural tissue involved. • Often asymptomatic *Meningocele* • Spinal opening with an exposed pouch of CSF • This sac contains none of the spinal cord, and there may or may not be only minimal nerve damage. *Myelomeningocele* • The most serious form of spina bifida • Part of the spinal cord and the adjoining nerves are in this sac. • There is nerve damage. • Sensorimotor problems at or below level of lesion • Paralysis of lower extremities • Physical abnormalities or deformities.[34] 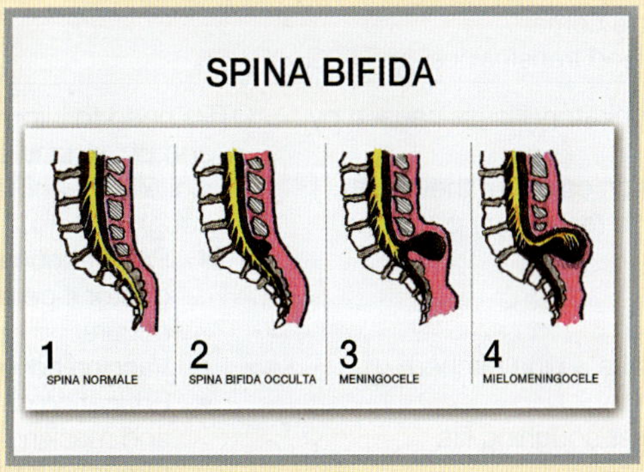	OT is typically referred when there are deficits. This is more likely to occur with *Myelomeningocele*. • Bowel and bladder programs may be indicated. • Because of interventions that may increase the chance of hydrocephalus, clients may or may not have cognitive and/or learning issues. • Educating the family and client on skin care, urology, and diet is always beneficial, including safe positioning during bathing, dressing, and feeding. • Use of assistive devices for mobility • Working to improve the child's access to meaningful activities
Down syndrome[35]	Caused by an extra copy of chromosome 21 Distinct facial features/physical characteristics: • Short stature • Low-set, small ears • Thick, protruding tongue with high-arched palate • Epicanthal folds in eyes • Shorter extremities • Broad, short fingers and toes • Smaller hands with a single palmar crease (lacks palmar arches) • Low muscle tone (hypotonicity) • Tiny white spots on the iris of the eye Common comorbidities: • Vision problems (i.e., strabismus, nystagmus) • Hearing loss • Sleep disturbances (i.e., sleep apnea) • Heart defects, cardiovascular anomalies • AAI • More likely to develop infections • Developmental delays • Cognitive deficits	Depending on the degree of severity and the specific conditions of the individual, the child or adult with Down syndrome could potentially benefit from: • Feeding support • Addressing developmental delays • Environmental and task modification • Family coaching and training • Education with self-help skills • Prevocational training • ADL/IADL interventions • School-based/educational interventions

(Continued)

TABLE 4.4 Conditions Affecting Physical Development Commonly Seen by OTPs—cont'd

Condition	Symptoms	Implications for Occupational Therapy Treatment
Jaundice[36] and kernicterus[37]	*Jaundice*: A yellow discoloration of the skin and the whites of the eyes caused by a build-up of bilirubin (a yellow pigment in red blood cells). It is seen most often in babies born before 38 weeks of gestation because their liver is not yet mature enough to filter the bilirubin from the blood. • Presents as yellow skin and eyes • Dark urine • Pale stool Some babies are born with jaundice (physiologic jaundice), which is very common and can be easily treated. Persistent or pathologic jaundice may be caused by various disorders (infectious, endocrine, genetic). *Kernicterus*: This is a complication from severe jaundice, resulting in brain damage from high levels of bilirubin in the blood. Can result in: • CP • Hearing loss • Intellectual disabilities • Permanent brain damage and possible coma • Interventions include phototherapy, blood transfusions, and IVIG.	• Notify the doctor if a child has jaundice. This may be an indication of a pathological cause and needs to be diagnosed and treated immediately to prevent the development of Kernicterus. Sometimes, the OTP is the first person to notice skin discolorations in a newborn infant receiving services for early intervention. Although this may be a minor episode of jaundice, it is always best to err on the side of caution. This is one place where OT advocacy comes into play and notifying the physician of this finding could save a life.
Pertussis[38]	Aka *whooping cough*, a very contagious respiratory illness caused by a bacteria called *Bordetella pertussis* • Symptoms at first look like the common cold, but the cough lasts weeks or months and can lead to respiratory problems. • Runny nose • Low-grade fever • Cough lasting for weeks or months • Inhaling after a coughing fit will make a high pitched, "whoop" sound • Vomiting and exhaustion during or after coughing fits • Breathing difficulties	OTPs need to inform the parents and physicians of their pediatric individuals who exhibit this type of cough pattern. • Parent education/notifying doctor if persistent cough occurs • Vaccine advocacy • Educating on hand washing and masking to prevent spread throughout the household
SIDS[39]	An unexplained death of an infant prior to their first birthday	The main focus of OT is to help with prevention, especially for at-risk clients. Factors making a child more at-risk include brain defects, low birth weight, and respiratory infection. • Parent education about positioning and safe sleeping habits • Encouraging parents to place their infant child on their back to sleep • Discuss support groups and stress management with parents

AAI, Atlantoaxial Instability; *CP*, cerebral palsy; *CSF*, cerebrospinal fluid; *IVIG*, intravenous immunoglobulin; *SIDS*, sudden infant death syndrome.

medical cause, it is referred to as nonorganic. This typically requires a nonmedical solution by modifying the environment in some way, like changing the formula or changing the way the baby is held during feeding. Inadequate nutrition, neglect, or abuse can be causes of nonorganic FTT.[25,26]

Large Intestinal Atresia/Stenosis

Large intestinal atresia/stenosis is a rare, congenital obstruction in the opening or the lumen of the colon.[27] This obstruction can be partial or complete. Because this is difficult to detect prenatally, most cases are not diagnosed until after the baby is born. The first symptom is the lack of meconium or stool. The baby might also have abdominal distention and/or vomiting. If the obstruction is partial and not complete, the baby might not be diagnosed until weeks after birth.[27]

Osteogenesis Imperfecta

Osteogenesis Imperfecta (OI), also called the brittle bone disease, is a genetic disorder affecting the bones, making them very soft and easy to break. Individuals with OI have one or two defective genes that were either inherited from one or both parents or formed as a mutation. These individuals are prone to frequent fractures, sometimes occurring in utero.[28] There are eight variations of this disorder, from type I, which is the mildest (about 50% of cases), to type II, which is the most severe (these babies usually die within 1 week of birth). Type III is the most severe type for babies who survive as newborns. Types IV through VIII vary in severity from mild to severe.[28]

Atypical Brain Development

There are many different types of congenital brain anomalies. The three discussed here are cerebral palsy (CP), autism, and Fragile X. Some other conditions affecting brain development in this age group that are commonly seen by OTPs in the clinical setting can be found in Table 4.5.

TABLE 4.5 Conditions Affecting Brain Development Commonly Seen by OTPs

Condition	Symptoms	Occupational Therapy Intervention
CP[40]	A group of disorders that appear during infancy or early childhood, characterized by motor impairments, typically caused by a brain injury (i.e., infarction, hemorrhage, infection, hypoxia) in utero, during birth, or in the first 2 years of life. Classification dependent on limbs involved and the quality of tone. All children with CP have problems with motor control and posture, but otherwise symptoms can vary greatly among individuals. Symptoms can include: • Decreased coordination • Stiff or rigid muscles • Variations in muscle tone from hypertonicity to hypotonicity • Weakness in one or more extremities • Random, involuntary movements called chorea (rapid and jerky) and athetosis (slow and writhing) Deficits may also include: • Language delay • Cognitive disability • Sensory problems • Psychosocial problems • Seizure disorders • Feeding disorders • Impaired vision • Hearing loss • Spinal deformities	There is an extensive scope for an OTP working with an individual with CP, including but not limited to: • Addressing developmental delays • Working toward the integration of primitive reflexes • Strengthening and ROM of affected extremity • Targeting upper extremity motor control • Working on bilateral coordination activities • Assisting with motor planning to address abnormal compensatory movement patterns • Increasing participation in ADLs, play, and other meaningful activities • Education and training on adaptive equipment and/or assistive technology for both the child and the caregiver
Fragile X[41]	An X-linked dominant inheritance caused by changes in the Fragile X messenger ribonucleoprotein 1 (FRM1) gene. It affects more males than females, but females can still be affected, only with milder symptoms. Symptoms include: • Developmental delays • Learning disabilities • Cognitive deficit • Social and behavioral problems	OTPs will often treat children with Fragile X with intervention aimed at the following: • Address developmental delays (gross motor, fine motor, social) • Utilize sensory integrative techniques • Parent education on behavioral strategies
ASD[42]	A spectrum of conditions characterized by (1) social interaction, learning, and communication impairments as well as (2) stereotypical, repetitive behaviors and interests. The abilities vary significantly from person to person, with some carrying on advanced conversations, while others may be nonverbal.These individuals might also have: • Self-stimulatory behaviors • Difficulties with sensory modulation • Language delays • Difficulty with learning • Delays in motor skills	OTPs will often work with individuals with ASD. Some of the interventions might include but are not limited to: • Addressing developmental delays • Utilizing sensory integrative therapy • Performing social skills training • Introducing visual supports

ASD, Autism spectrum disorder; *CP*, cerebral palsy.

Cerebral Palsy

CP is a group of disorders that result from damage to the developing brain, causing deficits in motor control, posture, and muscle tone.[29] Most cases of CP result from brain damage that happened before or during birth (congenital CP), but in a small percentage of cases, the damage occurs more than 28 days after birth (acquired CP).[30] About 75% to 85% of cases are considered to be spastic CP which means that the muscles have spasticity, but over 50% of children with CP can still walk independently.[30] Children with CP may or may not have signs of cognitive delay. The earliest signs of CP are seen when the child is not meeting the expected developmental motor milestones (see Fig. 4.2 and Table 4.3).

Autism Spectrum Disorder

Autism Spectrum Disorder (ASD) is a group of conditions related to brain development that impact how an individual perceives and interacts with others, causing challenges with socialization and communication.[31] Autistic individuals typically have difficulty with social interaction and will sometimes have set interests and/or repetitive behaviors. Autistic individuals interact and learn in ways that are different from most individuals.[32] There is a wide range of variation in the abilities of autistic people, with some able to conduct high-level conversations and others nonverbal.[32]

Fragile X

Fragile X is the most common type of inherited developmental and intellectual disability.[33] It is due to a mutated gene on the X chromosome inherited from a parent with the gene. Because it is on the X chromosome, a female with one X chromosome that carries a mutation and one healthy X chromosome might be asymptomatic but still a carrier. Since boys have only one X chromosome, they are more likely than girls to have symptoms. Fragile X affects a person's behavior and ability to learn. Communication skills, appearance, and sensitivity to light and sound are some of the more common symptoms.[33]

The OT Scope of Practice

Tables 4.4 through 4.6 provide a quick overview of some of the more common conditions seen by OTPs in this age group.

TABLE 4.6 Infections and Parasitic Conditions Commonly Seen by OTPs

Condition	Symptoms	Occupational Therapy Intervention
Chicken pox[43]	A very contagious disease caused by the Varicella-zoster virus, characterized by an itchy rash with fluid-filled blisters. The incidence of chicken pox has decreased significantly since the vaccine was developed in 1995. • Typically originates on face, chest, and back before spreading and turning into scabs • Blistering and scabbing rash • Fever • Tiredness • Headache • Loss of appetite	Much of an OTP's job is aimed at prevention, but the identification of suspicious symptoms in a client is always important. Not everyone has received the vaccine. • Vaccine advocacy • Know signs and symptoms in order to refer for diagnosis before severe complications arise
Toxoplasmosis[44]	Considered a "neglected" parasitic infection due to the high probability of carrying the single-celled parasite (*Toxoplasma gondii*). It is estimated that more than 40 million people in the United States carry this parasite without knowing it because the human immune system holds it at bay. Pregnant females and people with compromised immune systems should be cautious. This parasite comes from eating undercooked meat or shellfish and from contaminated food, water, or cat feces. Symptoms include: • Flu-like symptoms with swollen lymph glands and muscle aches and pains that last for about a month • Reduced or blurred vision, painful light sensitivity, redness, or tearing • Damage to the brain, eyes, or other organs • Unborn babies can remain asymptomatic at birth but have problems later in life, but some will have eye damage or brain damage at birth.	Again, prevention is always key. Warning people to avoid undercooked foods and to avoid cat litter box cleaning while pregnant can be helpful. • Education about meal preparation and food safety • Education regarding pet management IADLs • Education about hand hygiene • Know signs and symptoms in order to refer for diagnosis before severe complications arise
Pertussis (whooping cough)	See Table 4.4	

Application—Case Studies

CASE EXAMPLE 4.1

An OTP working in the school system is visited by a kindergarten teacher along with one of her students. He is a 5-year-old boy who is crying and holding his left forearm. The teacher claims nothing happened in the class and that he was crying when he walked into the school. The child has a history of fractures, his femur last year and his clavicle the year before, and the teacher thinks that although the parents seem to be "really nice," there may be abuse at home.

1. **Screen:** The OTP did a thorough screening of the child.
2. **Take a Closer Look:** Upon examination, the OTP discovered a malalignment of the radius and ulna in the mid-shaft region. The OTP was suspicious that this might be a fracture. The OTP talked to the boy to ask how this happened, and he informed her that he liked to play, and whenever he played, he would get hurt.
3. **Determine Flag Status:** Although this arm discomfort was not a life-or-death situation, the OTP decided that the child's pain required immediate intervention.
4. **Take Action if Needed:** The child was brought to the ER right away, and his arm was casted for a fracture of both the radius and ulna.
5. **Document the Findings:** The OTP described it in her documentation and decided to follow up on the child's progress to make sure things were really okay at home; but while in the hospital, the parents were questioned by hospital staff for possible abuse. The hospital staff was requesting that the parents be arrested.
6. **Take a Second Look:** The OTP contacted the child's physician to ask if it were possible that the child simply had low bone density and a mild type of Osteogenesis Imperfecta (OI) that had gone undiagnosed.
7. **Determine the Flag Status:** Because of the urgency of the situation with the parents being accused of a crime, the OTP felt it was important to check the child's bone density as soon as possible, and the physician agreed.
8. **Take Action if Needed:** The bone density was checked, and the child did have OI.
9. **Document the Findings**: The OTP again documented her findings and her phone calls and visits to the doctor for the medical record.

This is a true case. The child had OI. The hospital staff found out just before having the parents arrested for child endangerment and abuse. The mother broke down in tears thanking the physician who gave all the credit to the OTP.

References

1. Healthline. 3 Stages of parturition (childbirth). In: *Parenthood.* Healthline; 2018. https://www.healthline.com/health/parturition.
2. Huffman JW, Beck AC. *Birth: Biology*. Encyclopedia Britannica; 2022. https://www.britannica.com/science/birth.
3. Johns Hopkins. *What Is the Apgar Score?* Johns Hopkins All Children's Hospital; 2023. https://www.hopkinsallchildrens.org/Patients-Families/Health-Library/HealthDocNew/What-Is-the-Apgar-Score.
4. Boston. Brazelton Institute. *The Neonatal Behavioral Assessment Scale (NBAS)*. Boston Children's Hospital; 2023. https://www.childrenshospital.org/research/centers/brazelton-institute-research/nbas.
5. Brazelton TB, Nugent JK. *The Neonatal Behavioral Assessment Scale*. Mac Keith Press Cambridge; 2011.
6. Kilpatrick SJ, et al. Normal labor and delivery. In: Landon MB, ed. *Gabbe's Obstetrics: Normal and Problem Pregnancies*. 8th ed. Elsevier; 2021:204–225.e4.
7. Grieger JA, Hutchesson MJ, Cooray SD, et al. A review of maternal overweight and obesity and its impact on cardiometabolic outcomes during pregnancy and postpartum. *Ther Adv Reprod Health*. 2021;15:1–16. https://doi.org/10.1177/2633494120986544.
8. ACOG. Safe prevention of the primary cesarean delivery. American College of Obstetricians and Gynecologists (the College) and the Society for Maternal-Fetal Medicine. *Am J Obstet Gynecol.* 2014(123):693–711. https://doi.org/10.1016/j.ajog.2014.01.026.
9. Papalia DE, Martorell G. *Experience Human Development*. 5th ed. McGraw Hill; 2024.
10. CDC. Birthweight and gestation. In: *Birth Data for 2021*. National Center for Health Statistics. https://www.cdc.gov/nchs/fastats/birthweight.htm.
11. Karataşlı V, Kanmaz AG, Inan AH, Budak A, Beyan E. Maternal and neonatal outcomes of adolescent pregnancy. *J Gynecol Obstet Hum Reprod.* 2019;48(2019):347–350. https://doi.org/10.1016/j.jogoh.2019.02.011.
12. Polavarapu M, Klonoff-Cohen H, Joshi D, Kumar P, An R, Rosenblat K. Development of a risk score to predict sudden infant death syndrome. *Int J Environ Res Public Health*. 2022;19(16):1. https://doi.org/10.3390/ijerph191610270.
13. Ely DM, Driscoll AK. Infant mortality in the United States, 2020: data from the period linked birth/infant death file. *Natl Vital Stat Rep. 71*(5): 1–18. https://www.cdc.gov/nchs/products/index.htm.
14. Merriam Webster. *Neonate*. https://www.merriam-webster.com/dictionary/neonate.
15. CDC. *Data Table of Infant Weight-for-Age Charts*. National Center for Health Statistics. https://www.cdc.gov/growthcharts/html_charts/wtageinf.htm.
16. CDC. *Data Table of Infant Length-for-Age Charts*. National Center for Health Statistics. https://www.cdc.gov/growthcharts/html_charts/lenageinf.htm.
17. Udwin, N. *Primitive Reflexes*. Sprocket Therapy Solutions; 2015. https://www.sprockettherapy.com/primitive-reflexes.html.
18. Guy-Evans O. *Schwann Cells*. Simply Psychology. https://www.simplypsychology.org/schwann-cells.html.
19. Urban Child. *Baby's Brain Begins Now: Conception to Age 3*. The Urban Child Institute. http://www.urbanchildinstitute.org/why-0-3/baby-and-brain.
20. Shonkoff JP, Ohillips DA, eds. *From Neurons to Neighborhoods: The Science of Early Childhood Development. National Research Council Institute of Medicine, Committee on Integrating the Science of Early Childhood Development, Board on Children, Youth, and Families*. National Academy Press; 2000.
21. Freeborn DF, Trevino HM, Adler LC, Reviewers. *Newborn Senses. Health Encyclopedia*. Rochester Medical Center; 2023. https://www.urmc.rochester.edu/search.aspx?q=Newborn%20Senses.
22. Saluja G, Prakalapahorn SG, Saboo US. *Visual Acuity Assessment in Children*. The American Academy of Ophthalmology: EyeWiki; 2022. https://eyewiki.aao.org/Visual_acuity_assessment_in_children.

23. CDC. *Early Brain Development and Health*. Centers for Disease Control and Prevention; 2022. https://www.cdc.gov/ncbddd/childdevelopment/early-brain-development.html.
24. American Pregnancy Association. *Breastfeeding vs Bottle Feeding Formula*. American Pregnancy Association; 2023. https://americanpregnancy.org/healthy-pregnancy/breastfeeding/breastfeeding-vs-bottle-feeding-formula/.
25. Nationwide Children's Hospital. *Failure to Thrive in Infants*. Nationwide Children's Hospital; 2023. https://www.nationwidechildrens.org/conditions/failure-to-thrive-in-infants.
26. Raab CP. *Causes of Failure to Thrive in Children*. Merck Manual; 2023. https://www.merckmanuals.com/professional/pediatrics/miscellaneous-disorders-in-infants-and-children/failure-to-thrive-ftt?query=Failure%20to%20Thrive%20in%20children.
27. CDC. *Large Intestinal Atresia/Stenosis*. Centers for Disease Control and Prevention: Birth Defects Toolkit; 2021. https://www.cdc.gov/ncbddd/birthdefects/surveillancemanual/quick-reference-handbook/large-intestinal-atresia-stenosis.html.
28. Johns Hopkins. *Osteogenesis Imprefecta*. Johns Hopkins Health, 2023. https://www.hopkinsmedicine.org/health/conditions-and-diseases/osteogenesis-imperfecta.
29. Mayo Clinic. *Cerebral Palsy*. Mayo Clinic; 2023. https://www.mayoclinic.org/diseases-conditions/cerebral-palsy/symptoms-causes/syc-20353999.
30. CDC. *11 Things to Know About Cerebral* Palsy. Centers for Disease Control and Prevention; 2022. https://www.cdc.gov/ncbddd/cp/features/cerebral-palsy-11-things.html.
31. Mayo Clinic. *Autism Spectrum Disorder. Mayo Clinic*; 2023. https://www.mayoclinic.org/diseases-conditions/autism-spectrum-disorder/symptoms-causes/syc-20352928.
32. CDC. *What Is Autism Spectrum Disorder?* Centers for Disease Control and Prevention; 2022. https://www.cdc.gov/ncbddd/autism/facts.html.
33. NIH. Fragile X Syndrome. *Eunice Kennedy Shriver*. National Institute of Child Health and Human Development; 2023. https://www.nichd.nih.gov/health/topics/factsheets/fragilex#.
34. CDC. *What Is Spina Bifida?* Centers for Disease Control and Prevention; 2023. https://www.cdc.gov/spina-bifida/about/index.html.
35. CDC. *What Is Down Syndrome?* Centers for Disease Control and Prevention; 2023. https://www.cdc.gov/ncbddd/birthdefects/downsyndrome.html.
36. Mayo Clinic. *Infant Jaundice*. Mayo Clinic; 2022. https://www.mayoclinic.org/diseases-conditions/infant-jaundice/symptoms-causes/syc-20373865.
37. Cleveland Clinic. *Kernicterus*. Cleveland Clinic; 2023. https://my.clevelandclinic.org/health/diseases/25014-kernicterus.
38. CDC. *Pertussis (Whooping Cough)*. Centers for Disease Control and Prevention; 2022. https://www.cdc.gov/pertussis/about/signs-symptoms.html.
39. Mayo Clinic. *Sudden Infant Death Syndrome (SIDS)*. Mayo Clinic; 2023. https://www.mayoclinic.org/diseases-conditions/sudden-infant-death-syndrome/symptoms-causes/syc-20352800.
40. NIH. *Cerebral Palsy*. National Institute of Neurological Disorders and Stroke, Nationals Institutes of Health; 2023. https://www.ninds.nih.gov/health-information/disorders/cerebral-palsy.
41. CDC. *Fragile X Syndrome (FXS)*. Centers for Disease Control and Prevention; 2023. https://www.cdc.gov/ncbddd/fxs/facts.html.
42. CDC. *What Is Autism Spectrum Disorder?* Centers for Disease Control and Prevention; 2023. https://www.cdc.gov/ncbddd/autism/facts.html.
43. Cleveland Clinic. *Chickenpox*. Cleveland Clinic; 2023. https://my.clevelandclinic.org/health/diseases/4017-chickenpox.
44. CDC. *Toxoplasmosis*. Centers for Disease Control and Prevention; 2022. https://www.cdc.gov/parasites/toxoplasmosis/gen_info/faqs.html.

5

Typical Development and Pathophysiology During Early and Middle Childhood

OBJECTIVES

By the end of this chapter, the reader should be able to:

- Demonstrate a basic understanding of typical physiological development during early and middle childhood.
- List typical gross and fine motor skills for early and middle childhood.
- Demonstrate a basic understanding of typical grasp patterns and age of appearance.
- Differentiate between typical child development and atypical child development.
- List various pathophysiological conditions related to atypical child development.
- Compare and contrast various pathophysiological conditions that are common for this age group.

Typical Human Development

The terms *early childhood* and *middle childhood* have many different definitions in the literature. *Early childhood* in this textbook is defined as the developmental period from ages 1 to 5 years, and *middle childhood* is defined as the developmental period from ages 6 to 11 years. This chapter offers a brief review of the typical developmental progression of children in early and middle childhood, followed by some of the conditions typically seen in this population by occupational therapy professionals.

Early Childhood Development—Ages 1 to 5

During this period, a child's senses (i.e., what the child hears, sees, and touches) can motivate the child to move toward something interesting, which helps develop their motor skills. Sense enhances motor skills, and motor skills enhance sensation. Once children begin walking (typically around 12 months), they enter the stage of toddlerhood. As children move more, they sense more (i.e., the view of something from a different angle, the feel of a carpet on their palms and knees, or the muffled sound of music playing from another room). Gross motor skills, involving the larger muscles of the trunk and extremities, and fine motor skills, involving the smaller muscles of the hands and wrists, begin developing in infancy and continue to mature throughout early childhood as children engage in increasingly complex physical interactions with their environment (Table 5.1).[1]

Although bipedal functional ambulation (walking) typically begins at 12 months of age, this can vary greatly from anywhere between 6 and 18 months of age. Walking is one of the primary evaluative measures of gross motor ability. Delayed functional ambulation is not necessarily a sign of delayed development, as some children find other ways to get around, such as butt-scooting, crawling, or creeping. These alternative ways of movement can delay typical ambulation until around 2 years of age. When children initially begin the transition from cruising (using both arms on furniture or walls for support) to walking alone, they will often use a high-guard or middle-guard position of the upper extremities to assist with balance (Fig. 5.1).

The child in Fig. 5.1 is demonstrating a high-guard position for early functional ambulation. His upper extremities are slightly abducted and extended away from his body. This facilitates a broader base of support and allows for increased balance in the beginning stages of movement. The use of a high, middle, or even low-guard position of the arms has been found to be typical during the first 5 months of independent walking.[5] This use of the high- to middle-guard position typically starts to decrease at around age 2. As the child approaches 3 years of age, they can climb stairs, one at a time at first and then alternating feet by age 3 or 4 with the aid of a handrail (see Tables 5.1 and 5.2).

Children begin to demonstrate a strong preference for hand dominance between ages 3–4, and this is typically well-established between 5–6 years of age.[6] Handedness is

TABLE 5.1 Gross and Fine Motor Skills for Typically Developing Children Ages 1–3 Years Old

	1-Year-Old Milestones	2-Year-Old Milestones	3-Year-Old Milestones
Fine motor[1]	• Stack blocks • Eat with a spoon • Turn pages of a book • Scribble on paper • Drink from a cup • Pick objects up using thumb-to-index finger opposition	• Wash hands • Zip and unzip clothes • String beads • Remove and replace lids on canisters • Turn a doorknob	• Button and unbutton clothes • Use scissors to cut paper • Trace lines and shapes with a crayon on paper • Replicate a circle
Gross motor[2–4]	• Pull up to a standing position • Walk holding onto toys, walls, or furniture (by 18 months will take many steps independently but with a high-guard position of the arms) • Crawl up steps • Attempt to move from floor to stand without support • Attempt to walk independently	• Walk at a good pace independently, with less of a high-guard position of the arms • Climb stairs one step at a time (not alternating feet) • Kick a ball • Take a few steps on tip-toes • Walk up a few steps without assistance • Jump in place	• Climb stairs with alternating feet using a handrail • Balance on one foot for 3–5 seconds • Jump ahead 10–24 inches • Run fairly well • Peddle a tricycle • Catch a large ball
Language and cognition[2]	• Wave hello and goodbye • Say "mama" and/or "dada" • Understand the word "No" • Look for toys they see you hide	• Form two-word sentences • Point to 2 or more body parts when asked • Try to use buttons and switches on toys • Play with multiple toys at once	• Have a conversation with at least two back-and-forth interactions • Ask who, what, why, and where questions • State their first name • Avoid touching hot objects

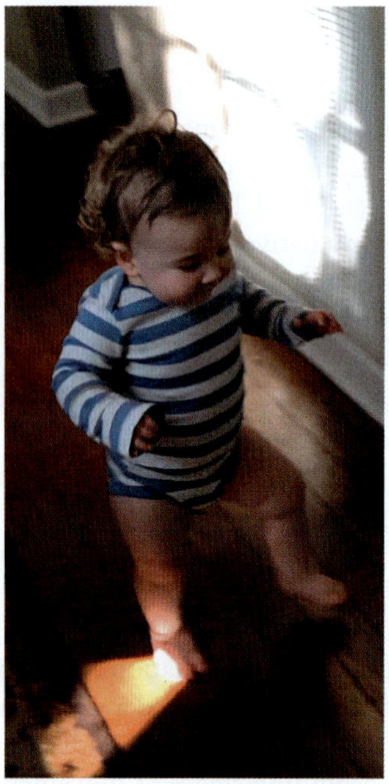

• **Fig. 5.1** Child ambulating with high-guard position.

one of the primary evaluative measures of fine motor ability, with right-handedness constituting the majority (approximately 70%–90%) of the population. A few decades ago, there was a theory that a gene existed for right-handedness, and if you inherited this gene, you would be right-handed. This was later changed to a belief that the gene was actually for left-handedness because it tends to run in families.[7] It is now known that left-handedness is definitely inherited, but there are an estimated 30 to 100 different genes that could possibly influence the likelihood of an individual having this trait.[8]

Fine motor milestones start to become more specific during early and middle childhood, especially with respect to grasp (Table 5.2). By the age of 3, a child can stabilize an object with one hand, allowing the other hand to manipulate the object (bilateral coordination). This skill enables a child to manipulate large buttons or string large beads.

At around 2.5 years of age, children begin to move objects from the palm to the fingers. This is called palm-to-finger translation and is considered one of several in-hand manipulation skills. Some of the typical fine and gross motor changes as well as development in language and cognition from ages 4 to 5 years can be found in Table 5.3.

Middle Childhood Development—Ages 6 to 11

Although physical growth slows considerably during middle childhood compared to the growth experienced during early childhood, children will continue to grow about 2 to 3 inches a year and double their weight during middle childhood.[4] Neurons in the brain are becoming more myelinated, and physical differences between boys and girls are becoming slightly more noticeable.

Nutrition is still a very important issue. Children in this age group need grains, fruits, and vegetables but tend to eat too much salt, fat, and sugar. This can affect a child physically, intellectually, and emotionally. Obesity is defined as a body mass index (BMI) of 30 or higher when talking about adults, but BMI categories for children and teens are based on sex and age-specific BMI percentiles (Table 5.4).

TABLE 5.2 Typical Grip/Grasp and Age of Appearance[9,10]

Grasp and Age	Grasp and Age
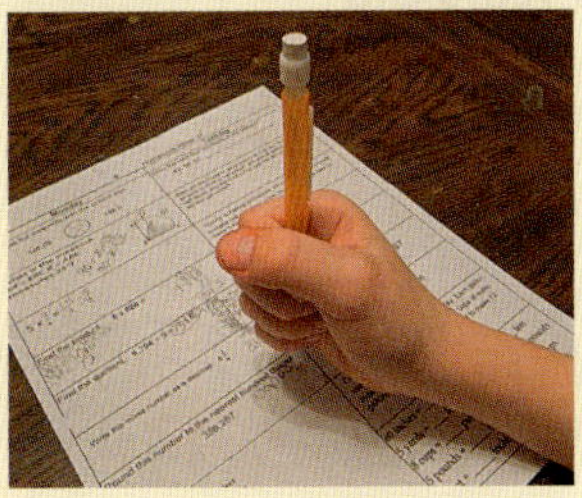 Fisted grasp, whole hand grasp, or palmar supinate grasp 1–2 years old	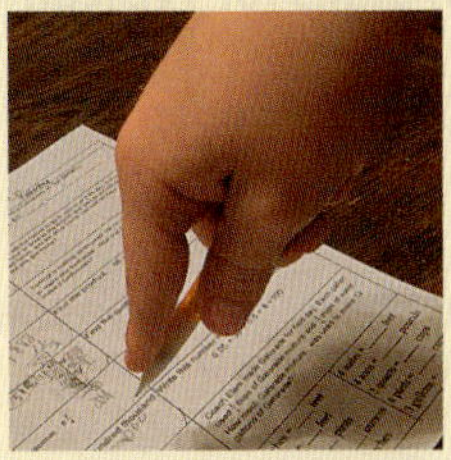 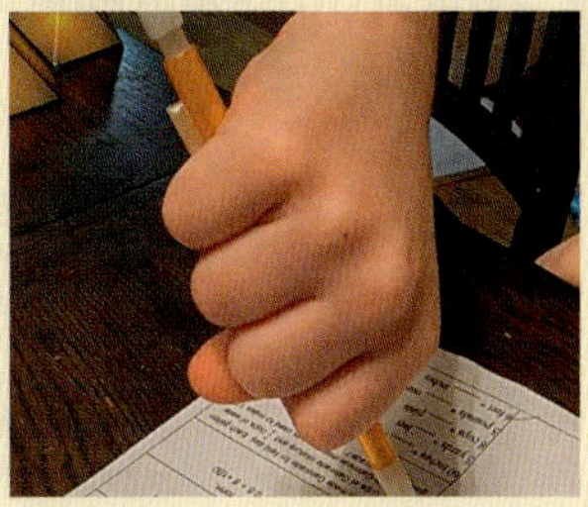 Digital pronate grasp 2–3 years old With index finger straight or with index finger bent.
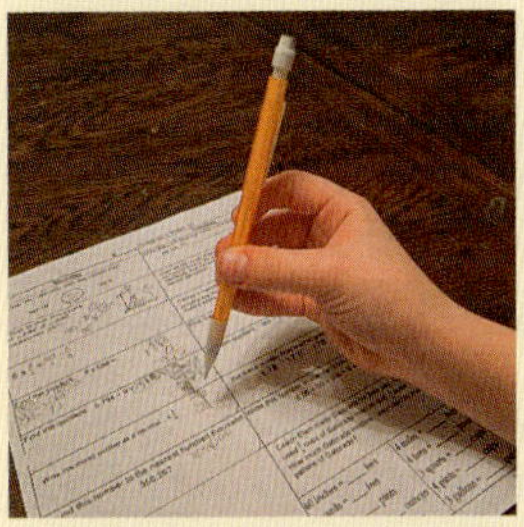 Quadrupod grasp or four-finger grasp 3–4 years old Note: The word "Quadrupod" can also refer to the use of four fingers instead of three to write and, although not typical, can be functional if used in adult years, especially if arthritis is present.	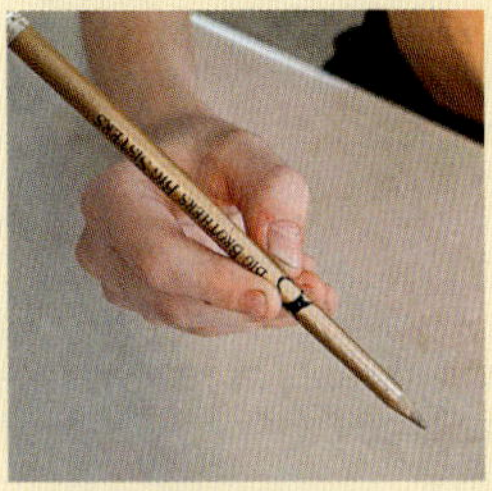 Static tripod grasp 3.5–4 years old The position of the fingers does not change when the pencil is moved. The arm is typically off the table.
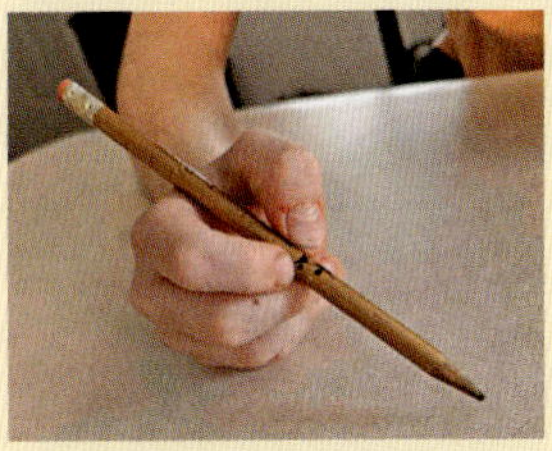 Dynamic tripod grasp 5–6 years of age. The position of the fingers changes and shifts when the pencil is moved. The thumb, index, and middle fingers as well as the hand itself manipulate the pencil. The arm is typically resting on the table.	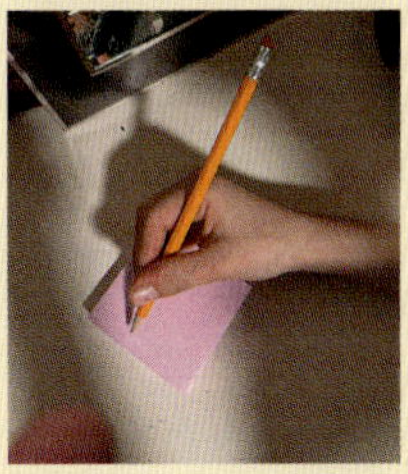 Lateral tripod grasp Like the dynamic tripod but instead of the thumb tip, the thumb pad is used (a "thumb wrap") to press the pencil against the side of the index finger, and the index and middle fingers manipulate the pencil. This grasp can cause increased fatigue.
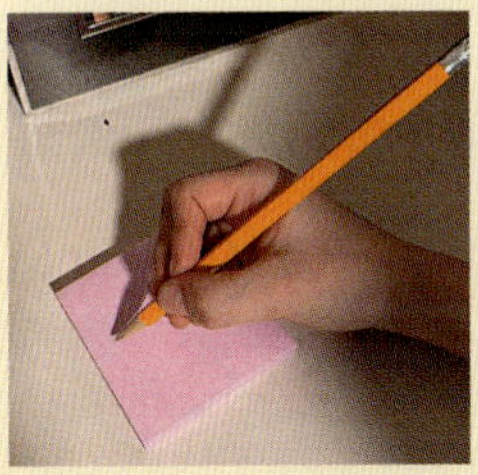 Dynamic quadrupod grasp The grasp is similar to the dynamic tripod, but the thumb, index, and middle fingers perform the opposition to the rest of the hand, which is stationary.	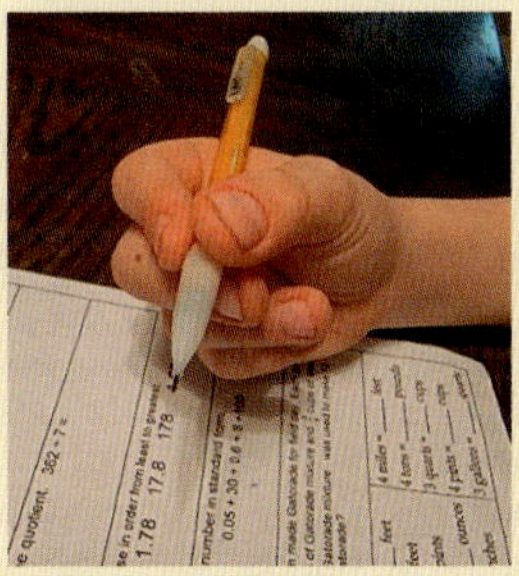 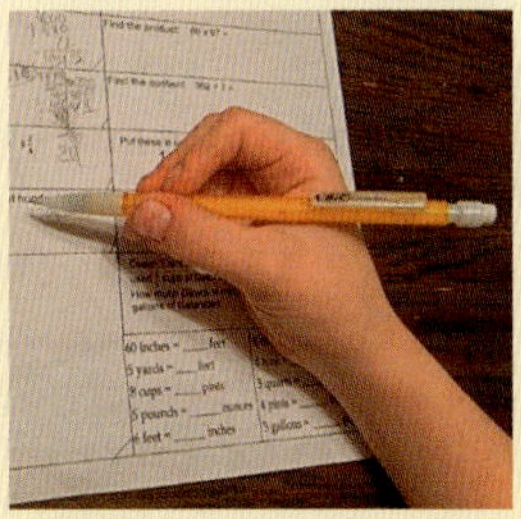 Lateral quadrupod grasp The grasp is similar to the lateral tripod, but the index, middle, and ring fingers manipulate the pencil.

Childhood obesity is a serious concern in the United States, with 1 out of every 5 children affected.[12,13] There are many factors involved, including genetics, behavior, certain medications, school environments, and access to healthy and affordable foods, to name a few.[13]

Motor development continues as children become more coordinated: learning to skip, jump rope, and ride bikes.[14] Children become more coordinated with practice, and opportunities to do this are important. A lack of adequate opportunities for physical fitness in our country is becoming more of an issue, some believe, because children are more interested in sedentary activities (such as computer games and applications) and often have less interest in outdoor play (Table 5.5).[15]

TABLE 5.3 **Typical Gross and Fine Motor Skills for Typically Developing Children Ages 4–5 Years Old**

	4-Year-Old Milestones	5-Year-Old Milestones
Fine motor[2]	• Draw a person with at least three body parts • Button clothing with front opening • Build a tower of 10 blocks • Begin to dress themselves • Imitate a square • Use scissors to cut along a straight line, followed by a curved line	• Use scissors to cut simple shapes • Draw a person with at least five body parts • Learn how to tie shoes • Draw to imitate a geometric shape
Gross motor[4,11]	• Catch a large ball • Jump as far as 24–33 inches • Walk downstairs alternating feet with some support • Hop on one foot	• Take a running jump as far as 28–36 inches • Walk downstairs alternating feet without assistance • Jump rope • Balance on one foot for 8 to 10 seconds
Language and cognition[2,11]	• Sing part of a song • Use sentences with four or more words • Answer simple questions, like "What is a hat used for?" or "What did you do today?"	• Tell a short story • Can keep a conversation going with more than three exchanges • Recognize and recite the alphabet • Answer simple questions related to a story they just heard

TABLE 5.4 **Child Body Mass Index (BMI) Categories and Their Corresponding Sex- and Age-Specific BMI Percentiles**

BMI Category	BMI Range
Underweight	Less than the 5th percentile
Healthy weight	5th percentile to less than the 85th percentile
Overweight	85th percentile to less than the 95th percentile
Obesity	95th percentile or greater
Severe obesity	120% of the 95th percentile or greater or 35 kg/m^2 or greater

From Centers for Disease Control and Prevention. *Defining Child BMI Categories*. 2023. https://www.cdc.gov/bmi/child-teen-calculator/bmicategories.html?CDC_AAref_Val=https://www.cdc.gov/obesity/basics/childhood-defining.html.

TABLE 5.5 **Typical Gross and Fine Motor Skills for Typically Developing Children Ages 6–11 Years Old**

	6- to 7 Year-Old Milestones	8- to 9-Year-Old Milestones	10- to 11-Year Old Milestones
Fine motor[14–16]	• Paint and draw more intricately • Tie shoelaces • Dress themselves completely • Brush their teeth • Catch a ball with two hands • Start learning to play a musical instrument	• Begin to use tools • Groom themselves • Do chores, like making their bed • Catch a small ball	• Use tools • Coordinate their movements (like dribbling before throwing a basketball)
Gross motor[14–16]	• Play hopscotch • Jump rope • Throw and kick a ball • Skip	• Take a running jump as far as 36–42 inches • Chase other kids • Ride a two-wheeled bike without training wheels	• Sometimes feel awkward in their new, taller body as they begin puberty • Learn to ice skate
Language and cognition[14,15]	• Can do simple addition and subtraction math equations • Start thinking about the future • Focus less on themselves and more on others	• Begin to experience more peer pressure • Start becoming more independent from parents • Interact better with friends	• Begin to form a body image • Start to form more complex friendships with peers

Pathophysiologic Conditions in This Age Group

There are many different disorders that can affect children in this age group. This section will briefly discuss a few of those disorders most likely encountered by occupational therapy practitioners (OTPs) in a typical setting in the continental United States.

Physical Anomalies

Most (more than 85%) children in the United States report they are in good health.[4] The most common acute illness in early and middle childhood still tends to be the common cold. Because the lungs are not yet fully developed in young children, the average child will catch at least 6 to 8 colds per year. These colds will become less frequent after age 6.[17] The most common chronic illness is asthma. Other chronic childhood conditions include diabetes, cystic fibrosis, and childhood hypertension.[4]

The incidence of many infectious childhood illnesses has declined since the advent of immunizations. Immunizations are strongly advised by the CDC to help provide immunity before children are exposed to diseases that could be potentially life-threatening.[18]

Accidents

Accidents (or unintentional injuries) are the major cause of death in this age group, including drownings, automobile accidents, and poisonings.[19] The CDC reports that more children between the ages of 1 and 4 years of age die from drowning than any other cause of death.[20] For children ages 5 to 14, drowning is the second leading cause of accidental death after motor vehicle accidents.[20] Medications (primarily narcotics and psychodysleptics) were responsible for most of the childhood deaths related to poisoning in the United States in 2020.[21] In addition, exposure to smoking is a preventable cause of childhood respiratory problems, illness, and death.[22]

There is a strong correlation between socioeconomic status (SES) and health in our country for all age groups. Individuals in impoverished conditions often have increased physical and psychosocial stressors with less opportunity for quality medical care, which contributes to poorer health outcomes and more frequent illnesses.[23] Childhood exposure to lead from contaminated food, water, or air (dust in homes where there is lead-based paint) can lead to impaired cognitive development and neurological problems.[24] Homelessness is also a concern with an estimated 1.2 million children in the public school system who experienced homelessness during the 2019–22 calendar years.[25]

Learning Disorders

There are many different types of learning disorders that appear in middle childhood. These have a wide range and vary in complexity and severity, from dyslexia (a cluster of symptoms that can include decoding, spelling, and word recognition problems associated with reading or even with spoken word)[26] to cognitive deficits (also called intellectual disability; begins in childhood and manifests as a significant limitation in the ability to learn with unknown etiology).[27] Hyperactivity is typically characterized by impulsivity and inappropriate overactivity, and attention-deficit disorder is characterized by inattention and distractibility.[28] ADHD is the acronym used for both attention deficit and hyperactivity, as these often occur together.

The OT Scope of Practice

Table 5.6 provides a quick overview of some of the more common conditions seen by occupational therapy practitioners in this age group.

TABLE 5.6 Conditions That Can Affect Physical Health in Early and Middle Childhood Often Seen by Occupational Therapy Practitioners (OTPs)

Condition	Symptoms	Occupational Therapy Intervention
Childhood cancer[29]	Cancer is typically hard to detect in children, but the American Society of Clinical Oncology uses the following acronym: • **C**ontinued weight loss with no explanation • **H**eadaches, sometimes with vomiting • **I**ncreased swelling or pain in the extremities • **L**ump or mass • **D**evelopment of bruising or rash • **C**onsistent or frequent infections • **A** white, colored ring behind the pupil • **N**ausea and/or vomiting • **C**onstant fatigue • **E**ye or visual changes • **R**ecurring fevers of unknown origin	Although many times an OTP will work with a child after cancer intervention has already begun, it is sometimes the OTP who notices the initial signs and symptoms of possible cancer. The OTP can be a valuable advocate for the child in these cases by: • Notifying the physician whenever there are signs and symptoms that fall outside the cluster of typical symptomatology you would expect to find in a child with their referring diagnosis After cancer has been diagnosed, OT intervention will be dependent on the type of cancer, the cancer interventions being done at the time of care, and the setting where the child is receiving services (acute care, home health, outpatient, palliative care, hospice care). Some areas addressed by OTPs with this population can include: • Endurance education after chemotherapy • Assistance with dressing and bathing, with respect to incision sites and overall weakness • Helping the family to cope with implications after receiving a diagnosis or while undergoing treatment • Encouraging engagement in meaningful occupations that are important to the child (i.e., hobbies, schoolwork, and independence with Activities of Daily Living [ADLs])

(Continued)

TABLE 5.6 Conditions That Can Affect Physical Health in Early and Middle Childhood Often Seen by Occupational Therapy Practitioners (OTPs)—cont'd

Condition	Symptoms	Occupational Therapy Intervention
Childhood asthma[30,31]	Asthma is a chronic lung disease affecting about 7.5 million children in the United States. During an asthma attack, the airways become inflamed when exposed to certain triggers. Symptoms include: • Frequent coughing spells • Rapid breathing • Shortness of breath • Chest pain or tightness • Wheezing • Retraction of ribs in order to better exhale • Fatigue	Although many times an OTP will work with a child after asthma has already been diagnosed, it is sometimes the OTP who notices the initial signs and symptoms. Notify the physician whenever there are signs and symptoms that fall outside the cluster of typical symptomatology you would expect to find in a child with their referring diagnosis. A child with previously diagnosed asthma will need to come to the OT clinic with their rescue inhaler in case it is needed. Some of the many possible interventions performed by OTPs include: • Endurance education • Breathing exercises or techniques • Family education on the importance of decreasing irritant exposure • Teaching stress management techniques or coping strategies • Energy conservation or pacing techniques • Encouragement and guidance to increase engagement in meaningful occupations that are important to the child (i.e., hobbies, schoolwork, and independence with ADLs)
Hemophilia[32]	A blood disorder characterized by the absence or reduction of blood clotting proteins called clotting factors. Because the recessive gene for this trait is located on the X chromosome (for the most common type of hemophilia), more males will present with symptoms than females, who would have another X to serve as dominant. Symptoms include: • Excessive bleeding from cuts and scrapes • Large deep bruises • Pain and swelling in the joints • Nosebleeds • Blood in the urine or stool • Longer bleeding time or bleeding episodes • If the child experiences double vision, weakness, headache, or convulsions, there may be bleeding into the brain. This is a red flag, and the child should go to the hospital immediately or call 911.	Typically, a child is diagnosed with hemophilia long before OT intervention is ordered. Still, being aware of the signs and symptoms can keep the OTP alert to changes in the child's condition. Some OT interventions include: • Endurance education • Exercise in a reduced-impact environment, such as an exercise bicycle or aquatic exercises (less prone to injury this way) • Instruction in safety/compensatory techniques used for occupations that may result in injury (i.e., cutting materials with scissors as part of schoolwork, leisure, or play; shaving; knife use during feeding or meal preparation) • Encouragement and guidance to increase engagement in meaningful occupations that are important to the child (i.e., hobbies, schoolwork, and independence with ADLs)
Muscular dystrophy[33]	Muscular dystrophy is a group of diseases that cause progressive loss of muscle mass and weakness. The most common type is Duchenne muscular dystrophy (DMD). This is more common in boys; although, girls can be carriers and have milder symptoms. • Frequent falls • Waddling gait • Walking on toes • Delayed growth • Muscle pain and stiffness • Learning disabilities • Enlarged calf muscles • Gower's sign (Fig. 5.2) Another type of muscular dystrophy is Becker, which is like DMD but symptoms are milder and progress more slowly. Myotonic muscular dystrophy is characterized by difficulty relaxing muscles after contraction. Limb-girdle muscular dystrophy affects the hips and shoulder muscles first.	OTPs working in pediatrics will typically see children with muscular dystrophy. Interventions are many and varied, but some are listed below: • Maximize and prolong independence in mobility and ADLs • Prevent deformity or contractures • Maintain strength and range of motion (ROM) • Provide psychosocial support • Educate and train on adaptive equipment • Encourage and provide guidance to increase engagement in meaningful occupations that are important to the child (i.e., hobbies, schoolwork, and independence with ADLs)

TABLE 5.6 Conditions That Can Affect Physical Health in Early and Middle Childhood Often Seen by Occupational Therapy Practitioners (OTPs)—cont'd

Condition	Symptoms	Occupational Therapy Intervention
Diabetes[34,35]	Diabetes mellitus (DM) is a disorder of the insulin that breaks down sugars in the human body. Type 1 DM involves the absence of insulin. Type 2 DM involves a peripheral insulin resistance. Type 1 is the most common type in children affecting 1 out of every 350 children in the United States. Type 2 was once rare but has increased with the child obesity epidemic. Symptoms include: • Increased hunger • Increased thirst • Fatigue • Polyuria • Dehydration • At risk for developing retinopathy Diabetes incipidus is rare, affecting only 1 out of every 30,000 children. With this disorder, too much water is released from the body through the kidneys. Children with diabetes incipidus will not only have many of the aforementioned symptoms but also delayed growth and sometimes a high fever.	OTPs working in pediatrics will typically see children with many comorbidities, and one of these will be diabetes. Interventions are many and varied, but some are listed below: • Endurance education • Creation of a medication schedule so that important injections are not missed • Instruction of self-management techniques (i.e., visual schedule/timers for insulin administration and choosing appropriate food choices) • Instruction of healthy habits, such as the elimination of sugar-containing drinks • Instruction to avoid unhealthy habits, such as skipping meals • Collaboration with the dietician to encourage increased fiber intake with fruits and vegetables • Encourage and guidance to increase engagement in meaningful occupations that are important to the child (i.e., hobbies, schoolwork, and independence with ADLs)
Attention-deficit/hyperactivity disorder (ADHD)	This is one of the most common neurodevelopmental disorders in childhood. These children have trouble focusing and behaving, to the extent that it causes difficulties at school, with friends, and at home. Symptoms include: • Daydreaming a lot • Squirming and fidgeting • Talking out of turn • Difficulty getting along with others • Difficulty paying attention to details or keeping attention during play • Difficulty listening to instructions or conversation • Difficulty with organization • Avoiding tasks that require a great deal of sustained attention • Blurting out answers and not being able to "filter" responses	OT interventions are many and varied, but some are listed below: • Instruction of cognitive-behavioral techniques • Instruction to modify behavior • Provide social skills training • Modify classroom environments to help with attention and focus • Teach self-management techniques • Use sensory modulation interventions • Encouragement and guidance to engage in meaningful occupations that are important to the child (i.e., hobbies, schoolwork, and independence with ADLs)
Long COVID-19[36]	This term is used to describe long-term symptoms or effects after having COVID-19, with causation unknown but may be related to viral load after contracting COVID-19, genetics, and/or overall health and well-being prior to contracting COVID-19. Some symptoms include: • Fatigue • Difficulty concentrating • Mood swings • Sensory disturbances (smell, taste) • Circulatory concerns • Musculoskeletal pain • Lingering cough or shortness of breath	OTPs will often work with children who exhibit these symptoms but might not have yet been diagnosed with long COVID-19. Asking the right questions related to recent illnesses can help zoom in on important information. Some OT interventions include: • Instruction in energy conservation • Provide education on compensatory strategies for concentration • Review sleeping habits and patterns with parents • Teach emotional regulation strategies • Assist with pain management

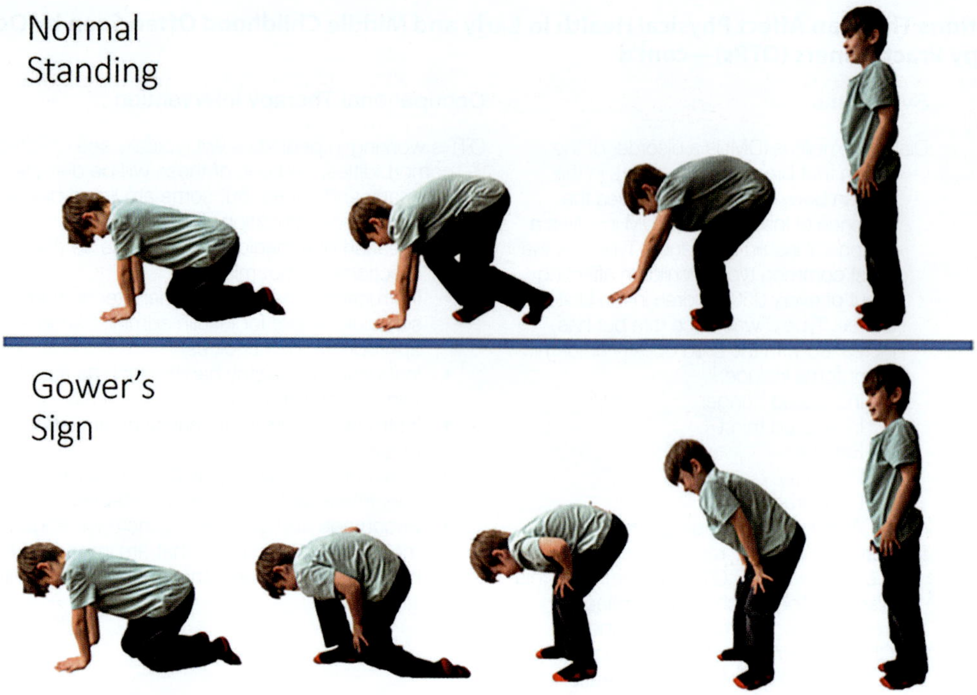

• **Fig. 5.2** Gower's sign in child with Duchene muscular dystrophy performing a sit-to-stand.

Application—Case Study

CASE EXAMPLE 5.1

A 4-year-old boy was referred by his teacher to the school occupational therapist to evaluate the child for "clumsiness."

1. **Screen:** The child demonstrated a strength grade of 3/5 (fair) in the hips and thighs and a strength grade of 4/5 (good) in the upper extremities.
2. **Take a Closer Look:** His calf muscles (gastrocsoleus) muscles were enlarged. The occupational therapist asked him to sit on the floor and then stand up again. She noticed that the child had to place his hands on his thighs and push to help him into a standing position (Gower's sign).
3. **Determine Flag Status:** Because of the gradual onset of weakness and positive Gower's sign, the occupational therapist decided this was a Yellow Flag.
4. **Take Action if Needed:** The occupational therapist contacted the child's pediatrician after parental consent. OTPs do not make a medical diagnosis, but the symptoms can be clearly explained to the pediatrican, enabling him or her to perform the appropriate tests needed to make the medical diagnosis.
5. **Document the Findings:** The occupational therapist documented the findings of the short examination as well as the phone call to the pediatrican.
6. **Take a Second Look:** The pediatrican consulted with specialists who performed a muscle biopsy and DNA testing. The test was positive for Duchenne Muscular Dystrophy.
7. **Determine the Flag Status:** With this new information, the occupational therapist and pediatrican changed this situation to a Red Flag.
8. **Take Action if Needed:** OT was again ordered in the school system and also in an outpatient clinic to work on gross and fine motor strengthening as well as bracing and other adaptive equipment as needed.

This is a true case. The child had the beginnings of Duchenne Muscular Dystrophy. The occupational therapist helped with an early diagnosis which can give the medical team and the family a head start on needed intervention.

References

1. Parenthood. *How to Help Your Child Develop Fine Motor Skills*. Healthline; 2023. https://www.healthline.com/health/fine-motor-skills.
2. CDC. *CDC's Developmental Milestones*. Centers for Disease Control and Prevention; 2022. https://www.cdc.gov/ncbddd/actearly/milestones/index.html.
3. NAPA. *Gross Motor Development for Infants and Toddlers*. NAPA; 2023. https://napacenter.org/gross-motor-development/.
4. Papalia DE, Martorell G. *Experience Human Development*. 15th ed. McGraw Hill; 2024.
5. Schrempf B, Looper J, Poole L, Gunselman A, Brett K. Arm positioning and walking styles of children during the first 5 months of independent walking. In: *Sound Ideas, Physical Therapy Research Symposium, 12. Fall*. 12. University of Puget Sound; 2015. http://soundideas.pugetsound.edu/ptsymposium/12.
6. D'Alessandro DM. *When Will I Know Which Hand She Will Use?* Pediatric Education; 2011. https://pediatriceducation.org/2011/02/28/when-will-i-know-which-hand-she-will-use/.
7. Ocklenburg S. Genetics of left-handedness: new breakthrough. *Psychology Today*. November 21, 2019. https://www.psychologytoday.com/us/blog/the-asymmetric-brain/201911/genetics-left-handedness-new-breakthrough.
8. McManus IC, Davidson A, Armour JAL. Multilocus genetic models of handedness closely resemble single-locus models in

explaining family data and are compatible with genome-wide association studies. *Ann New York Acad Sci.* 2013;1288:48–58. https://doi.org/10.1111/nyas.12102.

9. Shakibaie S. *4 Types of Tripod Grasp: Everything You Need to Know.* Ready Kids Occupational Therapy; 2023. https://ready-kids.com.au/tripod-grasp/.
10. Beck C. *Pencil Grasp Development.* The OT Toolbox; 2020. https://www.theottoolbox.com/pencil-grasp-development/.
11. CHOC. *Developmental Milestones: 4 to 5 Year Olds.* Children's Hospital of Orange County; 2023. https://www.choc.org/primary-care/ages-stages/4-to-5-years/.
12. CDC. *Defining Child BMI Categories.* Centers for Disease Control and Prevention; 2023. https://www.cdc.gov/bmi/child-teen-calculator/bmicategories.html?CDC_AAref_Val=https://www.cdc.gov/obesity/basics/childhood-defining.html.
13. CDC. *Childhood Overweight and Obesity.* Centers for Disease Control and Prevention; 2024. Childhood Obesity Facts | Obesity CDC.
14. CHOC. *Developmental Milestones: 6 to 12 Year Olds.* Children's Hospital of Orange County; 2023. https://www.choc.org/primary-care/ages-stages/6-to-12-years/.
15. CDC. *Child Development: Middle Childhood (6-8 Years of Age).* Centers for Disease Control and Prevention; 2021. https://www.cdc.gov/ncbddd/childdevelopment/positiveparenting/middle.html.
16. Morin A. *Coordination and Motor Skills: What to Expect at Different Ages.* Understood for All, Inc.; N.D. https://www.understood.org/en/articles/coordination-and-motor-skills-what-to-expect-at-different-ages.
17. Stanford. *Common Cold in Children.* Stanford Medicine; 2024. https://www.stanfordchildrens.org/en/topic/default?id=common-cold-in-children-90-P02966.
18. CDC. *Why Vaccinate.* Centers for Disease Control and Prevention; 2019. https://www.cdc.gov/vaccines/parents/why-vaccinate/index.html.
19. Child Stats. *Child and Adolescent Mortality.* Federal Interagency Forum on Child and Family Statistics; 2022. https://www.childstats.gov/americaschildren/mortality.asp.
20. CDC. *Drowning Facts.* Centers for Disease Control and Prevention; 2019. https://www.cdc.gov/drowning/facts/index.html.
21. CPSC. *Annual Report of Pediatric Poisoning Fatalities and Injuries.* United States Consumer Product Safety Commission; 2022. https://www.cpsc.gov/s3fs-public/AnnualReportonPediatricPoisoningFatalitiesandInjuries_January2022.pdf.
22. CDC. *Secondhand Smoke and Children.* Centers for Disease Control and Prevention; 2019. https://www.cdc.gov/global-health/infographics/tobacco/secondhand-smoke-and-children.html.
23. APA. *Work, Stress, Health & Socioeconomic Status.* American Psychological Association; 2022. https://www.apa.org/pi/ses/resources/publications/work-stress-health.
24. Mayo Clinic. *Lead Poisoning.* Mayo Clinic; 2023. https://www.mayoclinic.org/diseases-conditions/lead-poisoning/symptoms-causes/syc-20354717.
25. APA. *Exploring the Mental Health Effects of Poverty, Hunger, and Homelessness on Children and Teens.* American Psychological Association; 2022. https://www.apa.org/topics/socioeconomic-status/poverty-hunger-homelessness-children.
26. IDA. *Dyslexia Basics.* International Dyslexia Association; 2020. https://dyslexiaida.org/dyslexia-basics/.
27. Peacock G. *Cognitive Deficits.* eMedicine Health; 2022. https://www.emedicinehealth.com/cognitive_deficits/article_em.htm.
28. CDC. *What Is ADHD?* Centers for Disease Control and Prevention; 2022. https://www.cdc.gov/ncbddd/adhd/facts.html.
29. ASCO. *Childhood Cancer: Signs and Symptoms.* American Society of Clinical Oncology: Cancer.Net; 2023. https://www.cancer.net/cancer-types/childhood-cancer/symptoms-and-signs.
30. Mayo Clinic. *Childhood Asthma.* Mayo Clinic; 2023. https://www.mayoclinic.org/diseases-conditions/childhood-asthma/symptoms-causes/syc-20351507.
31. Cleveland Clinic. *Childhood Asthma.* Cleveland Clinic; 2023. https://my.clevelandclinic.org/health/diseases/6776-asthma-in-children.
32. Mayo Clinic. *Hemophilia.* Mayo Clinic; 2023. https://www.mayoclinic.org/diseases-conditions/hemophilia/symptoms-causes/syc-20373327.
33. Mayo Clinic. *Muscular Dystrophy.* Mayo Clinic; 2022. https://www.mayoclinic.org/diseases-conditions/muscular-dystrophy/symptoms-causes/syc-20375388.
34. Merck Manual. *Diabetes in Children and Adolescents.* Merck Manual; 2022. https://www.merckmanuals.com/professional/pediatrics/endocrine-disorders-in-children/diabetes-mellitus-in-children-and-adolescents.
35. BCH. *Diabetes Insipidus.* Boston Children's Hospital; 2024. https://www.childrenshospital.org/conditions/diabetes-insipidus.
36. Cleveland Clinic. *What to Know About Long COVID in Kids.* Cleveland Clinic: Health Essentials; 2022. https://health.clevelandclinic.org/long-covid-in-kids/.

6 Typical Development and Pathophysiology During Female Adolescence

OBJECTIVES

By the end of this chapter, the reader should be able to:

- Demonstrate a basic understanding of typical physiologic development during female adolescence.
- Differentiate between puberty and the adolescent growth spurt.
- Demonstrate an understanding of the effect of physical fitness, diet, and sleep on adolescent development in females.
- Differentiate between typical and atypical female adolescent development.
- List common pathophysiological disorders in female adolescence.
- Compare and contrast various pathophysiological conditions and eating disorders that are common for females in this age group.

Typical Female Adolescent Human Development

The definition of adolescence varies depending on the textbook, periodical, or other source because adolescence is a social construct (or a term defined by a particular society). Not all societies around the world consider adolescence to be a separate period of development. In recent literature, the term *adolescence* has been defined as the period from age 11 to 20 years or from 10 to 24 years (again, depending on the source).[1,2] According to Sawyer et al., trends over recent decades have shown an earlier onset of puberty, continued adolescent growth beyond age 20, and a delay in the timing of many of the roles of adulthood. This has led to a shift in perceptions of adolescence to more closely align with the age range of 10 to 24 years.[3] This definition of adolescence will be used throughout this text.

Two processes happen during the period of adolescence that greatly influence human physiological development: puberty and the adolescent growth spurt. These two occurrences need to be explained before one can truly understand the pathophysiological conditions that sometimes occur during this phase of development in females.

Puberty

The term *puberty* refers to the biological changes in growth and development that occur during adolescence, triggered by a cascade of various hormonal responses.[2] It is the phase of development where physiologic changes occur that enable reproduction.[4] During puberty, the pituitary gland sends a signal via gonadotropins that stimulate the testes in males and ovaries in females (Fig. 6.1), while the hypothalamus interacts with the pituitary to monitor the body's balance of these hormones. The rise in gonadotropins is responsible for many of the changes that take place during this phase of development, not only in the breasts and genitalia but also in the skin, muscle, and bones.[4]

Female Puberty

The typical age of puberty for girls is between the ages of 8 and 13.[5] For females, the most noticeable features of puberty include the development of the genitalia, the development of the secondary sex characteristics (like the breasts), and the appearance of menarche, or the first monthly period. The above-mentioned rise in gonadotropins causes an increase in the development of the ovaries, which then develop their first follicles.[6] During the *follicular phase* of the menstrual

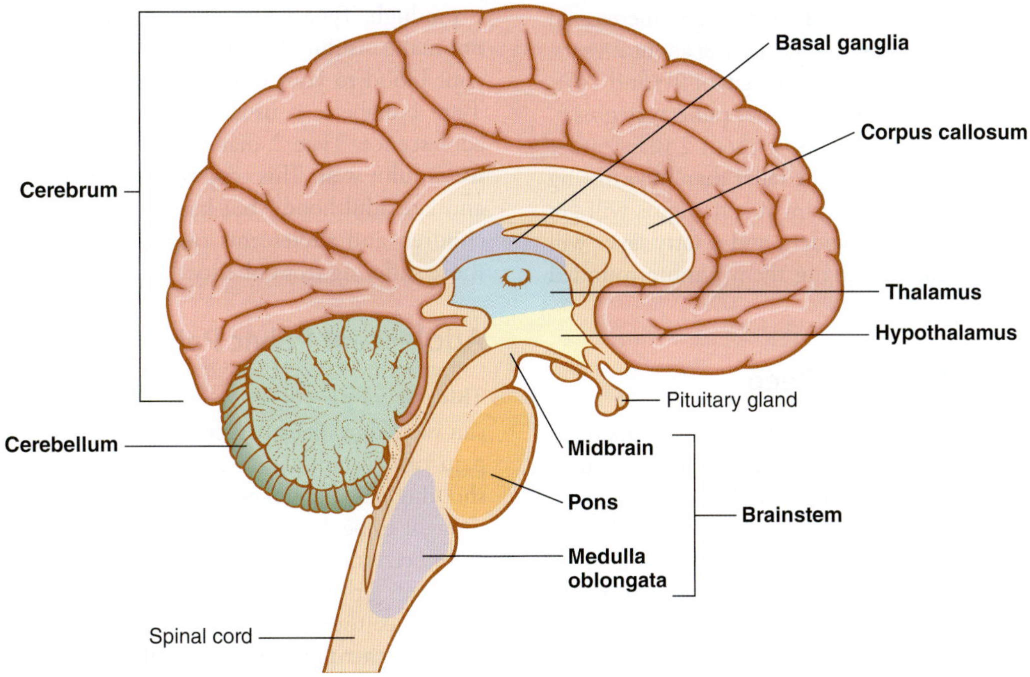

• **Fig. 6.1** The pituitary gland. (From Chabner D-E. Nervous system. In: *The Language of Medicine*. 13th ed. Elsevier; 2025.)

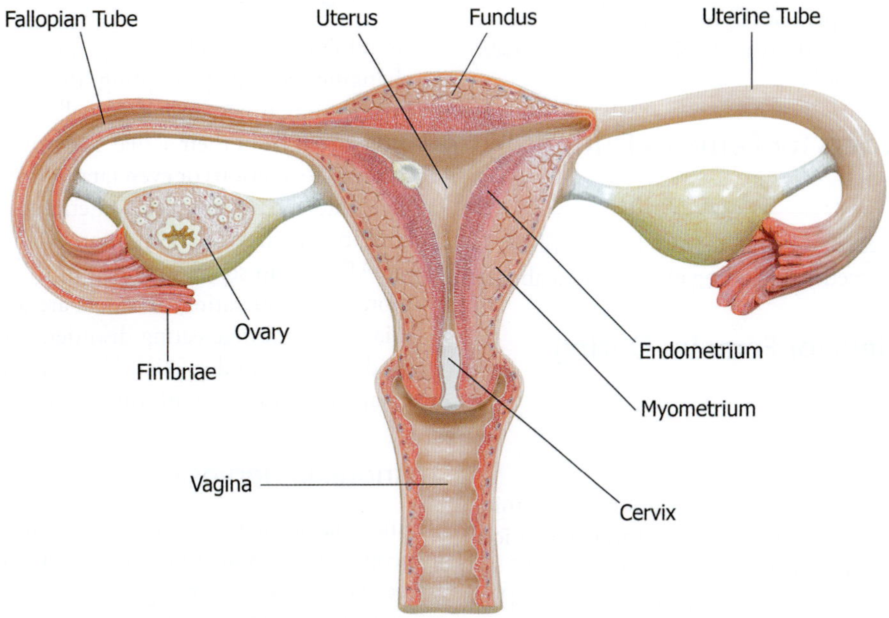

• **Fig. 6.2** The female uterus. (From https://www.iStock.com/kinwun.)

cycle, the body releases luteinizing hormone and follicle-stimulating hormone, which helps the egg inside the ovary to develop.[7] *Ovulation* is when the egg is released from the ovary to travel down the fallopian tube into the uterus (*the luteal phase* of the menstrual cycle) (Fig. 6.2). If the egg entering the uterus is not fertilized, the uterus will shed its lining (*the menses phase* of the menstrual cycle). This cycle will reset every 25 to 35 days.[6] The typical age of menarche is between ages 8 and 16, but the average age is about 12 to 13 years.[6,8]

The Adolescent Growth Spurt

The adolescent growth spurt is not the same as puberty. While puberty is the phase of human development, which includes the maturation of the reproductive organs, the adolescent growth spurt is the name for a rapid increase in height and weight during adolescence, lasting about 2 years. It begins in girls sometime between the ages of 9½ and 14½, typically around age 10, about a year after puberty begins.[2,9] Girls typically have their growth spurt about 2 years earlier than boys and, therefore, tend to be taller than boys during early adolescence.[2] During this growth spurt, girls will get taller, their hips will typically widen, and a fatty layer will accumulate under their skin giving them a more rounded appearance.[2]

Physical Fitness, Diet, and Sleep

The World Health Organization (WHO) has recommended an average of 60 minutes per day of moderate to vigorous exercise for adolescents.[10] Although the WHO has warned about the dangers of a sedentary lifestyle for this population, they have reported that over 80% of the world's adolescents do not get enough physical activity.[10] Being sedentary in this age group can increase the risk of obesity, diabetes, cardiometabolic problems, and even sleep disturbances. Physical activity, in moderation, with a good dietary program under a physician's supervision, can help decrease stress and improve sleep patterns. Adolescents who are sleep deprived can have problems physically, cognitively, psychosocially, and spiritually. They might also experience symptoms of depression, feelings of increased stress, decreased ability to concentrate, and poor grades in school.[11]

Common Disorders for Females During Adolescence

As stated earlier, a sedentary lifestyle can lead to physical problems during adolescence, including obesity and diabetes.

Physical Disorders for Females During Adolescence

Obesity

Obesity is currently considered to be a national epidemic. According to the Centers for Disease Control and Prevention (CDC), the obesity prevalence during the years 2017 to 2020 was 22.2% among adolescents ages 12 to 19.[12] This has been associated with conditions that used to be reserved for older adults, such as high blood pressure, high cholesterol, type 2 diabetes, and breathing problems like asthma.[12] A recent systematic review of prospective studies found evidence to support that there are genetic factors associated with adolescent obesity and that lower socioeconomic status can also play a part.[13]

Diabetes

The rates of newly diagnosed cases of type 2 diabetes have continued to rise in the adolescent population.[14] Diabetes is a disorder that happens when an individual's blood glucose is too high. Type 1 diabetes happens when your body does not make insulin, the hormone that transports glucose from your blood to your cells to make it usable in your body.[15] Type 1 diabetes is usually diagnosed during childhood or adolescence. Type 2 diabetes is when your body does not use insulin well. This type is typically diagnosed in middle and late adulthood[15] but has been seen more frequently in children and adolescents over the last 20 years, especially those suffering from obesity.[14]

Adolescent Pelvic Pain

This type of pain is very common in young girls. The causes can vary from menstrual cramps to bladder infections. Pelvic pain can come in waves, feel colicky, can be a stabbing or shooting pain, or can even be a dull ache. Menstrual cramps, thought to be due to the release of prostaglandins within the endometrium,[16] are common and typically cyclical. This pattern leads girls to be fairly certain that this is the cause of their pain, since they feel it every month. Still, it is important to rule out other potential causes, like appendicitis (see Chapter 15), kidney stones (see Chapter 17), endometriosis, ectopic pregnancy, or ovarian conditions.

Eating Disorders

As adolescents develop, they grow in awareness of their changing bodies, prompting the creation of their body image. Sometimes, an individual's perception of their body is distorted from their actual body type. This misperception can lead to a serious or even fatal eating disorder.[17] Although male adolescents are also sometimes diagnosed with these conditions, they are seen more commonly in those who are AFAB, and so are included in this chapter. Some of the more common eating disorders are anorexia nervosa, bulimia nervosa, binge-eating disorder, and avoidant-restrictive food intake disorder (ARFID). The reader can also refer to Chapter 27 for more information on eating disorders.

Anorexia Nervosa

Anorexia nervosa is a type of body image disorder in which people severely restrict their food intake. These individuals often see themselves as overweight even when they are dangerously underweight. There are two types: *Restrictive* (those who avoid food) and *Binge-Purge* (those who not only avoid food but also have episodes of eating followed by self-induced vomiting or use of laxatives or diuretics).[17] Symptoms include dry or yellowing of the skin, lanugo (fine hair) over most of the body, lethargy, slowed pulse and respiratory rate, and low blood pressure.[17]

Bulimia Nervosa

The symptoms of bulimia nervosa include uncontrollable binge eating followed by some form of purge (vomiting, laxatives, or diuretics). Symptoms include sore throat, worn tooth enamel, gastrointestinal problems, and electrolyte imbalance.[17] The individual might also demonstrate Russell's sign, which is the formation of calluses over the back of the metacarpophalangeal joints (knuckles) of the hand caused by forced vomiting.[18] This disorder can also lead to brain damage or death.

Binge-Eating Disorder

Binge-eating disorder is characterized by an individual's loss of control over their food intake, with the absence of purging. Individuals who struggle with binge-eating disorder tend to be overweight or obese. Symptoms include continued eating, even when full; eating alone to avoid embarrassment; frequent dieting without weight loss; and feeling ashamed or guilty about eating.[17]

Avoidant-Restrictive Food Intake Disorder

Avoidant-restrictive food intake disorder (ARFID) was once known as *selective eating disorder*. This may first appear during middle childhood. With ARFID, an individual restricts the intake of a type of food due to a fear of gaining weight. This is not the same as the picky eating phases that many children experience. With ARFID, the individual does not take in enough calories to grow properly (when a child) or to maintain healthy body functions (when an adolescent or adult). Symptoms include a lack of interest in food, a dramatic restriction of specific food types, upset stomach, and dramatic weight loss.[17]

As an occupational therapy practitioner (OTP), if an individual demonstrates symptoms that are outside of the typical cluster you expect to find with their diagnosis, it is important to report those symptoms to the referring physician. This includes possible symptoms of an eating disorder. If you, or anyone you know, exhibits symptoms of the above disorders, there is a helpline through the National Association of Anorexia Nervosa and Associated Disorders (ANAD) at (888) 375-7767 or hello@anad.org.

Psychosocial Disorders

During adolescence, individuals are beginning to investigate their role within society. It is a time of new experiences, challenges, and exploration. The psychological and social turbulence of this stage creates opportunity for psychosocial disorders to present themselves. The disorders covered in Chapter 7 are anxiety disorders, depression, and internet gaming disorder.

As previously stated, it is important for an OTP to report any client symptoms that are suspicious or outside of the typical cluster expected with a given diagnosis to the referring physician.

Death in Adolescence

Death in adolescence is typically due to accidents (especially car accidents), drowning, violence, and suicide.[2] Complications from pregnancy and childbirth are the leading cause of death for girls ages 15 to 19.[2]

The OT Scope of Practice

Table 6.1 provides a quick overview of some of the more common conditions seen by OTPs for females in this age group.

TABLE 6.1 Conditions Sometimes Seen in Occupational Therapy Specific to Adolescent Females

Condition	Symptoms	Occupational Therapy Intervention
46 XX DSD (Differences in Sex Development with 46, XX karyotype)[19,20]	An autosomal dominant genetic disorder in which a person with XX chromosomes presents with external genitalia that ranges from a typical male to ambiguous. These individuals are typically identified as male at birth. • Decreased testicular size with testosterone deficiency • Male hypogonadism • Polycystic ovaries • Gynecomastia • Infertility because of azoospermia (lack of sperm) • Additional health concerns associated with low testosterone	• Although this is usually diagnosed at birth, that is not always the case; therefore, having a basic understanding of normal human development can be key to facilitating physician referral if suspicion arises. • Provide support and stress management strategies to parents regarding child's medical condition • Address psychosocial impacts of condition as warranted, with the guidance of a psychiatrist, counselor, or social worker, whomever is part of the child's healthcare team • Utilize artistic and therapeutic techniques to improve self-esteem and body image

(Continued)

TABLE 6.1 Conditions Sometimes Seen in Occupational Therapy Specific to Adolescent Females—cont'd

Condition	Symptoms	Occupational Therapy Intervention
Turner syndrome[21]	Females born with only one X chromosome • Webbed neck • Large collections of fluid in the back of the neck, with swelling of the extremities, hands, and feet • Skeletal abnormalities • Broad chest and widely spaced nipples • Kidney problems • Congenital heart defects • Hormone imbalances • May lack secondary sex characteristics • Cognitive deficits	Some of the areas OTPs can address with this group of individuals, include but not limited to: • Improvement of motor planning, balance, and coordination • Development of skills to increase cognitive flexibility and improve affect/regulation during change(s) • Utilization of artistic and therapeutic techniques to improve self-esteem and body image • Enhancement of social skills, assistance with the understanding of social cues, and improvement regarding participation in same-aged peer activities
Amenorrhea[22]	An abnormal absence of menses in females of reproductive age. Typically one or two missed periods can qualify as amenorrhea. • Primary: a female who does not experience first menses by the age of 15 • Secondary: a menstruating female missing a period for 3 or more months • See Fig. 6.3 for some of the more common causes of amenorrhea	Individuals will often trust their OTP with this information when they have told no one else. This is why building rapport is important! Having the individual's permission to share this information with their physician is important before doing so. Informing the physician could be mandatory to ensure good care across the healthcare continuum. • Ensure thorough evaluation with health history well documented • With the individual's permission, inform the referring physician of any new symptoms or changes in their current condition
Precocious puberty[23,24]	This is when a child's body begins to undergo puberty too soon. Typically, puberty occurs after age 8 in girls and after age 9 in boys. Early puberty can be divided into two types: • Central precocious puberty: a gonadotropin-dependent type that occurs due to an abnormality in the brain (i.e., tumor, radiation, and infection), which signals the pituitary gland to start puberty prematurely. It is called "central" because it is due to a central nervous system problem • Peripheral precocious puberty: a gonadotropin-independent type that is caused by an abnormality in the ovaries or adrenal glands, which results in an overproduction of sex hormones (estrogens)	Adolescents and their parents will often trust their OTP with this information when they have told no one else. Having the primary caregiver's permission to share this information with the physician is important before doing so. Informing the physician could be mandatory to ensure good care across the healthcare continuum. • Ensure thorough evaluation with health history well documented • With the individual's permission, inform the referring physician of any new symptoms or changes in their current condition
Hypogonadism[25]	A medical condition, in which sex glands produce little to no hormones. Symptoms for females of menstrual age who do not secrete enough estrogen can include: • Hot flashes • Amenorrhea • Delayed breast bud development • Stunted growth in height • Weight gain • Irritability	Adolescents and parents will often trust their OTP with this information when they have told no one else. This condition might be embarrassing for the adolescent to discuss, yet they might begin to do so with their OTP. Offering to have another individual present, like their mother, might help them feel more comfortable. • Ensure thorough evaluation with health history well documented by knowing what questions to ask • With the individual's permission, inform the referring physician of any new symptoms or changes in their current condition

TABLE 6.1 Conditions Sometimes Seen in Occupational Therapy Specific to Adolescent Females—cont'd

Condition	Symptoms	Occupational Therapy Intervention
Anovulation[26]	Atypical failure of an egg (ovum) to release during a menstrual cycle. This results in an irregularity of periods or amenorrhea. In addition to menstrual irregularities, other symptoms can include: • Excessive bleeding with periods • Lack of cervical mucus • Irregular basal body temperature	Adolescents and parents will often trust their OTP with this information when they have told no one else. They might still feel a little embarrassed discussing this with others. • Ensure thorough evaluation with health history well documented. Know what questions to ask • With the individual's permission, inform the referring physician of any new symptoms or changes in their current condition
Polycystic ovary syndrome (PCOS)[27]	PCOS is when the ovaries produce an abnormally high amount of androgens (male sex hormones). This can stop or delay ovulation, which can result in the formation of numerous small cysts (fluid-filled sacs) in the ovaries. • Missed, irregular, or light periods • Painful ovarian cysts • Excessive body or facial hair • Acne • Formation of skin tags on the neck or armpits • Thinning hair	Adolescents and parents will often trust their OTP with this information when they have told no one else. • Ensure thorough evaluation with health history well documented by knowing what questions to ask • With the individual's permission, inform the referring physician of any new symptoms or changes in their current condition

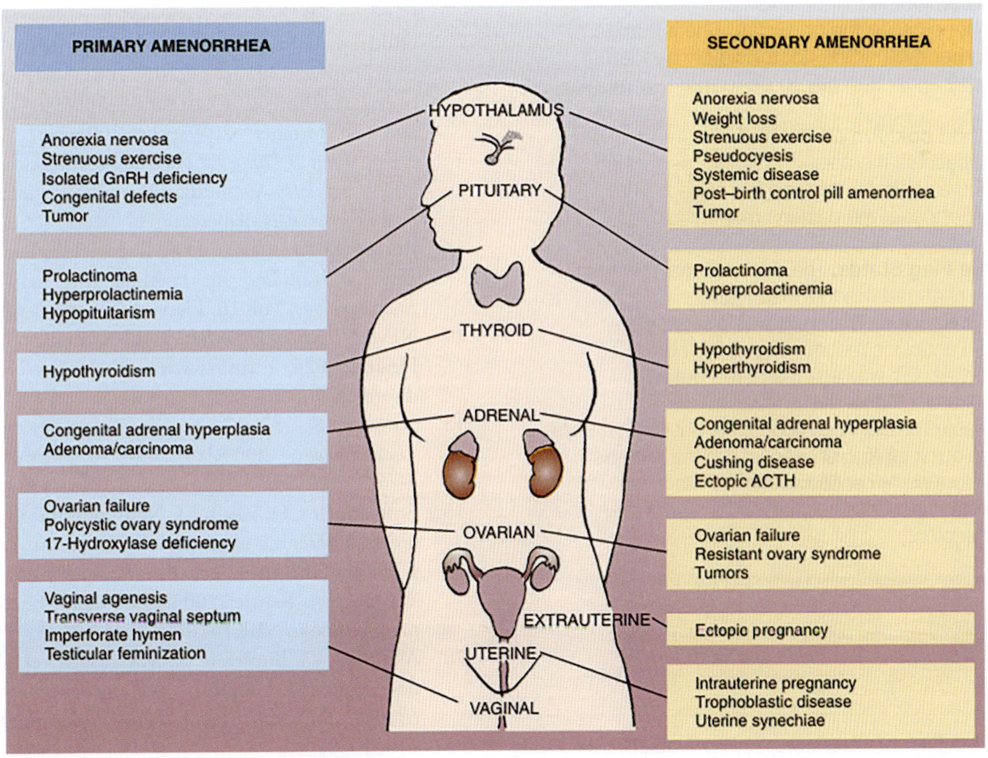

• **Fig. 6.3** Some of the more common causes of amenorrhea. (From Black JM, Hawks JH. Management of women with reproductive disorders. In: *Black's Adult Health Nursing I & II: Clinical Management for Positive Outcomes*. Elsevier; 2024.)

Application—Case Study

CASE EXAMPLE 6.1

A 16-year-old female was referred by her doctor to OT for upper extremity and abdominal weakness after a floor hockey injury at school.

1. **Screen:** She presented to the occupational therapist with a strength grade of 4/5 (good) for all muscles in both upper extremities but some inability to stabilize the trunk during reaching activities due to abdominal pain. The client reported that she had bilateral lower abdominal quadrant pain while performing these activities.
2. **Take a Closer Look:** The medical record showed this client had a possible strain of the abdominal muscles from a fall during a floor hockey game.
3. **Determine Flag Status:** The upper quadrant pain led the occupational therapist to consider this to be a Yellow Flag but wished for more information, so she asked if she could question the client without the mother present. During this time, the girl stated that this pain did not start after the fall but began before the game after she had sexual relations with a boy she knew from school. She also had painful urination and yellowish vaginal discharge. The occupational therapist was now leaning toward the possibility of a Red Flag situation.
4. **Take Action if Needed:** The occupational therapist contacted the physician immediately. OTPs do not make a medical diagnosis, but the symptoms can be clearly explained to the physician, enabling him or her to perform the appropriate tests needed to make the medical diagnosis.
5. **Document the Findings:** The occupational therapist documented the findings of the short examination as well as the phone call to the physician. She informed the client and her mother the doctor simply needed to see the client again that day to perform a few more tests.
6. **Take a Second Look:** Armed with this new information from the occupational therapist, the doctor performed a urinalysis and a vaginal swab and found bacterium *Neisseria gonorrhoeae*, the bacteria responsible for gonorrhea.
7. **Determine the Flag Status:** The occupational therapist and physician changed this to a Red Flag.
8. **Take Action if Needed:** The client was treated with ceftriaxone, an antibiotic recommended by the CDC to treat gonorrhea. OT was again ordered but for conditioning exercises after this illness.

This is a true case. The client had gonorrhea, but it was caught early, thanks to the quick thinking of her occupational therapist. The mother was informed by her daughter of her diagnosis while in the physician's office, and the occupational therapist upheld the confidentiality of her client.

References

1. Andrews JL, Foulkes L, Blakemore S. Peer influence in adolescence: public health implications for COVID-19. *Trends Cognit Sci.* 2020;24(8):585–587. https://doi.org/10.1016/j.tics.2020.05.001.
2. Papalia DE, Martorell G. *Experience Human Development.* 15th ed. McGraw Hill; 2024.
3. Sawyer SM, Azzopardi PS, Wickremarathne D, Patton GC. The age of adolescence. *Lancet Child Adolesc Health.* 2018;2(3):223–228. https://pubmed.ncbi.nlm.nih.gov/30169257/.
4. Wood CL, Lane LC, Cheetham T. Puberty: normal physiology (brief overview). *Best Pract Res Clin Endocrinol Metab.* 2019;33:101265. https://doi.org/10.1016/j.beem.2019.03.001.
5. Cleveland Clinic. *Puberty.* Cleveland Clinic; 2023. https://my.clevelandclinic.org/health/articles/22192-puberty.
6. Ali R, Rehman R. Reproductive cycle. In: Rehman R, ed. *Subfertility.* Elsevier; 2020. 65–75.
7. Marcin A. *What Is Ovulation? What to Know About Your Menstrual Cycle.* Healthlines; 2022. https://www.healthline.com/health/womens-health/what-is-ovulation.
8. Cleveland Clinic. *Menstrual Cycle.* Cleveland Clinic; 2022. https://my.clevelandclinic.org/health/articles/10132-menstrual-cycle.
9. Brennan D. *Stage of Puberty.* WebMD; 2023. https://www.webmd.com/children/ss/slideshow-puberty-stages.
10. WHO. *Physical Activity.* World Health Organization; 2022. https://www.who.int/news-room/fact-sheets/detail/physical-activity.
11. Kansagra S. Sleep disorders in adolescents. *Pediatrics.* 2020;145(Supplement_2):S204–S209. https://doi.org/10.1542/peds.2019-2056I.
12. CDC. *Childhood Obesity Facts.* Centers for Disease Control; 2022. https://www.cdc.gov/obesity/data/childhood.html#print.
13. Narciso J, Silva AJ, Rodrigues V, et al. Behavioral, contextual and biological factors associated with obesity during adolescence: a systematic review. *PLoS One.* 2018. https://doi.org/10.1371/journal.pone.0214941.
14. CDC. *Rates of New Diagnosed Cases of Type 1 and Type 2 Diabetes Continue to Rise Among Children, Teens.* Centers for Disease Control; 2022. https://www.cdc.gov/diabetes/research/reports/children-diabetes-rates-rise.html#:~:text=The%20rate%20of%20new%20cases%20%28or%20incidence%29%20of,issue%20of%20CDC%E2%80%99s%20Morbidity%20and%20Mortality%20Weekly%20Report.
15. NIH. *What Is Diabetes?* National Institutes of Health NIDDK; 2023. https://www.niddk.nih.gov/health-information/diabetes/overview/what-is-diabetes.
16. Rosenfield RL, Cooke DW, Radovick S. Puberty in the female and its disorders. In: Sperling MA, ed. *Sperling Pediatric Endocrinology.* Vol. 16. Elsevier; 2021:528–626.
17. NIMH. *Eating Disorders.* NIH: National Institute of Mental Health; 2024. https://www.nimh.nih.gov/health/topics/eating-disorders.
18. Strumia R. Skin signs in anorexia nervosa. *Dermato-Endocrinology.* 2009;1(5):268–270. https://doi.org/10.4161/derm.1.5.10193.
19. Emmanuèle CD, Vilain EJ. Nonsyndromic 46,XX testicular disorders/differences of sex development. In: Adam MP, Feldman J, Mirzaa GM, et al., eds. *GeneReviews® [Internet].* University of Washington, Seattle; 2003:1993–2024. https://www.ncbi.nlm.nih.gov/books/NBK1416/.
20. Alkhzouz C, Bucerzan S, Miclaus M, et al. 46, XX DSD: developmental, clinical, and genetic aspects. *Diagnostics (Basel).* 2021;11(8):1379. https://doi.org/10.3390/diagnostics11081379.
21. Mayo Clinic. *Turner Syndrome.* Mayo Clinic; 2022. https://www.mayoclinic.org/diseases-conditions/turner-syndrome/symptoms-causes/syc-20360782.
22. Cleveland Clinic. *Amenorrhea. Menstrual Cycle.* Cleveland Clinic; 2023. https://my.clevelandclinic.org/health/diseases/3924-amenorrhea.

23. Mayo Clinic. *Precocious Puberty*. Mayo Clinic; 2023. https://www.mayoclinic.org/diseases-conditions/precocious-puberty/symptoms-causes/syc-20351811.
24. NIH. *What Causes Normal Puberty, Precocious Puberty, and Delayed Puberty?* Eunice Kennedy Schriver National Institute of Child Health and Human Development; 2021. https://www.nichd.nih.gov/health/topics/puberty/conditioninfo/causes.
25. Gurarie M. *Symptoms of Hypogonadism*. Very Well Health; 2021. https://www.verywellhealth.com/hypogonadism-signs-symptoms-and-complications-5191935.
26. Johnson TC. *What Is Anovulation?* WebMD; 2023. https://www.webmd.com/infertility-and-reproduction/what-is-anovulation.
27. Johns Hopkins. *Polycystic Ovary Syndrome (PCOS)*. Johns Hopkins; 2024. https://www.hopkinsmedicine.org/health/conditions-and-diseases/polycystic-ovary-syndrome-pcos.

7

Typical Development and Pathophysiology During Male Adolescence

OBJECTIVES

By the end of this chapter, the reader should be able to:

- Demonstrate a basic understanding of typical physiologic development during male adolescence.
- Demonstrate an understanding of the effect of physical fitness and sleep on adolescent development in males.
- Differentiate between typical male adolescent development and atypical male adolescent development.
- List common pathophysiological disorders for male adolescence.
- Compare and contrast various pathophysiological conditions and various disorders affecting mental health that are common for males in this age group.

Typical Male Adolescent Human Development

As stated in Chapter 6, adolescence is typically defined as the period from ages 11 to 20 years or from ages 12 to 18 (depending on the source).[1,2] The definition of adolescence will depend on the text or article you are reading because adolescence is a social construct (or a term defined by a particular society). Not all societies around the world consider adolescence to be a separate period of development. For the purpose of this text, *adolescence* will be defined, in accordance with the suggestion made by Sawyer et al., as the period between 10 and 24 years of age.[3] This chapter will focus on individuals assigned male at birth (AMAB).

Male Puberty

Puberty has already been defined in Chapter 6 as the biological changes in growth and development that occur during adolescence, which are triggered by various hormones.[2] It is the process that enables the development of secondary sexual characteristics and the ability to reproduce.[4] After the pituitary gland secretes gonadotropin, leading to a rise in gonadal sex steroid production, there is growth of the genitalia, muscles, and bones.[5] This is not an isolated event but part of the continuous maturation of what is known as the hypothalamic-pituitary-gonadal axis.[6]

The typical age of puberty for boys is a little later than girls, typically occurring between the ages of 9 and 14.[7] For males, the most noticeable features of puberty include the development of genitalia and the development of secondary sex characteristics such as vocal changes, increased muscle mass, and the appearance of spermarche (the first ejaculation).[8] How is this different in males than in females? The above gonadotropins are released from the pituitary in a pulsating manner. An increase in frequency will favor the release of more luteinizing hormone (LH), whereas a lower frequency will favor the release of more follicle-stimulating hormone (FSH).[9] In females, LH is needed for ovulation, and FSH is needed for follicular growth. In males, however, the FSH binds to the Sertoli cells in the testes, supporting spermatogenesis, and LH works on the Leydig cells, also located in the testes, activating testosterone production[9] (Fig. 7.1).

The Adolescent Growth Spurt

As stated in Chapter 6, the adolescent growth spurt is not the same as puberty. It is a rapid increase in height and weight that lasts about 2 years and begins in boys sometime between the ages of 10½ and 16 (typically around age 12 or 13), about a year after puberty begins.[2,10] Girls typically have their growth spurt about 2 years earlier than boys.[2] During this growth spurt, boys will get taller, their shoulders will typically widen, and their forearms and legs will get longer, in relation to their trunk.[2]

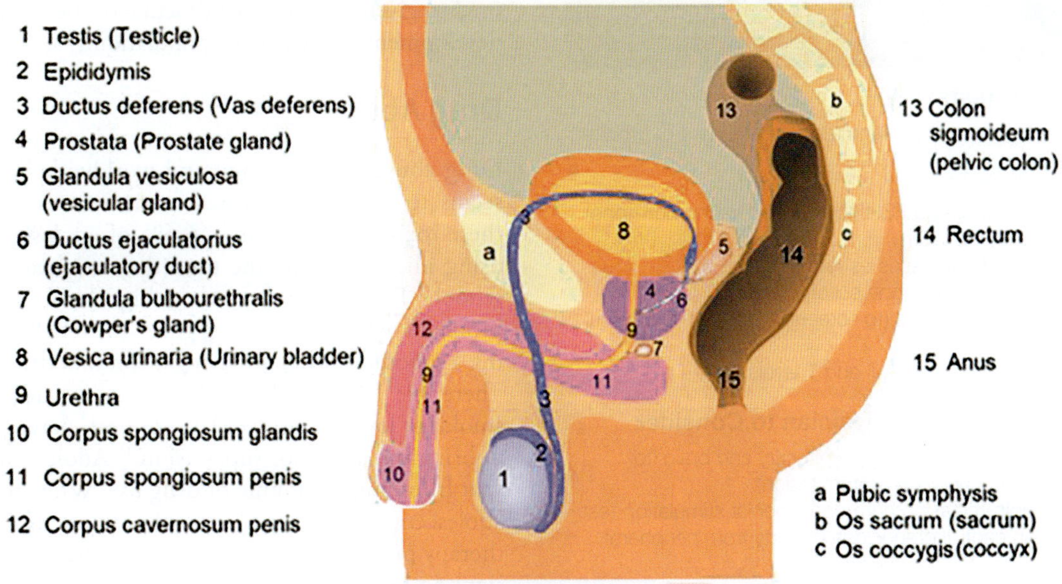

• **Fig. 7.1** The male reproductive system. (From https://commons.wikimedia.org/wiki/File:Male_anatomy_1.png.)

Physical Fitness and Sleep

Although this topic was already covered for adolescence in Chapter 6, the importance of adequate sleep during this stage of development cannot be overstated. Sleep deprivation during adolescence can lead to problems physically, cognitively, psychosocially, and spiritually.[11] Our body follows a melatonin secretion cycle that signals the most appropriate time for sleep. This is due to our circadian rhythm, a naturally occurring internal biological clock. Adolescents typically have a delayed secretion of these hormones, making their preferred sleep time later in the evening and their preferred wake time later in the day.[11] This is often not matched to the demands of a daily routine. This can be difficult for any adolescent, but if functional impairment is a result, the individual might be diagnosed with delayed sleep-wake phase disorder (DSPD).[11]

Identity and Sexuality

The development of sexuality takes on a "mature form" during adolescence and can be a source of stress, as physical, psychological, and cognitive development are all reaching their peak.[12] As previously stated in Chapter 6, girls will reach puberty about 12 to 18 months earlier than boys. Boys who mature early tend to have a better body image and are more confident than boys who reach puberty later.[12] Severe stress can result when the assigned sex at birth does not match the adolescent's gender identity. A mixed-method study by Hammock et al. surveyed 314 adolescents who were 14 to 18 years of age and found that 23.9% used nonbinary identity labels; yet, they reported facing challenges with respect to stigma and violence for transgender and nonbinary individuals.[13]

Death in Adolescence

The death rate of boys ages 15 to 19 in the United States is almost 2½ times the rate of girls.[2] For years, car accidents were the leading cause of death among this age group, but in 2020, it was surpassed by gun-related violence and accidents as the leading cause of death.[2]

Common Physical Disorders for Males During Adolescence

As stated earlier, a sedentary lifestyle can lead to physical problems during adolescence, including obesity and diabetes. These conditions were briefly discussed in Chapter 6, and diabetes will be covered again in Chapter 18. This chapter will briefly cover delayed puberty (DP) and drug abuse.

Precocious Puberty and Delayed Puberty

Precocious puberty is when the child begins to go through puberty earlier than expected (before 8 in girls and before 9 in boys).[14] This early puberty is sometimes referred to as central precocious puberty, and although most cases have no identifiable reason, in rare cases, it can be caused by brain injury, brain tumor, or various syndromes.[14] Palmert et al. have warned that many boys with sexual precocity have underlying causes and need to be carefully assessed (Box 7.1).

• BOX 7.1 Medical Testing for Sexual Precocity in Boys

Common Initial Tests

Careful history, physical examination, and assessment of growth velocity
Bone age
LH (luteinizing hormone) and FSH (follicle stimulating hormone) levels
Testosterone (and in some cases estradiol) levels
DHEA-S (dehydroepiandrosterone sulfate) levels
17-Hydroxyprogesterone levels (to screen for congenital adrenal hyperplasia)
TSH (thyroid-stimulating hormone) and T levels[4]

Secondary Tests for the Physician to Consider

MRI (magnetic resonance imaging) of pituitary and brain (to screen for a central nervous system lesion)
GnRH (gonadotropin-releasing hormone) agonist stimulation test (can distinguish central precocious puberty from peripheral precocity)
ACTH (adrenocorticotropin hormone) stimulation test (to diagnose congenital adrenal hyperplasia)[4]

Modified from Nathan BM, Palmert, MR. Regulation and disorders of pubertal timing. *Endocrinol Metab Clin North Am*. 2005;34:617–641.

DP is a delay in the development of the testicles, 2 to 2.5 standard deviations above the mean age in the population (usually around 14 years of age).[4] This can affect the adolescent's feelings of well-being, peer relationships, and participation in activities like sports.[4] Puberty plots are sometimes used to give practitioners a timeline of the stages of normal development in the general population.

Drug Abuse

Drug abuse is detrimental and worldwide.[15] Adolescence seems to be the time when many will experiment with these toxins. An alarming 46.6% of adolescents reported using illicit drugs by the time they graduated from high school.[2] Risk factors include a high level of impulsivity, problems with emotional regulation, rebelliousness, having a mood disorder, or having a conduct disorder (CD).[15] There are also familial risk factors including maternal smoking, low educational level of both parents, traumatic upbringing, and poor supervision.[15] Adolescents die every year from binge drinking or drug use. When working with adolescent populations, it is important, as occupational therapy practitioners (OTPs), that we are familiar with the signs and symptoms of drug abuse and misuse.

Testicular Cancer

Although testicular cancer is the most common type of cancer in young males between 18 and 39 years of age,[16] it is sometimes found in boys as young as 15 years of age and younger.[17,18] The testicles are egg-shaped glands held in the scrotum by the spermatic cord (Fig. 7.2). According to Johns Hopkins, the chance of developing this type of cancer is about 1-out-of-every-270 males, but the cure rate is high if caught

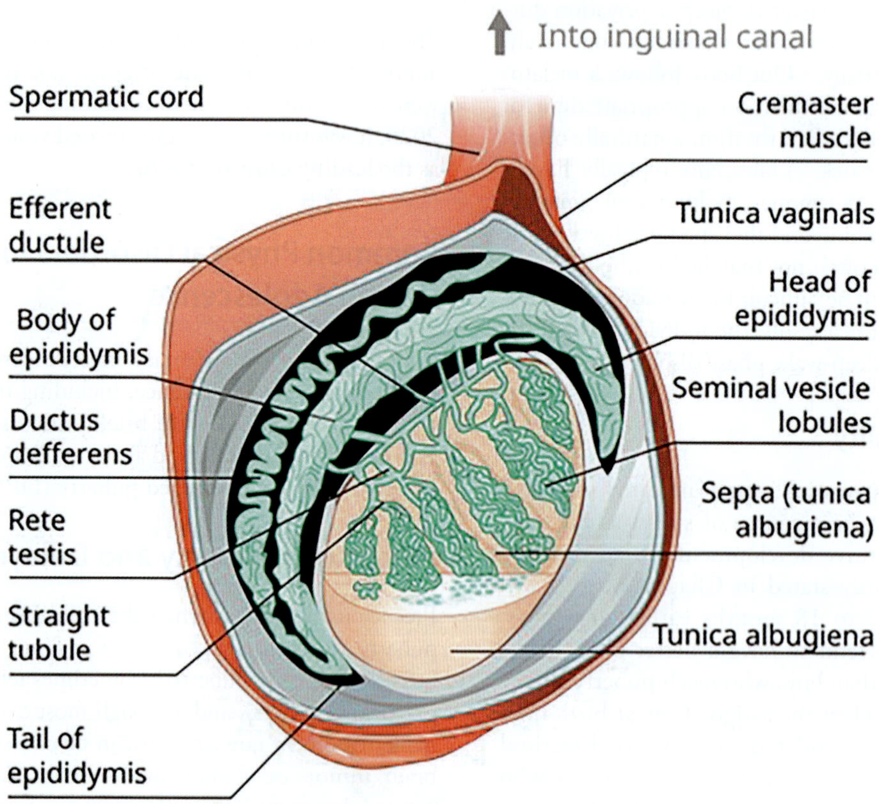

• **Fig. 7.2** The testicle. (From https://commons.wikimedia.org/wiki/File:Figure_28_01_03.JPG.)

TABLE 7.1 Conditions Sometimes Seen in Occupational Therapy That Are Specific to Adolescent Males

Condition	Symptoms	Occupational Therapy Intervention
Childhood testicular cancer[27,28]	A disease in which malignant cells are found in one or both testicles. Although more typical in males in their 20s and 30s, this disorder can occur during childhood. Symptoms of more advanced testicular cancer include: • A lump in the testicles that can be either painless or painful • Early puberty • Enlarged breasts • Dull ache in the lower abdomen or groin • Shortness of breath • Stomach pain • Headaches or confusion	Clients and parents will often trust their OTP with this information when they have told no one else. • Ensuring thorough evaluation and health history are documented and knowing what questions to ask • Communicating signs and symptoms to the referring physician, after receiving client and parent consent • Referring for education about testicular self-exams
Delayed puberty[29,30]	A delay in puberty, especially the development of the testicles that has not yet begun by age 14. Most will eventually go through puberty within a couple of years, but some may have inherited it from one or both parents. Symptoms include: • No enlargement of the penis or testicles • Less body and pubic hair compared to same-aged peers • Shorter stature due to a delayed growth spurt when compared to same-aged peers Certain comorbidities can lead to a delay in puberty in males like cystic fibrosis, celiac disease, inflammatory bowel disease, and diabetes mellitus.	Clients and parents will often trust their OTP with this information when they have told no one else. Some possible OT interventions could include: • Ensuring thorough evaluation and health history are documented and knowing what questions to ask • Communicating signs and symptoms to the referring physician, after receiving client and parent consent • Addressing gross motor and/or fine motor developmental delays • Improving social or leisure participation in same-aged peer activities • Encouraging engagement in meaningful occupations that are important to the adolescent (i.e., hobbies, schoolwork, and independence with ADLs) • Utilizing artistic and therapeutic techniques to improve self-esteem and body image
Klinefelter syndrome[31]	This is a fairly common chromosomal abnormality affecting about 1 out of every 600 people who are assigned male at birth, in which an extra X chromosome is present (47, XXY). Symptoms vary from person to person, and an individual might not have any symptoms until they are seen later in life for infertility. Those with symptoms might experience: • A smaller penis • Undescended testicles • Atypical proportions with long legs and a shorter trunk • Increased breast tissue • Flat feet • Coordination problems • Increase in the risk of blood clots • Osteopenia • ADHD • Impulsivity • Speech delays • Infertility	Clients and parents will often trust their OTP with this information when they have told no one else. Some possible OT interventions could include: • Ensuring thorough evaluation and health history are documented and knowing what questions to ask • Communicating signs and symptoms to the referring physician, after receiving client and parent consent • Addressing gross motor and/or fine motor developmental delays • Addressing coordination issues • Improving social or leisure participation in same-aged peer activities • Encouraging engagement in meaningful occupations that are important to the adolescent (i.e., hobbies, schoolwork, and independence with ADLs) • Utilizing artistic and therapeutic techniques to improve self-esteem and body image • Advocating for supports in school if limited due to learning difficulties and/or attentional difficulties

(Continued)

TABLE 7.1 Conditions Sometimes Seen in Occupational Therapy That Are Specific to Adolescent Males—cont'd

Condition	Symptoms	Occupational Therapy Intervention
DBDs[32]	DBDs are problems with emotions, self-control, and behavior that consistently interfere with a child's ability to function. The child with a DBD will disregard the rights of others and challenge the authority of adults There are five basic types: 1. *ODD* with frequent angry outbursts, refusal to follow the rules, blaming others for their own mistakes, or acting out in a vindictive way 2. *CD* with severe behaviors violating the rights of others, including aggression toward others and toward animals, destruction of property, stealing, lying, and breaking the law 3. IED with at least two violently unplanned explosive outbursts per week for three months, with temper tantrums and physical assaults 4. *Pyromania*, which is a rare condition in which the child has recurrent urges to start deliberate fires, with preceding anxiety, followed by pleasure after the fire has started 5. *Kleptomania*, which is a rare disorder characterized by impulsive, uncontrollable theft of things not needed for personal usage or gain. Stress is felt before stealing and is relieved after the theft	Clients and parents will often trust their OTP with this information when they have told no one else. Some possible OT interventions could include: • Ensuring thorough evaluation and health history are documented and knowing what questions to ask • Communicating signs and symptoms to the referring physician, after receiving client and parent consent • Addressing any accompanying gross motor and/or fine motor developmental delays • Addressing any accompanying coordination issues • Improving social or leisure participation in same-aged peer activities • Encouraging engagement in meaningful occupations that are important to the adolescent (i.e., hobbies, schoolwork, and independence with ADLs) • Utilizing artistic and therapeutic techniques to improve self-esteem • Advocating for supports in school if limited due to learning difficulties and/or attentional difficulties • Completing an emotional regulation curriculum to identify coping techniques • Trialing strategies to manage impulses or outbursts • Social skills training • Implementing behavioral strategies • Parent and teacher education/training to ensure carryover of socioemotional and behavioral strategies • Addressing any accompanying cognitive and executive functioning deficits

ADHD, Attention-deficit/hyperactivity disorder; *ADLs*, activities of daily living; *CD*, conduct disorder; *DBDs*, disruptive behavior disorders; *IED*, intermittent explosive disorder; *ODD*, oppositional defiant disorder; *OT*, Occupational therapy; *OTP*, Occupational therapy practitioner.
Modified from Nathan BM, Palmert MR. Regulation and disorders of pubertal timing. *Endocrinol Metab Clin North Am*. 2005;34:617–641.

early.[18] This cancer is four times more likely to occur in White males than in Black males, and a condition known as cryptorchidism (or an undescended testicle) increases the risk for this type of cancer.[19] Symptoms include a dull ache in the lower abdomen or groin, pain or discomfort in the testicle, and a lump or swelling in either testicle (with or without pain).[19] When caught early, this cancer can be cured, due to advances in chemotherapy, but this intervention is not without its side effects, which include cardiovascular disease, pulmonary toxicity, anxiety, and depression.[16]

Eating Disorders

Contrary to the belief of many, adolescent boys can be plagued with eating disorders as well as girls. Some of the more common eating disorders covered in Chapter 6 were anorexia nervosa, bulimia nervosa, binge-eating disorder, and avoidant-restrictive food intake disorder. See Chapter 27 for more information on eating disorders.

Common Psychosocial Disorders for Males During Adolescence

There are many different types of psychosocial disorders that can present themselves during this time period. The disorders covered in this chapter are anxiety disorders, depression, and internet gaming disorder (IGD).

Anxiety Disorders

These are the most common psychosocial disorders seen in adolescence. According to the CDC, they affect 9.4% of children and adolescents in the United States between the ages of 3 and 17.[20] Anxiety during adolescence, when compared to childhood anxiety, is associated with a higher chance of negative psychosocial outcomes by the age of 30, such as substance abuse, alcohol abuse, and adult anxiety.[21] Some anxiety is normal during teenage years, but it becomes a concern when the feelings become intense, lasting for weeks or even months, getting in the way of performing schoolwork or enjoying daily life. Symptoms include severe restlessness, irritability, and difficulty concentrating.[22] See Chapter 24 for more information on anxiety disorders.

Depression

Depression is a mood disorder. Although some sadness from time to time is normal, depression in adolescents can last months, making a teenager miss out on important events and milestones. Depression can affect energy levels, motivation, and sleep in teens.[23] Although depression is known to be biologically based with genetic links, it can be triggered by stressors. Symptoms include a persistent sad or empty feeling, loss of interest in typical activities, and irritability.[24] See Chapter 23 for more information on depression and other mood disorders.

Internet Gaming Disorder

IGD refers to excessive time spent playing internet games. This diagnostic condition was added to the DSM-5 in 2013.[25] There are nine criteria (symptoms), and five must be met within a 1-year time frame for this diagnosis. The nine categories are a high preoccupation for gaming, withdrawal, tolerance to gaming is high, inability to reduce gaming, loss of interest in other things, excessive time spent gaming even after negative consequences, deception toward others regarding gaming, use of gaming to escape negative mood or feelings, and lost relationships, jobs, or other opportunities.[26]

The OT Scope of Practice

As previously stated, when working as an occupational therapy practitioner (OTP), if a patient demonstrates symptoms that are outside of the typical cluster you expect to find with their diagnosis, it is important to report those symptoms to the referring physician. Table 7.1 provides a quick overview of some of the more common conditions seen by OTPs for males in this age group.

Application—Case Study

CASE EXAMPLE 7.1

An 18-year-old male was referred by his doctor to OT for body mechanics after a "groin tear" during football practice.

1. **Screen:** He presented to the occupational therapist with severe pain in the area of the right inguinal ligament. He was unable to stand straight and walked with a limp.
2. **Take a Closer Look:** The medical record showed that this client had a possible strain or tear in the area of the right groin.
3. **Determine Flag Status:** The possibility of a strain or tear led the occupational therapist to consider this to be a possible Yellow Flag, but she and her occupational therapy assistant wished for more information, so they asked the patient when it started. The OTPs expected the patient to say that it started suddenly after an accident, but instead, he reported that the only thing that helps decrease his pain is aspirin. The OTPs started to think this might be a Red Flag.
4. **Take Action if Needed:** The OTPs contacted the physician immediately. OTPs do not make a medical diagnosis, but the symptoms can be clearly explained to the physician, enabling them to perform the appropriate tests needed to make the medical diagnosis. In this case, the OTPs stated that the pain came on gradually (not suddenly), that the patient was awakened from sleep by this pain (indicative of potential system concerns and possible cancer), and that the pain is relieved with aspirin.
5. **Document the Findings:** The OTPs documented the findings of the short examination as well as the phone call to the physician. The occupational therapist informed the patient that the doctor simply needed to see the patient again that day to perform a few more tests.
6. **Take a Second Look:** Armed with this new information from the occupational therapist the doctor performed a proctologic examination and found a lump in the client's right testicle.
7. **Determine the Flag Status:** The OTPs and physician changed this to a definitive Red Flag.
8. **Take Action if Needed:** The client was sent to a surgeon. OT was again ordered but for conditioning exercises after this illness.

This is a true case. The client had testicular cancer, but it was caught early, thanks to the quick thinking of the OTPs. After surgery and a short bout of chemo, the client was diagnosed as cancer free.

References

1. Andrews JL, Foulkes L, Blakemore S. Peer influence in adolescence: public health implications for COVID-19. *Trends Cognit Sci.* 2020;24(8):585–587. https://doi.org/10.1016/j.tics.2020.05.001.
2. Papalia DE, Martorell G. *Experience Human Development.* 15th ed. McGraw Hill; 2024.
3. Sawyer SM, Azzopardi PS, Wickremarathne D, Patton GC. The age of adolescence. *Lancet Child Adolesc Health.* 2018;2(3):223–228. https://doi.org/10.1016/S2352-4642(18)30022-1.
4. Palmert MR, Chan Y, Dunkel L. Puberty and its disorders in the male. In: Sperling MA, ed. *Sperling Pediatric Endocrinology.* Elsevier; 2021;16:528–626.
5. Wood CL, Lane LC, Cheetham T. Puberty: Normal physiology (brief overview). *Best Pract Res Clin Endocrinol Metab.* 2019;33:101265. https://doi.org/10.1016/j.beem.2019.03.001.
6. Fechner PY. Gender differences in puberty. *J Adolesc Health.* 2002;30(4, suppl 1):44–48. https://doi.org/10.1016/S1054-139X(02)00357-9.
7. Cleveland Clinic. *Puberty.* Cleveland Clinic; 2023. https://my.clevelandclinic.org/health/articles/22192-puberty.
8. Kornhuber J, Lenz B. Markers of prenatal androgen exposure correlate with online sexual compulsivity and erectile function in men. *Front Psychiatry.* 2021;12:517411. https://doi.org/10.3389/fpsyt.2021.517411.
9. Spaziani M, Tarantino C, Tahani N, et al. Hypothalamo-pituitary axis and puberty. *Mol Cell Endocrinol.* 2021;520(2021):111094. https://doi.org/10.1016/j.mce.2020.111094.

10. Brennan D. *Stage of Puberty.* WebMD; 2023. https://www.webmd.com/children/ss/slideshow-puberty-stages.
11. Kansagra S. Sleep disorders in adolescents. *Pediatrics.* 2020; 145(suppl 2):S204–S209. https://doi.org/10.1542/peds.2019-2056I.
12. Kar SK, Choudhury A, Singh A. Understanding normal development of adolescent sexuality: a bumpy ride. *J Hum Reprod Sci.* 2015;8(2):70–74. https://doi.org/10.4103/0974-1208.158594.
13. Hammock PL, Hughes SD, Atwood JM, Cohen EM, Clark RC. Gender and sexual identity in adolescence: a mixed-methods study of labeling in diverse community settings. *J Adolesc Res.* 2022;37(2):167–220. https://doi.org/10.1177/07435584211000315.
14. Mayo Clinic. *Precocious Puberty. Patient Care and Health Information.* Mayor Clinic; 2023. https://www.mayoclinic.org/diseases-conditions/precocious-puberty/symptoms-causes/syc-20351811.
15. Nawi AM, Ismail R, Ibrahim F, et al. Risk and protective factors of drug abuse among adolescents: a systematic review. *BMC Public Health.* 2021;21:2088. https://doi.org/10.1186/s12889-021-11906-2.
16. Fung C, Dinh PC, Fossa SD, Travis LB. Testicular cancer survivorship. *J Natl Compr Cancer Netw.* 2019;17(12):1557–1568. https://doi.org/10.6004/jnccn.2019.7369.
17. Simone G. Urologic Cancers. In: Barber N, Ahmed A, eds. *The Epidemiology of Testicular Cancer.* Exon Publications; 2022.
18. John Hopkins. Testicular cancer statistics. In: *Health.* John Hopkins; 2024. https://www.hopkinsmedicine.org/health/conditions-and-diseases/testicular-cancer/testicular-cancer-statistics.
19. NIH. *Testicular Cancer Screening (PDQ®)—Patient Version.* NIH: National Cancer Institute; 2021. https://www.cancer.gov/types/testicular/patient/testicular-screening-pdq.
20. CDC. *Data and Statistics on Children's Mental Health.* Centers for Disease Control; 2023. https://www.cdc.gov/childrensmentalhealth/data.html.
21. Essau CA, Lewinsohn PM, Olaya B, Seeley JR. Anxiety disorders in adolescents and psychosocial outcomes at age 30. *J Affect Disord.* 2014;163(2014):125–132. https://doi.org/10.1016/j.jad.2013.12.033.
22. Katzenstein J. Anxiety and stress in teens. In: *Health.* Johns Hopkins; 2023. https://www.hopkinsmedicine.org/health/conditions-and-diseases/anxiety-disorders/anxiety-and-stress-in-teens.
23. Miller L. Debunking myths of teen depression. In: *Health.* Johns Hopkins; 2023. https://www.hopkinsmedicine.org/health/wellness-and-prevention/debunking-myths-of-teen-depression.
24. John Hopkins. Depression in children. In: *Health.* Johns Hopkins; 2023. https://www.hopkinsmedicine.org/health/conditions-and-diseases/depression-in-children.
25. Darvesh N, Radhakrishnan A, Lachance CC, et al. Exploring the prevalence of gaming disorder and internet gaming: a rapid scoping review. *Syst Rev.* 2020;9:68.
26. Jo YS, Bhang SY, Choi JS, et al. Clinical characteristics of diagnosis for internet gaming disorder: comparison of DSM-5 IGD and ICD-11 GD diagnosis. *J Clin Med.* 2019;8(7):945. https://doi.org/10.3390/jcm8070945.
27. NIH. *Childhood Testicular Cancer Treatment (PDQ®)S—Patient Version.* National Cancer Institute: National Institutes of Health; 2021. https://www.cancer.gov/types/testicular/patient/child-testicular-treatment-pdq.
28. ACS. *Signs and Symptoms of Testicular Cancer.* American Cancer Society; 2018. https://www.cancer.org/cancer/types/testicular-cancer/detection-diagnosis-staging/signs-and-symptoms.html.
29. PES. *Delayed Puberty – Boys.* Pediatric Endocrine Society; 2024. https://pedsendo.org/patient-resource/delayed-puberty-boys/.
30. MedLinePlus. *Delayed Puberty in Boys.* Medline Plus; 2022. https://medlineplus.gov/ency/article/007695.htm.
31. Cleveland Clinic. *Klinefelter Syndrome.* Cleveland Clinic; 2023. https://my.clevelandclinic.org/health/diseases/21116-klinefelter-syndrome.
32. Kumar K. What are the types of disruptive behavior? *Med Net.* 2022. https://www.medicinenet.com/what_are_the_types_of_disruptive_behavior/article.htm.

8 Typical Development and Pathophysiology During Early and Middle Adulthood

OBJECTIVES

By the end of this chapter, the reader should be able to:

- Demonstrate a basic understanding of typical physiologic development during early and middle adulthood.
- List signs and symptoms for various physical disorders sometimes present during early and middle adulthood.
- Demonstrate an understanding of the psychological disorders sometimes present during early and middle adulthood.
- Differentiate between typical adult development and atypical adult development.
- List common pathophysiological disorders for early and middle adulthood.
- Compare and contrast various pathophysiological conditions and various disorders affecting mental health that are common during early and middle adulthood.

Normal Adult Development

The line of demarcation depicting exactly when a person becomes an "adult" depends in part on culture, timing, and many other factors. What used to be a specific age in years is now varied depending on circumstances. It is for this reason that the phase of young adulthood is often referred to as *emerging adulthood*.[1] Still, for the purposes of this text, young (early) adulthood will be defined in accordance with the definitions proposed by the APA Dictionary of Psychology as roughly ages 20 to 35, and middle adulthood will be defined in this text as ages 36 to 64.[2] Although human development is generally a gradual process, each phase includes specific developmental tasks (Table 8.1).

Early Adult Development—Ages 20 to 35

Most young adults in the United States consider themselves to be in good health.[1] In our country, young adults who identify as White or Asian are more likely to be in good health when compared to those who identify as Black or Latino. This is believed to be primarily due to obesity.[1] According to a report by Hales et al., 40.0% of young adults in the United States were considered to be obese in 2018.[5] There are also numerous reports of negative health outcomes due to implicit biases from healthcare providers regarding client care. A common example of this is when doctors, nurses, and/or therapists are less likely to take symptoms seriously from those of marginalized genders and racial backgrounds, especially Black females.[6] This is important for OTPs to consider in order to better understand obstacles they might face when attempting to build trust with clients in this age group and older.

In light of the sometimes overwhelming demands placed on this age group, such as graduating from college, entering the workforce, and starting a family, there is a need for educational, emotional, and social supports among this age group and among the medical community that serves them.[7] This could be an important niche for occupational therapy.

Young adults are at their physical peak with respect to visual acuity, taste, and smell. The mid-20s also marks the peak in muscular strength, but the sense of hearing begins to decline in the 30s. In fact, the National Institute on Deafness and Other Communication Disorders found that about 15% of Americans ages 18 and over report some age-related hearing loss, also known as prebyscus.[8] Although many young adults are at their peak physically, they have twice the mortality rate of adolescents and are at a higher risk for violence, injury, sexually transmitted diseases, and substance abuse.[9]

TABLE 8.1 Developmental Tasks for Young Adulthood and Middle Adulthood

Criteria	Young Adulthood[3] (Age 20–35)	Middle Adulthood[4] (Age 36–64)
Erikson's Stage	Intimacy versus isolation (ages 19–40)	Generativity versus stagnation (ages 40–65)
Autonomy	Establishing oneself as independent	Adjusting to home life without children
Identity	Confirming likes and dislikes	Preparing for what is to come
Stability	Developing emotional stability	Adjusting to home life without children
Career	Establishing a career	Polishing up career and getting ready for retirement
Intimacy	Finding intimacy and long-term relationships	Acting as partner and caregiver
Community	Becoming involved in community activities	Becoming involved in community activities
Residence	Learning how to manage a household	Gradually planning where to live after retirement
Parenting	Becoming a parent and raising children	Dealing with adult children who still live at home and becoming grandparents
Marriage	Making adjustments to support the marriage and family	Acting as caregivers for aging parents and spouses

Middle Adult Development—Ages 36 to 64

Middle age can be not only a time of decline but can also be a time of gain and growth.[1] Most middle-aged people in our society consider themselves to be in good health, but middle age is filled with many responsibilities, along with multiple demanding roles. Although not studied as thoroughly as young and older adulthood, middle adulthood has been called a pivotal period with an interplay of generativity, which includes a balance of multiple roles.[10]

There are many physical changes, and studies continue to find that the more people do, the more they can do. Exercise in this age group has been found to be a highly effective way to not only live longer but to have more years without pain or disabling conditions.[11] Yet, there will still be some natural signs of aging during this time period. The most common visual deficit during middle adulthood is *Presbyopia* (farsightedness), which causes people to attempt reading from a greater distance because they cannot focus on objects that are too close to the eyes.[12] Another decline that sometimes occurs is *Myopia*, or nearsightedness, but this typically occurs during childhood and adolescence, becoming more stable during the 20s and 30s.[13] *Presbycusis*, the gradual loss of hearing, accelerates after age 55 and typically involves the loss of sounds at higher frequencies.[8,14] Bone mass starts a gradual decline during middle adulthood (*osteopenia*), especially for females after menopause (the age-related cessation of ovulation and menses).[15] During menopause, a female's hormone levels will decline quickly over a short period of time over several months. Males also have a decline in testosterone, sometimes called andropause, but this occurs over a period of many years (at a rate of about 1% per year), and the symptoms vary.[16] Muscular strength and coordination, which both peaked during the mid-20s, will typically show decline during middle adulthood, due in part to atrophy of muscle fibers as well as accumulation of lipofuscin (age-related pigment) and fatty deposits in the muscle tissue.[15] Endurance holds up much better but begins to decline in the 60s due to the gradual decline of basal metabolic rate (the way we use energy for vital bodily functions).[17]

Death in Early and Middle Adulthood

The leading cause of death in the United States across all age groups continues to be heart disease followed by cancer.[18] Accidents, however, are the leading cause of death during young adulthood, followed by homicide and suicide.[9] The primary causes of death during middle adulthood used to be accidents, but from 2010 to 2017, it changed to alcohol-related liver disease, drug overdoses, and suicide, with an increase in midlife mortality and a resultant decrease in the overall life expectancy in the United States.[19] This is believed to be due to the opioid epidemic, obesity, and healthcare system deficiencies affecting people in this age group.[20]

Common Disorders During Early and Middle Adulthood

As stated above, a sedentary lifestyle can lead to physical problems, including obesity and diabetes. These conditions were briefly discussed in Chapter 6, and diabetes will be covered again in Chapter 18. This chapter will briefly cover hyperlipidemia, heart disease, kidney stones, clinical depression, and drug dependency.

Physical Disorders During Early and Middle Adulthood

Most diseases during young and middle adulthood are multifactorial with both a genetic (nature) and an environmental (nurture) component. Some examples of this are hyperlipidemia, heart disease, and kidney stones.

Hyperlipidemia. Cholesterol levels in the blood can be related to both genetics and nutrition. Low-density lipoproteins (LDLs) are considered to be more harmful and are therefore dubbed the "bad" cholesterol, as opposed to the high density lipoproteins (HDLs), or "good" cholesterol, which some believe help to flush out LDLs in the bloodstream. High cholesterol can lead to the formation of plaque in the vasculature and result in atherosclerotic heart disease.[20]

Heart disease. The term *heart disease*, or more specifically cardiovascular disease, consists of many conditions that affect the heart or vasculature including arrhythmias, high blood pressure, heart attack, and stroke.[21] While many risk factors play a role in the development of cardiovascular disease, one key mechanism is believed to be inflammation. A marker of this inflammation is C-reactive protein (CRP).[22] CRP is created in the liver whenever there is infection or inflammation.[23] A simple blood test can check a person's CRP level to help assess cardiovascular risk. Once this risk of inflammation is identified, it can be treated with diet, exercise, and use of one of the statin drugs (e.g., Lipitor).[23] Eating regular meals, exercising moderately under the supervision of your physician, sleeping regularly, and not smoking can make one less likely to become ill later.

Kidney stones. Also known as renal calculi, urolithiasis, or nephrolithiasis, kidney stones are solid pebbles of salts and minerals that form within one or both kidneys or in the passageways leading to and from the kidneys.[24] These typically form when the urine becomes concentrated and the minerals in the urine stick together. Symptoms include a sharp pain in the back, typically on one side or the other, in the area of the latissimus dorsi over or near the kidneys.[25] Some of these stones pass through the urinary tract and do not require any treatment. Although some may be asymptomatic, passing of these stones can be very painful. Larger stones can be broken apart with shock wave lithotripsy (using high-energy sound waves in multiple, short pulses) or surgically removed.[26,27]

Psychological Disorders That Sometimes Present During Early and Middle Adulthood

Major Depression

Major depression is currently the second-leading cause of disability throughout the world. During 2018, approximately 6.7% of adults in the United States reported having had at least one episode of major depression. This can affect quality of life and participation in meaningful occupations, increasing the risk for substance abuse and suicide.[28] In 2019, the American Psychological Association released its new *Clinical Practice Guideline for the Treatment of Depression Across Three Age Cohorts* in an effort to help practitioners identify this condition and offer treatment options.[29]

Substance Use Disorders

Although the APA replaced the use of the terms *addiction* and *dependence* with the term *substance use disorder (SUD)* to cover both terms in the 2013 Diagnostic and Statistical Manual of Mental Disorders, *addiction* is not the same as *dependence*.[30] A person can be *dependent* on a medication (i.e., the medication is needed to control a chronic medical condition such as diabetes), yet not *addicted* to the medication. Addiction, however, can be a factor that leads to dependence.[30] According to the Substance Abuse and Mental Health Services Administration 2020 National Survey, alcohol use disorder (UD) affected 15.6% of adults ages 18 to 25 and 10.3% of those over age 26, marijuana UD affected 13.5% of adults ages 18 to 25 and 4.0% of those over age 26, and opioid UD affected 0.9% of adults ages 18 to 25 and 1.1% of those over age 26.[31] Even though the numbers for opioid UD appear on the low side, more than 42,000 people in the United States died from opioid overdoses in 2016, leading the US Department of Health and Human Services to declare a 2017 health emergency on the US opioid epidemic.[32]

The OT Scope of Practice

It cannot be overstated that when working as an occupational therapy practitioner (OTP), if a client demonstrates symptoms that are outside of the typical cluster you expect to find with their diagnosis, it is important to report those symptoms to the referring physician. Table 8.2 provides a quick overview of some of the more common conditions seen by OTPs for individuals in this age group.

TABLE 8.2 Conditions Sometimes Seen in Occupational Therapy That Typically Appear During Young and Middle Adulthood

Condition	Symptoms	Occupational Therapy Intervention
High cholesterol[33]	A buildup of fatty deposits in the blood vessels due to too much cholesterol, with genetic (family history) and/or environmental causes (inactivity, poor diet, smoking, etc.) • No symptoms but can be detected through a blood test • Can lead to angina, heart attack, blood clots, or heart disease	While an OTP may work with clients after high cholesterol has already been diagnosed, it is sometimes the OTP who initially notices risk factors and various other signs and symptoms. Some possible OT interventions include: • Ensuring thorough evaluation and health history to educate on predisposition to condition • Communicating findings clearly to the referring physician • Helping the individual to establish healthy habits to manage weight • Teaching the individual to establish new lifestyle routines or habits (i.e., low-salt diet, limit fats in diet, exercise/physical activity, quit smoking, limit alcohol intake) • Teaching stress management techniques • Assisting with medicine management if needed
Osteopenia[34]	This is a weakened BMD, most frequently affecting postmenopausal females, typically those over the age of 50 and those with poor nutrition. A BMD score of −1 to +1 is considered to be a "normal bone density examination." With osteopenia, the BMD is somewhere between −2.5 and −1 • Typically presents with no symptoms except for occasional bone pain • Can lead to osteoporosis (more severe outcome with associated symptoms)	While an OTP may work with clients after osteopenia has previously been diagnosed, it is sometimes the OTP who initially notices risk factors and various other signs and symptoms, such as bone pain or already diagnosed fractures. Some possible OT interventions include: • Ensuring thorough evaluation and health history to educate on predisposition to condition • Communicating findings clearly to the referring physician • Helping the individual to establish healthy habits to exercise and eat healthy • Supporting physician's treatment and assisting with medication/supplement management if needed • Establishing new lifestyle routines or habits (i.e., quit smoking, limit alcohol and caffeine intake, participate in weight-bearing exercise, improve diet to include a variety of vitamins/minerals)
MS[35]	MS is included in this section because it is a neurological condition that typically appears in an individual between the ages of 20 and 50, although MS can occur in those younger and older than this age range. Close to 1 million people are afflicted with this condition in the United States alone. It is more than three times more common in females than in males. The disorder causes demyelination of the nerves in the central nervous system (brain and spinal cord) with sclerotic plaques. The most common symptoms include: • Fatigue • Gait disturbances • Spasticity • Vision problems, often with blurred or double vision • Sexual problems • Paresthesia (numbness or tingling) • Weakness • Depression • Dizziness • Bladder problems • Emotional problems Other difficulties might arise in time such as: • Speech problems • Breathing difficulties • Tremor • Seizures	While an OTP may work with clients after MS has already been diagnosed, it is sometimes the OTP who initially notices risk factors and various other signs and symptoms outside the scope of what is expected for the client's current diagnosis. Some possible OT interventions include: • Ensuring thorough evaluation and health history to educate on predisposition to condition • Communicating findings clearly to the referring physician • Providing exercises to help improve strength and endurance • Providing balance activities and education in fall prevention • Practicing gait and safe stair climbing with assistive devices as needed • Assisting as the disease progresses to ensure continued safety of movement • Assisting as the disease progresses to help continue healthy habits to exercise and eat healthy • Supporting physician's treatment and assist with medication/supplement management if needed

TABLE 8.2 Conditions Sometimes Seen in Occupational Therapy That Typically Appear During Young and Middle Adulthood—cont'd

Condition	Symptoms	Occupational Therapy Intervention
Obesity[36]	Obesity is considered by the Mayo Clinic to be "a complex disease" in which an individual has too much body fat with BMI of 30.0 or higher. It is a medical problem that increases the risk of other disorders and diseases. It can be caused by genetic, physiological, and/or environmental causes. Although a BMI of 30 or higher is required for obesity, a BMI of 25 or higher can still lead to increased health risks. **BMI Range – Category** Less than 18.5 – Underweight 18.5–24.9 – Healthy weight 25.0–29.9 – Overweight 30.0 or higher – Obesity	Some possible OT interventions could include: • Establishing new lifestyle routines or habits (i.e., limit screen time; quit smoking; limit alcohol, sugary drinks, and caffeine intake; participate in daily physical activity; improve diet) • Establishing healthier sleeping habits • Teaching stress management techniques • Addressing psychosocial impacts of condition • Teaching energy conservation techniques as it relates to maximizing participation in Activities of Daily Living (ADLs) and other meaningful occupations • Assisting with the prevention of secondary comorbidities, such as diabetes and cellulitis

Heart disease[37,38]	Heart disease is the leading cause of death in the United States. The term itself refers to several different heart conditions, including:
	• Heart attack. Symptoms are varied but include:
	  • Chest pain
	  • SOB
	  • Pain in neck, jaw, throat, abdomen, or back pain
	  • Dizziness
	  • Weakness
	  • Sensation changes in upper extremities or lower extremities
	• Arrhythmia. Examples include tachycardia, bradycardia, and atrial fibrillation.
	  • Irregular heartbeats
	  • Palpitations
	  • Fluttering
	• Heart failure. When the heart has difficulty pumping enough blood to other parts of the body. Symptoms include:
	  • SOB
	  • Fatigue
	  • Edema in the legs and feet, abdominal area, or neck veins
		While an OTP may work with clients after heart disease has previously been diagnosed, it is sometimes the OTP who initially notices risk factors and various other signs and symptoms outside the scope of what is expected for the client's current diagnosis. Some possible OTP interventions include:
		• Ensuring thorough evaluation and health history to educate on predisposition to condition
		• Communicating findings clearly to the referring physician
		Once a diagnosis has been established, OTPs will often see these individuals to help them continue meaningful activities. Some possible OT interventions include:
		• Encouraging exercises to help improve strength and endurance
		• Establishing healthy habits to manage weight, blood pressure, cholesterol, diabetes, etc.
		• Teaching stress management techniques
		• Helping the client to explore healthy lifestyle routines or habits (i.e., quit smoking; low-fat, low-salt diets; participate in daily physical activity; good sleep habits)
		• Assisting with medication management if needed

(Continued)

TABLE 8.2 Conditions Sometimes Seen in Occupational Therapy That Typically Appear During Young and Middle Adulthood—cont'd

Condition	Symptoms	Occupational Therapy Intervention
Drug addiction (substance use disorder)[39]	Drug addiction (substance use disorder) is a disease affecting an individual's brain and their behavior, leading to an inability to control their use of a legal or illegal drug or medication. Symptoms include: • Feeling that you must use the drug regularly • Having intense urges to take the drug that interferes with other thoughts • Taking more of the drug than originally intended • Making certain that there is always a supply of the drug • Doing things to get the drug that you normally would not do • Not meeting work responsibilities or other obligations because of the drug use • Continuing to use the drug even though it is causing problems in one's life • Withdrawal symptoms begin when the drug is stopped	While an OTP may work with clients after drug addiction has been established, it is sometimes the OTP who initially notices risk factors and various other signs and symptoms outside the scope of what is expected for the client's current diagnosis. Some possible OT interventions include: • Ensuring thorough evaluation and health history to educate on predisposition to condition • Communicating findings clearly to the referring physician Other OT interventions can include: • Teaching the client to identify and utilize healthy coping techniques • Helping the individual start a daily journal to identify triggers, emotions, etc. • Teaching stress management skills • Helping the individual to create structure and routine in daily life by reestablishing roles and engagement in meaningful occupations • Helping the client to focus on skills training (life skills, vocational skills). • Encouraging participation in OT-led groups and other support groups held by the interdisciplinary team

ADL, Activities of daily living; *BMD*, bone mineral density; *MS*, multiple sclerosis; *OT*, occupational therapy; *OTP*, occupational therapy practitioner; *SOB*, shortness of breath.

Application—Case Study

CASE EXAMPLE 8.1

A 30-year-old female was referred by her doctor to OT for exercises for carpal tunnel syndrome in the right wrist.

1. **Screen:** She presented to the occupational therapist with severe pain in the right upper extremity that comes and goes and lately has also been in the left wrist as well. She also reports all over body aches and extreme fatigue.
2. **Take a Closer Look:** The medical record indicated carpal tunnel syndrome alone, as the client had been reasonably healthy until her carpal tunnel symptoms began. She just gave birth to a baby girl, about 2 months before her symptoms appeared. Otherwise, there was nothing else atypical about her case.
3. **Determine Flag Status:** The occupational therapist felt that there was more going on here and determined this to be an orange flag (he was still deciding).
4. **Take Action if Needed:** The occupational therapist pulled in the occupational therapy assistant, and together, the OTPs found that the client had tingling and numbness in her left arm and sometimes in her left leg. She also complained of double vision and of an electric shock sensation when bending her neck forward (Lhermitte sign). The occupational therapist contacted the physician, asking for a neurological consult for this individual.
5. **Document the Findings:** The occupational therapist documented the findings of his examination as well as the phone call to the physician. He informed the client that he and the occupational therapy assistant were requesting a neurological consult to gain more information about the possible cause of her pain.
6. **Take a Second Look:** Armed with this new information from the OTPs, the doctor requested a neurological consult. The neurologist simply performed a nerve conduction study and confirmed carpal tunnel syndrome. The occupational therapist called the neurologist and gave him the information regarding the double vision and the positive Lhermitte sign and asked for testing to rule out multiple sclerosis. The doctor ordered a lumbar puncture and a brain MRI. The MRI showed multiple sclerotic lesions, and the lumbar puncture was positive for abnormal antibodies.
7. **Determine the Flag Status:** The occupational therapist and physician changed the client's plan of care. This was not life threatening but definitely needed to be addressed. The OT proceeded with this as a yellow flag once the client's condition was known.
8. **Take Action if Needed:** The client was sent to a neurologist who specialized in multiple sclerosis. OT was again ordered for exercises and work on in-home safety and ADLs.

This is a true case. The client had multiple sclerosis and needed to have treatment in accordance with the condition. The OTPs realized that there was more going on and wanted to treat the whole person, not just her arm.

References

1. Papalia DE, Martorell G. *Experience Human Development.* 15th ed. McGraw Hill; 2024.
2. APA. *The APA Dictionary of Psychology.* 2023. https://dictionary.apa.org/adulthood.
3. LibreTexts. Developmental tasks of early adulthood. In: *Lifespan Development.* Chapter 8.3. https://socialsci.libretexts.org/Bookshelves/Human_Development/Lifespan_Development_Lumen)/08%3A_Early_Adulthood/8.03%3A_Developmental_Tasks_of_Early_Adulthood.
4. LibreTexts. Psychosocial development in middle adulthood. In: *Lifespan Development.* Chapter 9.2. https://socialsci.libretexts.org/Courses/Foothill_College/Psych_40%3A_Lifespan_Development_(Pilati)/09%3A_Middle_Adulthood/9.02%3A_Psychosocial_Development_in_Middle_Adulthood.
5. Hales CM, Carroll MD, Fryar CD, Ogden CL. Prevalence of obesity and severe obesity among adults in the United States, 2017–2018. In: *NCHS Data Brief.* 2020:360. https://www.pfizer.com.sg/files/db360-h.pdf.
6. Harvard TH. Chan. *How Discrimination Can Harm Black Women's Health.* Harvard T.H. Chan: School of Public Health; 2018. https://www.hsph.harvard.edu/news/hsph-in-the-news/discrimination-black-womens-health/.
7. Committee on Improving the Health, Safety, and Well-Being of Young Adults; Board on Children, Youth, and Families; Institute of Medicine; National Research Council. In: Bonnie RJ, Stroud C, Breiner H, eds. *Investing in the Health and Well-Being of Young Adults.* National Academies Press (US); 2015. https://www.ncbi.nlm.nih.gov/books/NBK284776/.
8. NIH. *Age-Related Hearing Loss (Presbycusis).* National Institute on Deafness and Other Communication Disorders. https://www.nidcd.nih.gov/health/age-related-hearing-loss.
9. Park MJ, Mulye TP, Adams SH, Brindis CD, Irwin CE. *J Adolesc Health.* 2006;39:305–317. https://doi.org/10.1016/j.jadohealth.2006.04.017.
10. Inferna FJ, Gerstorf D, Lachman ME. Midlife in the 2020s: opportunities and challenges. *Am Psychologist.* 2020;75(4):470–485. https://doi.org/10.1037/amp0000591.
11. NIH. *What Do We Know About Healthy Aging?* National Institute on Aging; 2022. https://www.nia.nih.gov/health/what-do-we-know-about-healthy-aging.
12. Mayo Clinic. *Presbyopia.* Mayo Clinic; 2021. https://www.mayoclinic.org/diseases-conditions/presbyopia/symptoms-causes/syc-20363328.
13. Mayo Clinic. *Nearsightedness.* Mayo Clinic; 2022. https://www.mayoclinic.org/diseases-conditions/nearsightedness/symptoms-causes/syc-20375556.
14. Mayo Clinic. *Hearing Loss.* Mayo Clinic; 2023. https://www.mayoclinic.org/diseases-conditions/hearing-loss/symptoms-causes/syc-20373072.
15. Medline. *Aging Changes in the Bones – Muscles – Joints.* Medline Plus; 2023. https://medlineplus.gov/ency/article/004015.htm.
16. Mayo Clinic. *Male Menopause: Myth or Reality?* Men's Health. Mayo Clinic; 2022. https://www.mayoclinic.org/healthy-lifestyle/mens-health/in-depth/male-menopause/art-20048056.
17. Stanford FC, Anekwe C. *Surprising Findings About Metabolism and Age. Staying Healthy.* Harvard Health Publishing; 2021. https://www.health.harvard.edu/blog/surprising-findings-about-metabolism-and-age-202110082613.
18. CDC. *Leading Cause of Death.* National Center for Health Statistics, Centers for Disease Control and Prevention; 2023. https://www.cdc.gov/nchs/fastats/leading-causes-of-death.htm.
19. NIH. *Deaths in Middle-Aged Adults Drive Decrease in U.S. Life Expectancy. NIH Research Highlights.* 2019. https://www.nia.nih.gov/news/deaths-middle-aged-adults-drive-decrease-u-s-life-expectancy.
20. Su L, Mittal R, Ramgobin D, Jain R, Jain R. Current management guidelines on hyperlipidemia: the silent killer. *J Lipids.* 2021;2021:9883352. https://doi.org/10.1155/2021/9883352.
21. NIH. *Heart and Vascular Diseases.* National Heart, Lung, and Blood Institute, NIH. https://www.nhlbi.nih.gov/science/heart-and-vascular-diseases.
22. Cozlea DL, Farcas DM, Nagy A, et al. The impact of C reactive protein on global cardiovascular risk on patients with coronary artery disease. *Curr Health Sci J.* 2013;39(4):225–231. https://www.ncbi.nlm.nih.gov/pmc/articles/PMC3945266/.
23. Johns Hopkins. Assessing cardiovascular risk with C-reactive protein. In: *Health.* Johns Hopkins; 2023. https://www.hopkinsmedicine.org/health/treatment-tests-and-therapies/assessing-cardiovascular-risk-with-c-reactive-protein.
24. Mayo Clinic. *Kidney Stones.* Mayo Clinic Diseases and Conditions; 2022. https://www.mayoclinic.org/diseases-conditions/kidney-stones/symptoms-causes/syc-20355755.
25. NIH. *Kidney Stones.* National Institute of Diabetes and Digestive and Kidney Diseases, NIH. https://www.niddk.nih.gov/health-information/urologic-diseases/kidney-stones.
26. NIH. *Treatment for Kidney Stones.* National Institute of Diabetes and Digestive and Kidney Diseases, NIH. https://www.niddk.nih.gov/health-information/urologic-diseases/kidney-stones/treatment.
27. Uroweb. *Shock-wave Lithotripsy.* Uroweb Patient Information; 2023. https://patients.uroweb.org/treatments/shock-wave-lithotripsy/.
28. Weir K. APA offers new guidelines for treating depression. *Monit Psychol.* 2019;50(8):34. https://www.apa.org/monitor/2019/09/ce-corner-depression.
29. APA. *Clinical Practice Guidelines for the Treatment of Depression Across Three Age Cohorts.* American Psychological Association; 2019. https://www.apa.org/depression-guideline.
30. Seiner M. *Drug Dependence.* Healthline; 2018. https://www.healthline.com/health/drug-dependence.
31. Substance Abuse and Mental Health Services Administration (SAMHSA). *Key Substance Use and Mental Health Indicators in the United States: Results From the 2020 National Survey on Drug Use and Health.* In: HHS Publication No. PEP21-07-01-003, NSDUH Series H-56. Center for Behavioral Health Statistics and Quality, Substance Abuse and Mental Health Services Administration; 2021. https://www.samhsa.gov/data/sites/default/files/reports/rpt35325/NSDUHFFRPDFWHTMLFiles2020/2020NSDUHFFR1PDFW102121.pdf.
32. Ignaszewski MJ. The epidemiology of drug abuse. *J Clin Pharmacol.* 2021;61(S2):S10–S17. https://doi.org/10.1002/jcph.1937.
33. Mayo Clinic. *High Cholesterol.* Mayo Clinic; 2023. https://www.mayoclinic.org/diseases-conditions/high-blood-cholesterol/symptoms-causes/syc-20350800.
34. Cleveland Clinic. *Osteopenia.* Cleveland Clinic; 2021. https://my.clevelandclinic.org/health/diseases/21855-osteopenia.

35. MS. *MS Signs & Symptoms*. National Multiple Sclerosis Society; 2024. https://www.nationalmssociety.org/Symptoms-Diagnosis/MS-Symptoms.
36. Mayo Clinic. *Obesity*. Mayo Clinic; 2023. https://www.mayoclinic.org/diseases-conditions/obesity/symptoms-causes/syc-20375742.
37. CDC. *Heart Disease*. Centers for Disease Control and Prevention; 2024. https://www.cdc.gov/heartdisease/index.htm.
38. CDC. *About Heart Disease*. Centers for Disease Control and Prevention; 2023. https://www.cdc.gov/heartdisease/about.htm.
39. Mayo Clinic. *Drug Addiction (Substance Use Disorder)*. Mayo Clinic; 2023. https://www.mayoclinic.org/diseases-conditions/drug-addiction/symptoms-causes/syc-20365112.

9

Typical Development and Pathophysiology During Late Adulthood

OBJECTIVES

At the end of this chapter, the reader will be able to:

- Demonstrate a basic understanding of typical physiologic development during late adulthood.
- List signs and symptoms for various physical disorders sometimes present during late adulthood.
- Demonstrate an understanding of the psychological disorders sometimes present during late adulthood.
- List common pathophysiological disorders for late adulthood.
- Differentiate between typical older adult development and atypical older adult development.
- Compare and contrast various pathophysiological conditions and various disorders affecting mental health that are common during late adulthood.

Normal Human Development

The term "Graying of America" is a phrase that is sometimes given for the growing number of people in our country who are over the age of 65.[1] According to the US Census, approximately 17.1% of the population was over the age of 65 in 2021.[2] The year 2030 marks a milestone because this is when all baby boomers (those born between 1946 and 1964[3]) will be over the age of 65.[1] It is estimated that by the year 2030, approximately 20% of all Americans will be over the age of 65, that is, one out of every five people in this country.[1]

There are two types of aging that are typically mentioned in the literature: *primary aging* (gradual inevitable decline due to normal aging, such as graying of hair and wrinkled skin) and *secondary aging* (decline from the environment, disuse, or disease, such as Parkinson's disease or Alzheimer's disease).[4] A person's *functional age* is a measure of an individual's capability based on norm-referenced standards.[5] An individual's actual chronological age might be 60, but they may have a functional age of 25, or a functional age of 84, depending on their health and ability.

Life expectancy is the age an individual can expect to live based on their health and cohort. A baby born in the early 1900s in the United States was expected to only live to be about 48 years old.[6] The average life expectancy is now 78.7 years.[1] This is due to a decline in the nation's death rate.[6] The term *longevity* refers to the actual length of an individual's life, and the term *lifespan* is the longest period that members of a species can live. The lifespan of humans is typically listed as about 110 years, but there have been reported cases of people who have lived longer.[6] There are also regional and ethnic differences depending on overall health of the population, metabolism, and level of stress in different environments. There are also sex differences, with females in our country typically living longer than males. The average life expectancy in our country is currently 76.3 years for males and 81.1 years for females.[1]

Why do we age? There are many different theories. One perspective is called *Genetic Programming*. This is a group of theories that contend that we age because of programming in our chromosomes. Leonard Hayflick found that human cells will divide in a protected environment in a laboratory only about 50 times, and then, they begin to age and die.[7] This is called the Hayflick Limit and estimates human life (free of disease) to be about 110 years. Although this theory received some criticism during the time it was initially presented in the 1960s, it encouraged further research, especially research related to telomeres.[7] Telomeres are repetitive sequences of DNA that protect the ends of the chromosomes. They stop replicating with cellular division over time, resulting in cell death.[7]

Another perspective is the *Variable-Rate Perspective*. These theories contend that, although there may be genetic changes that cause us to age, there are also environmental factors and

TABLE 9.1 Some of the Developmental Tasks for Early and Middle Older Adulthood and for Later Older Adulthood[10,11]

Criteria	Early and Middle Older Adulthood (Ages 65–84)	Later Older Adulthood (Ages 85 and Up)
Erikson[10]	Ego integrity versus despair (age 65 to death)	Ego integrity versus despair (age 65 to death)
Identity[10]	Taking on new family and work roles	Acceptance of one's life
Stability[10]	Adequate income with bills paid and vacations possible	Adequate income
Focus on the independent self[11]	Focus on one's own goal and agenda with some effort to influence others with positive enthusiasm (stressed more in the United States)	This can have a more negative impact over time if not rectified
Focus on the interdependent self[11]	Focus is on adjusting to the age-graded roles in relation to age-related decline (stressed more in East Asian cultures)	This can have a more positive impact over time, with an acceptance of those things that cannot be changed
Career versus retirement[10]	Career focused but readying for retirement	More focused on leisure
Community[10]	Meaningful identity and social status	Focused relationships with the most meaningful people
Residence[10]	Acceptable living conditions	Comfortable living conditions
Companionship[10]	Focus on good companionship	Caring for older spouse and grief work for loss
Acceptance[10]	Life review begins	Acceptance of one's life

other random experiences that will vary for each person.[6] Two examples are the *wear-and-tear theory* that contends that we age because of accumulated damage from use and disuse, and the *free radical theory* that contends that we age because of a buildup of free radicals (highly unstable oxygen atoms and molecules that result from metabolism in our bodies).[6]

Late adulthood constitutes approximately 40 years, and there are many changes that occur, including things such as retirement and great-grandchildren. Adding to that are all the physical changes that occur during this time period, and as a result, the range of individual differences becomes extremely broad.[8] Many texts divide this long stage of development into four sections of time: young-old (ages 60–74), old-old (ages 75–84), oldest-old (ages 85–99), and centenarians (those over the age of 100).[9] This text has divided late adulthood into two sections of chronological age: early and middle older adult (ages 65–84) and later older adult (ages 85 and above). Some of the typical developmental tasks for people in this age group is found above (Table 9.1), but it cannot be overstressed that each individual is unique, and many people in this chronological age group may not be in the same functional age group.

Early and Middle Older Adult Development—Ages 65 to 84

It cannot be overstated how rapidly the population of people over the age of 65 is growing in the United States. It is estimated that by the year 2060, the number of people over the age of 65 will outnumber the number of people under the age of 5, and 25% of people who are currently over the age of 65 will live into their 90s.[9]

Although individuals in their mid-60s and 70s are much healthier overall than they would have been 30 years ago, they are still at a much higher risk of having chronic health problems such as osteoporosis and diabetes.[12]

As people age, they typically experience some osteopenia or osteoporosis, some lessening of height due to shrinkage of the vertebral discs, and loss of muscle strength and endurance. Some of these things are partially reversible with a proper diet, enough water, and exercise.[13] The heart's rhythm at rest will stay about the same, but the heart rate may not increase during activity like it did when the person was younger, resulting in higher than normal blood pressure.[13] This leads to a decline in reserve capacity (the ability to put forth additional effort under extreme stress).[14] Individuals in this age group will typically have some visual changes, with presbyopia (farsightedness) and decreased night vision.[9] In addition, about 25% of adults over the age of 65 and 50% of adults over the age of 75 have hearing impairment.[9] With changes in equilibrium and reaction time, it is easier to see why many (about one in three) of the individuals in this age group will experience at least one fall during the next year.[12]

There is still an advantage among this population. Individuals over the age of 65 have more knowledge from experience that has accumulated over time. This is called crystallized intelligence. Many older adults can outperform younger individuals who require this accumulated knowledge.[9] New skills that require a more fluidized intelligence can still be learned as people age, it may just take a little longer to learn than it would for a younger person, and wisdom and creativity will often remain strong for life.[9]

Later Older Adult Development—Ages 85 and Up

As people enter into the later years of older adulthood, the range of individual differences becomes even more widely spread. Most of the physiological changes mentioned above continue into these older adult years. However, it is the cognitive changes that occur during these years that seem to concern people the most. As stated above, some of these changes are expected as we age such as slower reaction time and some difficulties learning new skills that require fluid intelligence.[9,15]

A very famous research project called "The Seattle Longitudinal Study of Adult Intelligence" measured six primary mental abilities in adults over time. This study began in 1956 with 500 randomly chosen participants: 25 males and 25 females in each age bracket from ages 22 to the 80s. Every 7 years, the original participants were retested, and new participants were added, until about 5000 people were being studied. The most recent report from this study was in 2010, and Schaie concluded that cognition does slow, and there is a great deal of variation. Some people show decline as early as their 40s, while others were functioning fully until their later years.[6,16,17] This study also found that the variables that seemed to be associated with a reduction of risk of cognitive decline included: the absence of any cardiovascular or other type of chronic disorder, better living conditions due to a higher socioeconomic status, an intellectually stimulating environment, a more flexible personality style, an intelligent spouse, and participation in activities that help maintain a higher speed of perceptual processing.[16]

Although 25% of older adults live with a mental health problem such as anxiety or depression, most report that they feel they have good mental health.[9] The rate of suicide for males over the age of 85, however, is higher than any other age group,[9] and according to the 2020 Substance Abuse and Mental Health Services Administration report, 39% of older adults have used illicit drugs sometime during their lifetime, with 7.9% having used during the past year.[18]

Death in Older Adulthood

The most common causes of death during late adulthood are heart disease, stroke, and cancer.

Common Disorders During Late Adulthood

Chronic physical conditions in late adulthood are many and varied, but some of the conditions that lean toward primary aging include osteoarthritis (OA), osteoporosis, and hypertension. Chronic psychological conditions in late adulthood are becoming more and more prevalent and include depression, anxiety, and dementia.

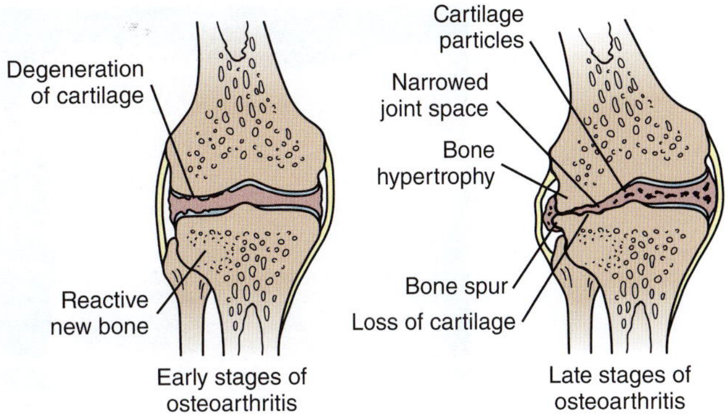

• **Fig. 9.1** Osteoarthritis in the knee. (From Magee DJ, et al., eds. *Pathology and Intervention in Musculoskeletal Rehabilitation*. 2nd ed. Elsevier; 2016.)

Physical Disorders During Late Adulthood

Osteoarthritis. OA is the most common type of arthritis in the older adult population.[19] OA is mostly due to secondary aging but also wear and tear. OA arises from inflammation of the joints, typically the larger joints of the body (such as the hips and knees) but can also affect the smaller joints of the spine, hands, and feet. OA occurs when the tissues that protect and cushion the ends of the bones in the joints break down or degenerate over time due to normal wear and tear.[19] The changes will typically develop slowly over the course of one's life, causing pain, swelling, and stiffness (Fig. 9.1). Movement, heat, weight control, and anti-inflammatory medications can help elevate the discomfort.

Osteoporosis. Osteoporosis is a softening of the bone that happens over time and might not even be recognized until after an individual has broken a bone. Because of this, it is considered to be a "silent disease."[20] According to the 2017–18 CDC report, females (18.8%) are more than four times more likely to have osteoporosis than males (4.2%) because females tend to lose bone mass during menopause (Fig. 9.2).[21]

To diagnose this potential problem, a bone density scan is done, typically of the hip and lumbar spine (two of the major weight-bearing areas in the body).[22] A *T*-score is then calculated from this scan. This is simply the number of standard deviations that a person's density is away from the mean. This mean is the average bone density of a healthy 30-year-old person.[22] A standard deviation of +1 is about a 10%–12% difference from the mean and implies that an individual's bone mass is about 10%–12% stronger than the mean. A *T*-score of −1 to +4 is considered to be normal.[22] A *T*-score of −1 to −2.5 is low bone mass otherwise known as *osteopenia*, and anything below −2.5 is

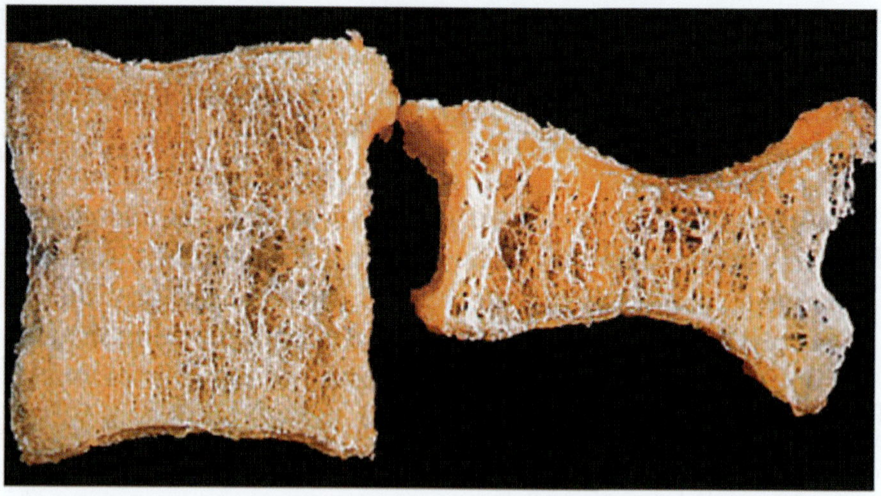

• **Fig. 9.2** Bone density depicting normal bone on the left, and bone with osteoporosis after sustaining prolonged compressive forces on the right. (From Kumar V, et al. *Robbins & Cotran Pathologic Basis of Disease*. 10th ed. Elsevier; 2021.)

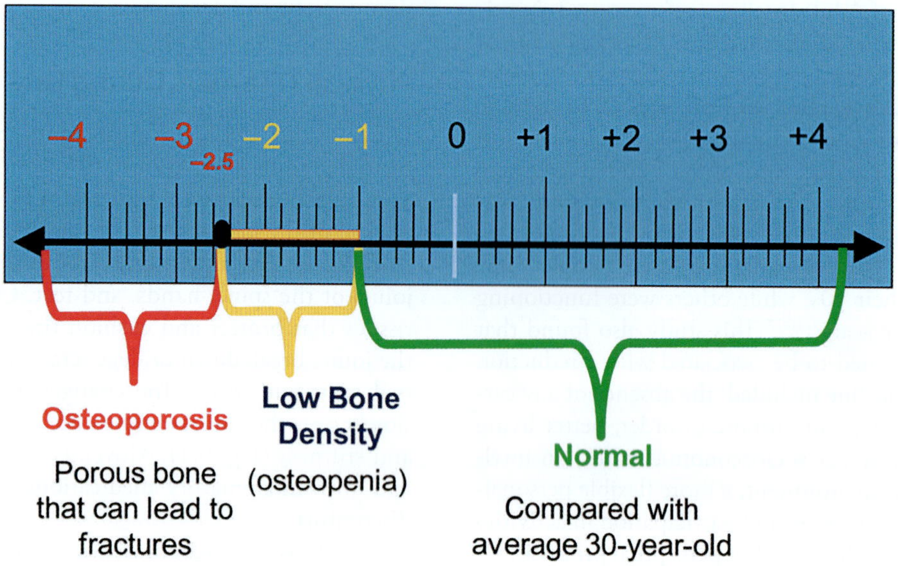

• **Fig. 9.3** Scale defining *T*-scores for osteopenia and osteoporosis.[22] (From https://americanbonehealth.org/bone-density/understanding-the-bone-density-t-score-and-z-score/.)

considered to be osteoporosis (Fig. 9.3).[22] Regular exercise and a good diet can slow the progression of osteoporosis.[17] Medications such as calcitonin and estrogen replacement can help slow the loss of bone. There is a synthetic version of the parathyroid hormone that might also help to rebuild bone.[1,20]

Hypertension. Hypertension, also known as high blood pressure, affects almost half of all adults living in the United States.[23] Many complications can arise from this, including heart attack, stroke, or even kidney disease. Although there are medications to treat this disorder, healthy eating, regular exercise, and management of stress can also be of benefit.[23] More information on hypertension can be found in this text in Chapter 12.

Psychological Disorders During Late Adulthood

Depression. Although depression was previously discussed in Chapter 8 regarding young and middle adulthood, it has relevance here for the older adult. Depression is a chronic condition seen in many elderly individuals and can lead to lack of motivation to thrive, starvation, self-neglect, and not taking essential medications.[24] It is a serious condition and is not a part of normal aging. Most older adults report feeling satisfied with their lives, but if a person had depression when younger, they are more likely to have depression when older.[24] Life events, such as the death of a spouse, can make this more likely. Depression in the elderly can sometimes be masked by physical illness and often requires focused medical attention.[21] Depression will be covered in more detail in Chapter 23.

Anxiety. Excessive anxiety that interferes with a normal daily routine is not a part of normal aging.[25] It is estimated that approximately 3% to 14% of older adults meet the criteria for a specific anxiety disorder, but an estimated 27% of those under the care of aging service providers have symptoms that do not qualify for a diagnosis but still significantly impact their functioning.[25] Some anxiety disorders include panic disorder, obsessive-compulsive disorder, and phobia. Anxiety disorders will be covered in more detail in Chapter 24.

Dementia. The term *dementia* refers to a group of symptoms that affect cognition, memory, and social abilities, and in turn, interfere with daily life.[26] Simple episodes of forgetfulness or losing the car key are not indications of dementia, and dementia is not a part of normal aging. Dementia occurs when there is a gradual loss of ability due to the damage of nerve cells or loss of connection to various areas of the brain.[26] Care must be considered when a doctor makes this diagnosis, as a simple bladder infection or certain medications can sometime mimic dementia. The type of dementias that become worse over time and are not reversible are referred to as progressive dementias. The most common type is Alzheimer's disease. This disorder is caused by neurofibrillary tangles, amyloid plaques, and there is thought to be a genetic predisposition.[26] Dementia will be covered in more detail in Chapter 21.

The OT Scope of Practice

Once again when working as an OTP, if a client demonstrates symptoms that are outside of the typical cluster you expect to find with their diagnosis, it is important to report those symptoms to the referring physician. Table 9.2 provides a quick overview of some of the more common conditions seen by occupational therapy practitioners (OTPs) for individuals in this age group.

TABLE 9.2 Conditions Sometimes Seen by Occupational Therapy Practitioners That Typically Appear During Late Adulthood

Condition	Symptoms	Occupational Therapy Intervention
Cerebrovascular accident or CVA (stroke)[27]	A CVA occurs when there is an interruption in the blood supply to a part of the brain leading to a depletion of needed oxygen. Brain cells will begin to die in minutes. Another type of stroke is due to hemorrhage, occurring when a blood vessel leaks or bursts in the brain. Symptoms include: • Difficulty speaking • Numbness or paralysis on one side of the body or face • Problems seeing in one or both eyes • Headache • Difficulty walking • Confusion	Although many times, an OTP will work with a client after a recent CVA has been diagnosed, it is sometimes the OTP who first notices risk factors and various other signs and symptoms outside the scope of what is expected for the client's current diagnosis. If a stroke is suspected, immediate action is required. This is a definitive **RED** flag and cannot be taken lightly. • Call 911 if in an outside clinic. Report directly to the ER if in a hospital setting. • Ensure thorough evaluation and health history to educate on predisposition to condition. • Communicate findings clearly to the referring physician. Once a diagnosis has been established, OTPs will often see these clients to help them continue meaningful activities. Some possible OT interventions include: • Encouraging exercises to help improve strength, ROM, and activity tolerance as needed for ADLs • Assistance with cognitive tasks using strategies and tools for easier communication • Family education for safety and fall prevention
Parkinson's disease[28]	Parkinson's disease is a brain disorder that causes uncontrolled movements and rigidity. It is caused by death of the cells in the basal ganglia that are responsible for the production of dopamine (Fig. 9.4). Symptoms include: • Tremors in the hands, legs, jaw, and head. It may be hard to show facial expressions • Stiffness and rigidity • Slowed movement • Impaired balance and coordination • Depression • Difficulty swallowing or speaking • Possible mental and behavioral problems	Although many times an OTP will work with a client after Parkinson's disease has previously been diagnosed, it is sometimes the OTP who first notices risk factors and various other signs and symptoms outside the scope of what is expected for the client's current diagnosis. • Ensure thorough evaluation and health history to educate on predisposition to condition. • Communicate findings clearly to the referring physician. Once a diagnosis has been established, OTPs will often see these clients to help them continue meaningful activities. Some possible OT interventions include: • Encouraging exercises to help improve strength, ROM, and activity tolerance as needed for ADLs • Assistance with cognitive tasks using memory strategies and tools for easier communication • Family education for safety and fall prevention

(Continued)

TABLE 9.2 Conditions Sometimes Seen by Occupational Therapy Practitioners That Typically Appear During Late Adulthood – cont'd

Condition	Symptoms	Occupational Therapy Intervention
Type 2 Diabetes[29]	• Type 2 diabetes is the most common type of diabetes, mainly affecting older adults but can occur in younger adults and in children. The body is unable to use insulin properly, resulting in high blood sugar levels or hyperglycemia. More can be found about diabetes in Chapter 18. • Symptoms include: ° Increased thirst ° Increased hunger ° Fatigue ° Blurred vision ° Sudden weight loss ° Numbness or tingling in the toes or fingers ° Slow healing of cuts and sores • Diabetic Hypoglycemia[30] ° This is an event of lower than normal blood sugar. It can occur after insulin or after exercise. ° Pale, confused, shaking, difficulty speaking, problems with coordination	• Although many times an OTP will often work with diabetic clients, it is sometimes the OTP who first notices risk factors and various other signs and symptoms outside the scope of what is expected for the client's current diagnosis. If diabetes is suspected, it is a yellow flag but needs to be addressed by the physician as soon as possible. If diabetic hypoglycemia is suspected, it is a **RED** flag and needs to be addressed immediately (See Case study 9.1). • OTPs working in an older adult setting will often have clients with diabetes. ° Encouraging exercises to help improve strength, ROM, activity tolerance, and participation in ADLs ° Help set up a medication schedule and reminders for the client to use their insulin ° Encourage daily activity outdoors and with family and friends ° Family education for safety and fall prevention
Osteoarthritis[31]	This is the most common form of arthritis, with millions of individuals affected worldwide. It is caused by the normal wear and tear of the protective cartilage cushioning the ends of bones over time, and it is irreversible. Symptoms include: • Pain, typically in the weight-bearing joints such as the hips and knees • Stiffness • Decreased ROM • Crepitus or a grating sensation on movement • Bone spurs • Swelling	Although many times an OTP will work with a client after osteoarthritis has previously been diagnosed, it is sometimes the OTP who first notices risk factors and various other signs and symptoms outside the scope of what is expected for the client's current diagnosis. • Ensure thorough evaluation and health history to educate on predisposition to condition • Communicate findings clearly to the referring physician • Encouraging exercises to help improve strength, ROM, and activity tolerance as needed for ADLs • Pain management • Teach healthy eating and exercise habits • Help promote participation in meaningful occupations
Clinical depression[32]	A common but serious mood disorder. Also known as major depression, clinical depression, or major depressive disorder. Symptoms include some, but often not all, of the following: • Depressed mood and a loss of interest that interferes with daily activities • Feelings of hopelessness • Irritability, restlessness • Difficulty concentrating • Difficulty sleeping • Changes in appetite • Physical aches and pains with no clear physical cause • Thoughts of death or suicide • Easily angered • Isolating from family and friends	Again, there are many times that an OTP will work with a client after a diagnosis of depression has been previously made, but there will be times when the OTP is the one who first notices risk factors and various other signs and symptoms outside the scope of what is expected for the client's current diagnosis. • Ensure thorough evaluation and health history to educate on predisposition to condition • Communicate findings clearly to the referring physician • OTPs will often see clients who have a diagnosis of depression as a comorbidity. Some interventions include: • Helping the individual to identify and utilize healthy coping techniques (such as writing in a daily journal of completing an "Interest Checklist") • Teach stress management skills • Create structure and routine in daily life by prioritizing self-care activities • Focus on skills training (life skills, vocational skills, self-management skills) • Participate in OTP-led groups, especially expressive activities • Encourage participation in meaningful occupations

CVA, Cerebral vascular accident; *OTP*, occupational therapiy practitioner; *ROM*, range of motion.

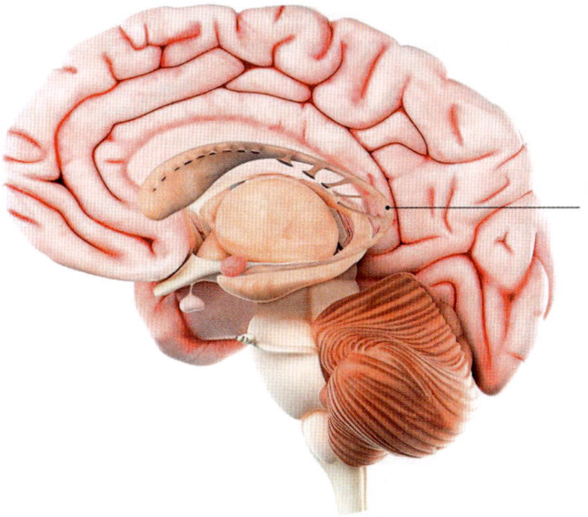

• **Fig. 9.4** The basal ganglia of the brain responsible for the production of dopamine. (From https://www.nia.nih.gov/health/parkinsons-disease/parkinsons-disease-causes-symptoms-and-treatments.)

Application—Case Study

CASE EXAMPLE 9.1

A group of occupational therapy students were performing a service activity with their professor at an older adult living community. They were performing aquatic exercises to music with the residents in waist-deep water. Things were going well, but after the music ended, one individual continued dancing in the water. The resident was a 78-year-old male, in no apparent distress, but smiling and singing the song. His wife was standing next to him.

1. **Screen:** The students noticed this right away, notifying the professor who immediately jumped into the water. His wife informed him that the music had ended, but he continued to dance.
2. **Take a Closer Look:** The professor noticed that the resident couldn't speak, just sing in a mumbled voice, and that he lacked his typical coordination. The students were close by and all gently guided the resident out of the water.
3. **Determine Flag Status:** Knowing the medical history of each resident before beginning the program, the professor asked about his diabetes. The wife said that he used his insulin right before the exercise. The professor asked his wife if this had ever happened before. She said yes, sometimes after his insulin. The professor determined this to be hypoglycemia and a possible red flag situation.
4. **Take Action if Needed:** The professor asked one of the students to immediately run to the front desk to get some orange juice, candy, or something sweet. One of the other residents in the pool had an unopened can of cola and recommended that they use that. After a few sips, the resident started acting a little more like himself. The professor asked one of the students to contact the facility's on-call nurse, while she stayed with the resident, and called the individual's doctor to inform him of the situation.
5. **Document the Findings:** The professor documented the events and asked that the facility's on-call nurse also document the occurrence.
6. **Take a Second Look:** After informing the doctor of the incident, the professor gave the phone to the resident's wife so she could take down new instructions in the use of his insulin.
7. **Determine the Flag Status:** The client visited the physician the next day, and changes in medication dosage were ordered, but the physician also requested that the aquatic exercises continue after the resident's sugar levels were stabilized.
8. **Take Action if Needed:** The following week, the resident returned for water exercises with a clearance from his doctor. His wife seemed very happy, thanking the professor for her quick action. The professor admitted that she couldn't have done it without her occupational therapy students.

This is a true case. The client had diabetes, and exercise can lower blood sugar, especially when insulin levels need to be adjusted. The resident and his wife both returned to aquatic exercises the following week and did well with no more occurrences.

References

1. Overstreet L. *The "Graying" Population and Life Expectancy*. LibreTexts Social Sciences. UC Davis; 2023. https://socialsci.libretexts.org/@go/page/60535?pdf
2. U.S. Census. *The Older Population in the United States*. United States Census; 2021. https://www.census.gov/data/tables/2021/demo/age-and-sex/2021-older-population.html.
3. Hecht E. What years are Gen X? A detailed breakdown of when each generation was born. *USA Today*. 2023. https://www.usatoday.com/story/news/2022/09/02/what-years-gen-x-millennials-baby-boomers-gen-z/10303085002/.
4. Anstey K, Stankov L, Lord S. Primary aging, secondary aging, and intelligence. *Psychol Aging*. 1993;8(4):562–570. https://doi.org/10.1037/0882-7974.8.4.562.
5. APA. *Functional Age*. APA Dictionary of Psychology; 2023. https://dictionary.apa.org/functional-age.
6. Papalia DE, Martorell G. *Experience Human Development*. 15th ed. McGraw Hill; 2024.
7. Bartlett Z. *The Hayflick Limit*. The Embryo Project Encyclopedia; 2014. https://embryo.asu.edu/handle/10776/8237.
8. APA. *Older Adults: Health and Age-Related Changes*. American Psychological Association; 2021. https://www.apa.org/pi/aging/resources/guides/older.
9. Portland State. Late adulthood. In: *Human Development*. Portland State; 2020. https://pdx.pressbooks.pub/humandevelopment/chapter/late-adulthood/.
10. Levine D. Developmental tasks in late adulthood. *Navigating Change*. 2012. http://www.debilevine.com/?p=840.
11. Kitayama S, Berg M, Chopik W. Culture and wellbeing in late adulthood: theory and evidence. *Am Psychol*. 2020;75(4):567–576. https://psycnet.apa.org/doi/10.1037/amp0000614.
12. OASH. Older adults. In: *Healthy People 2030*. 2020. https://health.gov/healthypeople/objectives-and-data/browse-objectives/older-adults.
13. Mayo Clinic. *Healthy Aging Healthy Lifestyle 2022*. Mayo Clinic; 2023. https://www.mayoclinic.org/healthy-lifestyle/healthy-aging/in-depth/aging/art-20046070.
14. Lakatta EG. Changes in cardiovascular function with aging. *Eur Heart J*. 1990;11(suppl_C):22–29. https://doi.org/10.1093/eurheartj/11.suppl_C.22.
15. Parkin AJ, Java RI. Deterioration of frontal lobe function in normal aging: influences of fluid intelligence versus perceptual

speed. *Neuropsychology.* 1999;13(4):539–545. https://doi.org/10.1037/0894-4105.13.4.539.
16. Schaie KW, Willis SL. The Seattle Longitudinal Study of adult cognitive development. *ISSBD Bull.* 2010;57(1):24–29. PMID: 23536918; PMCID: PMC3607395. https://www.ncbi.nlm.nih.gov/pmc/articles/PMC3607395/.
17. Schaie KW. The Seattle Longitudinal Study: a thirty-five-year inquiry of adult intellectual development. *Z für Gerontologie.* 1993;26(3):129–137. PMID: 8337905. https://pubmed.ncbi.nlm.nih.gov/8337905/.
18. SAMHSA. *National Survey of Drug and Health (NSDUH) Releases.* Substance Abuse and Mental Health Services Administration; 2020. https://www.samhsa.gov/data/release/2020-national-survey-drug-use-and-health-nsduh-releases.
19. NIH. *Osteoarthritis.* National Institute on Aging; 2022. https://www.nia.nih.gov/health/osteoarthritis.
20. NIH. *Osteoporosis.* National Institute on Aging; 2022. https://www.nia.nih.gov/health/osteoporosis.
21. CDC. *Osteoporosis.* Centers for Disease Control and Prevention; 2022. https://www.cdc.gov/nchs/fastats/osteoporosis.htm.
22. ABH. *Understanding Bone Density Results.* American Bone Health; 2020. https://americanbonehealth.org/bone-density/understanding-the-bone-density-t-score-and-z-score/.
23. NIH. *Hypertension (High Blood Pressure).* National Center for Complimentary and Integrative Health; 2018. https://www.nccih.nih.gov/health/hypertension-high-blood-pressure.
24. NIH. *Depression and Older Adults.* National Institute on Aging; 2021. https://www.nia.nih.gov/health/depression-and-older-adults.
25. MHA. *Anxiety in Older Adults.* Mental Health America; 2023. https://www.mhanational.org/anxiety-older-adults.
26. Mayo Clinic. *Dementia.* Mayo Clinic; 2022. https://www.mayoclinic.org/diseases-conditions/dementia/symptoms-causes/syc-20352013.
27. Mayo Clinic. *Stroke.* Mayo Clinic; 2024. https://www.mayoclinic.org/diseases-conditions/stroke/symptoms-causes/syc-20350113.
28. NIH. *Parkinson's Disease: Causes, Symptoms, and Treatments.* National Institute on Aging, NIH; 2022. https://www.nia.nih.gov/health/parkinsons-disease/parkinsons-disease-causes-symptoms-and-treatments.
29. Cleveland Clinic. *Type 2 Diabetes: What It Is, Causes, Symptoms & Treatment.* Cleveland Clinic; 2023.
30. Mayo Clinic. *Diabetic Hypoglycemia - Symptoms & Causes.* Mayo Clinic; 2022.
31. Mayo Clinic. *Osteoarthritis.* Mayo Clinic; 2021. https://www.mayoclinic.org/diseases-conditions/osteoarthritis/symptoms-causes/syc-20351925.
32. NIH. *Depression.* National Institute of Mental Health, NIH; 2023. https://www.nimh.nih.gov/health/topics/depression.

SECTION II

Pathophysiology by System

Introduction to Section II

We were honored to have Charlene Marshall, BS, PTA, executive editor of *Pathology for the Physical Therapist Assistant*,[1] co-author of *Recognizing and Reporting Red Flags for the Physical Therapist Assistant*,[2] and Director of Rehabilitation at Edgewater Haven Nursing Home serve as the executive reviewer for Section II of this textbook.

Much of the information in Section II comes from the mind and research of an incredible scholar, Dr. Catherine C. Goodman, MBA, PT, formerly known as Catherine Goodman. Catherine C. Goodman is a prolific writer, authoring several physical therapy textbooks focusing on pathophysiology and differential diagnosis. A book entitled *Differential Diagnosis for Physical Therapists: Screening for Referral, 7th edition*[3] is referenced frequently in the pages that follow, especially in Chapter 20. We are very grateful to Catherine C. Goodman for sharing her knowledge over the years and motivating thousands of students to study the field of pathology. We also wish to thank her for her inspiration and support.

Section II examines pathophysiology utilizing a systems approach. Chapter 10 covers pathophysiology and neoplasms on a cellular level. Chapter 11 summarizes hematologic pathophysiology, and Chapter 12 covers integumentary pathophysiology. The systemic approach in this section continues with Chapters 13–19. Chapter 20 summarizes the information by discussing neuromuscular pathophysiology and how systemic illnesses can present as neuromuscular problems and vice versa. Each of the chapters in Section II of this book begins with a quick overview of a healthy system, followed by signs and symptoms of possible disorders related to that system, ending with the occupational therapy scope of practice and case studies for application.

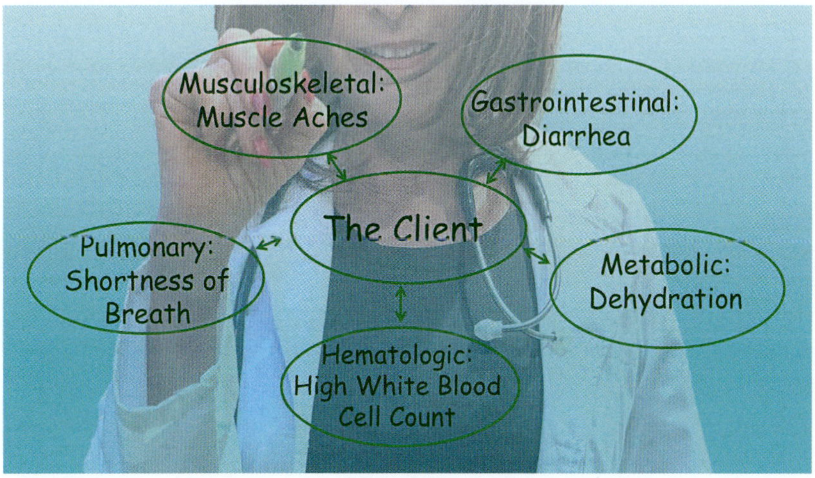

Critical thinking strategy for a patient with a possible stomach virus. (Courtesy Natalie Norman Michaels.)

References

1. Marshall C. *Goodman and Fuller's Pathology for the Physical Therapist Assistant*. 3rd ed. Elsevier; 2023.
2. Goodman CC, Marshall C. *Recognizing and Reporting Red Flags for the Physical Therapist Assistant*. Elsevier; 2014.
3. Heick J, Lazaro RT. *Goodman and Snyder's Differential Diagnosis for Physical Therapists: Screening for Referral*. 7th ed. Elsevier; 2023.

10 Cellular Pathophysiology and Neoplasms

OBJECTIVES

By the end of this chapter, the reader should be able to:

- Demonstrate a basic understanding of normal change over time on a cellular level.
- Demonstrate a basic understanding of various types of cellular pathology.
- Differentiate between basic elements of normal versus pathological cellular change.
- Categorize what causes endogenous cell injury, exogenous cell injury, or cellular necrosis.
- Diagram neoplasms and their potential metastatic path.

Normal Cellular Changes

Before we can understand human pathophysiology, it is important to first gain a better understanding of how a healthy system works. The best way to gain this understanding is to start with the smallest element: the human cell. Depending on the type of cell, the cycle of life involves regulated stages of cell growth and eventually cell division. Interphase is the period when the cell gets larger, and the DNA within the cell is replicated.[1] The mitotic phase is when the replicated DNA and contents of the cell separate into two parts, and the cell divides.[1]

Human cells grow and divide at different rates; some divide continuously, such as certain cells in the gastrointestinal system, while others divide only occasionally or may enter a dormant state known as quiescence.[2] Oocytes, for example, will form in females prenatally but remain dormant until after a girl has reached puberty.[2] There are also some cells in the human body that do not replicate at all, such as skeletal muscle cells, red blood cells, and most of the body's neurons.[3,4] Skeletal muscle fibers get larger with exercise, but they do not replicate.[4] Red blood cells do not contain nuclei and therefore lack the DNA and centrioles (protein organelles) needed for cellular division.[5] Early in human development, neurons that do not yet have a determined function have centrioles that enable them to divide, but once they become differentiated (with a determined function), they no longer have these centrioles, so division is no longer possible.[6]

Why We Age

There are many different theories pertaining to cellular aging.[7] These theories are typically broken up into either program theories, damage theories, or a combination of both.[8] Program theories contend that we age because of programming on a molecular or cellular level.[8] Leonard Hayflick found that human cells will divide in a protected environment in a lab only about 50 times and then will begin to age and die.[9] This is called the Hayflick limit, and it estimates human life (free of disease) to be about 110 years. Programmed senescence is the belief that aging is purposely caused by biological mechanisms that have evolved in a species over time.[10] Another theory is the telomere aging clock theory, which contends that our telomeres (protective tips on our chromosomes) begin to shorten and that this programmed erosion coincides with the point when cell division stops.[11]

Damage theories contend that we age primarily due to environmental factors, implying that it could be prevented.[8] One such theory, the free radical theory, contends that we age because of a buildup of free radicals (highly unstable oxygen atoms and molecules that result from metabolism in our bodies). These free radicals cause DNA damage and oxidative stress in the cells, resulting in aging.[7,12] The wear-and-tear theory contends that we age because of accumulated damage from use and disuse.[12] The rate of living theory is the belief that we only have a certain amount of work in our bodies, and the greater our metabolisms, the faster we use up what we have and the sooner we begin to age.[2] Regardless of the reason for aging, many cellular changes are typical and therefore not considered to be pathological. Some of the less typical and possibly more pathological cellular changes are described in the following sections.

Cellular Pathology

A normal cell is comprised of a cellular membrane and smaller units called organelles (Fig. 10.1).[13] These membranes and organelles can become injured by either what occurs within the cell (endogenous factors) or what occurs outside of the cell (exogenous factors).

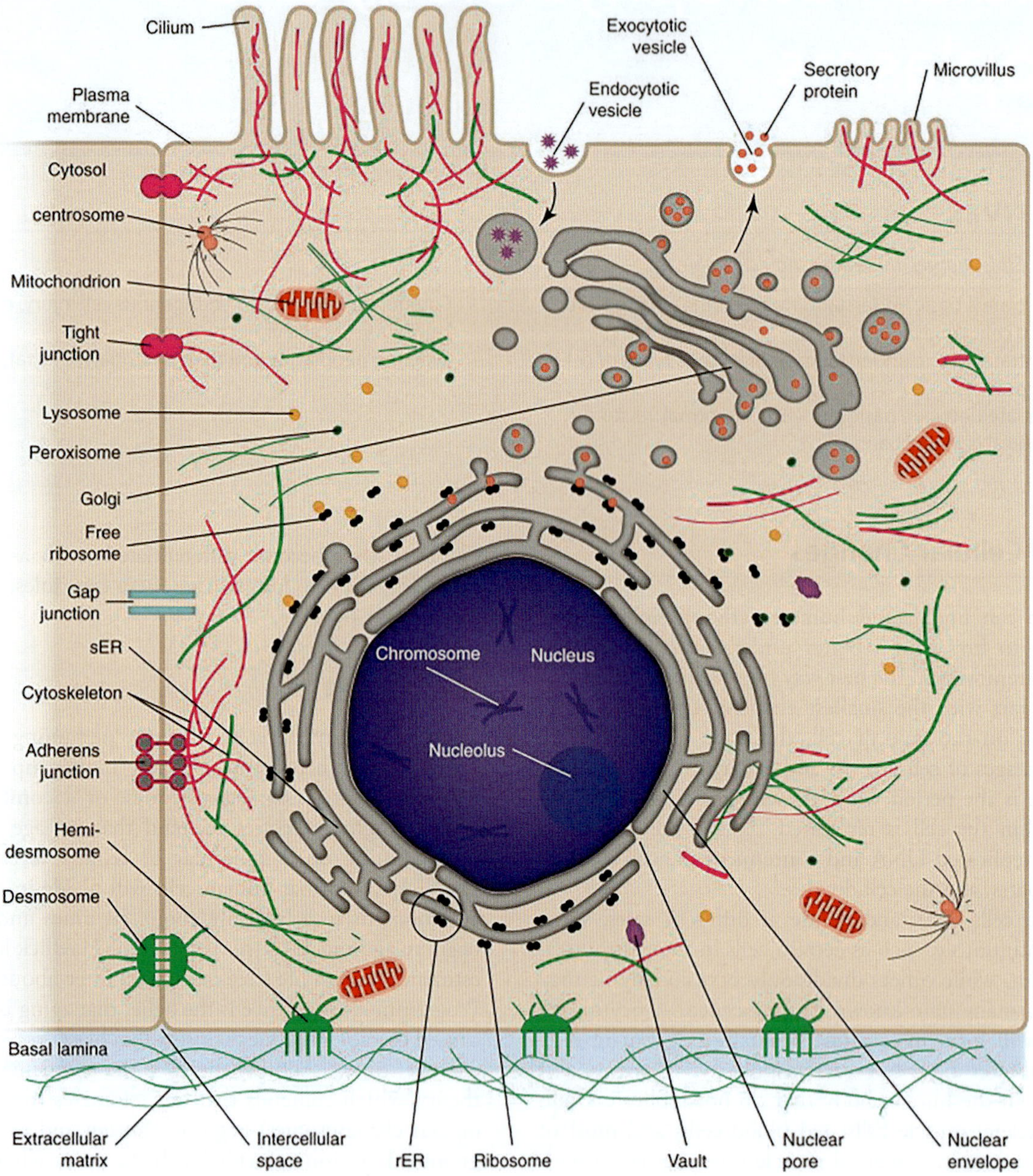

• **Fig. 10.1** The organelles of a living cell. (Courtesy Dr. M.A. Miller, College of Veterinary Medicine, Purdue University; and Dr. J.F. Zachary, College of Veterinary Medicine, University of Illinois.)

Although some cell injury is reversible, the cellular adaptations that can occur in chronic conditions are often irreversible.

Endogenous Cell Injury

Endogenous cell injury occurs from conditions within the cell itself. Atrophy is a physiological process resulting in the reduction of cell size. This term is used most often when describing a reduction in muscle mass due to inactivity, genetic factors, lack of proper nutrition, or certain medical conditions.[14] Apoptosis, derived from the Latin phrase *to fall off* (like a leaf falls from a tree), is the term for programmed cell death. This is our body's way of eliminating unwanted cells.[15] This can not only be valuable during embryologic development but can also be a response to severe injury.[13] Hypertrophy is an increase in cell size that can be due to a normal stressor causing an increased demand on tissue (like with weight lifting), or it can be due to an abnormal stressor, like a thickening of the left ventricular wall when a person has congestive heart failure.[16] Hyperplasia is an increase in the number of cells, typically caused by a compensatory mechanism for increased demands, resulting in an increase in the size of the tissues.[16] This can also be due to a normal stressor, like breastfeeding, or due to an abnormal stressor, like a hormonal imbalance.

Metaplasia occurs when one mature cell type is replaced by another mature cell type within the same tissue germline.[17] Cells sometimes change their characteristics to help protect the body against an insult from abnormal external stimuli, like smoking. Metaplasia is sometimes reversible, but it can slowly transform into dysplasia.[17] Dysplasia occurs when cells vary so much in size and shape that they appear less mature, and the change is no longer reversible. Growth becomes disordered with dysplasia, which can lead to cancer (Fig. 10.2).[18]

Anaplasia refers to cells that are undifferentiated, less specified, and more immature with variable nuclear and cellular structures.[19] These cells tend to divide quickly. Neoplasia means "new growth." The terms *benign* and *malignant* are often used to describe the progression of a neoplasm.[16] A collection of these cells is called a tumor. A tumor is benign if it is slow growing and does not metastasize (travel) to other body tissues. A tumor is considered malignant if it grows rapidly, invades surrounding tissues, and is often capable of metastasizing.[16]

Autophagy is when cells "eat" their own damaged, altered, or mutated cellular structures. The cells take their own damaged components and send them to another part of the cell called a lysosome.[20] Here, the parts are "digested," and newer components are released into the cell. The cell then uses these components to make new cellular structures. It is a way for healthy cells to eliminate damaged organelles and recycle older parts into fully functioning components.[20]

Neoplasm

As stated earlier, neoplasms are tumors or collections of cells that are similar in varying degrees to the tissues where they originate. Benign tumors are closer to normal cells without metastasis, and malignant cells are closer to abnormal cells.[21] Most malignant tumors will metastasize to other areas, but not all of them will. For example, primary brain tumors, although rare, typically do not metastasize outside the central nervous system (Fig. 10.3). They

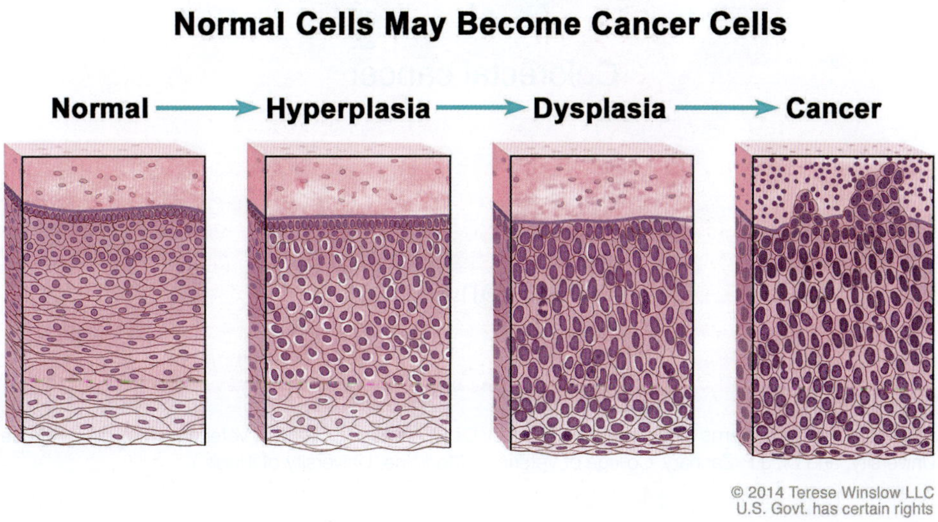

• **Fig. 10.2** The progression from normal cells to cancer. (From https://www.cancer.gov/publications/dictionaries/cancer-terms/def/hyperplasia.)

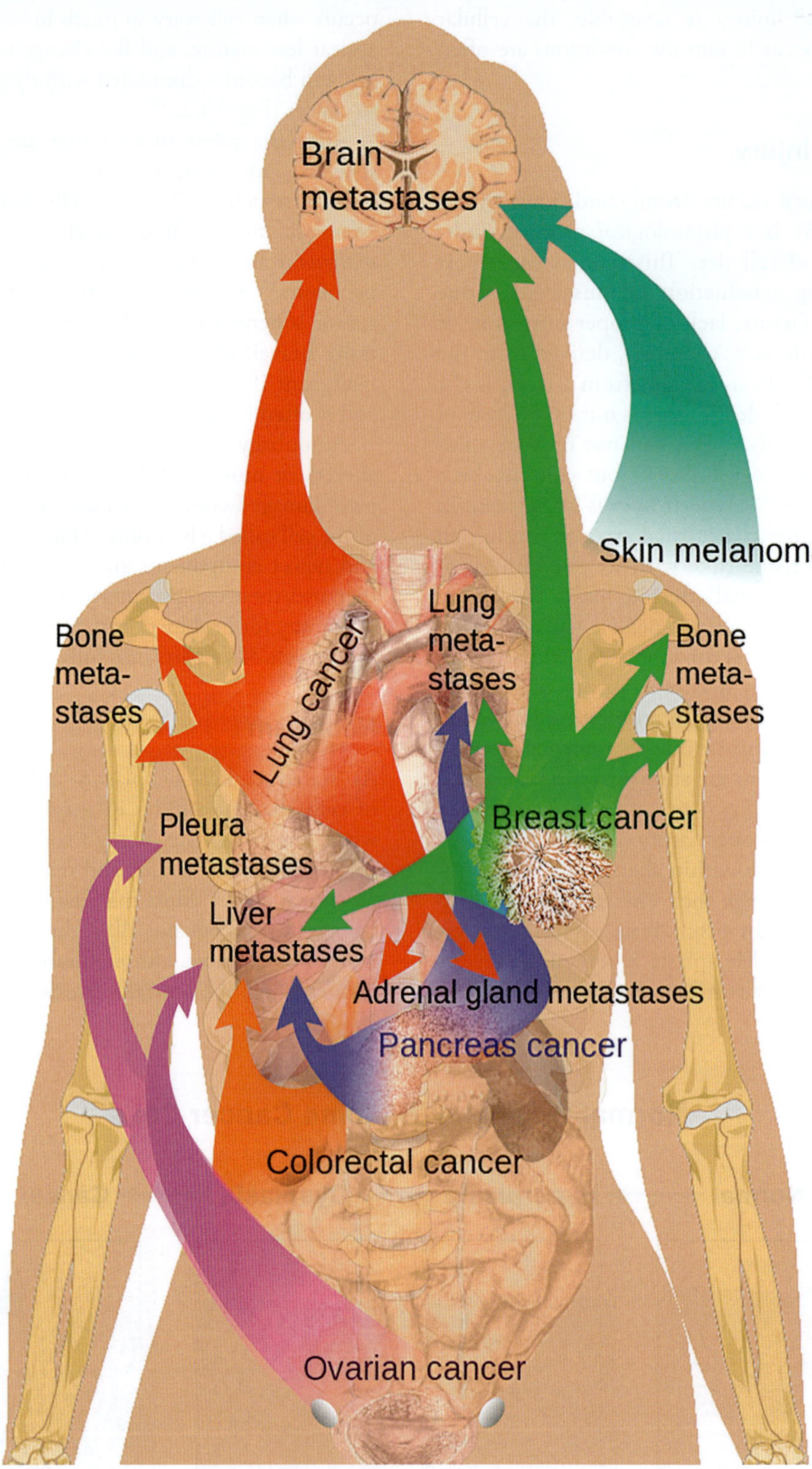

• **Fig. 10.3** Typical patterns of metastasis. (Courtesy Dr. M.A. Miller, College of Veterinary Medicine, Purdue University; and Dr. J.F. Zachary, College of Veterinary Medicine, University of Illinois.)

remain in situ (in one place). The term *primary cancer* means that the cancer is located in the original site where it first began. A *secondary cancer* is typically from the metastasis of a primary cancer.[22]

Some warning signs of possible cancer in the body include unusual bleeding or discharge; a fever of unknown origin; waking at night because of pain; persistent or worsening pain; changes in bowel or bladder habits; changes in a wart or mole; unexplained weight loss; a solid lump (often painless) in the breast, testes, or elsewhere in the body; and severe fatigue or paraneoplastic syndrome.[23]

Cellular Trauma or Exogenous Cell Injury

Exogenous cell injury occurs from conditions outside of the body that result in changes or damage to the cell membrane and/or the cellular organelles. Some examples of this include hydropic swelling, ischemic cell injury, and oxidative stress.[21] Hydropic swelling occurs when there is an increased amount of fluid in the cells. This can result from many factors including external toxins, infections, and excessive temperature changes. Ischemic cell injury occurs when there is a decrease in necessary oxygen to the cells, typically from an interruption in blood flow.[21] Oxidative stress results when there is an increase in reactive oxygen species and free radicals. These are very reactive chemical compounds that can accumulate when there are problems with mitochondrial functions or when there is acute inflammation.[21] Some other examples of exogenous cell injury include ionizing radiation, viral cytotoxicity, chemical cytotoxicity, and neoplasms.

Cellular Necrosis

Cellular necrosis refers to the death of a cell or cells in a tissue or structure. This is not the same as programmed cell death; rather, it results from irreversible damage.[22] When damage to the cell leads to a loss of function, this damage might still be reversible until morphological changes begin to appear within the cell itself. Once these changes occur, the damage is more likely to become irreversible.[24] Typically, the cell will swell and rupture, releasing destructive enzymes from the lysosomes. This then causes inflammation that can damage nearby cells and their ability to function.[24]

The OT Scope of Practice

It would be difficult to choose a case study or specific application scenario for this chapter since everything we treat revolves around our cellular health. This will become more evident in the following chapters. This chapter is important, however, as a conduit for the information in the chapters that follow.

Application—Case Study

CASE EXAMPLE 10.1

A 17-year-old male was playing on his high school football team when he began to experience severe groin pain. The physician diagnosed him with a groin muscle strain and ordered OT intervention to help him safely navigate through his environment to get dressed, reach for objects, and so forth.

1. **Screen:** The occupational therapist (OTR) screened the client and, at first, it did appear that this individual had a strain of the muscles in the groin area.
2. **Take a Closer Look:** During the examination, the client asked the OTR if he could tell her something that was personal and "a little embarrassing." The OTR was very professional, actively listening to the client. She reminded the client that he did not need to feel embarrassed. He then told the OTR that he had a bump on his testicle, and he was afraid that this could be the problem.
3. **Determine Flag Status:** The OTR asked when he first noticed the bump and the status of the pain. He said he noticed it months ago, but it was gradually becoming larger. He added that the pain was also becoming more severe, and during the last football game, he "really felt it." The OTR concluded that this could be a red flag situation.
4. **Take Action if Needed:** The OTR contacted the physician immediately for a prompt reexamination. Occupational therapy practitioners do not make a medical diagnosis, but the symptoms can be clearly explained to the physician, enabling them to perform appropriate tests needed to make the medical diagnosis.
5. **Document the Findings:** The OTR documented the findings of the short examination as well as the phone call to the physician.
6. **Take a Second Look:** The physician performed a testicular ultrasound, which revealed that the individual had testicular cancer.
7. **Determine the Flag Status:** This was definitely a red flag.
8. **Take Action if Needed:** The physician referred the individual for oncology and surgery.

This is a true case. The physician diagnosed him with testicular nonseminoma, but it was caught early, and the client responded well to intervention. There was no metastasis.

References

1. Fowler S, Roush R, Wise J. The cell cycle. In: *Concepts of Biology*. Chapter 6. OperStax; 2023. https://openstax.org/books/concepts-biology/pages/6-2-the-cell-cycle.
2. Davis N. To divide or not to divide? *MIT News*; 2019. https://news.mit.edu/2019/divide-or-not-divide-cell-division-0821.
3. Oregon State. Cell growth and division. In: *Anatomy & Physiology*. Chapter 3.5. Oregon State University; 2019. https://open.oregonstate.education/aandp/chapter/3-5-cell-growth-and-division/.
4. MRL. How often do skeletal muscle cells go through mitosis? In: *UCSB Science Line*. Materials Research Laboratory; 2017. http://scienceline.ucsb.edu/getkey.php?key=5873.
5. U.C. Davis. *RBC Anatomy*. LibreTexts. Chapter 16.2A. https://med.libretexts.org/Bookshelves/Anatomy_and_Physiology/Anatomy_and_Physiology_ (Boundless)/16%3A_Cardiovascular_System_-_Blood/16.2%3A_Red_Blood_Cells/16.2A%3A_RBC_Anatomy.

6. Slaughton J. *Why Don't Brain Cells Undergo Mitosis?* Science ABC. https://www.scienceabc.com/humans/dont-brain-cells-undergo-mitosis.html.
7. Goodman CC, Fuller KS. *Goodman and Fuller's Pathology: Implications for the Physical Therapist.* 5th ed. Elsevier; 2022.
8. da Costa JP, Vitorino R, Silva GM, Vogel C, Duarte AC, Rocha-Santos T. A synopsis on aging-Theories, mechanisms and future prospects. *Ageing Res Rev.* 2016;29:90–112. https://doi.org/10.1016/j.arr.2016.06.005.
9. Shay JW, Wright WE. Hayflick, his limit, and cellular ageing. *Nat Rev Mol Cell Biol.* 2000;1(1):72–76. https://doi.org/10.1038/35036093.
10. Goldsmith TC. Evolution of aging theories: why modern programmed aging concepts are transforming medical research. *Biochem (Mosc).* 2016;81(12):1406–1412. https://doi.org/10.1134/S0006297916120026.
11. Razgonova MP, Zakharenko AM, Golokhvast KS, et al. A. Telomerase and telomeres in aging theory and chronographic aging theory (Review). *Mol Med Rep.* 2020;22(3):1679–1694. https://doi.org/10.3892/mmr.2020.11274.
12. Jin K. Modern Biological theories of aging. *Aging Dis.* 2010;1(2):72–74. https://www.ncbi.nlm.nih.gov/pmc/articles/PMC2995895/.
13. Miller M, Zachary JF. Mechanisms and morphology of cellular injury, adaptation, and death. In: *Pathologic Basis of Veterinary Disease.* Elsevier; 2017. https://doi.org/10.1016/B978-0-323-35775-3.00001-1.
14. Eske J, Morrison W. What to know about muscle atrophy. *Medical News Today.* October 18, 2023. https://www.medicalnewstoday.com/articles/325316.
15. NIH. *Apoptosis.* National Human Genome Research Institute; 2023. https://www.genome.gov/genetics-glossary/apoptosis.
16. Kemp WL, Burns DK, Brown TG. *Pathology: The Big Picture.* McGraw Hill; 2008. https://accessmedicine.mhmedical.com/content.aspx?bookid=499&sectionid=41568284.
17. Giroux V, Rustgi AK. Metaplasia: tissue injury adaptation and a precursor to the dysplasia-cancer sequence. *Natl Rev Cancer.* 2017;17(10):594–604. https://doi.org/10.1038/nrc.2017.68.
18. NIH. *Fibromuscular Dysplasia.* National Institute of Neurological Disorders and Stroke; 2023. https://www.ninds.nih.gov/health-information/disorders/fibromuscular-dysplasia.
19. Cancer Ca. *Anaplasia.* The Canadian Cancer Society; 2023. https://cancer.ca/en/cancer-information/resources/glossary/a/anaplasia.
20. Cleveland Clinic. *Autophagy.* Cleveland Clinic; 2022. https://my.clevelandclinic.org/health/articles/24058-autophagy.
21. VanMeter KC, Hubert RJ. *Gould's Pathology for the Health Professions.* 7th ed. Elsevier; 2023.
22. Fayed L. *Differentiating Between Primary and Metastatic Tumors.* Verywell Health; 2022. https://www.verywellhealth.com/primary-and-metastatic-brain-tumors-513566.
23. Rubin E, Reisner HM. *Principles of Rubin's Pathology.* 7th ed. Wolters Kluwer; 2019.
24. American Cancer Society. *Signs and Symptoms of Cancer.* American Cancer Society; 2020. https://www.cancer.org/cancer/diagnosis-staging/signs-and-symptoms-of-cancer.html.

11

Hematologic Pathophysiology

OBJECTIVES

By the end of this chapter, the reader should be able to:

- Depict the elements of whole blood on a cellular level.
- Demonstrate a basic understanding of various types of hematological pathology.
- Categorize the various symptoms associated with leukocyte, thrombocyte, and erythrocyte disorders.
- Demonstrate a basic understanding of a healthy immune system.
- Explain and/or predict the possible symptoms resulting from the pathophysiology of various autoimmune disorders.
- Assess and justify whether a specific hematologic or autoimmune symptom could constitute a yellow or red flag.

Healthy Physiology

The term *hematology* (sometimes spelled haematology) refers to the branch of medicine that studies the blood and the treatment of disorders that affect either the blood or its various components.[1] It is important for an occupational therapist or occupational therapy assistant (together identified in this book as occupational therapy practitioners or OTPs) to be able to identify symptoms outside of the norm for the client's condition. Pathology related to the hematological system can be due to many factors, including chemotherapy or radiation, pernicious anemia, or even the use of non-steroidal anti-inflammatory medications (NSAIDs).[2]

Histology: The System on a Cellular Level

Before we can understand human pathophysiology, it is important to first gain a better understanding of how a healthy system works, and the best way to gain this understanding is to start with the smallest element: the human cell. Blood contains three primary cell types: erythrocytes (red blood cells [RBCs]), leukocytes (white blood cells [WBCs]), and thrombocytes (platelets). These cells are suspended in a fluid known as plasma. Whole blood composition is made up of about 55% plasma and 45% formed elements (Fig. 11.1).

All blood cells originate from multipotent (or pluripotent) stem cells within the marrow of bones (Fig. 11.2). As the cells divide, they eventually differentiate into the three main blood cell types, with WBCs forming various subtypes.

Each of the formed elements has a specific job, and it all works in harmony, as long as there is no impeding pathology. The erythrocytes (RBCs) carry oxygen to the tissues, the thrombocytes (platelets) are responsible for blood clotting and tissue repair, and the various types of leukocytes (WBCs) work to fight infection.[3,4]

Leukocytes consist of granulocytes (neutrophils, eosinophils, and basophils) and agranulocytes (with two subtypes: lymphoid cells and monocytes).[2] Neutrophils fight off bacteria and fungi, eosinophils help destroy parasites, and basophils play a big part in wound healing and allergic reactions.[5] Lymphocytes Lymphocytes have many functions, but they primarily protect the body from viral infections. Monocytes help rid the body of dead or damaged tissue (Table 11.1).[5]

Signs and Symptoms of Hematological Disorders

The signs and symptoms of blood disorders depend on the cell type involved and how those cells are affected. Some helpful hints with nomenclature can be seen in Table 11.2. Signs and symptoms of hematological disorders include those associated with exertion (e.g., dyspnea, palpitations, chest pain, weakness, and fatigue), those associated with the nervous system (e.g., dizziness, headache, or syncope), those associated with the integumentary system (e.g., pallor or cyanosis of the hands, lips, face, and nail beds, easy bruising, or clubbing of the fingernails), and those associated with various medications (e.g., steroids and NSAIDs can upset a stomach leading to a bleeding peptic ulcer and subsequent anemia, and certain chemotherapy agents for cancer can cause thrombocytopenia).

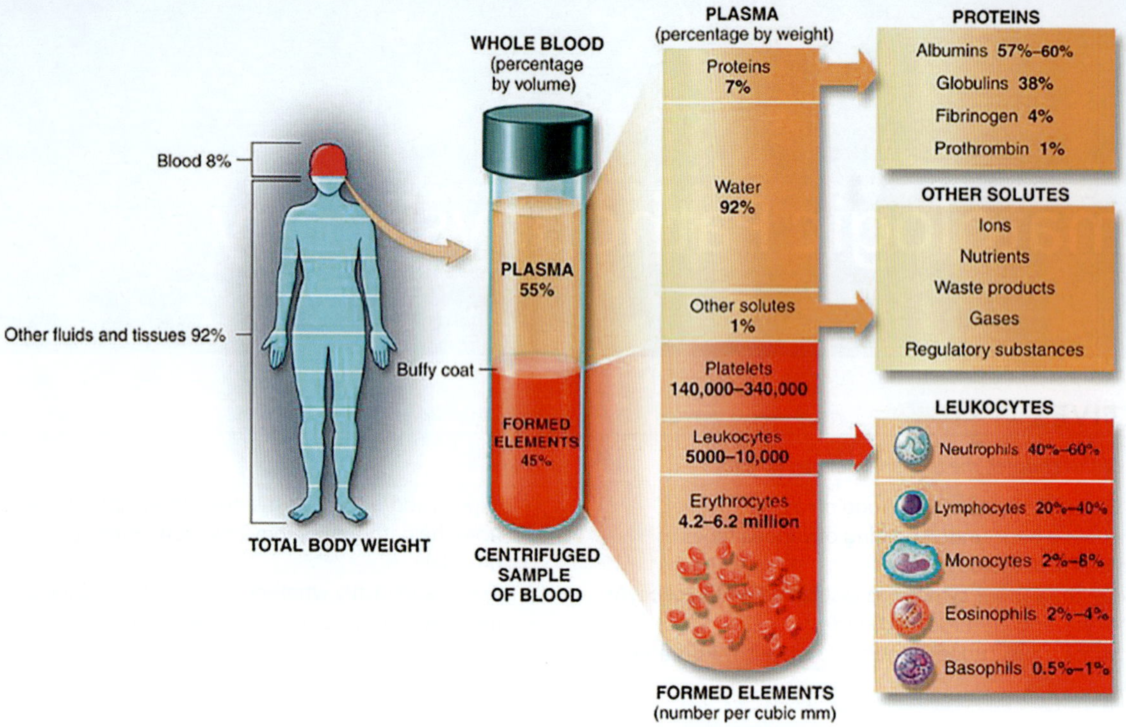

• **Fig. 11.1** The composition of whole blood. (From Patton KT, Bell F, Thompson T, Williamson PL. *Anatomy & Physiology*. 11th ed. Mosby; 2022.)

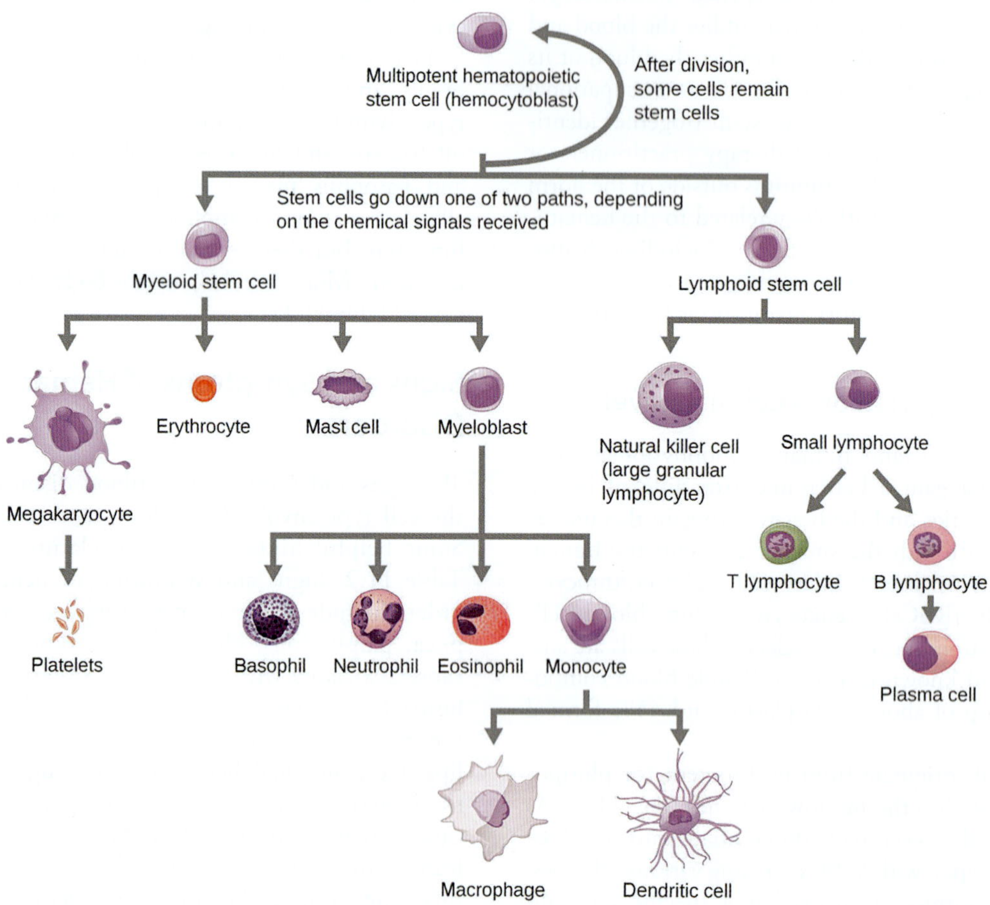

• **Fig. 11.2** Differentiation of the stem cells into the various blood cell types. (From Schatz P. *Microbiology*. OpenStax; 2023. https://openstax.org/books/microbiology/pages/1-introduction.)

TABLE 11.1 The Formed Elements of the Blood and the Various Subtypes of Leukocytes

Formed Element	Number of Cells Present/ Microliter[a]	Functions[b]
Red blood cells (RBCs) or erythrocytes 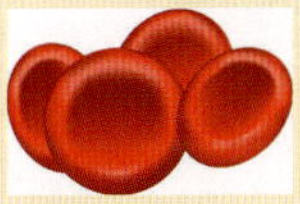	4.6–6.2 million	RBCs obtain oxygen from the lungs and carry it to all parts of the body.
Platelets or thrombocytes 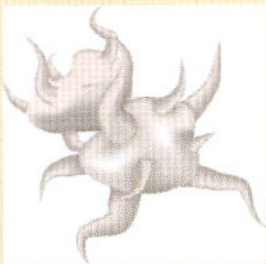	14,000–450,000	These cells aid in the clotting of blood by sticking together.
Lymphocytes (a type of white blood cell [WBC]) 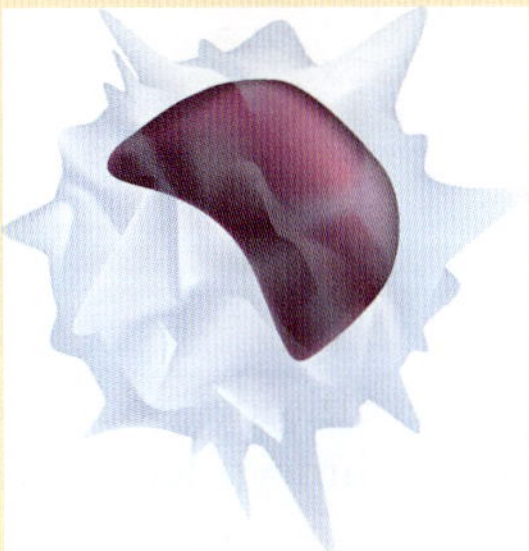	Total WBC count is around 4500 to around 11,000. For lymphocytes, the number is 1000–4000.	These cells make antibodies to help fight against infection.
Monocytes (WBC) 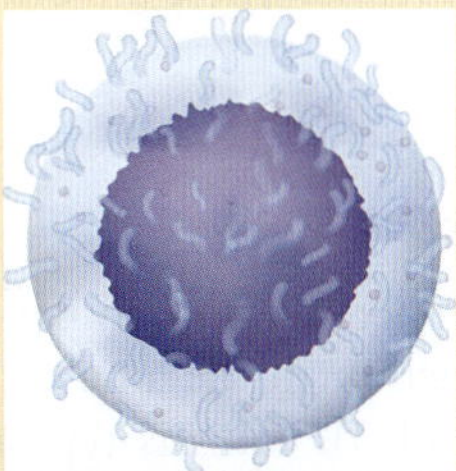	200–1000	These cells help remove damaged tissue, bacteria, and viruses.
Basophils (WBC) 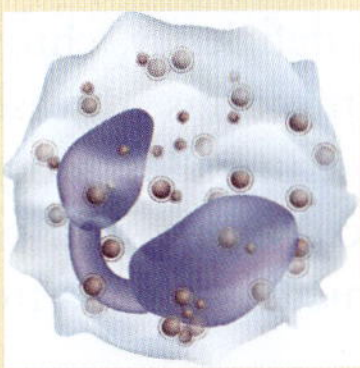	0–200	These release histamine when allergic and help to prevent blood clots.
Neutrophils 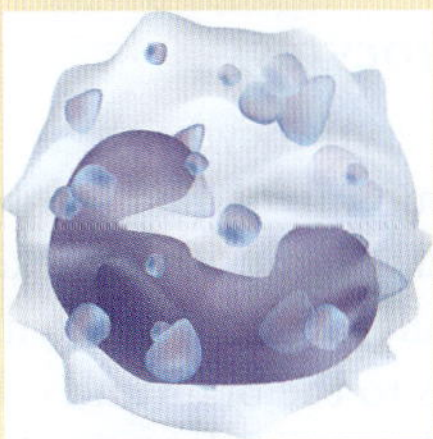	1500–8000	These cells help to remove infection and tissue that is damaged.

(Continued)

TABLE 11.1 The Formed Elements of the Blood and the Various Subtypes of Leukocytes—cont'd

Formed Element	Number of Cells Present/ Microliter[a]	Functions[b]
Eosinophils 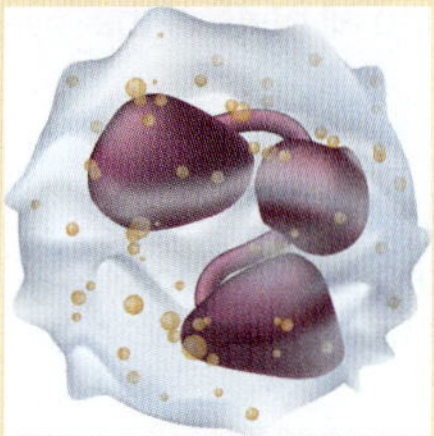	0–500	These kill parasites, help the immune system, and help destroy cancerous cells.

[a]NIH. *Normal and Abnormal Complete Blood Count with Differential*. NIH: National Library of Medicine, Stats Pearls; 2024. https://www.ncbi.nlm.nih.gov/books/NBK604207/.
[b]American Red Cross. *What Do Blood Cells Do?* American National Red Cross; 2024. https://www.redcrossblood.org/local-homepage/news/article/function-of-blood-cells.html.
Adapted from www.istockphoto.com/ikryannikovgmailcom.
From Schatz P. *Microbiology*. OpenStax; 2023. https://openstax.org/books/microbiology/pages/1-introduction.

TABLE 11.2 Some of the More Common Terms Seen When Talking About Various Hematological Disorders

Term	Meaning
Leukocytes	White blood cells
Erythrocytes	Red blood cells
Thrombocytes	Platelets
...emia	In the blood
...penia	Too few
...cythemia	Too many
...cytosis	Abnormally shaped
Anemia	Too few erythrocytes in the blood
Polycythemia	Too many erythrocytes
Poikilocytosis	Abnormally shaped erythrocytes
Thrombocytopenia	Not enough thrombocytes

Erythrocyte Disorders

Erythrocytes, also known as RBCs, consist primarily of hemoglobin with a supporting framework to transport oxygen to the tissues and carbon dioxide from the tissues.[2] About 40% of the blood volume consists of these RBCs with males having more than females. An increase in physical activity will require more oxygen and more erythrocytes to supply that oxygen.[2] Altitude is also important because there is less oxygen in the air at higher altitudes, so this will require more erythrocytes. Normal erythrocyte levels can be found in Table 11.3.

Some examples of erythrocyte disorders include anemia, polycythemia, and sickle cell anemia. These are briefly described below.

Anemia (Too Few Erythrocytes)

Anemia is an abnormally low number of properly working erythrocytes resulting in a reduction in the amount of oxygen carried by the blood (Fig. 11.3).[2] This is typically caused by a large amount of blood loss, a low production of erythrocytes, and/or an increase in the destruction of the erythrocytes. This can result from iron deficiency, chronic diseases, neurologic conditions, or infectious diseases.[2] Signs and symptoms of anemia include skin pallor, fatigue, dyspnea on exertion, decreased diastolic pressure, and possible nervous system manifestation (pernicious anemia from low vitamin B12).[2]

Polycythemia (Too Many Erythrocytes)

Polycythemia (sometimes called erythrocytosis) is an increased number of RBCs and amount of hemoglobin, which causes an increase in the blood volume. This thickening of the blood makes it more difficult for the blood to flow freely, and therefore, not enough gets to the brain and other organs of the body, increasing the chance of thrombosis or embolism.[2] Primary polycythemia is an uncommon disease of the bone marrow. Secondary polycythemia is the result of the decreased oxygen supply to the tissue and is linked to

TABLE 11.3 Normal RBC Count, Hematocrit, Hemoglobin, and Sedimentation Rate[2]

	RBC Count	Hematocrit	Hemoglobin	Sedimentation Rate
Adult female	4.2–5.4 million/mm³	37%–47%	12.2–16 g/dL	<20 mm/h
Adult male	4.7–6.1 million/mm³	42%–52%	14–18 g/dL	<20 mm/h

1 cubic millimeter (mm³) = 1 microliter (μL).
1 cubic centimeter (cm³) = 1 milliliter (mL) = 1/1000 L.
Values are from Heick J, Lazaro RT. *Goodman and Snyder's Differential Diagnosis for Physical Therapists: Screening for Referral*. 7th ed. Elsevier; 2023: Inside cover.

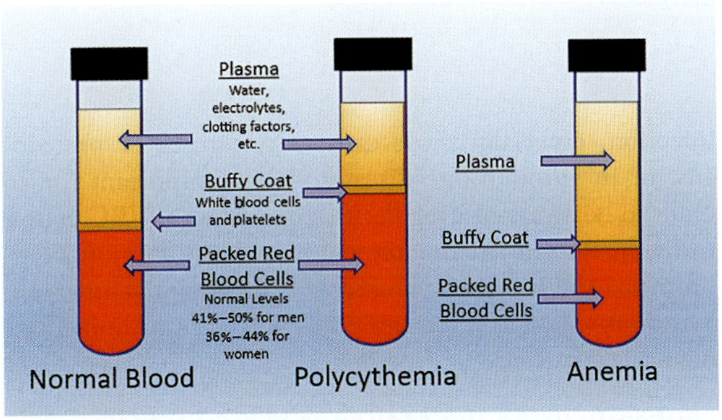

• **Fig. 11.3** Anemia. (Based on https://www.redcrossblood.org/donate-blood/dlp/hematocrit.html.)

high altitude, smoking, sleep apnea, and chronic heart and lung conditions.[2]

Signs and symptoms of polycythemia include constitutional symptoms (malaise and fatigue) as well as headache, dizziness, shortness of breath, decreased mental acuity, weight loss, easy bruising, gout (primary polycythemia), blurred vision, and possible cyanosis.[2]

Sickle Cell Anemia (Sickle-Shaped Erythrocytes)

Sickle cell anemia (i.e., sickle cell disease) is a label for a group of disorders caused by an autosomal recessive gene that results in an amino acid substitution in hemoglobin, causing the hemoglobin to group into long chains, which change the shape of the cell (Fig. 11.4).[2] This new sickle-shaped cell has a harder time passing through small vessels, resulting in the tissue losing its blood supply and leading to chroming hemolytic anemia and vaso-occlusion.[2] This disorder affects about 1 out of every 365 African American births, and 1 out of every 16,300 Hispanic American births.[6] Severity of symptoms varies a great deal from person to person, with some having only a few symptoms and others more affected, possibly even with a shorter lifespan. The primary symptom is pain in the tissues, bone and joint

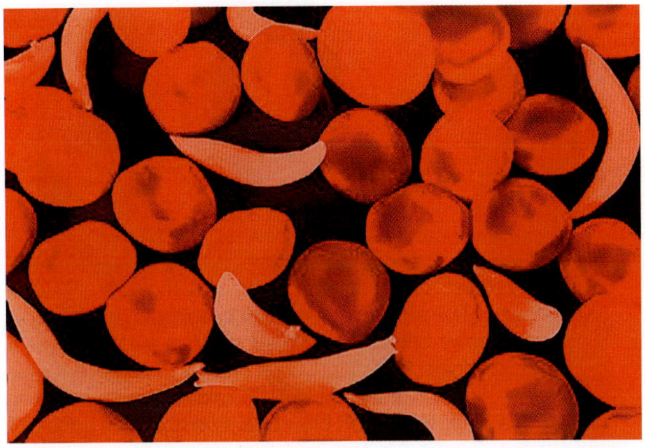

• **Fig. 11.4** Sickle cell disease showing a mix of healthy red blood cells mixed with sickle cells. (From the National Human Genome Research Institute. https://www.genome.gov/news/news-release/Systematic-review-study-supports-that-sickle-cell-trait-increases-risk-for-some-health-conditions.)

pain, dyspnea, vascular complications, episodes of ischemic tissue damage, and seizures.[2]

Leukocyte Disorders

The bone marrow produces about 70% of the body's leukocytes, with the thymus, spleen, and lymph nodes producing the rest.[7] Leukocytes, also known as WBCs, include the following types: granulocytes, monocytes, and what is known as lymphoid cells (lymphocytes and plasma cells). Granulocytes protect the body from infection by using phagocytosis (ingesting the foreign substance).[2] Monocytes (the largest group of all the leukocytes) are immature cells while in the blood, but once they leave the blood and enter the tissues, they become macrophages that can engulf and ingest foreign substances.[2] As previously stated, lymphocytes also help fight infection. They do this by producing antibodies that react with an antigen, and this initiates an immune response in the body.[2] Plasma cells are derived from a leukocyte known as B cells. These cells produce antibody molecules that are released into the blood and lymph

TABLE 11.4 Normal White Blood Cell (WBC) Count[2]

Cell Type	Normal Values
Total WBC count	5000–10,000/mm³ (4.5–11.0 × 10^3) (WBC <1000: protective isolation)

1 cubic millimeter (mm³) = 1 microliter (µL).
1 cubic centimeter (cm³) = 1 milliliter (mL) = 1/1000 L.
From Heick J, Lazaro RT. *Goodman and Snyder's Differential Diagnosis for Physical Therapists: Screening for Referral*. 7th ed. Elsevier; 2023.

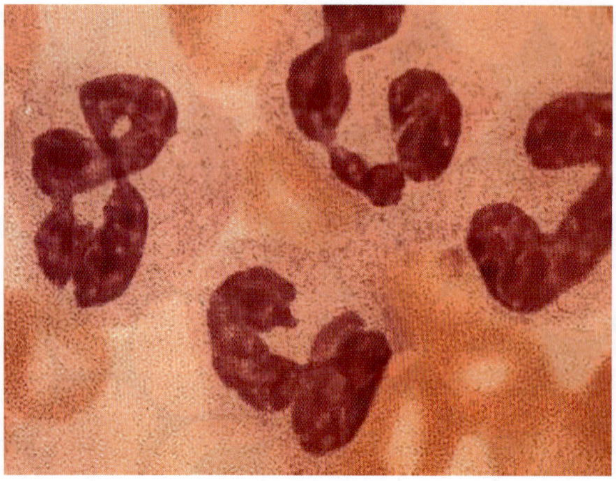

• **Fig. 11.5** Leukocytosis. (From CDC. https://phil.cdc.gov/Details.aspx?pid=6048.)

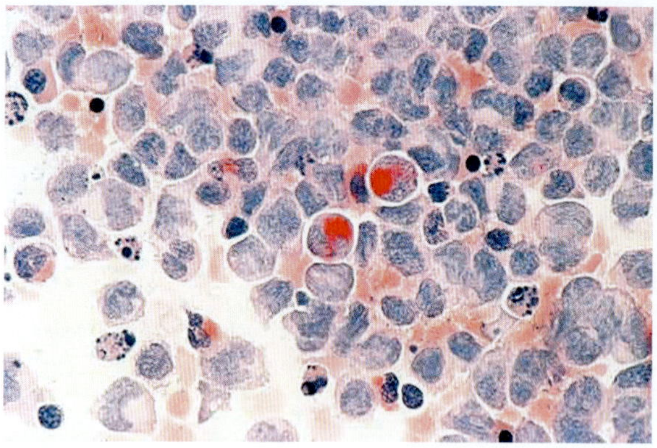

• **Fig. 11.6** Acute myelocystic leukemia. (From NIH. https://www.cancer.gov/types/leukemia/research.)

to neutralize foreign substances.[7] Normal leukocyte levels can be found in Table 11.4.

Some examples of leukocyte disorders are leukocytosis, leukopenia, leukemia, and multiple myeloma. These are briefly described below.

Leukocytosis (An Abnormally High Number of Leukocytes in the Blood)

When the number of leukocytes exceeds 10,000 per cubic millimeter (mm³) or microliter (µL) of blood, it is called leukocytosis (Fig. 11.5).[8] This happens as a response to infection, strenuous exercise, or convulsions. Typically, when a person has leukocytosis, they also have a fever, symptoms of either localized or systemic infection, or tissue inflammation.[2]

Leukopenia (Not Enough Leukocytes)

When the number of leukocytes is less than 5000 per cubic centimeter (cm³), also known as a milliliter (mL) of blood, it is called leukopenia (see Table 11.4).[2] Leukopenia is typically a symptom of bone marrow failure and can occur with chemotherapy, radiation therapy, dietary deficiencies, as a side effect of some medications, after an overwhelming infection, especially those caused by viruses or protozoans, or in autoimmune diseases.[2,9] It is important for an OTP to be aware of irregularities in a client's WBC count. Individuals with leukopenia will be severely immunocompromised and need to be protected from potential infection. Symptoms such as fever and chills will warrant immediate medical attention.

Leukemia (Irregular Malignant Leukocytes)

The term *leukemia* represents not one disorder, but a group of malignant blood disorders affecting the blood and bone marrow (Fig. 11.6).[10] These disorders are cancerous and life threatening. Leukemia is most common in adults over the age of 55, but it is also the most common cancer in children under the age of 15.[11] Leukemias are grouped according to the speed of disease development (acute or chronic).[12] The most common type of acute leukemia in children is called acute lymphoblastic leukemia, with the peak incidence between 2 and 5 years of age, and the most common type in adults is acute myeloid leukemia.[10] Symptoms of leukemia will vary depending on the type of leukemia but typically include fever, chills, fatigue, weakness, loss of appetite, weight loss, easy bruisability, sweating at night, and bone or joint pain.[12]

Multiple Myeloma (Cancer of the Plasma Cells)

As stated earlier, healthy plasma cells are needed to fight infection via the creation of antibodies. When an individual has multiple myelomas, the plasma cells become cancerous and accumulate in the marrow of the bones, making it harder for healthy cells to function properly (Fig. 11.7).[13] The symptoms of multiple myeloma are similar to those of leukemia and other cancers and include bone pain, nausea, loss of appetite, weight loss, excessive thirst, constipation, and weakness or numbness in the legs.[13] This can be diagnosed by a blood test that detects M-proteins produced by the myeloma cell.[14] These proteins can also sometimes be detected in the urine and are then referred to as Bence Jones proteins.[14]

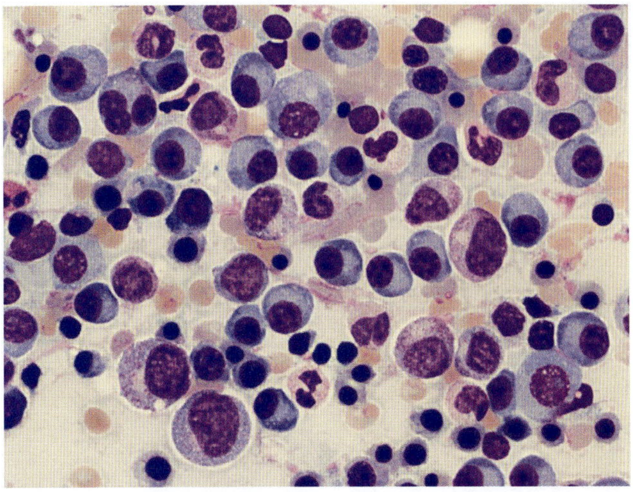

• **Fig. 11.7** Multiple myeloma. (From Young B, Woodford P, O'Dowd G. *Wheater's Functional Histology: A Text and Color Atlas*. Elsevier; 2023.)

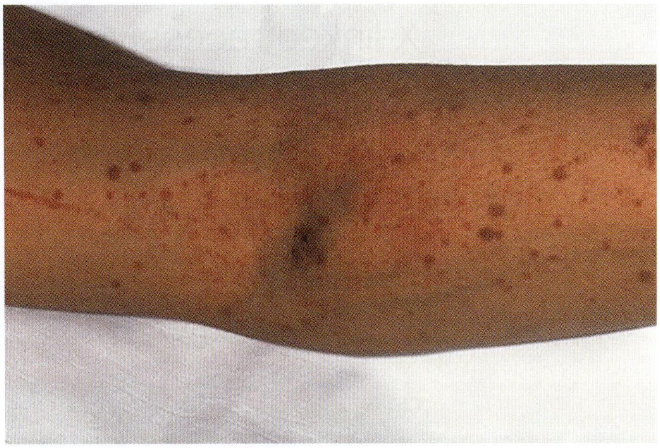

• **Fig. 11.8** Petechiae and purpura. (From NIH. https://www.nhlbi.nih.gov/health/thrombocytopenia.)

TABLE 11.5 Thrombocyte Count[2,15]

Cell Type	Normal Values
Platelet count	150,000–400,000/µL

1 cubic millimeter (mm^3) = 1 microliter (µL).
1 cubic centimeter (cm^3) = 1 milliliter (mL) = 1/1000 L.
Values are from Heick J, Lazaro RT. *Goodman and Snyder's Differential Diagnosis for Physical Therapists: Screening for Referral*. 7th ed. Elsevier; 2023: Inside cover.
NIH. Thrombocytopenia. *National Heart, Lung, and Blood Institute*. 2025. https://www.nhlbi.nih.gov/health/thrombocytopenia.

Thrombocyte Disorders

Thrombocytes, or platelets, are small cell fragments responsible for hemostasis (blood clotting).[2] The name "platelet" was used because scientists thought the cell resembled the shape of a plate.[6] Platelets have sticky proteins on their exterior surface. During hemostasis, the platelet extends filaments that look similar to the legs of a spider, which stick to the injured tissue to stop the bleeding.[6] Normal thrombocyte levels can be found in Table 11.5.

Some examples of thrombocyte disorders are thrombocytopenia, thrombocytosis, and hemophilia.

Thrombocytopenia (Low Platelet Count)

A low platelet count is typically defined as less than 150,000 per microliter of blood, although sources vary on what is considered to be a critical low value (anywhere from 20,000 to 30,000/mm^3).[2,15] Because platelets are necessary for blood clotting, having too few can be life threatening.[15] Symptoms include bleeding for a longer amount time than usual with even small cuts, petechiae (small, flat, red spots under the skin from small bleeds) and purpura (red, purple, or brownish spots on the skin from small bleeds) (Fig. 11.8), nosebleeds, blood in the urine, or heavy menstrual periods.[15]

Thrombocytosis (High Platelet Count)

When thrombocytosis is due to abnormal cell development in the bone marrow, causing the production of too many platelets, it is called primary or essential thrombocytosis.[2,16] This is extremely rare.[16] When thrombocytosis is caused by other factors, such as surgery, splenectomy, infection, iron deficiency, or lung cancer, it is called secondary or reactive thrombocytosis.[2,16] This is typically only a temporary increase in platelet count.[16] This will typically be asymptomatic until the platelet count reaches 1 million per cubic millimeter.[2] This increase in platelets will increase clotting, which could result in thrombosis, with fingers and toes most affected. The person might also have an enlarged spleen and easy bruisability.[2]

Hemophilia (Deficient Clotting Factor)

This is an inherited blood clotting disorder in which the individual has an abnormality of plasma-clotting proteins (factors VIII and IX).[2] Hemophilia is caused by a mutation of the gene that produces these factors,[17] which is inherited from the parents via a recessive gene on the X chromosome. A male (XY) only has one possible allele for the trait, but a female (XX) has two alleles, so a healthy gene can override a hemophilia gene.[17] Although it is a recessive trait, if a male has the gene, it will typically be expressed as hemophilia, whereas a female would need two alleles, one on each X, for the trait to be expressed. She can, however, still be a carrier (Fig. 11.9).[17]

Some predisposing factors of hemophilia include a family history of hemophilia, a family history of bleeding, any unexplained deaths in the family, and a tendency to bleed for longer than usual periods with even small cuts.[18] Babies with a known family history of hemophilia are typically diagnosed at birth. Hemophilia can cause bleeding into joint spaces (called hemarthrosis), which can damage the joint tissues.[2] Symptoms of hemarthrosis include decreased joint range of motion, swelling, joint pain, and heat felt on palpation of the affected joint.[18]

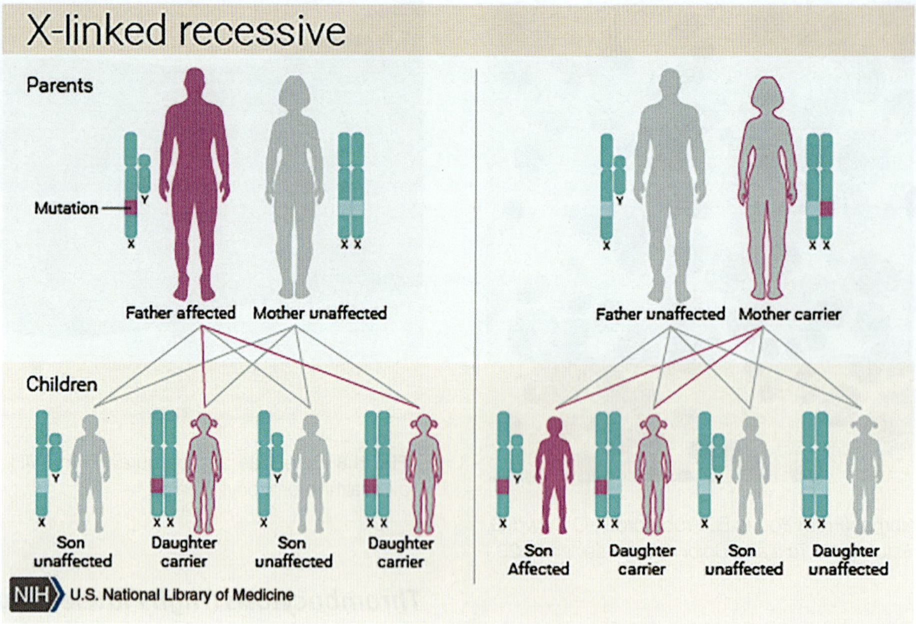

• **Fig. 11.9** X-linked recessive. (From NIH U.S. National Library of Medicine.)

Autoimmune Disorders

So far, this chapter has covered hematological pathophysiology. This next section ties several systems together, including hematology, to discuss autoimmune disorders. The body's immune system consists of a network of various organ systems, proteins, blood cells, and chemicals.[19] These entities work together to help protect the body from environmental pathogens like bacteria and viruses and to help heal the body after injury.[19] Sometimes, however, this system will begin to attack its own tissues, leading to various autoimmune disorders.

Physiology of the Healthy Immune System

The first line of defense against infection is the skin.[20] Skin cells secrete antimicrobial proteins to guard against infection, and there are immune cells found in various layers of the skin. More information on the integumentary system can be found in Chapter 12. The body's bone marrow is responsible for the production of cells that act as the first line of defense against infection. These include neutrophils, basophils, eosinophils, monocytes, mast cells, and macrophages. T cells are produced in the thymus. These are white blood cells (lymphocytes) that help fight off pathogens, such as bacteria, viruses, and other cells that could be harmful like cancer cells.[21] There are two types of T cells: cytotoxic T cells ($CD8^+$ cells), also known as T-killer cells because they kill cells that are infected, and helper T cells ($CD4^+$ cells) that coordinate an attack against invaders (Fig. 11.10).

The lymphatic system helps by acting as a conduit between the bloodstream and the bodily tissues. Immune cells travel through the lymphatic system and congregate in the lymph nodes until they are needed.[20] The spleen acts to enrich immune cells by processing information from the bloodstream, helping cells recognize bloodborne pathogens. Immune hubs located in the mucosal lining of the respiratory tract and gastrointestinal system (like Peyer patches in the small intestine) also help to combat infection.[20]

Autoimmune Disorders

The immune system, when working properly, will help guard against infection. A dysfunction of the system, however, can result in the body conducting an attack against its own tissues and organ systems. This typically results in the client acquiring one or more of the over 100 different autoimmune disorders currently identified.[22] Some of the more common autoimmune disorders seen by OTPs can be found in Table 11.6 below.

The OT Scope of Practice

Once again when working as an OTP, if a client demonstrates symptoms that are outside of the typical cluster you expect to find with their diagnosis, it is important to report those symptoms to the referring physician. Case Example 11.1 provides an example of how advocacy from a quick-thinking OTP can save a person's life.

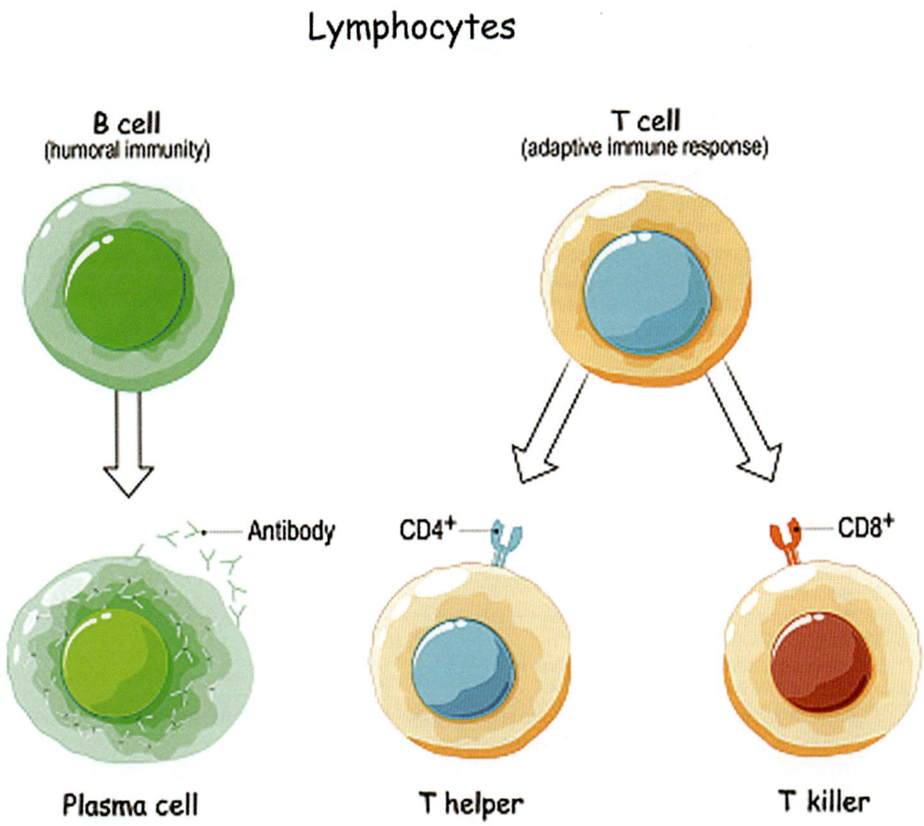

• **Fig. 11.10** Types of lymphocytes: T and B cells. (From iStock.)

TABLE 11.6 Some of the More Common Autoimmune Disorders Often Seen by Occupational Therapy Practitioners

Disorder	Pathophysiology	Symptoms
Rheumatoid arthritis[23]	This is a chronic inflammation, typically of the smaller joints of the wrist, fingers, and toes, but over time it can affect the larger joints of the body as well as other organ systems.	Symptoms include: • Joint pain and stiffness that is usually worse in the morning • Fever and fatigue • Loss of appetite • Over time, symptoms might involve the skin, lungs, heart, kidneys, etc.
Fibromyalgia[24]	This complicated but highly prevalent syndrome is somewhat mysterious in origin but is thought to be due to a problem with the brain's ability to process pain, causing a heightened response. This is believed to be due to difficulties with monoaminergic neurotransmission.	Symptoms include: • Chronic musculoskeletal pain that is widespread • Heightened response to nociceptive (pain-producing) stimulation • Possible joint stiffness • Anxiety • Fatigue • Sleep disturbances
Meniere's disease[25,26]	A benign disorder of the inner ear that varies in severity and can either be lifelong or have a spontaneous remission. It typically starts in individuals between the age of 40 and 60 years.	Symptoms include: • Periodic sensations of vertigo (dizziness) lasting 20 minutes to 12 hours • Some hearing loss in the low- to mid-frequency • Tinnitus (ringing in the ears) • Endolymphatic hydrops (increase in hydrostatic pressure)
Addison's disease[27,28]	Another name for this is adrenal insufficiency, with insufficient amounts of cortisol and sometimes insufficient amounts of aldosterone. This is a **red flag** situation because it can be fatal if it goes undiagnosed.	Symptoms include: • Extreme fatigue • Sweating • Hypoglycemia (low blood sugar) • Stomach cramps • Muscle cramps • Diarrhea • Vomiting • Depression • Salt cravings

(Continued)

TABLE 11.6 Some of the More Common Autoimmune Disorders Often Seen by Occupational Therapy Practitioners—cont'd

Disorder	Pathophysiology	Symptoms
Ehlers-Danlos syndrome[29]	A disorder that affects the body's collagen. It has been classified into six different types: classical hypermobile, vascular, kyphoscoliotic, arthrochalasis, and dermatosparaxis. It can be focused primarily on the joints (hypermobile type) but can also affect every organ system, making it a possible **red flag** situation.	Individuals with this disorder vary widely with respect to symptoms, but most have the following: • Hyperextensibility of the skin • Skin that feels soft, doughy, and velvety • Delayed wound healing • Shoulder dislocations • Muscle weakness • Possible Parsonage-Turner syndrome[30] (another autoimmune disorder: inflammation of the brachial plexus leading to intense shoulder pain followed by arm and hand weakness or paralysis)
Ankylosing spondylitis[31]	This disorder causes inflammation in the spine making it appear bamboo-like in appearance on X-ray. It can affect the ankles, knees, and hips, and there may be symptoms of an eye disorder called uveitis, skin psoriasis, and intestinal disorders.	Symptoms include: • Joint pain and stiffness • Fatigue • Visual problems • Skin rashes • Kyphotic posture • Abdominal discomfort
Multiple sclerosis[32,33]	This is a condition that occurs when the immune system causes interruptions in the myelin sheath covering of the neurons in the brain and spinal cord, leading to a slowing or interruption of nerve impulses.	Symptoms include: • Visual problems • Balance problems • Numbness or weakness in the arms and legs • Muscle stiffness • Depression • Fatigue • Sexual dysfunction • Problems with urination
Type 1 diabetes[34]	Once known as insulin-dependent diabetes, or juvenile diabetes, this condition is caused by problems in the pancreas, leading to a decreased production of insulin. This can be life threatening if the sugar levels in the blood become too high, making this a possible **red flag** situation. There is no known cure, and intervention typically consists of insulin administration with diet and lifestyle changes.	Symptoms include: • Increased thirst • Bed wetting • Increased urination • Hunger • Weight loss • Fatigue • Blurry vision • Irritability
Lupus erythematosus[35,36]	This is a chronic condition consisting of inflammation and damage to various organ systems. It is believed that there are environmental triggers for this disorder such as infections or exposure to ultraviolet light.	Symptoms may include: • Fever • Edema (swelling) in the joints • Arthralgia (achy joints) • Fatigue • Skin rashes, most characteristically a butterfly-shaped rash on the face over the nose and cheeks (butterfly rash) • Hair loss • Pain in the chest when breathing (pleurisy) • Ankle swelling • Mouth or nose sores • Raynaud phenomenon (purple or blue fingers when stressed or cold)
Hashimoto's thyroiditis[37]	In this disorder, the body develops antibodies: thyroglobulin (Tg) and/or thyroid peroxidase (TPO) that damage or destroy parts of the thyroid gland. This can lead to inflammation causing goiter (enlarged thyroid gland) or cause the gland to wither away.	Symptoms include: • Fatigue • Abnormal weight gain • Constipation • High sensitivity to cold • Muscle aches • Difficulty exercising • Dry skin • Heavy or irregular menstrual periods • Slowed height in children

Application: Case Study

CASE EXAMPLE 11.1

A 16-year-old male was referred by his doctor to OT for help with dressing and transfers, after an episode of hemarthrosis in his left knee. The medical record reported that the client had hemophilia, but the hemarthrosis was under control, and the client needed to rest his leg and remain non–weight bearing (NWB) for another 2 weeks.

1. **Screen:** At the time of the first visit, the client presented to the OTR in good spirits with knee pain reported to be 3 out of 10. Although the knee had normal color and temperature on palpation, the OTR thought it might be beneficial to get a circumferential measure of the knee at the mid-patellar level during this visit. It measured 14¼ in (roughly 36.2 cm). He performed the light activities and NWB transfers with the OTR, and the OTR scheduled a return visit to check on the client's status 2 days later.
2. **Take a Closer Look:** The OTR had a COTA with her during the return visit. Both the OTR and the COTA were surprised that the client's reported pain level had increased to 6 out of 10. The knee appeared to be a bit more red in color and was warm on palpation. A new circumferential measurement was found to be 16 in (40.7 cm).
3. **Determine Flag Status:** Because of the client's diagnosis of hemophilia, the OTR felt that this was a red flag.
4. **Take Action if Needed:** The OTR contacted the doctor immediately and informed them of the situation. The client was asked to leave the OT clinic and proceed directly to the ER where his doctor would be waiting.
5. **Document the Findings:** The OTR documented the findings of the examination as well as the phone call to the physician.
6. **Take a Second Look:** Armed with this new information from the OTR, the doctor ordered an infusion of the missing clotting factor to stop the bleeding in this client's knee. After this stopped, draining techniques were initiated. Two days later, OT was again ordered for NWB transfers. The client was now in a protective knee brace.
7. **Determine the Flag Status:** The OTR and COTA proceeded with this as a yellow flag.
8. **Take Action if Needed:** Within 2 weeks, the client's knee was no longer swollen, the pain level was 2 out of 10, and he was able to upgrade his weight-bearing status and perform partial weight-bearing transfers with the OTR.

This is a true case. The client had a relapse of a recent hemarthrosis. Thanks to the careful observations of the OTR, and the circumferential measurements taken, the OTR was able to depict the amount of swelling to the physician, enabling the doctor to act quickly to not only prevent further damage to the knee but quite possibly to save the client's life.

References

1. Hopkins. *Hematology*. Johns Hopkins Medicine; 2023. https://www.hopkinsmedicine.org/health/treatment-tests-and-therapies/hematology.
2. Heick J, Lazaro RT. *Goodman and Snyder's Differential Diagnosis for Physical Therapists: Screening for Referral*. 7th ed. Elsevier; 2023.
3. Schatz P. *Microbiology*. OpenStax; 2023. https://openstax.org/books/microbiology/pages/1-introduction.
4. Cleveland Clinic. *Platelets*. Cleveland Clinic; 2023. https://my.clevelandclinic.org/health/body/22879-platelets.
5. Mayo Clinic. *Pediatric White Blood Disorders*. Mayo Clinic; 2023. https://www.mayoclinic.org/diseases-conditions/pediatric-white-blood-cell-disorders/symptoms-causes/syc-20352674?p=1.
6. CDC. *Sickle Cell Disease (SCD)*. Centers for Disease Control; 2023. https://www.cdc.gov/ncbddd/sicklecell/data.html.
7. Rogers K. *Plasma Cell: Biology*. Britannica; 2023. https://www.britannica.com/science/plasma-cell.
8. Tikkanen A. *Leukocytosis*. Britannica; 2023. https://www.britannica.com/science/leukocytosis.
9. Rogers K. *Leukocytosis*. Britannica; 2023. https://www.britannica.com/science/leukopenia.
10. Dong Y, Shi O, Zeng Q, et al. Leukemia incidence trends at the global, regional, and national level between 1990 and 2017. *Exp Hematol Oncol*. 2020;9(14):1–11. https://doi.org/10.1186/s40164-020-00170-6.
11. NIH. *Leukemia—Patient Version*. National Cancer Institute; 2023. https://www.cancer.gov/types/leukemia.
12. CDC. *Questions and Answers About Leukemia*. Centers for Disease Control and Prevention; 2023. https://www.cdc.gov/nceh/radiation/phase2/mleukemi.pdf.
13. Mayo Clinic. *Multiple Myeloma*. Mayo Clinic; 2022. https://www.mayoclinic.org/diseases-conditions/multiple-myeloma/symptoms-causes/syc-20353378.
14. Mayo Clinic. *Multiple Myeloma. Diagnosis and Treatment*. Mayo Clinic; 2022. https://www.mayoclinic.org/diseases-conditions/multiple-myeloma/diagnosis-treatment/drc-20353383multiple.
15. NIH. *Thrombocytopenia*. National Heart, Lung, and Blood Institute; 2022. https://www.nhlbi.nih.gov/health/thrombocytopenia.
16. Cleveland Clinic. *Thrombocytosis*. Cleveland Clinic; 2023. https://my.clevelandclinic.org/health/diseases/13350-thrombocytosis.
17. CDC. *How Hemophilia Is Inherited*. Centers for Disease Control and Prevention; 2022. https://www.cdc.gov/ncbddd/hemophilia/inheritance-pattern.html.
18. CDC. *Diagnosis of Hemophilia*. Centers for Disease Control and Prevention; 2022. https://www.cdc.gov/ncbddd/hemophilia/diagnosis.html.
19. Cleveland Clinic. *Immune System*. Cleveland Clinic; 2023. https://my.clevelandclinic.org/health/body/21196-immune-system.
20. NIH. *Overview of the Immune System*. National Institute of Allergy and Infectious Diseases, NIH; 2013. https://www.niaid.nih.gov/research/immune-system-overview.
21. Cleveland Clinic. *T Cekks*. Cleveland Clinic; 2023. https://my.clevelandclinic.org/health/body/24630-t-cells.
22. Autoimmune Association. *Autoimmune Disease List*. Autoimmune Association; 2025. https://www.niaid.nih.gov/diseases-conditions/autoimmune-diseases.
23. Mayo Clinic. *Rheumatoid Arthritis*. Mayo Clinic; 2023. https://www.mayoclinic.org/diseases-conditions/rheumatoid-arthritis/symptoms-causes/syc-20353648.
24. Jurado-Priego LN, Cueto-Ureña C, Ramírez-Expósito MJ, Martínez-Martos JM. Fibromyalgia: a review of the pathophysiological mechanisms and multidisciplinary treatment strategies. *Biomedicines*. 2024;12(7):1543. https://doi.org/10.3390/biomedicines12071543.
25. Rizk HG, Mehta NK, Qureshi U, et al. Pathogenesis and etiology of Ménière disease: a scoping review of a century of evidence. *JAMA Otolaryngol Head Neck Surg*. 2022;148(4):360–368. https://doi.org/10.1001/jamaoto.2021.4282.
26. Mayo Clinic. *Meniere's Disease*. Mayo Clinic; 2024. https://www.mayoclinic.org/diseases-conditions/menieres-disease/symptoms-causes/syc-20374910.

27. Røyrvik EC, Husebye ES. The genetics of autoimmune Addison disease: past, present and future. *Nat Rev Endocrinol.* 2022;18:399–412. https://doi.org/10.1038/s41574-022-00653-y.
28. Mayo Clinic. *Addison's Disease*. Mayo Clinic; 2024. https://www.mayoclinic.org/diseases-conditions/addisons-disease/symptoms-causes/syc-20350293.
29. Miklovic T, Sieg VC. Ehlers-Danlos syndrome. In: *StatPearls*. NIH; 2023. https://www.ncbi.nlm.nih.gov/books/NBK549814/.
30. Cleveland Clinic. *Parsonage-Turner Syndrome*. Cleveland Clinic; 2023. https://my.clevelandclinic.org/health/diseases/15390-parsonage-turner-syndrome.
31. NIH. *Ankylosing Spondylitis Basics*. NIH, National Institute of Arthritis and Musculoskeletal and Skin Diseases; 2023. https://www.niams.nih.gov/health-topics/ankylosing-spondylitis/basics/symptoms-causes.
32. Caporuscio J. MS lesions on the spine: what do you need to know? *Medical News Today*; 2022. https://www.medicalnewstoday.com/articles/ms-lesions-on-spine.
33. WHO. *Multiple Sclerosis*. World Health Organization; 2023. https://www.who.int/news-room/fact-sheets/detail/multiple-sclerosis.
34. Mayo Clinic. *Type 1 Diabetes*. Mayo Clinic; 2024. https://www.mayoclinic.org/diseases-conditions/type-1-diabetes/symptoms-causes/syc-20353011.
35. Arnaud L, Chasset F, Martin T. Immunopathogenesis of systemic lupus erythematosus: an update. *Autoimmun Rev*. 2024;23(10): https://doi.org/10.1016/j.autrev.2024.103648. 103648.
36. Gopal A. *Lupus: Causes and Treatments*. WebMD; 2024. https://www.webmd.com/lupus/arthritis-lupus.
37. ATA. *Hashimoto's Thyroiditis*. American Thyroid Association; 2025. https://www.thyroid.org/hashimotos-thyroiditis/.

12

Integumentary Pathophysiology

OBJECTIVES

By the end of this chapter, the reader should be able to:

- Demonstrate a basic understanding of various types of a healthy integumentary system.
- Demonstrate a basic understanding of various changes in the skin that could be due to underlying causes, not expected with the client's diagnosed condition.
- Categorize the various integumentary symptoms associated with hematologic, gastrointestinal, and other systemic disorders.
- Classify possible rashes and skin lesions associated with various disorders.
- Differentiate between a skin lesion that is benign and one that could be cancerous.
- Assess and justify whether a specific integumentary symptom could constitute a yellow or red flag.

Healthy Physiology

Human skin is the largest organ of the body, protecting the individual from hazards in the environment, working to regulate the body's temperature, storing water and fat, and manufacturing vitamin D with the help of the sun.[1] Many disorders of the human body are manifested by changes in the skin that can be detected by an observant occupational therapy practitioner (OTP).

Histology—The System on a Cellular Level

The skin is composed of three layers, namely, the epidermis, the dermis, and the subcutaneous layer (i.e., the hypodermis)[1] (Fig. 12.1)

Epidermis. This layer is the protective layer that makes new skin and provides skin color.[2] It consists of two cell types: keratinocytes (that make up about 90% of the epidermis) and melanocytes (found at the base of the epidermis).[1] Keratinocytes play an essential role not just in the protection of the body but also in tissue repair. These cells begin the reepithelialization process, by traveling to the wound, replicating, and differentiating to rebuild the skin.[3] These cells also help contract the wound together and host the immune response during wound healing.[3] Melanocytes originate from neural crest cells and have the ability to produce melanin.[4] They are found in what is called the basal layer of the epidermis.[4] Melanin is a pigment with a high refractive index (enabling control of electromagnetic wavelengths offering protection against UV rays) and stiffness (which enhances the strength of the skin).[5] The melanin produced is stored in the melanosomes in the keratinocytes (Fig. 12.2).

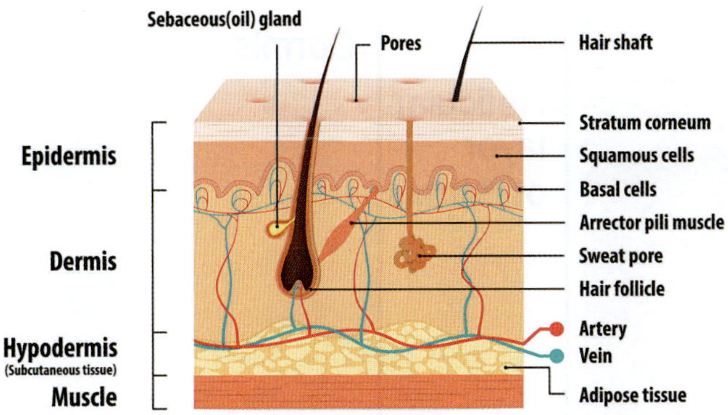

• **Fig. 12.1** The three layers of human skin. (From iStock.com/Paladjai.)

Dermis. The dermis is the second layer, held together by collagen protein, containing the blood vessels, hair follicles, sweat glands, lymph vessels, and nerves (Fig. 12.3).[1] This layer also offers protection for the body. It supports the epidermis and allows for different sensations via receptors as well as the production of sweat and hair.[6] The deeper layer of the dermis is called the reticular dermis. It is a thick layer containing blood vessels, nerves, glands, hair follicles, and fat cells. The more superficial layer of the dermis is called the papillary dermis. It is a thin layer made up of collagen fibers, fat cells, fibroblast cells (these produce collagen), Meissner corpuscles (touch receptors), and phagocytes (cells that fight bacteria).[6]

Subcutaneous Layer (Hypodermis). This layer of the skin connects the dermis to the underlying muscles and bones. It insulates your body, protects, and produces adipocytes (fat cells) that store energy.[7] The hypodermis contains adipose

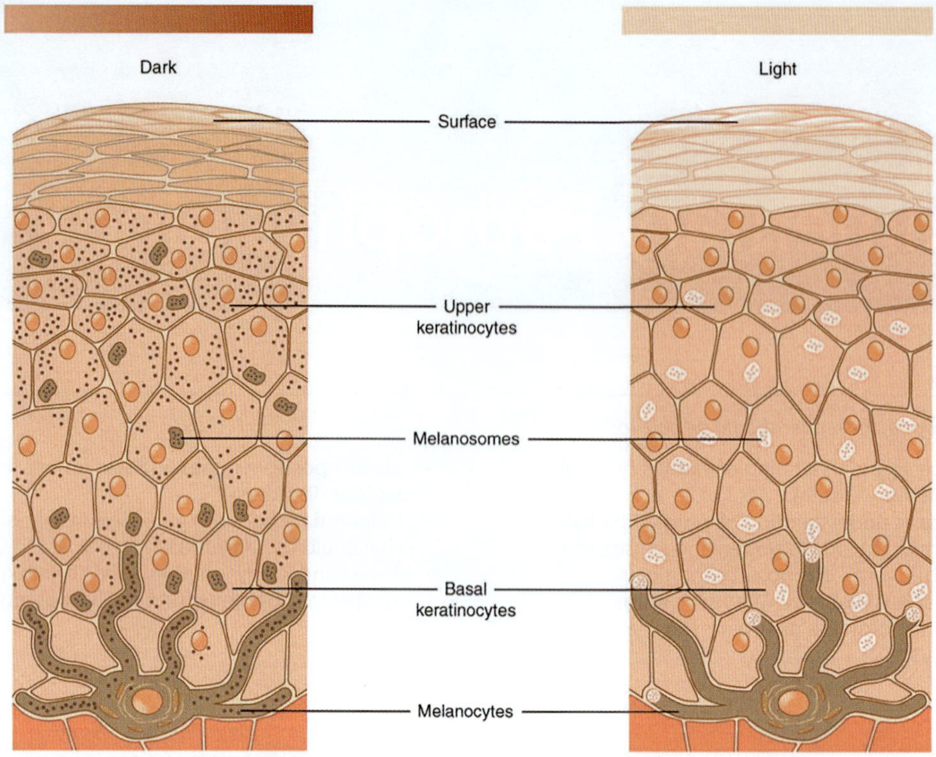

• **Fig. 12.2** The epidermis depicting the keratinocytes and melanocytes. (From https://courses.lumenlearning.com/wm-biology2/chapter/pigmentation/.)

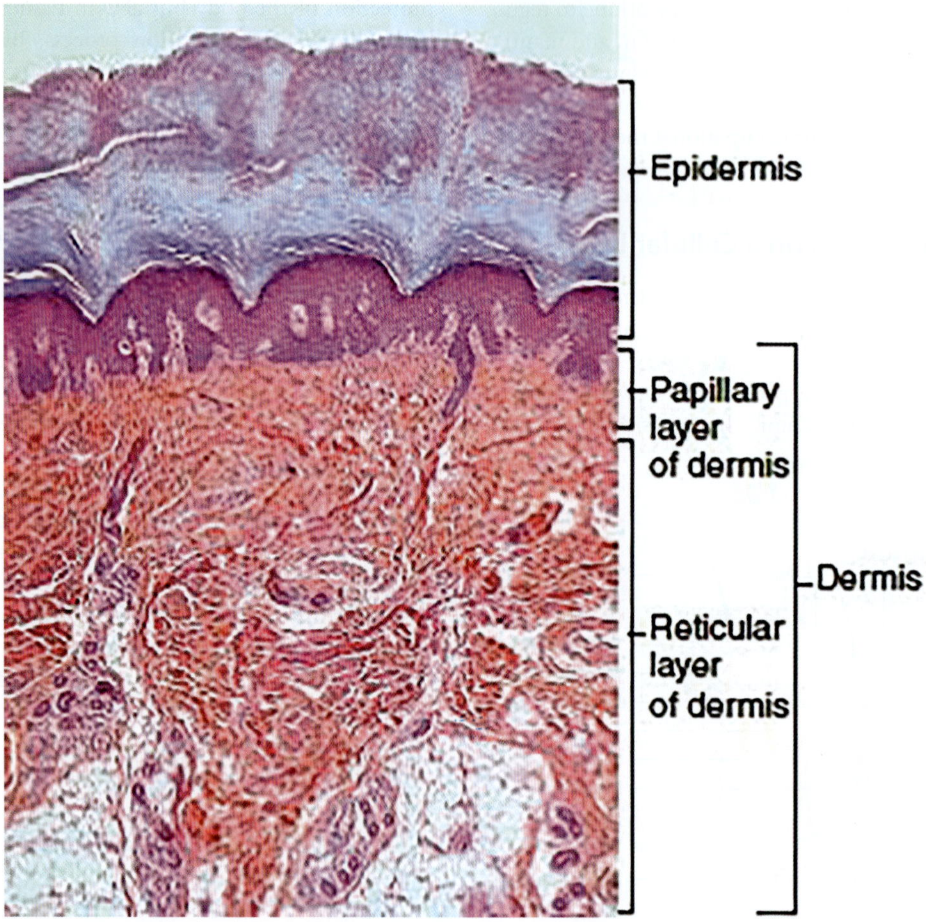

• **Fig. 12.3** The dermis. (From http://encyclopedia.lubopitko-bg.com/structureofskin.html.)

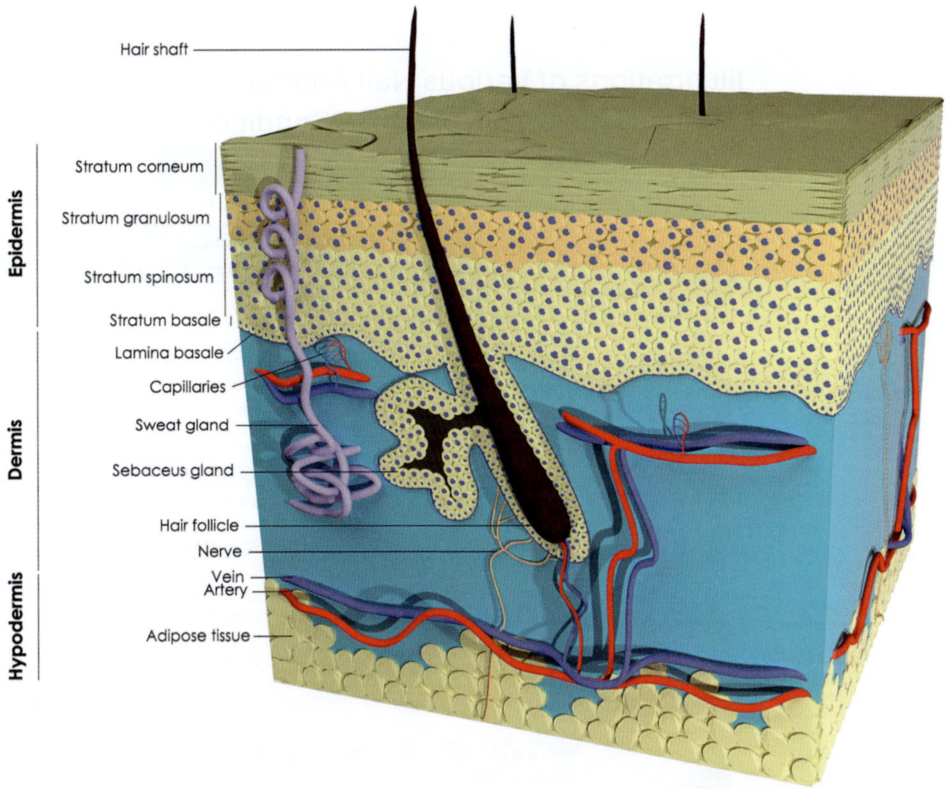

• **Fig. 12.4** The hypodermis. (From iStock.com/MeletiosVerras.)

tissue (fatty tissue), connective tissue, fibroblasts, hair follicles, sweat glands, nerves, macrophages (white blood cells that attack microbes), and lymphatic vessels[7] (Fig. 12.4).

Signs and Symptoms of Skin Disorders

An OTP can learn a great deal about a client's health by closely observing the skin. In Chapter 11, some of the skin changes that can accompany hematological conditions were discussed. A few more details follow, along with possible skin changes associated with other bodily systems.

Skin Changes due to Hematological Conditions

A close look at the client's hands can give some important clues to possible hematological conditions. It is advised that the hands are warm and held at heart level during this observation.[8] If the skin is light yellow in color, it could be an indication of pernicious anemia. If hands are pale, it could mean anemia, but if hands are white and waxy in appearance, it could be an indication of severe anemia.[8] A gray-green yellow color indicates chronic blood loss, but a gray tint alone could mean leukemia. Brittle and/or concave nail beds (i.e., spoon nails) could mean iron-deficiency anemia.[8] Some common nail changes and associations with various disorders can be found in Fig. 12.5. More about hematological conditions can be found in Chapter 11.

Skin Changes due to Cardiopulmonary Conditions

Pressure ulcers, loss of body hair, and cyanosis (bluish discoloration of the lips and nail beds) could be indicative of a possible cardiovascular problem.[8] Cyanosis is also a possible indicator of pulmonary issues as is clubbing of the fingers and toes (widening of the distal phalanges to look like a club, see Fig. 12.5).[8] More about cardiopulmonary conditions can be found in Chapters 13 and 14.

Skin Changes due to Gastrointestinal, Hepatic, and Biliary Conditions

Hyperesthesia (extra sensitive skin to sensory stimulation) and hyperalgesia (increased sensitivity to noxious stimulation) can be indicators of a gastrointestinal problem.[8] This is due to a problem in the viscera causing afferent impulses that trigger a sympathetic nervous response, leading to itching,

Illustrations of Various Nail Anomalies Potentially Indicative of Other Conditions

Picture	Name	
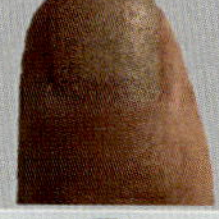	Nail Pitting*– Small round notches or depressions in the nails.	This is more common in individuals with various types of skin disorders like psoriasis or eczema.
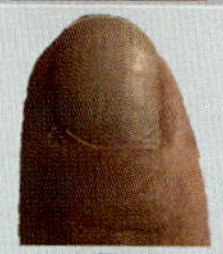	Clubbing of the Nails*– When the nail curves around the fingertips.	This is more common in individuals with low blood oxygen levels, heart or lung disease, or gastrointestinal problems.
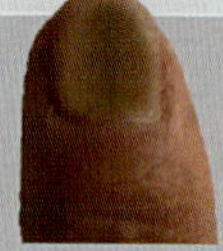	Koilonychia*– Also called spoon nails, when the nails are indented and curled up along the edges.	This can be a symptom of iron deficiency or a condition of the liver called hemochromatosis.
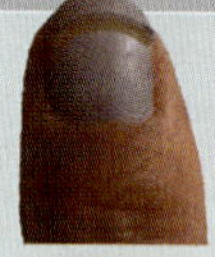	Terry's Nails**– Most of the nail appears white except for a thin band of brown or pink near the tip.	This can be a sign of normal aging or possibly a sign of liver disease.
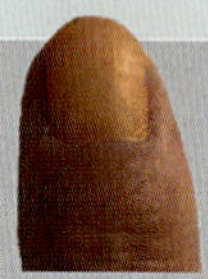	Yellow Nails ***- Yellowish nail discoloration.	This is typically caused by a fungal infection but can also be due to thyroid disease, diabetes, lung disease, or psoriasis.
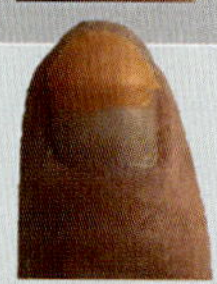	Onycholysis ****– The separation of the nail from the nail bed.	This can be a sign of psoriasis, hyperthyroidism, infection, trauma, or a connective tissue disorder.
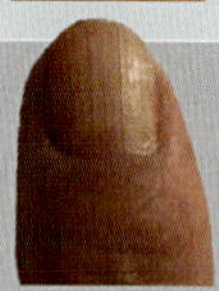	Beau's Lines **** - Lines or grooves that run from the base of the nail toward the tip.	This can be caused by any systemic illness that can disrupt nail growth, trauma, or Raynaud's disease.

• **Fig. 12.5** Nail changes and associations with various conditions. (*Information is from: The Mayo Clinic. https://www.mayoclinic.org/healthy-lifestyle/adult-health/in-depth/7-fingernail-problems-not-to-ignore/art-20546860. **Information is from: The Cleveland Clinic. https://my.clevelandclinic.org/health/symptoms/22890-terrys-nails. ***Information is from Wed MD. https://www.webmd.com/skin-problems-and-treatments/ss/slideshow-nails-and-health. ****Information is from AAFP. https://www.aafp.org/pubs/afp/issues/2004/0315/p1417.html.)

perspiration, or other sudomotor changes. Because the viscera do not perceive pain, these sympathetic sudomotor changes help inform a person that something is wrong.[8] Skin changes associated with the hepatic and biliary system include jaundice (yellowing of the whites of the eyes and/or the skin, Fig. 12.6), which is due to a buildup of bilirubin levels in the blood. Pruritus (itching) and bruising might also occur. Spider angiomas (branched dilated superficial capillaries, Fig. 12.7) and palmar erythema (redness) can be signs of liver disease.[8] More about this can be found in Chapters 15 and 16.

Skin Changes due to Urogenital Conditions

Pruritus (itchy skin), ecchymosis (bruises under the skin), thin brittle nails, smell of urine on the skin, uremic frost (the appearance of white urea crystals on the face and upper trunk, Fig. 12.8), and pallor can all be signs of kidney disease.[8]

Chancres (painless sores) can be an indication of syphilis (Fig. 12.9), and Kaposi sarcoma (a type of cancer that can form red, brown, or purple blotchy lesions on the skin) can

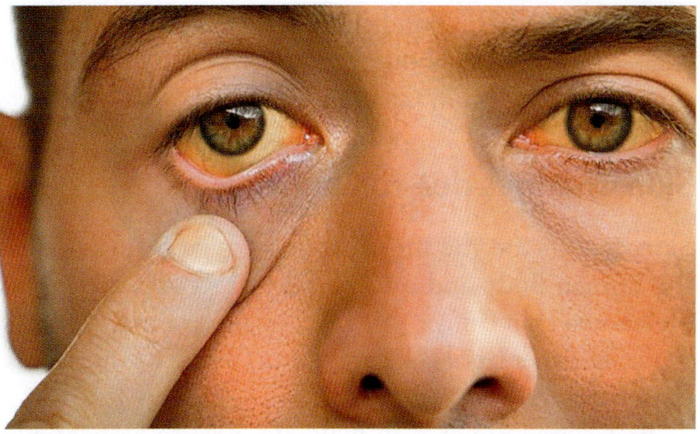

• **Fig. 12.6** Jaundice. (From Daria Kulkova/iStock via Getty Images.)

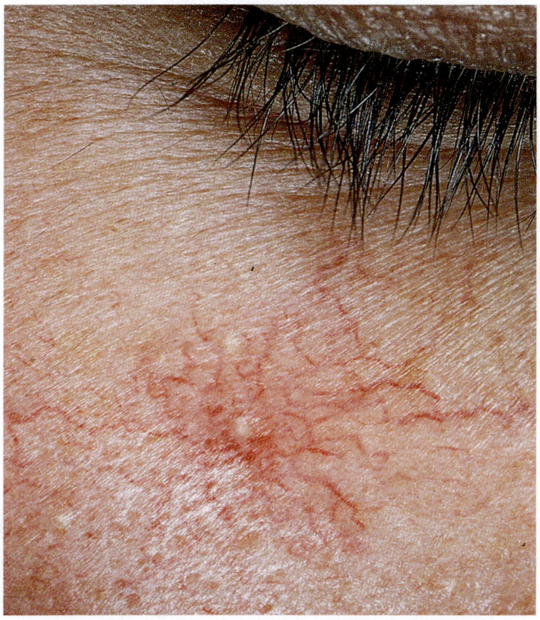

• **Fig. 12.7** Spider angioma. (From Dinulous JGH. *Habif's Clinical Dermatology: A Color Guide to Diagnosis and Therapy*. 7th ed. Elsevier; 2021.)

sometimes be found on clients with AIDS (Fig. 12.10). More about urogenital conditions can be found in Chapter 17.

Skin Changes due to Endocrine and Metabolic Conditions

There are many skin changes that can be associated with metabolic or endocrine conditions. Heat intolerance, easy hair breakage, increased skin pigmentation, and onycholysis (separation of the nails from the nail beds) can be indicators of hyperthyroidism.[8] A purple hardened area over the anterior tibia (thyroid dermopathy), although rare, can also be indicative of hyperthyroidism, and when this is present, the client will almost always have some sort of ophthalmic pathology (eye disease) (Fig. 12.11).[9]

Myxedema (boggy swelling and possible thickening of the skin that can be life-threatening), scaly skin, coarse thinning hair, intolerance to cold, non-pitting edema, and thick, cool, dry skin can all be indicative of hypothyroidism.[8] Dry scaly skin, thinning of the hair, and brittle finger nails can be indicative of hypoparathyroidism. Xanthomas (small fatty lumps under the skin) and fat deposits with yellow patches on the eyelids can be indicative of hyperlipidemia

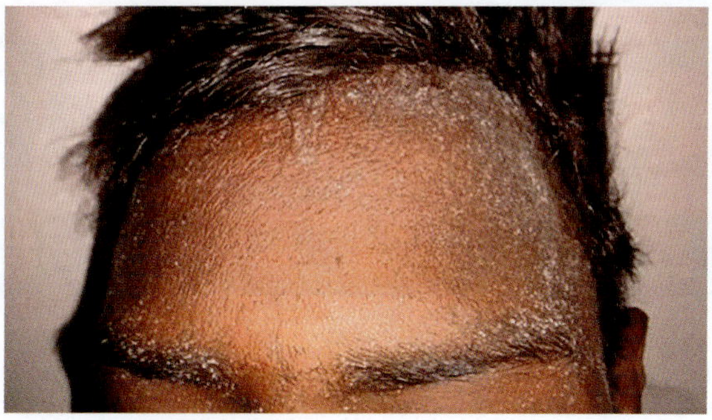

• **Fig. 12.8** Uremic frost. (From Mathur M, et al. Uremic frost. *Clin Kidney J*. 2014;7(4):418–419.)

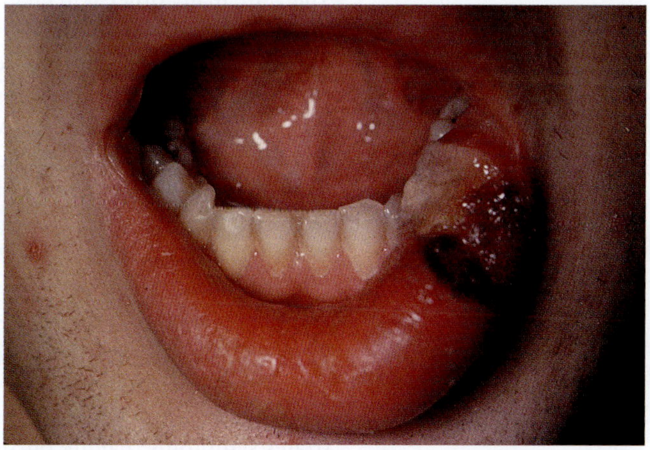

• **Fig. 12.9** Chancre from syphilis. (From Elston, DM, et al. Cutaneous signs and diagnosis. In: *Andrew's Diseases of the Skin*. 14th ed. Elsevier; 2026.)

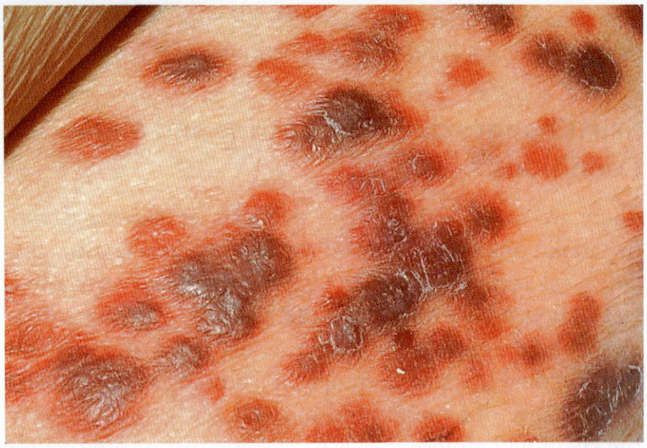

• **Fig. 12.10** Kaposi sarcoma. (From https://en.wikipedia.org/wiki/Kaposi%27s_sarcoma.)

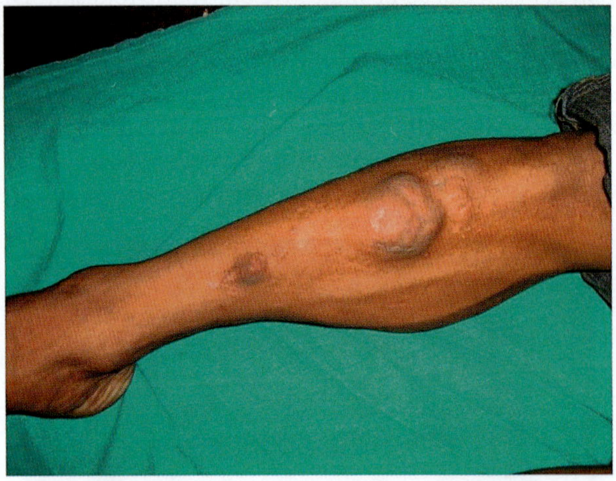

• **Fig. 12.11** Thyroid dermopathy: nodules and tumors over the skin of the anterior tibia. (From Dhali TK, Chahar M. Thyroid dermopathy—a diagnostic clue of hidden hyperthyroidism. *Dermato-Endocrinology*, 2014;6(1):e981078. https://doi.org/10.4161/19381980.2014.981078.)

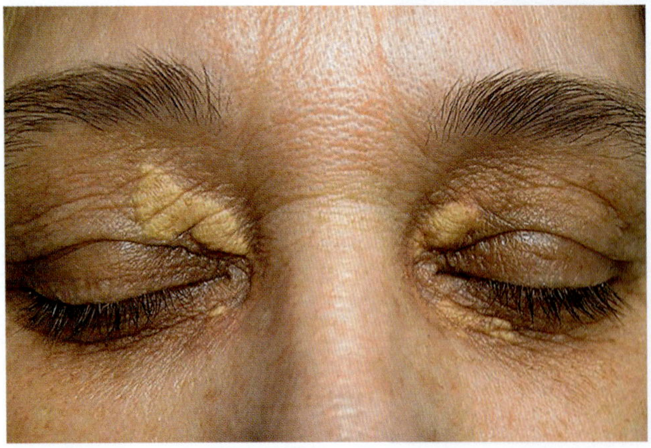

• **Fig. 12.12** Xanthelasma. (Image used with permission from AllAboutVision.com, http://www.allaboutvision.com.)

from diabetes.[8] This condition is also known as xanthelasma (Fig. 12.12). More about endocrine and metabolic conditions can be found in Chapter 18.

Skin Changes due to Cancer

Skin cancers are the most common type of malignancy in the human body and are typically classified as either non-melanoma skin cancer (NMSC) or melanoma. NMSCs are typically either basal cell carcinoma (BCC) or squamous cell carcinoma (SCC) (Fig. 12.13).[10]

BCCs are estimated to make up 50% to 80% of all skin cancers. They are slow-growing, rarely metastasize, and found in the more sun-exposed areas of the skin, such as the head, neck, and back.[10] SCCs are estimated to make up about 20% to 50% of all skin cancers. These are also slow-growing and found in the more sun-exposed areas of the skin, but they are more likely to metastasize than BCCs.[10] Melanomas make up only about 1% of all skin cancers.[10] Although melanoma is the most fatal type of skin cancer, there is a 92.5% survival rate if caught early before any metastasis (a spread to other parts of the body) has occurred.[8] If it has already spread, however, there is only a 25% chance of a 5-year survival.[8] Melanomas can be found anywhere on the body regardless of sun exposure.[10] Merkel cell carcinoma can also occur but is extremely rare, highly aggressive, and found in the more sun-exposed areas of the skin.

The OTP needs to be aware of potential skin changes that could be cancerous. A changing mole, or the appearance of a new mole, merits attention. The Skin Cancer Foundation advocates for the use of the "ABCDE method" of early detection of melanoma (Fig. 12.14).

Risk factors for skin cancer include advanced age, a family history of skin cancer, moles with the ABCDE features, fair complexion, skin that is easily sunburned, use of tanning beds or lamps, short intense bouts in the sun, or transplant recipients.[8]

Skin Changes due to Other Conditions

There are many other skin changes that can occur with various infections or disorders. Rheumatoid nodules (firm lumps under the skin near affected joints) can sometimes occur with rheumatoid arthritis. Shingles (herpes zoster) produces a painful rash (Fig. 12.15).[11] When a Lyme-infected deer tick bites, the result can be a bull's-eye rash, also called erythema migrans (Fig. 12.16). Shiny, silvery patches can be seen with psoriasis (Fig. 12.17), and a red rash over the nose and cheeks can be seen with systemic lupus erythematosus (Fig. 12.18).

The OT Scope of Practice

Once again, when working as an OTP, if a client demonstrates symptoms that are outside of the typical cluster you expect to find with their diagnosis, it is important to report those symptoms to the referring physician.

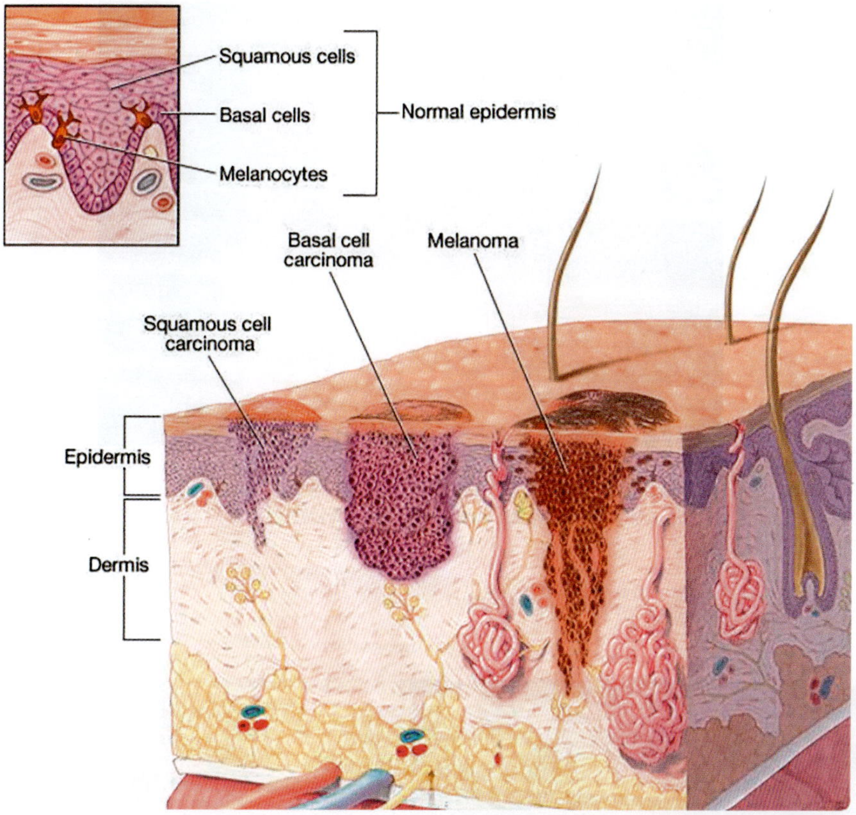

• **Fig. 12.13** Types of skin cancer. (From https://www.mayoclinic.org/diseases-conditions/basal-cell-carcinoma/symptoms-causes/syc-20354187, used with permission of Mayo Foundation for Medical Education and Research. All rights reserved.)

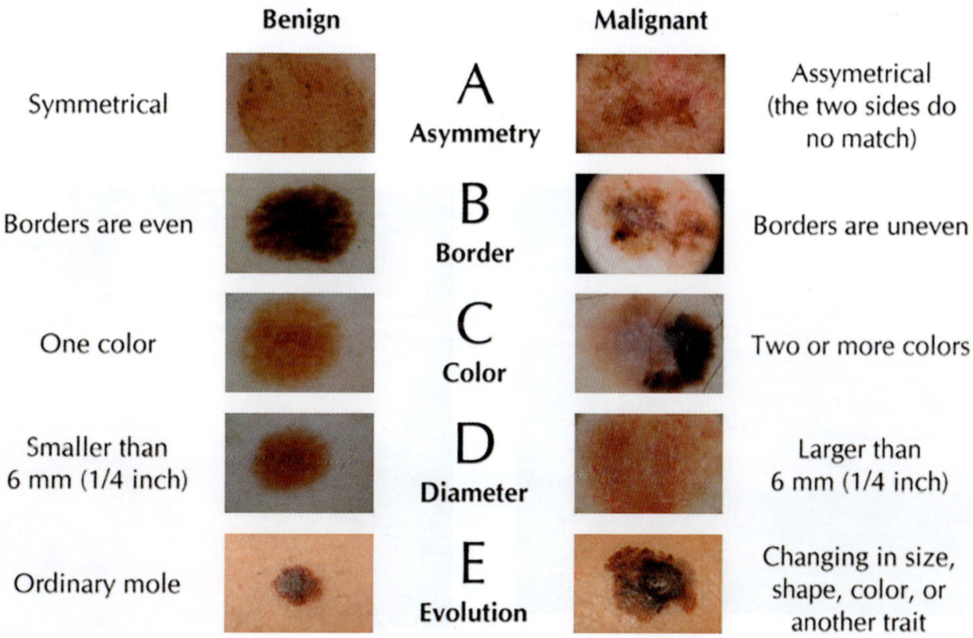

• **Fig. 12.14** The ABCDE method of melanoma detection. (© AIM at Melanona Foundation.)

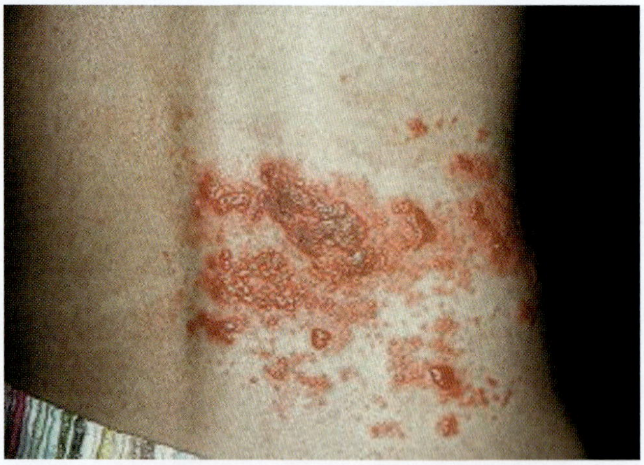

• **Fig. 12.15** Shingles (herpes zoster). (From Whitley RJ. Chickenpox and herpes zoster. In: Bennett JE, Dolin R, Blaser MJ, eds. *Mandell, Douglas, and Bennett's Principles and Practice of Infectious Diseases*. 8th ed. Elsevier; 2015.)

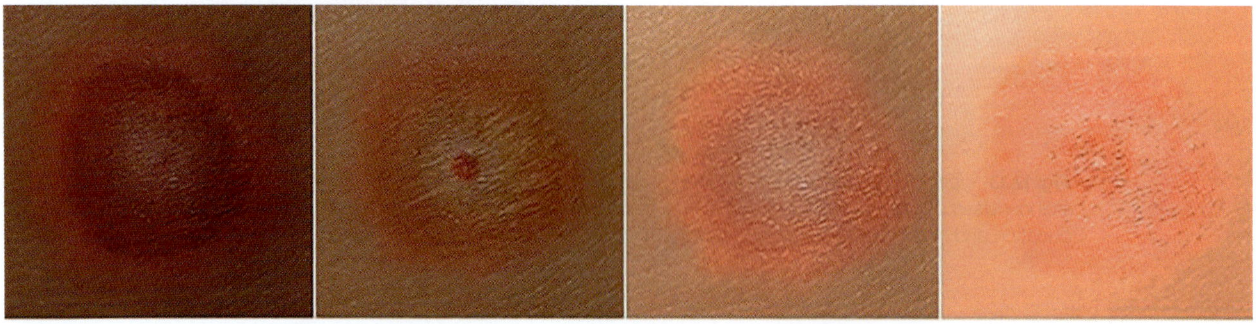

• **Fig. 12.16** Bull's-eye rash (erythema migrans) from Lyme-infected tick bite. (From https://www.mayoclinic.org/diseases-conditions/lyme-disease/symptomscauses/syc-20374651, used with permission of Mayo Foundation for Medical Education and Research. All rights reserved.)

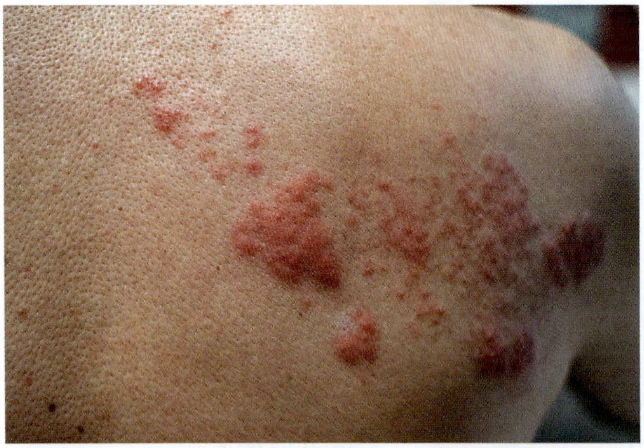

• **Fig. 12.17** Psoriasis. (From https://iStock.com/Mumemories.)

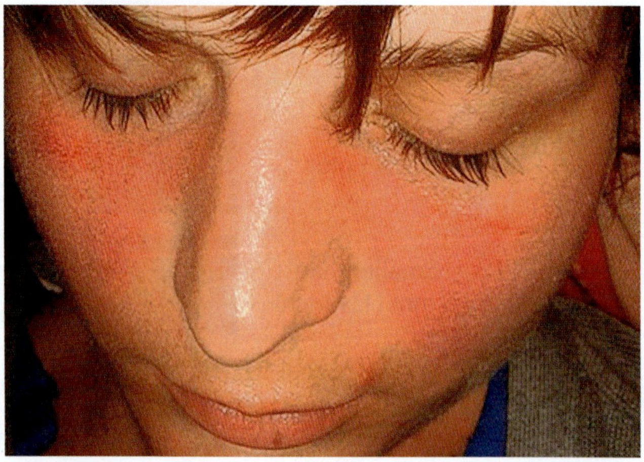

• **Fig. 12.18** Systemic lupus erythematosus. (From Doktorinternet, CC BY-SA 4.0, via Wikimedia Commons.)

Application—Case Study

CASE EXAMPLE 12.1

An OTP was performing ergonomic screenings for desk workers in a local business. One of the employees, a 45-year-old male, showed the OTP a mole on his left forearm that had changed over the past 2 months, getting bigger and "mottled."

1. **Screen:** The OTP measured the mole to be 7 mm in diameter, with uneven borders.
2. **Take a Closer Look:** The OTP took a picture of the mole and requested that the client allow her to send the picture to his physician. The client agreed. The OTP sent it to the doctor with a note documenting size, asymmetry, and mottled colors.
3. **Determine Flag Status:** Not having seen the individual prior, the OTP had no basis for comparison, but based on the individual's statement of recent change, the OTP considered this to be a potential red flag.
4. **Take Action if Needed:** The physician was able to see the client the next day and took a biopsy for the mole.
5. **Document the Findings:** The OTP documented the interaction with the physician and sent all relevant information to the physician's office with client consent.
6. **Take a Second Look:** The biopsy came back positive for melanoma, and the mole was removed by the physician.
7. **Determine the Flag Status:** The physician agreed with the OTP's determination that this was definitively a red flag, but the OTP's quick action may have saved the man's life.
8. **Take Action if Needed:** The client was extremely grateful needing no other intervention after the mole was removed. He stopped into the OTP's clinic with roses and a thank you card from his wife.

This is a true case and another example of occupational therapy advocacy, demonstrating the importance of thinking outside the box and the potential to save a life.

References

1. Hopkins. *Anatomy of the Skin*. Johns Hopkins Medicine; 2023. https://www.hopkinsmedicine.org/health/skin/anatomy-of-the-skin.
2. Cleveland Clinic. *Skin*. Cleveland Clinic; 2021. https://my.clevelandclinic.org/health/articles/10978-skin.
3. Piipponen M, Li D, Landén NX. The immune functions of keratinocytes in skin wound healing. *Int J Mol Sci*. 2020;21:8790. https://doi.org/10.3390/ijms21228790.
4. Cichorek M, Wachulska M, Stasiewicz A, Tymińska A. Skin melanocytes: biology and development. *Postepy Dermatol Alergol*. 2013;30(1):30–41. https://doi.org/10.5114/pdia.2013.33376.
5. D'Alba L, Shawkey MD. Melanosomes: biogenesis, properties, and evolution of an ancient organelle. *Physiol Rev*. 2018;99:1–19. https://doi.org/10.1152/physrev.00059.2017.
6. Cleveland Clinic. *Dermis*. Cleveland Clinic; 2022. https://my.clevelandclinic.org/health/body/22357-dermis.
7. Cleveland Clinic. *Hypodermis (Subcutaneous Tissue)*. Cleveland Clinic; 2021. https://my.clevelandclinic.org/health/body/21902-hypodermis-subcutaneous-tissue.
8. Heick J, Lazaro RT. *Goodman and Snyder's Differential Diagnosis for Physical Therapists: Screening for Referral*. 7th ed. Elsevier; 2023.
9. Dhali TK, Chahar M. Thyroid dermopathy—a diagnostic clue of hidden hyperthyroidism. *Dermatoendocrinology*. 2014;6(1):e981078. https://doi.org/10.4161/19381980.2014.981078.
10. Poon D. *Skin Cancer in Singapore—When the Most Visible Shows up in Camouflage*. Dr. D.H.Y Poon Associates; 2017. https://dyhpoon.com/skin-cancer-in-singapore-when-the-most-visible-cancer-shows-up-in-camouflage/.
11. MedLine. *Shingles*. MedLine Plus; 2023. https://medlineplus.gov/shingles.html.

13

Cardiovascular Pathophysiology

OBJECTIVES

By the end of this chapter, the reader should be able to:

- Demonstrate a basic understanding of a healthy cardiovascular system.
- Demonstrate a basic understanding of pathophysiological conditions affecting the heart, the heart's valves, vasculature, and nervous system.
- Identify possible symptoms associated with various cardiovascular disorders.
- Assess and justify whether a specific cardiovascular symptom could constitute a yellow or red flag.
- Categorize the various symptoms associated with the heart, the valves, vasculature, and nervous system.
- Explain and/or predict the possible symptoms resulting from the pathophysiology of various cardiovascular disorders.

Healthy Cardiovascular Physiology

The cardiovascular system consists of the heart and the vascular network. The following is a very brief overview of the physiology of the healthy heart.

Gross Anatomy of the Heart

The adult heart consists of four chambers, with blood circulating from the superior and inferior vena cava, into the right atrium, then through the tricuspid valve, and into the right ventricle. From there, the blood is passed through the pulmonary valve into the pulmonary artery to the lungs. After the blood is oxygenated in the lungs, it returns via the pulmonary veins into the left atrium of the heart, then through the bicuspid valve (mitral valve) to the left ventricle, and finally from the aortic valve to the rest of the body via the aorta (Fig. 13.1).[1,2] The term *heart rate* refers to the number of times your heart beats per minute, and the *stroke volume* is the amount of blood that is pumped to the body with each heartbeat.[1] When you multiply these together, you get the amount of blood pumped by the ventricle each minute, or the *cardiac output*.[3]

Stimulation for cardiac contraction in the adult heart begins at the sinoatrial node (the heart's pacemaker),[4] travels to the autonomic nerve and ganglion cells, and next to the atrioventricular (AV) node, which delays the impulse slightly to allow the atria some time to empty before ventricular contraction.[5,6] The impulse is then sent from the AV node to the bundle of His, which stimulates the right and left bundle branches, and onto the ventricles, where the stimulus is picked up by the Purkinje fibers, which innervate the ventricles and causes them to contract. Then, the cycle begins again[7] (Fig. 13.2).

Histology of the Human Heart

The heart is located in an area of the thoracic cavity known as the mediastinum.[8] The human heart has three layers: the endocardium, the myocardium, and the pericardium. The endocardium is the thin inner lining of the heart chambers and the surface of the heart valves.[2] This layer consists of simple squamous epithelium and some vascularized connective tissue.[8] The myocardium is the thicker middle layer consisting of muscle cells called cardiomyocytes. These cells are branched in a linear manner, and the layer is well vascularized.[2,8] The pericardium is a saclike structure that covers the outside of the heart.[2] It consists of a two-layered connective tissue sheath. The innermost layer of the pericardium, called the epicardium, is lubricated with adipocytes to enable smooth motion of the heart (Fig. 13.3).

The Vasculature

The vascular system consists of arteries that take blood from the heart to the body and veins that return blood from the body back to the heart. There are three types of arteries: elastic (or conducting), muscular (or distributing), and arterioles.[9,10] The elastic arteries have characteristically more elastic tissue than muscle tissue, enabling them to expand and contract more easily to allow for surges of blood. Examples of elastic arteries are the aorta and the pulmonary artery, the ones closest to the heart.[9,10] The muscular arteries

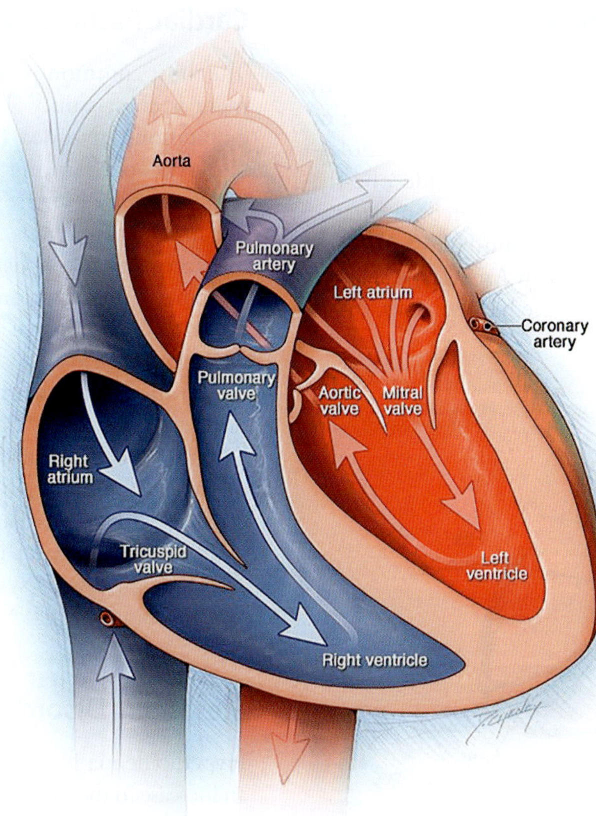

• **Fig. 13.1** The flow of blood in the heart. (From https://www.mayoclinic.org/chambers-and-valves-of-the-heart/img-20007497, used with permission of Mayo Foundation for Medical Education and Research. All rights reserved.)

consist of more muscular tissue than elastic, which helps them control blood flow more easily. Examples of muscular arteries include the femoral arteries and the coronary arteries.[9,10] These larger arteries eventually branch into smaller vessels called arterioles that distribute blood to the tissues via even smaller microscopic blood vessels called capillaries. Capillaries have very thin walls, consisting of a single endothelial layer, so this is the ideal environment for diffusion to take place, the passage of metabolites and nutrients between the blood and the body (Figs. 13.4 and 13.5).[11]

Each artery has three layers: the tunica intima, the tunica media, and the tunica adventitia. The tunica intima is the innermost layer with elastic membranes to enable the blood to flow more easily. The tunica media is the thickest layer consisting of elastin and smooth muscle fibers. The tunica adventitia is the outermost layer that consists of elastin and collagen fibers for added strength to help control blood pressure (BP) (Fig. 13.6).

There are four types of veins: deep veins, superficial veins, perforating veins, and venules. The deep veins are typically found deep in the muscles of the body and run alongside the bones. The deep veins in the lower extremities hold about 90% of the blood returning to the heart.[12] These veins have valves that keep the blood traveling in the correct direction. Superficial veins are typically smaller and can be found just underneath the skin. Perforating veins are short veins that carry blood from the superficial veins to the deep veins.[12] Venules, the smallest veins, receive blood from the capillaries to initiate the return to the heart. Venules are very thin, fragile, and permeable, and can help assist in the exchange of oxygen and nutrients[11] (Fig. 13.5).

Each vein also has three layers: the tunica intima, the tunica media, and the tunica adventitia. Their function is very similar to that of the arteries with some notable differences. Veins contain valves that prevent the back flow of blood and keep it moving in one direction.[12] Veins also have thinner and less muscular walls with a lower resultant pressure. Arteries will beat and contract with the rhythm of the heart, but veins simply guide blood flow return via the arterial BP and the one-way valves.[12]

In a healthy cardiovascular system, the blood goes from the aorta to the elastic and muscular arteries, to the arterioles, to the capillaries, to the venules, to the veins, to the inferior and superior vena cava, and back through the chambers of the heart.[12]

Cardiovascular Pathophysiology

Cardiovascular disease (CVD) is the leading cause of death in the United States, and 47% of Americans have one or more of the three high-risk factors: high BP, high cholesterol, and smoking.[13] Other risk factors include obesity, advanced age, sedentary lifestyle, excessive alcohol intake, oral contraceptive use, tobacco use, family history, and race (with African Americans, Mexican Americans, Native Americans, and Pacific Islanders at the highest risk).[13]

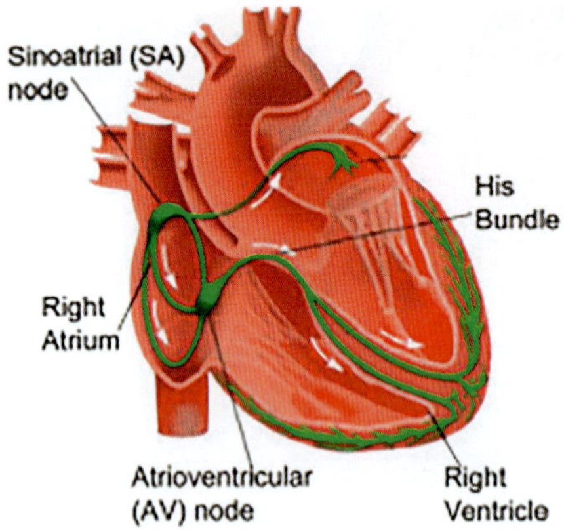

• **Fig. 13.2** The electrical stimulation of the heart. (From Jiang Z, et al. *Modeling and Verification of a Dual Chamber Implantable Pacemaker*. Springer Nature. https://link.springer.com/chapter/10.1007/978-3-642-28756-5_14.)

Cardiac Pathology

The most common presenting symptom of cardiac involvement is chest pain.[13] The individual might also experience palpitations, dyspnea (shortness of breath, or SOB), cardiac syncope (fainting or lightheadedness), fatigue, cough (aggravated by exercise or the supine position), cyanosis of the nail beds and lips, edema (a weight gain of 3 pounds or more over a few days, with swelling in the ankles and abdomen), claudication (pain in the lower extremities with movement), abnormal heart rate, or a systolic BP that falls during exercise.[13]

Cardiac muscle pathology is typically caused by obstruction (coronary artery disease, or CAD), inflammation (pericarditis), or dilation/distention (aneurysms).[13] Disorders that affect the heart valves include rheumatic fever, endocarditis, mitral valve prolapse, and congenital deformities that will be discussed later in this chapter. Disorders that affect the cardiac nervous system include arrhythmias, tachycardia, and bradycardia.[13]

Metabolic Disorders Affecting the Heart

Hyperlipidemia is a group of metabolic disorders that lead to an increase in the low-density lipoproteins (LDLs) in the blood. These LDLs cause a sludgy buildup in the walls of the arteries.[13] High-density lipoproteins (HDLs) can help to scrape away that sludge and clear the arteries for blood to pass through; unfortunately with a high level of LDLs, this is less possible, and thus

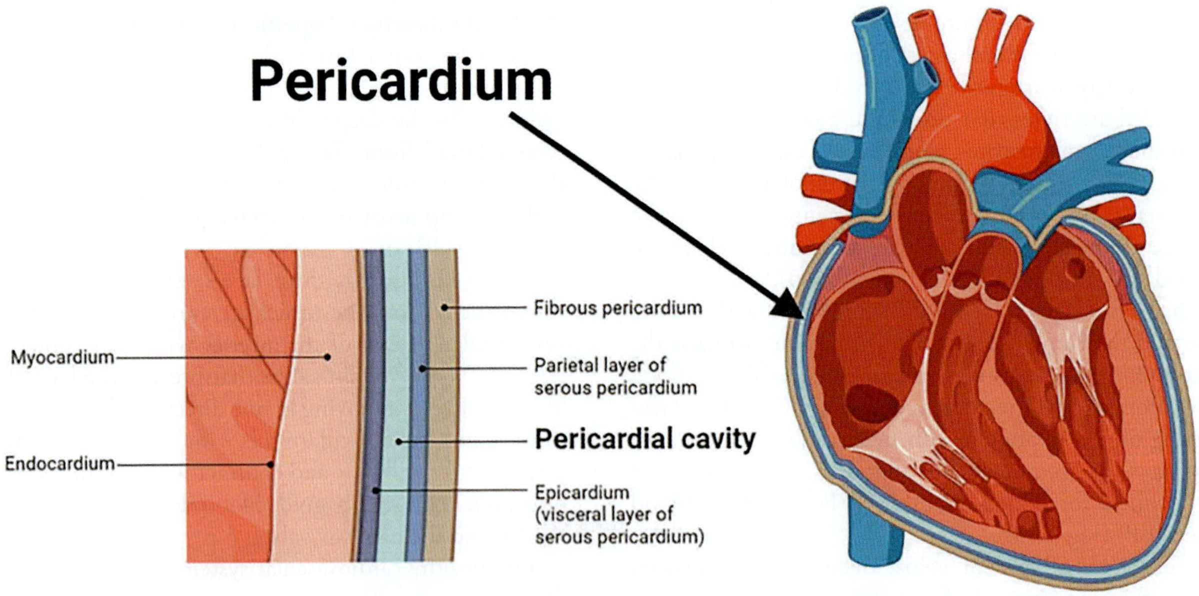

• **Fig. 13.3** The layers of the human heart. (From https://microbenotes.com/pericardium-structure-functions/.)

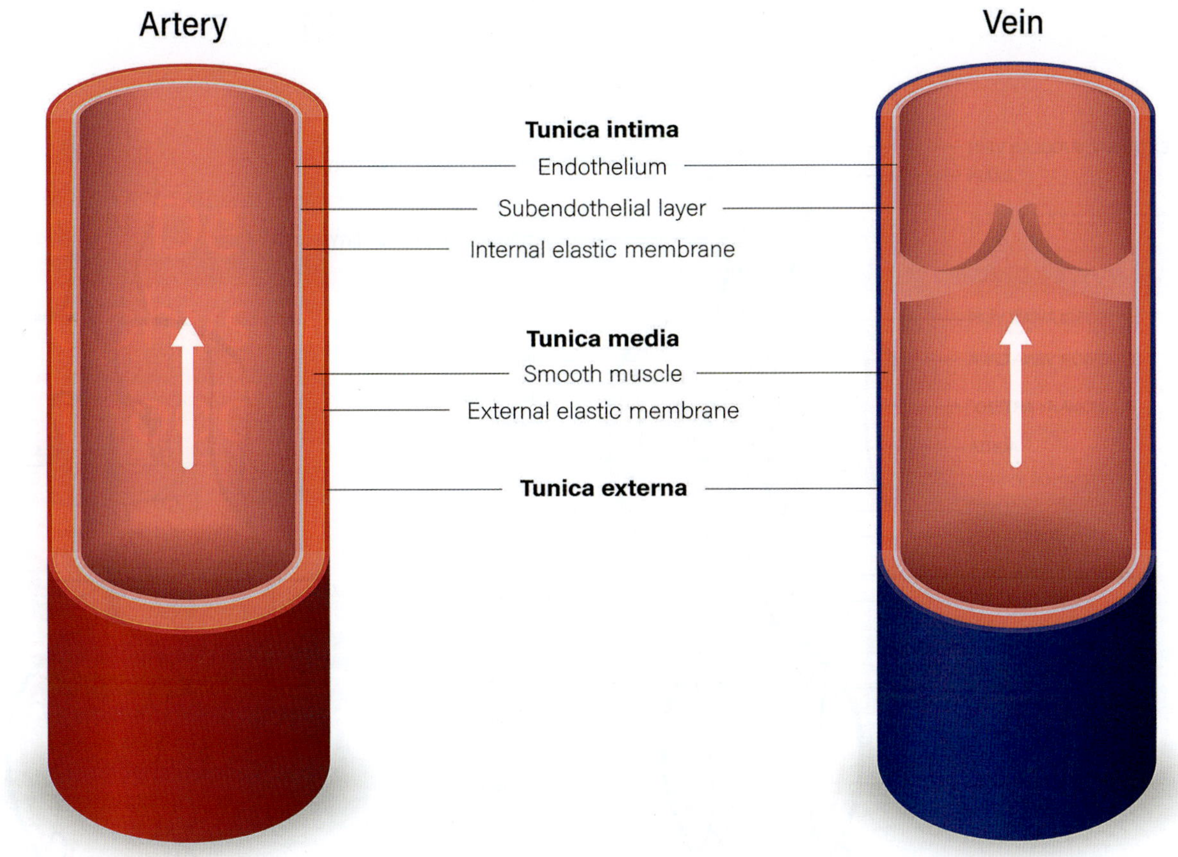

• **Fig. 13.4** Layers of tissue in the blood vessel walls. (From iStock.com/RujiratBoonyong.)

results in atherosclerosis or CAD.[13] Statin medications can help decrease the levels of LDLs in the blood. These medications can be lifesaving, but they are not without side effects. Statin-associated muscle symptoms are one of the more common myotoxic side effects of statins.[13] When muscles break down (rhabdomyolysis) due to a toxic substance, the myocytes release creatinine phosphokinase (CPK) into the blood, so it is important to check an individual's CPK levels periodically while they are taking a statin medication. Because statin medications are metabolized in the liver, monitoring for serum liver enzymes is also important.[13]

Coronary Artery Disease

When a person has arteriosclerosis, or "hardening of the arteries," the vessels carrying oxygen and nutrients become thick and stiffen up, restricting blood flow. Atherosclerosis is a specific type of arteriosclerosis.[14] With atherosclerosis, there is a buildup of fats, especially the LDLs mentioned above. This buildup can eventually form a plaque, which over time will restrict blood flow[14] (Fig. 13.7).

When a coronary artery becomes blocked, it is called CAD. This can cause angina pectoris or myocardial infarction (MI), also known as a heart attack. There are different types of anginas, including stable, resting, unstable, and nocturnal. The typical pain pattern is slightly different for males compared to females (Fig. 13.8 for male pain patterns and Fig. 13.9 for female pain patterns). When the plaque builds up in the artery enough to form a clot, it is called a thrombus. If it dislodges and travels to another area of the body, it is called an embolism.

The rate of CAD is rising for females in the United States. Although males typically get CAD at a younger age than females, females make up for this after menopause. Because of this, females are 10 times more likely to die of CVD than of breast cancer. CVD is now the leading cause of death in females in the United States.[13] Diabetes poses the highest risk when predicting cardiovascular problems in females, with a sevenfold increase in likelihood of having cardiovascular problems and roughly a 50% chance of death from CAD[13] (Table 13.2).

Vascular Disorders

Hypertension is the most common condition affecting the circulatory system. Normal BP is a systolic pressure of less than

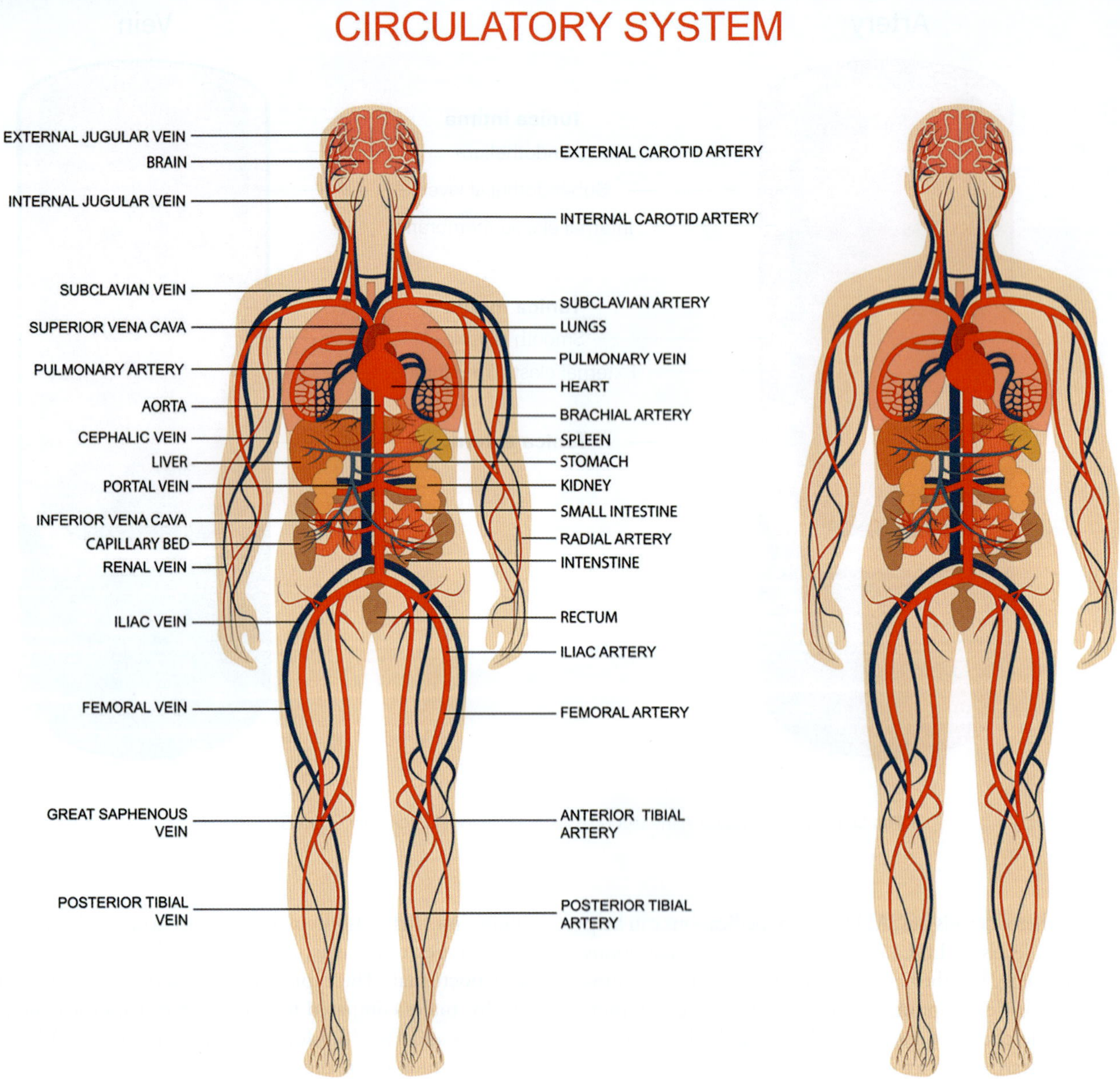

• **Fig. 13.5** The circulatory system. (From iStock.com/kowalska-art.)

120 mm Hg and a diastolic pressure of less than 80 mm Hg (120/80). The line of demarcation for a diagnosis of hypertension (high BP) was a BP above 140/90 in the guidelines released in 2003, but in 2017, this changed to a consistent BP above 130/80 mm Hg. Some of the conditions that affect the cardiovascular system can be found in Table 13.2.

Disorders Affecting the Cardiac Nervous System

Disorders that affect the cardiac nervous system will typically cause an arrhythmia, or an irregularity in the heartbeat. Some of these arrhythmias are listed in Table 13.3.

Disorders Affecting the Heart Valves

As discussed earlier in this chapter, the heart has four valves: the aortic valve, the pulmonary valve, the bicuspid (or mitral) valve on the left side of the heart, and the tricuspid valve on the right side of the heart. Some disorders that can affect the valves can be found in Table 13.4.

Embryological Development and Congenital Anomalies

The prenatal circulation of blood through the heart looks a little different from that of the adult depicted earlier in this chapter. The blood does not go from the right ventricle to

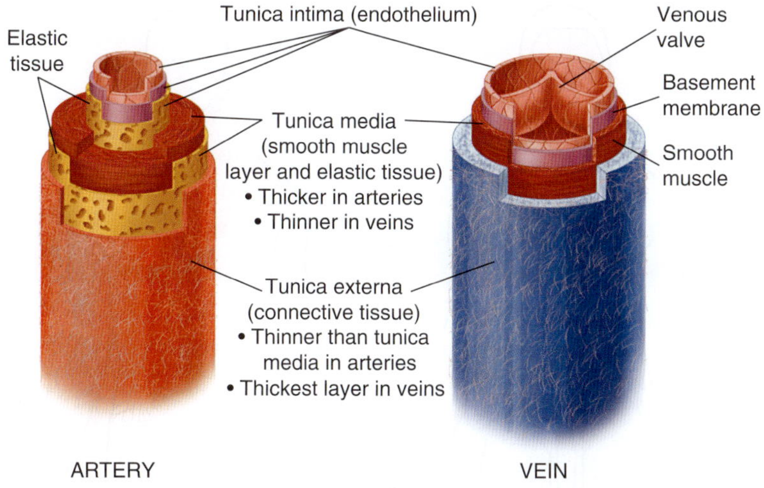

• **Fig. 13.6** The different layers of arteries versus veins. (From Giddens, JF, Wilson, SF, Klenke-Borgmann, L, Goegel, SK, Yamane SS. *Health Assessment for Nursing Practice*. 8th ed. Elsevier; 2026.)

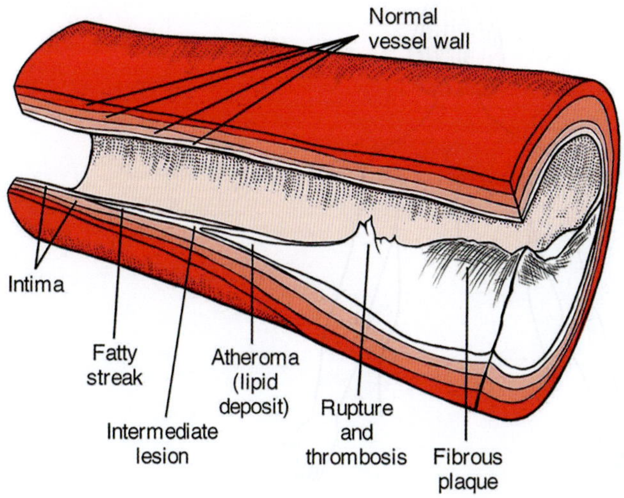

• **Fig. 13.7** Atherosclerosis. (From Heick J, Lazaro RT. *Goodman and Snyder's Differential Diagnosis for Physical Therapists: Screening for Referral*. 7th ed. Elsevier; 2023:257.)

the lungs in the prenatal heart because the embryo is not yet using the lungs. The blood bypasses the lungs so the gas exchange can occur in the placenta, and it does this through three shunts: the ductus venosus, the foramen ovale, and the ductus arteriosus (Fig. 13.13).[36] The foramen ovale shunts blood from the right ventricle directly to the left ventricle and bypasses the lungs.[36] The ductus arteriosus shunts blood from the beginning of the pulmonary artery directly to the aorta, and the ductus venosus carries oxygenated blood from the umbilical vein to the inferior vena cava. Thus, the highly oxygenated blood mingles with the deoxygenated blood from the lower body of the embryo and travels to the right atrium.[36] These three shunts will begin to close immediately after the newborn's first breath.

The newborn's resting heart rate is about 120 BPM (range: 110–160). By age 6, it will decrease to about 80 BPM (range: 60–100), and when we reach adulthood, the typical heart rate decreases to about 70 BPM.[37] Congenital defects of the heart occur in about 1 out of every 100 infants born in the United States.[13] Fig. 13.14 depicts some of the congenital defects that often require surgery shortly after birth.

The OT Scope of Practice

Once again, when working as an OTP, if an individual demonstrates symptoms that are outside of the typical cluster you expect to find with their diagnosis, it is important to report those symptoms to the referring physician.

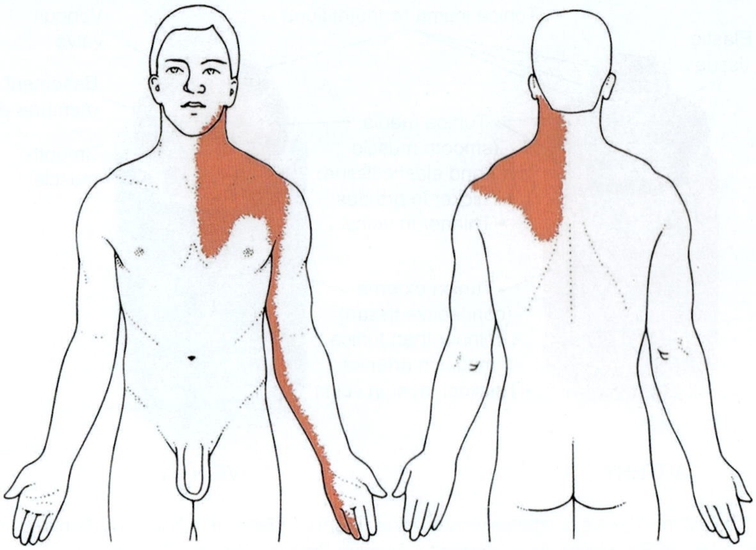

• **Fig. 13.8** Angina typical pain distribution for men. (From Heick, J., and Lazaro, R.T. *Goodman and Snyder's Differential Diagnosis for Physical Therapists: Screening for Referral*. 7th ed. Elsevier; 2023:289.)

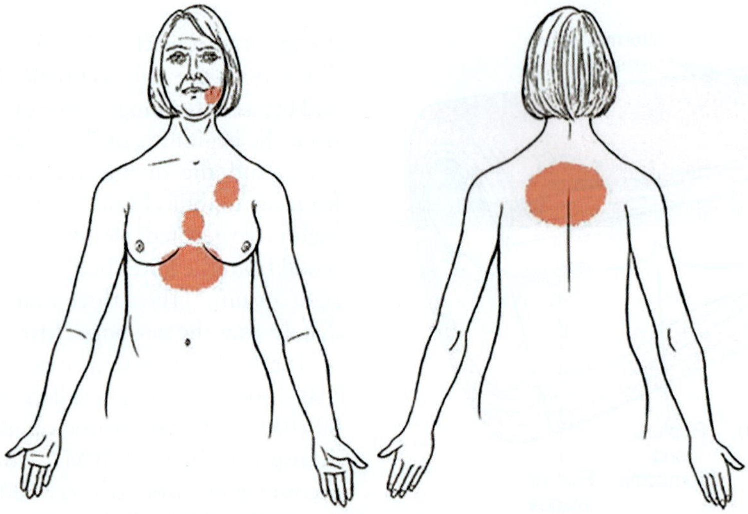

• **Fig. 13.9** Angina typical pain distribution for women. (From Heick, J., and Lazaro, R.T. *Goodman and Snyder's Differential Diagnosis for Physical Therapists: Screening for Referral*. 7th ed. Elsevier; 2023:260.)

TABLE 13.1 **Conditions Affecting the Heart Muscle**

Disorder	Pathophysiology	Common Symptoms
Myocardial infarction (MI)	Also known as a heart attack, MI occurs whenever the blood flow to the heart is severely reduced. Even when temporary, this lack of blood flow can damage the heart muscle.[15]	Chest pain, dyspnea, cardiac syncope (fainting), and cyanosis are only a few of the symptoms of MI (Fig. 13.10).
Pericarditis	Pericarditis is inflammation of the pericardium. The cause is typically unknown but can be postviral.[16]	Debilitating pleuritic chest pain that increases with inspiration or when lying in the supine position, along with neck, back, and shoulder pain, dry cough, palpitations, and dyspnea.[16]
Congestive heart failure (CHF)	This happens when the heart is not pumping enough blood to the body, resulting in fluid back up.[17]	*Left-sided heart failure* is a result of the fluids backing up in the lungs. Symptoms include constant coughing, weight gain, edema in the abdomen, ankles, and lower extremities, as well as shortness of breath (SOB). *Right-sided heart failure* usually happens because of left-sided heart failure. Symptoms include fluid in the feet and ankles, lower back, and abdomen (ascites) as well as chest pain, breathlessness, and palpitations. *High output failure* is rare but occurs when the heart cannot pump enough blood to meet the body's needs. It is usually due to medication or to an underlying condition.[17]
Left ventricular hypertrophy	This is when the walls of the left ventricle thicken, making the chamber of the left ventricle smaller in size, and can lead to a stiffening of the ventricular wall (Fig. 13.11).[18]	SOB, chest pain (typically when exercising), swelling of the lower extremities, syncope or lightheadedness, and a feeling of either heart fluttering or pounding heartbeats.[18]
Abdominal aortic aneurysm (AAA)	AAA is a weakness in the aortic wall that results in a bulging of the artery in that area (Fig. 13.12).[19]	Many people have no symptoms at all, but those who do experience pain in the abdomen, chest, groin, or lower back. It can be found on x-ray, MRI, or CT scan.[1]

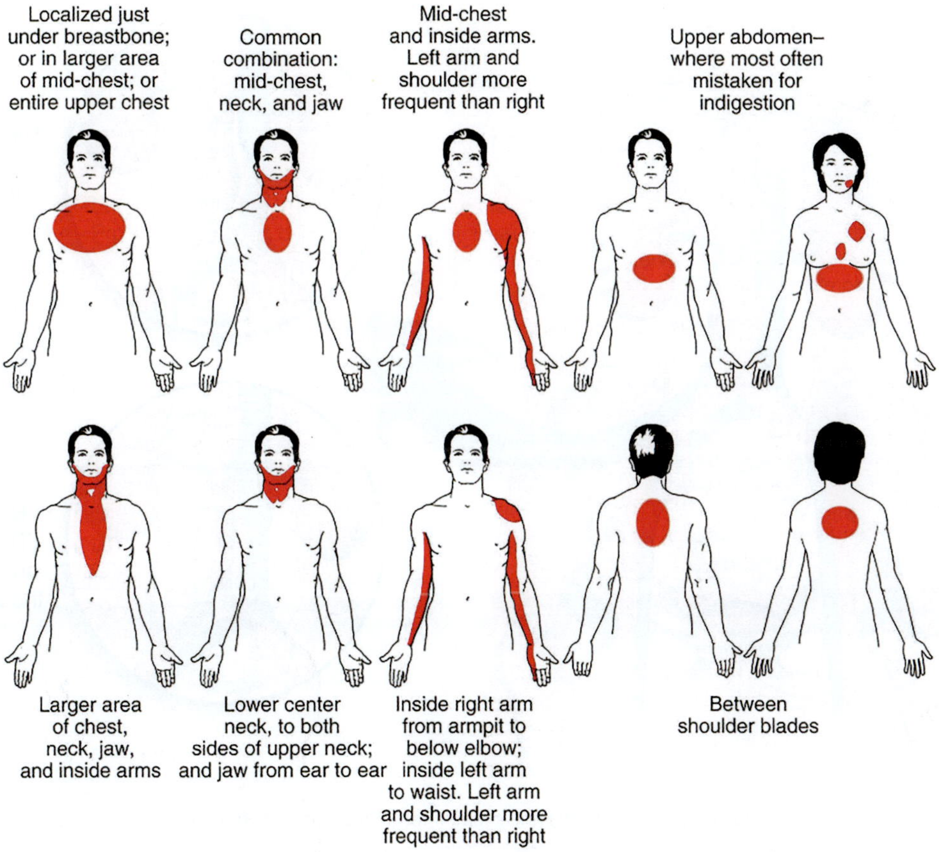

• **Fig. 13.10** Signs and symptoms of a myocardial infarction. (From Goodman CC, Fuller K. *Pathology: Implications for the Physical Therapist*. 3rd ed. WB Saunders; 2009.)

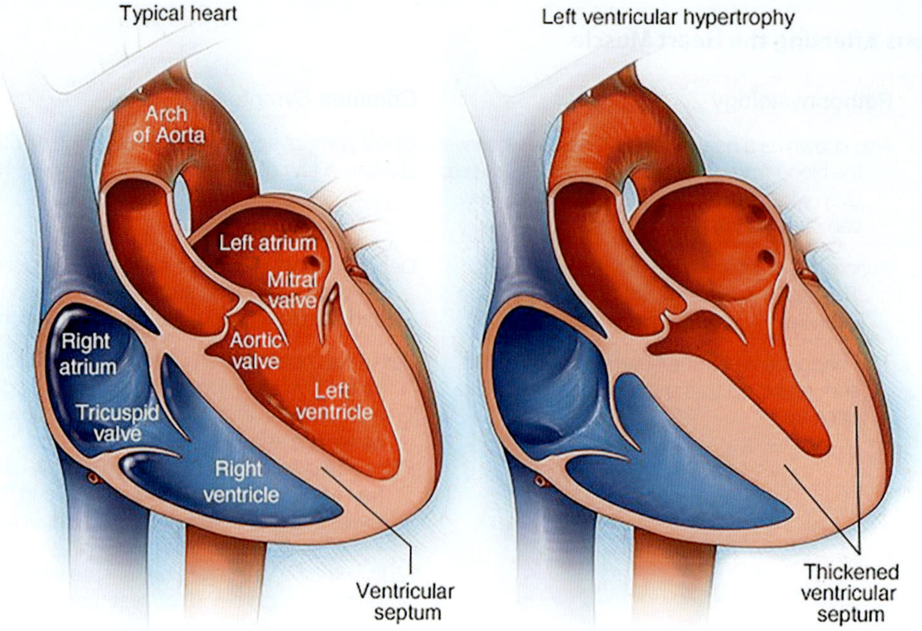

• **Fig. 13.11** Ventricular hypertrophy. (From https://www.mayoclinic.org/diseases-conditions/left-ventricularhypertrophy/symptoms-causes/syc-20374314, used with permission of Mayo Foundation for Medical Education and Research. All rights reserved.)

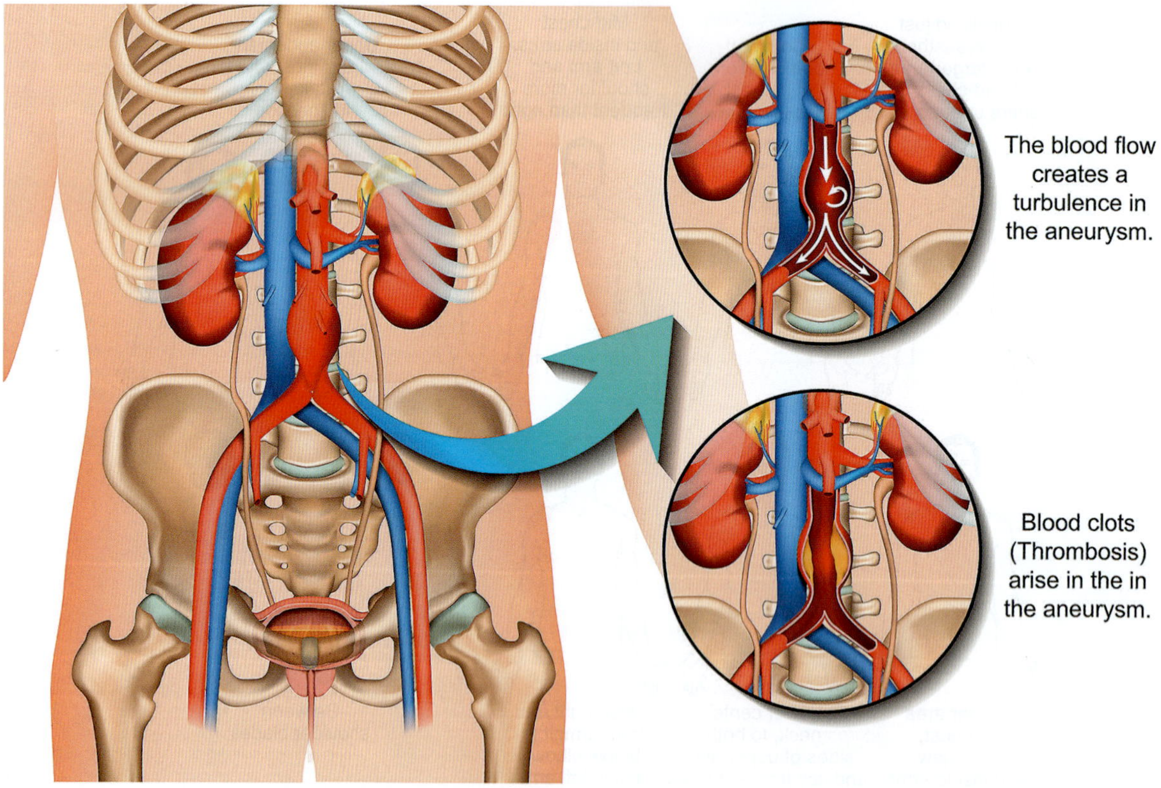

• **Fig. 13.12** Abdominal aortic aneurysm. (From iStock.com/medicalstocks.)

TABLE 13.2 **Conditions Affecting the Cardiovascular System**

Disorder	Pathophysiology	Common Symptoms
Coronary artery disease (CAD)	This is a common condition, and it occurs when the coronary arteries have difficulty supplying blood to the heart because of cholesterol deposits and plaque.[20]	Symptoms can include angina, fatigue, and SOB. CAD can also lead to a myocardial infarction.[20]
Hypertension (HTN)	A consistent BP above 130/80 mm Hg.[21]	There are typically no symptoms for high BP, but hypertension puts a person at a higher risk of heart disease and stroke.[21]
Orthostatic hypotension (OH)	Also known as postural hypotension, OH is when a person's BP suddenly drops when going from a seated or supine position to a standing position.[22]	This can cause lightheadedness or even fainting and is a common cause of falls in the elderly.[22]
Peripheral vascular disease—arterial (PAD) or arterial insufficiency	This is a narrowing of the arteries and is typically felt more in the lower extremities (LEs) than in the upper extremities (UEs).[23]	Claudication (a cramping sensation in the LEs that comes on gradually during exercise but stops with rest), coldness in one LE compared with the other, a weak pulse in the LEs or feet, painful cramping, skin color changes, erectile dysfunction, and hair loss on the LEs are all possible symptoms.[23] There can also be rubor (redness) when the LEs are in a dependent position and pallor (paleness) when the LEs are elevated.[24]
Peripheral vascular disease—chronic venous insufficiency (CVI)	CVI is caused by damage to the veins in the LEs and damage to the valves that keep the blood from backing up into the feet and enable venous return to the heart.[25]	LE edema, achy and tired LEs, discolored skin, cramping in the LEs at night, full or heavy feeling in the LEs, or open ulcers typically near the ankles.[25]
Lymphedema	This is an accumulation of fluid that leads to swelling in the UEs or LEs, caused by inadequate drainage of fluids via the lymphatic system.[26]	Swelling of a UE or LE, with decreased range of motion, thickening of the skin, recurring infections, and a feeling of heaviness or tightness of the skin.[26]
Deep vein thrombosis (DVT)	This is a clot in a deep vein, typically in the pelvis, thigh, or LE, but it can also occur in the UE.[27] The biggest danger with a DVT is that it can lead to a PE.	The individual will often have pain and swelling with redness of the skin.[27] There may be differences in temperature on palpations when comparing the skin above and below the clot.

TABLE 13.3 **Conditions Affecting the Cardiac Nervous System**

Disorder	Pathophysiology	Common Symptoms
Bradycardia	This is a slow heart rate: less than 60 BPM.[28]	Fatigue, dizziness, confusion, chest pain, and SOB.[28]
Tachycardia	This is a fast heart rate: more than 100 BPM.[29]	Fainting, lightheadedness, fluttering in the chest, SOB, fatigue, and palpitations.[29]
Premature contractions	These are contractions that happen a bit too early and usually are of no consequence. They can either be PACs or PVCs.[30]	There may be a sudden feeling that your heart skipped a beat.[30] You may also have a fluttering or pounding feeling.[31] PVCs in someone without heart disease is typically not a concern, but PVCs are watched more closely in those with heart disease.[31]
Ventricular fibrillation	This is when the heart chambers quiver in response to disordered electrical activity. This is the most serious of the arrhythmias because it can lead to sudden death from cardiac arrest.[32]	Symptoms include loss of consciousness, sudden collapse, no pulse, and not breathing. This is a medical emergency requiring 911 and CPR.[32]

BPM, Beats per minute; *CPR*, cardiopulmonary resuscitation; *PACs*, premature atrial contractions; *PVCs*, premature ventricular contractions.

TABLE 13.4 Conditions Affecting the Heart Valves

Disorder	Pathophysiology	Common Symptoms
Rheumatic fever	This is an infection caused by streptococcal bacteria.[13] This can sometimes cause mitral valve stenosis (narrowing of the opening) and increasing resistance of blood flow from the left atrium to the left ventricle.[33]	Initial cold or sore throat, with a gradual onset of painful joints, palpitations, and SOB. There may also be subcutaneous nodules or a flat, painless skin rash.[13]
Endocarditis	Endocarditis is a common heart infection and inflammation of the heart endothelium, leading to damage to the valves.	Arthralgia, arthritis, back pain, petechiae, and constitutional symptoms.[13]
Aortic valve stenosis	Aortic valve stenosis is a decreased blood flow from the left ventricle to the aorta, occurring more frequently in the older adult population.[34]	An irregular heart sound (murmur), SOB, inadequate food intake, feeling faint or dizzy, and fatigue.[34]
Pulmonary valve stenosis	This is usually a congenital condition in which the right ventricle must work harder to get blood to flow to the pulmonary artery, causing right ventricular hypertrophy.[35]	A whooshing sound (murmur), fatigue, SOB, chest pain, and syncope.[35]
Mitral valve prolapse	The mitral valve will have a bulging of its leaflets, so the valve will not close properly, thus causing some blood to leak backward.[13] There is typically a clicking sound heard with a stethoscope.[13]	This can be asymptomatic, but occasionally there will be dysautonomia (or an imbalance in the autonomic nervous system), profound fatigue, SOB, and cold hands and feet.[13]

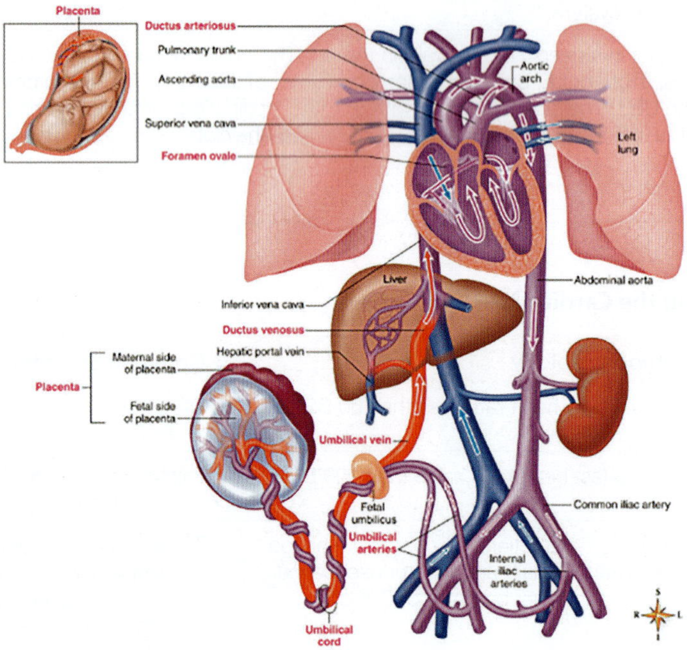

• **Fig. 13.13** Prenatal blood flow. (From Thibodeau GA, Patton KT. *Anatomy & Physiology*. 11th ed. Elsevier; 2022.)

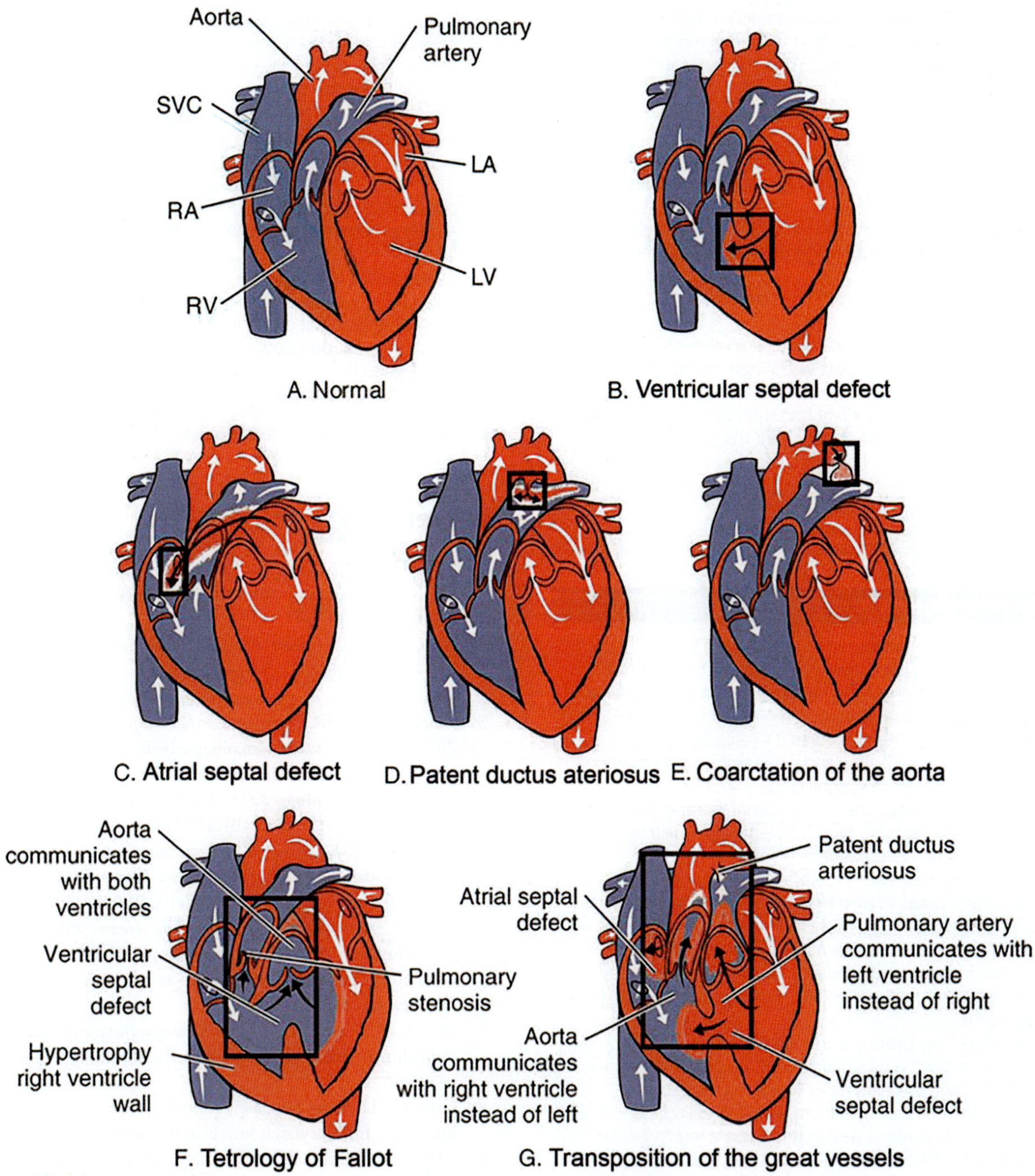

• **Fig. 13.14** Congenital heart anomalies. *LA*, Left atrium; *LV*, left ventricle; *RA*, right atrium; *RV*, right ventricle; *SVA*, superior vena cava. (From Heick J, Lazaro RT. *Goodman and Snyder's Differential Diagnosis for Physical Therapists: Screening for Referral*. 7th ed. Elsevier; 2023:290.)

Application—Case Study

CASE EXAMPLE 13.1

A 64-year-old female presented to an OT clinic for strengthening, range of motion, and assist with functional movement of her right upper extremity during ADLs (activities of daily living), IADLs (instrumental activities of daily living), and leisure participation after a recently healed humerus fracture.

1. **Screen:** During the screening process, the OTP noticed that the client was out of breath and extremely tired.
2. **Take a Closer Look:** The OTP asked how long this fatigue had been going on, and the client reported that it started the day of the fracture. She had become dizzy and fell, and that is how she had broken her arm. The OTP then took a second look at the client's medical record to see if there had been any recent changes in medications or any other risk factors that may be contributing to these symptoms.
3. **Determine Flag Status:** Since she was concerned, the OTP determined this to be a yellow flag situation. She called the doctor to see if there might have been a reason for the client's fatigue and dizzy spell the day of the injury.

4. **Take Action if Needed:** The doctor found that the only change had been an increase in her statin medications about 2 weeks before her fall. The OTP requested that the doctor perform a blood test called a CPK level to see if the statin medication might be causing a breakdown of the muscle fibers.
5. **Document the Findings:** The OTP documented the findings of her examination as well as the phone call to the physician.
6. **Take a Second Look:** Armed with this new information from the OTP, the doctor ran the bloodwork, and the client did have elevated levels of CPK.
7. **Determine the Flag Status:** This had quickly become a red flag.
8. **Take Action if Needed:** The statin medication was reduced back to the prior dosage by the physician, and the client returned to the OT clinic 2 weeks later, feeling much better.

This is a true case. The client had rhabdomyolysis caused by the increase in statin medication, but this was another OT success story, since it had been caught early. If not for the quick thinking of her OTP, this might have become much worse, even lethal.

CASE EXAMPLE 13.2

An 81-year-old male presented to an OT clinic for strengthening, range of motion, and assist with functional movement of his left shoulder during yardwork IADLs after a rotator cuff repair.

1. **Screen:** Although the client was 81 years of age, he looked remarkably healthy and was talking about how he hurt his shoulder while weightlifting.
2. **Take a Closer Look:** The occupational therapy assistant (COTA) carefully looked over the client's pain distribution, and although he did present with some of the normal pain you would expect to see after a rotator cuff repair, he had other areas of pain that did not quite fit the normal cluster of symptoms. His pain radiated from his left 4th and 5th digits up the lateral aspect of his arm, to the left anterior chest, and even into his jaw. The pain was aggravated by breathing and felt worse when he was lying supine.
3. **Determine Flag Status:** Although this seemed like it might be "making a mountain out of a molehill" to the COTA, she had a feeling more was going on, so she informed the occupational therapist, who called the physician right away, believing this to be a red flag.
4. **Take Action if Needed:** The doctor thought that the client was "more than likely fine," but if the occupational therapist was worried, then she should instruct the client to go to the emergency room (ER).
5. **Document the Findings:** The occupational therapist documented the findings of her examination as well as the phone call to the physician.
6. **Take a Second Look:** Not wanting to alarm the client unnecessarily, the COTA and the occupational therapist asked the client to go to the ER "just to be on the safe side and to rule out anything suspicious, so we can begin OT intervention." The client reluctantly went to the ER, insisting all the while that he was fine.
7. **Determine the Flag Status:** The ER performed an electrocardiogram (ECG), followed by a blood workup to check troponin levels (proteins known as cardiac markers). The client was indeed having a heart attack. He was admitted to the hospital, where he was treated, and a few days later, was evaluated and treated by an acute care occupational therapist to ensure a safe discharge home. This had quickly become a red flag, but the COTA and occupational therapist had acted immediately, saving the client's life.
8. **Take Action if Needed:** The client continued to receive outpatient occupational therapy services as follow-up for the original rotator cuff surgery but requested a different occupational therapist or COTA, still believing that he did not have a heart attack and his hospital visit had been a waste of time.

This is a true case. The client was having a heart attack, and his OTPs, working well together as a team, may have saved his life. Still, the client was not happy with the OTPs. Although they felt bad about it, they were okay knowing it is better to let a client "fire" you than to fail to advocate for a client when they need it most.

References

1. Mayo Clinic. *Chambers and Valves of the Heart.* Mayo Clinic; 2023. https://www.mayoclinic.org/chambers-and-valves-of-the-heart/img-20007497.
2. NIH. *What the Heart Looks Like.* National Heart Lung and Blood Institute; 2022. https://www.nhlbi.nih.gov/health/heart/anatomy.
3. King J, Lowery DR. *Physiology, Cardiac Output.* StatPearls Publishing; 2023. https://www.ncbi.nlm.nih.gov/books/NBK470455/.
4. Kashou AH, Basit H, Chhabra L. *Physiology, Sinoatrial Node.* StatPearls Publishing; 2023. PMID: 29083608. https://www.ncbi.nlm.nih.gov/books/NBK459238/.
5. Markowitz AM, Lerman BB. A contemporary view of atrioventricular nodal physiology. *J Interv Card Electrophysiol.* 2018;52(3):271–279. https://doi.org/10.1007/s10840-018-0392-5.
6. Health. *Anatomy and Function of the Heart's Electrical System.* John Hopkins; 2023. https://www.hopkinsmedicine.org/health/conditions-and-diseases/anatomy-and-function-of-the-hearts-electrical-system.
7. Patra C, Zhang X, Brady MF. *Physiology, Bundle of His.* StatPearls Publishing; 2023. https://www.ncbi.nlm.nih.gov/books/NBK531498/.
8. Crumble L. *Heart Histology.* KenHub; 2023. https://www.kenhub.com/en/library/anatomy/histology-of-the-heart.
9. Cleveland Clinic. *Arteries.* Cleveland Clinic; 2023. https://my.clevelandclinic.org/health/body/22896-arteries.
10. DePietro M. *What to Know About Arteries.* Medical News Today; 2022. https://www.medicalnewstoday.com/articles/arteriesv.
11. Tucker WD, Arora Y, Mahajan K. *Anatomy, Blood Vessels.* StatPearls Publishing; 2023. PMID: 29262226. https://pubmed.ncbi.nlm.nih.gov/29262226/.
12. Cleveland Clinic. *Veins.* Cleveland Clinic; 2023. https://my.clevelandclinic.org/health/body/23360-veins.
13. Heick J, Lazaro RT. *Goodman and Snyder's Differential Diagnosis for Physical Therapists: Screening for Referral.* 7th ed. Elsevier; 2023.
14. Mayo Clinic. *Arteriosclerosis/Atherosclerosis.* Mayo Clinic; 2023. https://www.mayoclinic.org/diseases-conditions/arteriosclerosis-atherosclerosis/symptoms-causes/syc-20350569.
15. Mayo Clinic. *Heart Attack.* Mayo Clinic; 2023. https://www.mayoclinic.org/diseases-conditions/heart-attack/symptoms-causes/syc-20373106.

16. Heart of Inflammation. *About Recurrent Pericarditis*. Heart of Inflammation; 2023. https://www.heartofinflammation.com/recurrent-pericarditis-overview.
17. Cleveland Clinic. *Congestive Heart Failure*. Cleveland Clinic; 2023. https://my.clevelandclinic.org/health/diseases/17069-heart-failure-understanding-heart-failure.
18. Mayo Clinic. *Left Ventricular Hypertrophy*. Mayo Clinic; 2022. https://www.mayoclinic.org/diseases-conditions/left-ventricular-hypertrophy/symptoms-causes/syc-20374314.
19. Hopkins. *Abdominal Aortic Aneurysm. Health*. Johns Hopkins Medicine. https://www.hopkinsmedicine.org/health/conditions-and-diseases/abdominal-aortic-aneurysm.
20. Mayo Clinic. *Coronary Artery Disease*. Mayo Clinic; 2022. https://www.mayoclinic.org/diseases-conditions/coronary-artery-disease/symptoms-causes/syc-20350613.
21. CDC. *High Blood Pressure*. Centers for Disease Control and Prevention; 2023. https://www.cdc.gov/bloodpressure/index.htm.
22. Mayo Clinic. *Orthostatic Hypotension (Postural Hypotension)*. Mayo Clinic; 2022. https://www.mayoclinic.org/diseases-conditions/orthostatic-hypotension/symptoms-causes/syc-20352548.
23. Mayo Clinic. *Peripheral Artery Disease*. Mayo Clinic; 2022. https://www.mayoclinic.org/diseases-conditions/peripheral-artery-disease/symptoms-causes/syc-20350557.
24. Gey DC, Lesho EP, Manngold J. Management of peripheral arterial disease. *Am Fam Physician*. 2004;69(3):525–532. https://www.aafp.org/pubs/afp/issues/2004/0201/p525.html.
25. Cleveland Clinic. *Chronic Venous Insufficiency*. Cleveland Clinic; 2022. https://my.clevelandclinic.org/health/diseases/16872-chronic-venous-insufficiency-cvi.
26. Mayo Clinic. *Lymphedema*. Mayo Clinic; 2022. https://www.mayoclinic.org/diseases-conditions/lymphedema/symptoms-causes/syc-20374682.
27. NTTW. *Some Things to Know About Deep Vein Thrombosis and Pulmonary Embolism*. No Time to Wait; 2023. https://www.notimetowait.com/dvt-pe-explained?cid=sem_1521314&gclid=eba16c5a9310167653e708850b7c0fa9&gclsrc=3p.ds.
28. AHA. *Bradycardia: Slow Heart Rate*. American Heart Association; 2022. https://www.heart.org/en/health-topics/arrhythmia/about-arrhythmia/bradycardia--slow-heart-rate.
29. AHA. *Tachycardia: Fast Heart Rate*. American Heart Association; 2022. https://www.heart.org/en/health-topics/arrhythmia/about-arrhythmia/tachycardia--fast-heart-rate.
30. AHA. *Premature Contractions: PACs and PVCs*. American Heart Association; 2022. https://www.heart.org/en/health-topics/arrhythmia/about-arrhythmia/premature-contractions-pacs-and-pvcs.
31. Mayo Clinic. *Premature Ventricular Contractions (PVCs)*. Mayo Clinic; 2022. https://www.mayoclinic.org/diseases-conditions/premature-ventricular-contractions/symptoms-causes/syc-20376757.
32. AHA. *Ventricular Fibrillation*. American Heart Association; 2022. https://www.heart.org/en/health-topics/arrhythmia/about-arrhythmia/ventricular-fibrillation.
33. Hopkins. *Heart Valve Diseases. Health*. Johns Hopkins Medicine. https://www.hopkinsmedicine.org/health/conditions-and-diseases/heart-valve-diseases.
34. Mayo Clinic. *Aortic Valve Stenosis*. Mayo Clinic; 2022. https://www.mayoclinic.org/diseases-conditions/aortic-stenosis/symptoms-causes/syc-20353139.
35. Mayo Clinic. *Pulmonary Valve Stenosis*. Mayo Clinic; 2022. https://www.mayoclinic.org/diseases-conditions/pulmonary-valve-stenosis/symptoms-causes/syc-20377034.
36. Stanford. *Fetal Circulation*. Stanford Medicine Children's Health. https://www.stanfordchildrens.org/en/topic/default?id=fetal-circulation-90-P01790.
37. Cleveland Clinic. *What You Need to Know About Infant and Children's Vital Signs*. Health Essentials, Cleveland Clinic; 2022. https://health.clevelandclinic.org/pediatric-vital-signs/.

14

Pulmonary Pathophysiology

OBJECTIVES

By the end of this chapter, the reader should be able to:

- Demonstrate a basic understanding of a healthy pulmonary system.
- Demonstrate a basic understanding of pathophysiological conditions affecting the lungs, the pulmonary tree, and the vasculature.
- Demonstrate a basic understanding of the genetic pathophysiological conditions affecting respiration.
- Identify possible symptoms associated with various pulmonary disorders.
- Identify signs and symptoms of pulmonary inflammation and/or infection.
- Compare and contrast respiratory acidosis and respiratory alkalosis.
- Explain and/or predict the possible symptoms resulting from the pathophysiology of various pulmonary disorders.
- Assess and justify whether a specific pulmonary symptom could constitute a yellow or red flag.

Healthy Pulmonary Physiology

When a client complains of pain in the neck, shoulder, or back that increases or decreases with inspiration and expiration, their pain might be due to a pulmonary condition.[1] Many pulmonary conditions can mimic musculoskeletal conditions, including pulmonary embolism (PE), pneumonia (PNA), or pneumothorax.[1]

Development of the Lungs

The pulmonary system develops primarily from the endoderm of the developing blastocyst. The bronchial buds begin to appear at the end of the laryngotracheal tube during weeks 3 to 6 of gestation.[2,3] By 42 days of gestation (week 6), airway conducting branches appear, and between 42 and 56 days of gestation, this branching continues into two respiratory bronchioles.[3] This generation of the bronchial tree continues up until about the 17th week of gestation. From this point, the development of the terminal respiratory units continues along with the development of primitive alveoli, the terminal sacs needed for gas exchange (Fig. 14.1).[3] For some premature infants, survival is possible if born after week 25, because of the development of some of the alveoli, but those born after 32 weeks have a higher chance of survival because of the development of more alveoli and the addition of pulmonary surfactant.[3] Surfactant reduces surface tension and increases pulmonary compliance, reducing the chance of atelectasis (collapse of the alveoli).[4]

Fetal breathing movements, through contraction of the muscles that cause inhalation and exhalation of the amniotic fluid, begin at around 20 to 21 weeks of gestation.[2] Although the lungs are filled with amniotic fluid before birth, much of the fluid is expelled as the fetus is squeezed through the birth canal. Any remaining fluid is absorbed by the body shortly after birth.[2]

After the baby is born and takes their first breath, gas exchange begins to occur in the infant's lungs. The lungs become filled with oxygen, and the arterioles in the lungs dilate, increasing pulmonary blood flow.[5] The baby's breathing is not extremely efficient because of the shape of the chest, the position of the diaphragm, and limitations in movement of the muscles (such as the diaphragm) that are pulling from a more compliant, flexible thorax.[6,7]

As the baby learns to move through space, this efficiency increases. The child's ribcage will approximate the adult shape by around age 2 and become more rigid around age 3. Along with the child's physical growth, the diaphragm will be pulled into its dome shape.[8] There will also be the development of collateral ventilation systems that will begin to develop from what is known as the alveolar pores of Kohn. These pores begin to develop in humans at around 4 years of age.[9] The alveoli present at birth equate to about 150 million, which is only about half of that seen in adulthood.[10] New alveoli continue to develop into adolescence, when the adult number of alveoli (about 300 million) is attained.[11]

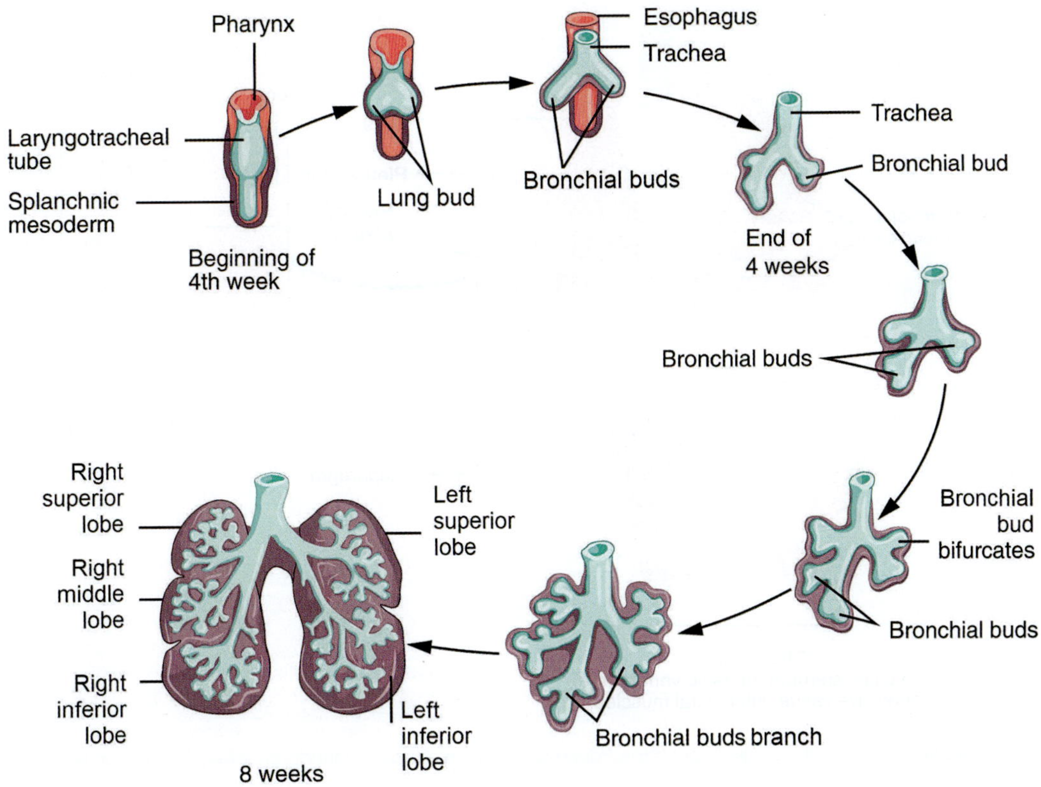

• **Fig. 14.1** Embryologic development of the lungs. (Image credit "Development of the Lower Respiratory System" by Julie Jenks.)

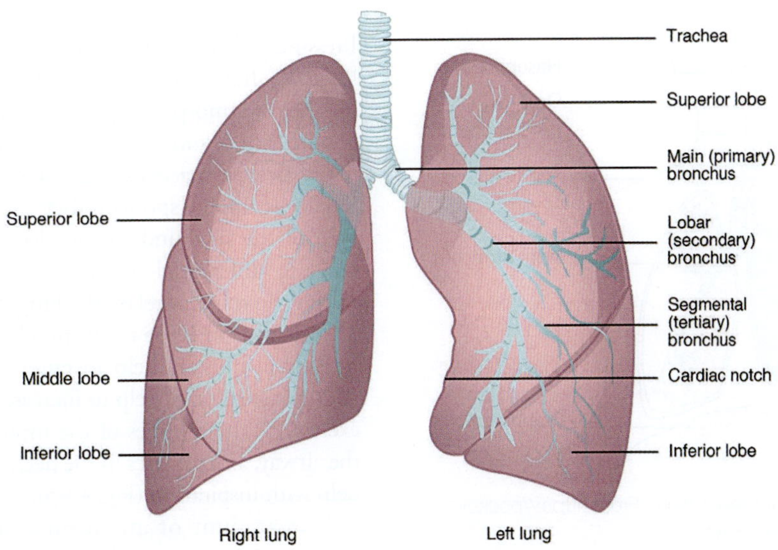

• **Fig. 14.2** The lungs. (From https://open.oregonstate.education/aandp/chapter/22-2-the-lungs/.)

Gross Anatomy of the Lungs

The primary function of the lungs is to deliver oxygen into the blood circulation and remove carbon dioxide (CO_2) from the body into the atmosphere across an epithelial surface area of about 70 m^2.[12] The lungs are a pair of pyramid-shaped organs on each side of the chest cavity, connected to the trachea by the right and left bronchi.[12] The left lung has what is called the cardiac notch on the inferior-medial border for the heart (Fig. 14.2).

The lungs are covered with a translucent, glistening, and protective tissue called pleura.[13] There are two layers of pleura. The innermost layer, just superficial to the lungs, is called the *visceral pleura*. The outermost layer, called the *parietal pleura,* connects to the thoracic wall to the mediastinum (the central part of the thoracic cavity) and the diaphragm (Fig. 14.3).[12]

The right lung consists of three lobes, and the left lung has two lobes. Each lobe consists of multiple bronchopulmonary segments, and some disorders will attack just one or more of

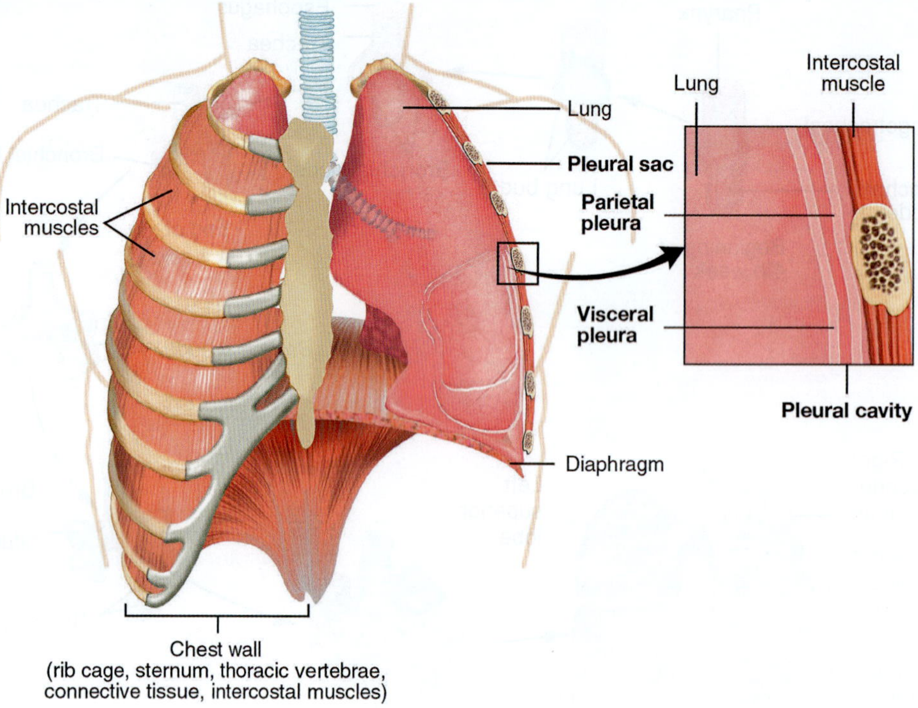

• **Fig. 14.3** Pleura of the lungs. (From https://open.oregonstate.education/aandp/chapter/22-2-the-lungs/.)

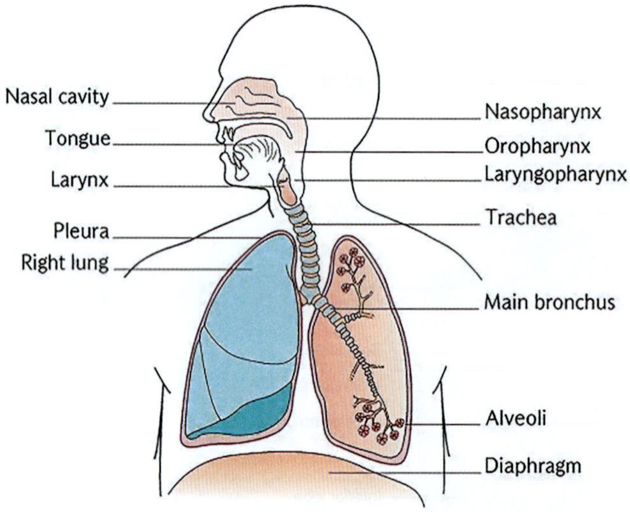

• **Fig. 14.4** The passage of air for respiration. (From https://pocket-dentistry.com/5-the-respiratory-system/.)

these segments.[12] When we breathe, air passes through the conducting portion of the respiratory system (the nose and mouth), into the pharynx (consisting of the nasopharynx, the oropharynx, and the laryngopharynx), and then into the larynx, the trachea, and lastly into the bronchial tree (Fig. 14.4).

Physiology of Respiration

Pressure differences cause air to move either into or out of the lungs. Air flows into the lungs when the air in the alveolar spaces falls below atmospheric pressure, and the larynx is open.[14] This is called inspiration. Expiration occurs when the air pressure in the alveolar spaces exceeds atmospheric pressure.[14] Although the lungs are like sponges, they cannot get bigger without the help of the surrounding muscles, which contract to create a pressure differential around the lungs, causing inspiration. When the muscles relax, the lungs can deflate on their own.[15] The diaphragm is the main muscle used for breathing, but the intercostal muscles help to raise and lower the ribs, and the abdominal muscles help to increase the respiratory rate during exercise.[15] The muscles of the mouth and pharynx help open the airway, and muscles in the neck and around the clavicle also help with inspiration (Fig. 14.5).[15]

The amount of air inspired and expired during normal respiration is called the tidal volume (TV). The functional residual capacity (FRC) is the amount of air remaining in the lungs after a normal TV expiration. This amount cannot be measured with spirometry.[15] More of these volumes and their definitions can be found in Figs. 14.6 and 14.7. Doctors consider an individual's medical history when performing their physical examination and related diagnostic pulmonary tests, in which they search

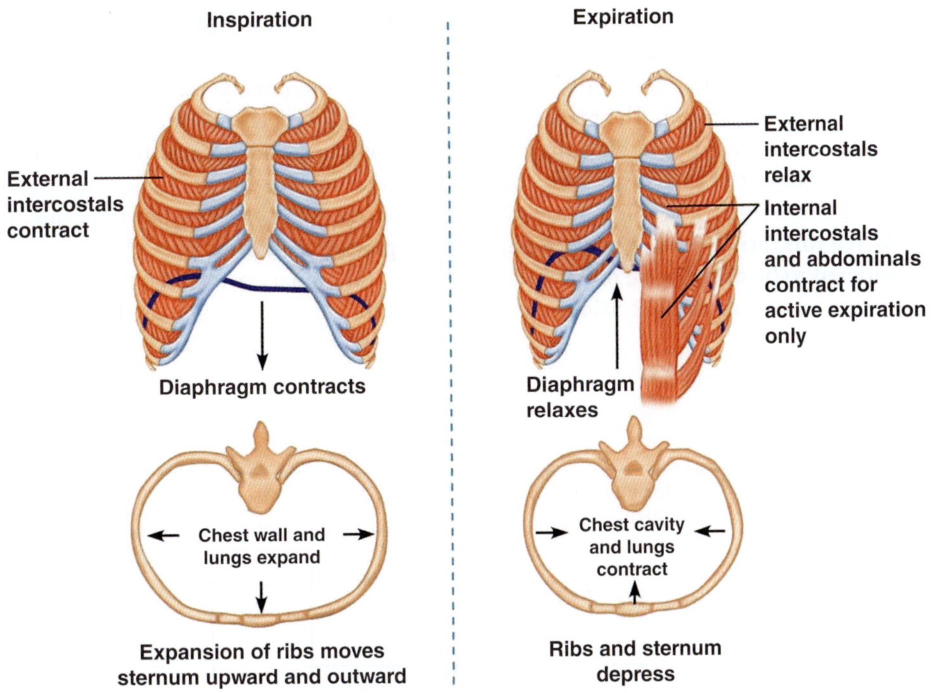

• **Fig. 14.5** The muscles of respiration. (From Shankar N. *Textbook of Applied Anatomy for Nurses*, Volume 1, 3rd ed. Elsevier; 2025.)

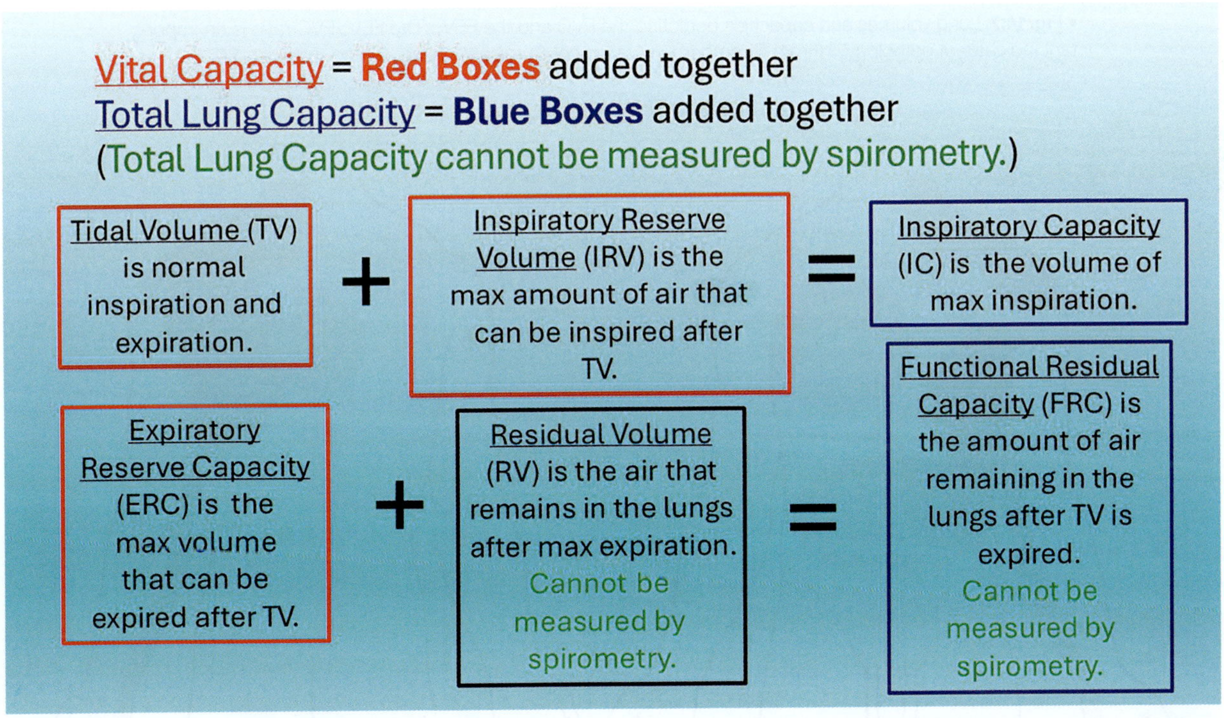

• **Fig. 14.6** Lung volumes and capacities.[16] (Created by Natalie Norman Michaels.)

for patterns and determine if the problem can be labeled as *obstructive* or *restrictive*.[16] The forced vital capacity (FVC) is the amount of air that can be forcefully exhaled by an individual after a deep inhalation. The forced expiratory volume in 1 second (FEV_1) is the amount of air exhaled during the first 1 second of the FVC. The ratio of FEV_1/FVC tells us if the individual's problem is obstructive or restrictive. When this ratio is lower than the norm, the problem is considered to be obstructive in nature, but when it is over the norm, the problem is considered to be restrictive (see Fig. 14.7).[16]

Pulmonary Pathophysiology

Many pulmonary conditions mimic the symptoms of the musculoskeletal system, including PNA, PE, pleurisy, pneumothorax, and pulmonary artery hypertension.[1] The most common sites for referred pain from the pulmonary system are the chest, ribs, upper trapezius, shoulder, and thoracic spine (Fig. 14.8).

Pulmonary pain will typically increase on inspiration and with movements such as laughing, coughing, sneezing, or deep breathing. Palpation and movements against resistance

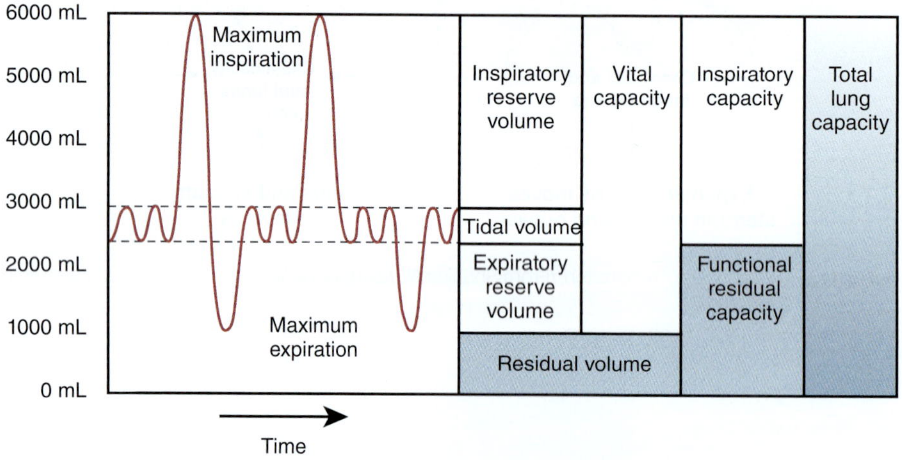

• **Fig. 14.7** Lung volumes and capacities depicting the FVC and the FEV_1. The FEV_1/FVC ratio is an important indicator of pathology.[16] (From Stromberg HK. *Medical-Surgical Nursing*. 6th ed. Elsevier; 2026.)

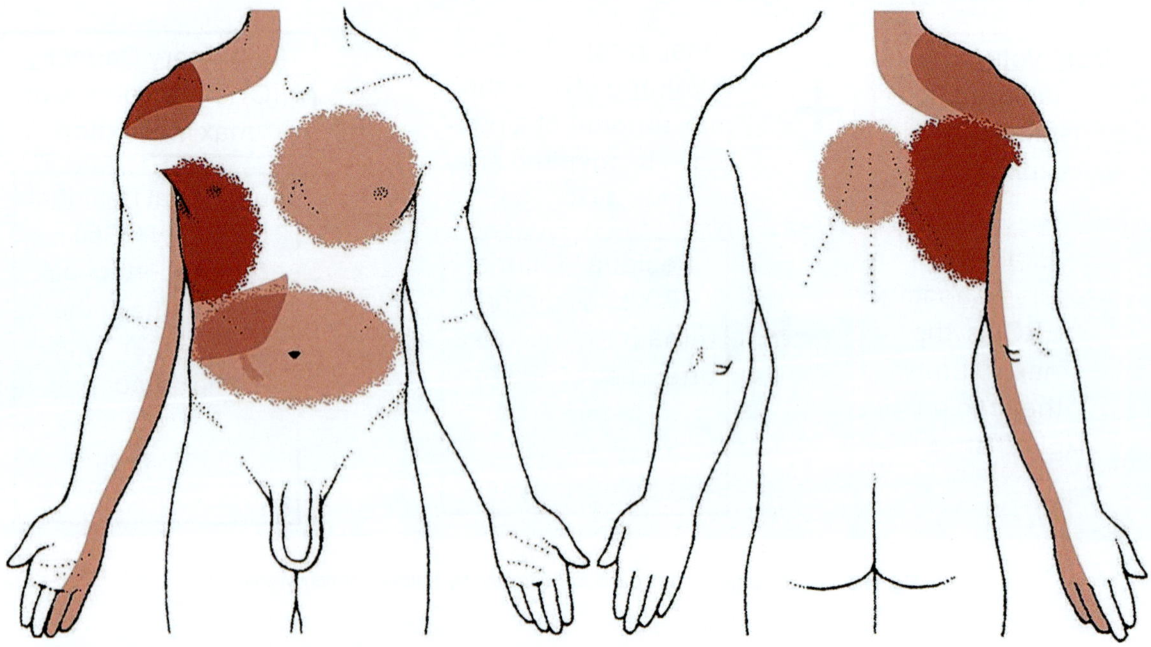

• **Fig. 14.8** Possible pulmonary pain patterns. (From Heick J, Lazaro RT. *Goodman and Snyder's Differential Diagnosis for Physical Therapists: Screening for Referral*. 7th ed. Elsevier; 2023:301.)

Hyperventilation
- Anxiety
- Acute head injury
- Hypoxemia
- Fever

Hypoventilation
- Fibromyalgia syndrome
- Chronic fatigue syndrome
- Sleep disorder
- Muscle fatigue
- Muscle weakness
- Malnutrition
- Neuromuscular disease
  - Guillain-Barré
  - Myasthenia gravis
  - Poliomyelitis
  - Amyotrophic lateral sclerosis (ALS)
- Pickwickian or obesity hypoventilation syndrome
- Severe kyphoscoliosis

Kussmaul
- Strenuous exercise
- Metabolic acidosis

Cheyne-Stokes
- Congestive heart failure
- Renal failure
- Meningitis
- Drug overdose
- Increased intracranial pressure
- Infants (normal)
- Older people during sleep (normal)

Apneustic
- Midpons lesion
- Basilar artery infarct

Biot Respiration (Ataxia)
- Exercise
- Shock
- Cerebral hypoxia
- Heat stroke
- Spinal meningitis
- Head injury
- Brain abscess
- Encephalitis

• **Fig. 14.9** Altered breathing patterns.[1] (From Ikeda B, Goodman CC, Fuller K. The respiratory system. In: Goodman CC, ed. *Pathology: Implications for the Physical Therapist*. 3rd ed. Elsevier; 2009.)

will not reproduce the pain symptoms, and the pain might get worse on recumbency.[1] Other signs and symptoms of pulmonary pathology include a cough, dyspnea, cyanosis (blue discoloration of the lips and nails), clubbing of the fingers and toes (a widening at the distal phalanges), and altered breathing patterns (Fig. 14.9).[1]

Pleural Pain

As previously mentioned, there are two layers of pleura lining the thoracic cavity. The visceral layer covers the lungs, and although there is sensation to stretch and chemical irritants, it is insensitive to pain.[17] The parietal layer that lines the rib cage, however, has sensation to temperature, localized pressure, and pain.[17] Pathology of the lungs can be pain-free until the condition becomes severe enough to move more superficially, pressing on the parietal pleura. When this happens, the pain is often described as sharp and localized and aggravated by any movement of respiration. The pain often decreases when lying on the affected side or when autosplinting.[1] Autosplinting is when an individual protects their own body by pressing a pillow or their hands against the rib cage to immobilize or cushion their movements as well as reduce the pain felt with inspiration and expiration. Parietal pleural pain is often evident in pulmonary diseases, such as pleurisy, pulmonary infarct, PNA, pneumothorax, and cancer.[1] Diaphragmatic pleural pain occurs via the phrenic and intercostal nerves, is described as a sharp pain along the margins of the ribs, and can be referred to the upper trapezius on the ipsilateral side. Pain from the diaphragm and from the heart is often felt in the shoulder because they are both supplied by the C5-C6 spinal segment.[1]

Acid-Base Regulation

The healthy exchange of air through the lungs, along with the body's chemical buffer systems and the renal system, works to maintain proper blood pH levels. Body fluid pH (which is determined by the hydrogen ion concentration in body fluids) must stay between 7.35 and 7.45 for our cells to remain healthy.[1]

Respiratory Acidosis

Respiratory acidosis is caused by any condition that decreases pulmonary ventilation (or breathing), resulting in an increase in the number of hydrogen ions and a subsequent decrease in body fluid pH to less than 7.35. When respiratory ventilation becomes severely compromised, CO_2 levels can become high, resulting in hypoxia.[1] Conditions that can result in a decrease in efficiency of the respiratory system causing respiratory acidosis include damage to the neurological system that controls breathing (medulla oblongata), neoplasms, chronic obstructive pulmonary disease (COPD), Guillain-Barré syndrome, or overdose of drugs that cause respiratory depressant effects.[1] Symptoms of respiratory acidosis include cyanosis, shallow rapid breathing, diaphoresis (excessive sweating), confusion, sleepiness, or unconsciousness. These symptoms constitute a **RED** flag issue. Any client demonstrating inadequate ventilation requires immediate referral.[1]

Respiratory Alkalosis

Respiratory alkalosis is caused by an increase in respiratory rate and an increase in the depth of inspiration, with a subsequent decrease in CO_2 and hydrogen ion concentration and an increase in body fluid pH to above 7.45.[1] It is typically due to hyperventilation but can also be caused by anxiety, pain, neurologic conditions, or physiologic conditions. Symptoms of respiratory alkalosis include shortness of breath, lightheadedness, dizziness, paresthesia, syncope (fainting), or numbness in the face, fingers, or toes. When severe, respiratory alkalosis can result in muscular tetany and convulsions. Treatment often consists of training in slow, relaxed breathing techniques, sedation, and/or pain control. Although this is typically a **YELLOW** flag when caused by pain or anxiety, this could be a **RED** flag issue. Any client demonstrating hyperventilation in the absence of pain or anxiety could have a serious systemic problem, and immediate referral will be necessary.[1]

When either respiratory acidosis or respiratory alkalosis persists in a less aggressive manner for several hours to days, the kidneys will begin to assist in the restoration of normal body fluid pH using a process called renal compensation.

Obstructive Lung Disease

Individuals with obstructive lung disease have difficulty exhaling all of the air from their lungs due to narrowing of the airways or damage to the lungs.[18] Chronic obstructive pulmonary disease, bronchitis, emphysema, bronchiectasis, and asthma are examples of obstructive lung disease.[18]

Chronic Obstructive Pulmonary Disease

COPD is a term that refers to a number of disorders that cause abnormal airway structures resulting in airway obstruction, such as obstructive bronchitis and emphysema.[1] COPD is the leading cause of mortality among cigarette smokers, rarely occurring in nonsmokers. In COPD, the obstructed airways cause air to become trapped in the bronchioles and alveoli, which increases the resistance to airflow and hinders normal gas exchange, causing the alveoli to distend.[1] In a healthy person, the bottom of the diaphragm sits at about T9, and when we inspire, it lowers to T11 to let in the new air, but in a person with COPD, the lower margin of the lower lobes of the lungs already sits at T11 because of overexpansion, resulting in a decreased ability to expand further during inspiration.[1]

Acute Bronchitis

Acute bronchitis is an inflammatory condition of the trachea and the bronchi, typically of short duration and self-limiting. Symptoms include mild fever, malaise, sore throat, cough and wheezing, and possible laryngitis. Chronic bronchitis is typically associated with exposure to bronchial irritants (e.g., cigarette particles, pollutants, dust, or pollen). There is hyperexcretion of mucus and structural changes in the bronchi, leading to partial or complete blockage of the airways and insufficient oxygenation to the alveoli. Treatment is directed toward methods to clear the airways.[1] These clients have an increased susceptibility toward infections with associated wheezing, reduced chest expansion, persistent productive cough that is worse in the morning and evening (with slight midday relief), dyspnea (or shortness of breath), decreased activity or exercise tolerance, and possible cyanosis.[1]

Emphysema

Emphysema occurs when the alveolar walls are destroyed, leading to a permanent overdistention of alveolar air spaces and loss of the lung's normal elastic tension.[1] This condition, which can develop after chronic bronchitis, results in obstruction of the air passages and collapse of the alveoli. When the alveoli collapse, there are resultant air spaces in the alveolar area (called blebs) and in the lung parenchyma (called bullae).[1] With this dead space, breathing becomes more difficult, resulting in low arterial oxygen levels and a characteristic barrel chest.[1]

Bronchiectasis

Bronchiectasis is a type of bronchitis that is progressive and occurs after an infection (typically cystic fibrosis [CF] or a poorly treated childhood PNA). It is characterized by abnormal permanent dilation of the bronchi and destruction of the bronchial walls. This results in a vicious cycle of bacterial infection and inflammation of the bronchial walls with loss of ventilation and irreversible lung damage. In advanced cases, the individual might develop cor pulmonale. Cor pulmonale is a change in structure and function of the heart's right ventricle resulting from a respiratory disorder.[19] Symptoms of bronchiectasis include dyspnea, chronic wet cough, hemoptysis (bloody sputum), weight loss, anemia, malaise, recurrent fever, and chills.[1]

Asthma

Asthma is a reversible obstructive disease of the lungs.[1] Asthma can become a chronic inflammatory condition with life-threatening exacerbations, if poorly controlled. It is believed that in people with asthma, an inflammatory reaction to allergens or other triggers occurs, extending beyond the upper airways and into the lungs, causing airway constriction due to underlying inflammation.[1] The cause of asthma is believed to be both genetic (nature) and environmental (nurture). In the United States alone, there are as many as 24 million people of all ages who suffer with asthma.[1] Status asthmaticus is a life-threatening complication of asthma, characterized by severe bronchospasms, trapped air, a paradoxic pulse, and a drop in blood pressure. Pneumothorax can develop and eventually lead to acidosis. Status asthmaticus is a **RED** flag requiring immediate medical attention. The key symptom is a decrease in blood pressure of more than 10 mm Hg during inspiration.[1] The occupational therapist or occupational therapy assistant should also listen for wheezing, clearing of the throat, irregular breathing with prolonged expiration, flexed body posture, flaring of the nostrils, sweating, pallor, and skin retraction over the clavicles, ribs, and sternum.[1]

Restrictive Lung Disease

Individuals with restrictive lung disease have difficulty filling their lungs with air during inhalation.[18] The lungs are restricted from fully expanding. Interstitial lung disease, sarcoidosis, amyotrophic lateral sclerosis (ALS), and various morphological conditions can be examples of restrictive lung disease.[18]

Interstitial Lung Disease

Interstitial lung disease is a group of disorders caused by the accumulation of both cells and/or noncellular material in the alveoli of the lungs. This accumulation can lead to stiffening and scarring in the tissues, making it difficult to breathe.[20] Symptoms include shortness of breath on exertion and a nagging dry cough. Some examples of interstitial lung disease include chronic eosinophilic PNA, rheumatoid lung, scleroderma lung, idiopathic pulmonary fibrosis, and sarcoidosis.[20]

Sarcoidosis

Sarcoidosis occurs when there are tiny collections of granulomas anywhere in the body, especially in the lungs and lymph nodes, but also sometimes found in the eyes, heart, skin, and other organs.[21] Although the cause is unknown, some suspect an autoimmune origin. There is no known cure, but for some individuals, this disorder goes away on its own.

Amyotrophic Lateral Sclerosis

ALS, also known as Lou Gehrig's disease, is a neurological disorder affecting communication between the spinal cord and the voluntary muscles of the body, including those that help with breathing, swallowing, and chewing food.[22] This is a progressive disorder that greatly restricts breathing. More on ALS can be found in Chapter 20.

Morphological Restrictions

Anything that limits movement of the rib cage or expansion of the lungs can lead to restrictive lung disease. Examples of this include obesity, pregnancy, ankylosing spondylitis (a disorder of the joints in the spine), and scoliosis.[18]

Inflammation and Infection

There are many various infections and inflammatory processes that can lead to either pulmonary restriction or obstruction. Some examples include PNA, tuberculosis (TB), and Long COVID.

Pneumonia

PNA is lung inflammation that may be caused by food aspiration, inhalation of toxic substances, or infection.[1] Risk factors include smoking, exposure to pollutants, upper respiratory infection, malnutrition, dehydration, age (very young or elderly), and long-term bed rest.[1] Symptoms of PNA include sudden, sharp pleuritic chest pain, shoulder pain, a productive cough (with rust-colored or green sputum), dyspnea, cyanosis, fever, and chills.[1]

Tuberculosis

TB is a bacterial infectious condition caused by *Mycobacterium tuberculosis*.[1] There was a decline in the number of TB cases after the development of medications with anti-TB properties in the 1940s; however, there was a rise again in 1980, secondary to an increase in immigrants from Third World countries, an increase in the homeless population, and the development of new drug-resistant strains of TB.[1] People at risk include healthcare workers, older adults, and people with diabetes or renal disease. Symptoms include fatigue, malaise, anorexia, weight loss, night sweats, dyspnea, and dull chest pain with tightness or discomfort.[1] TB skin testing will determine the differential diagnosis by checking the body's immune response to see if it has been activated by the presence of the bacillus.[1]

Long COVID

In 2019, a new coronavirus that could cause severe acute respiratory syndrome (SARS) was identified. It was named SARS-CoV-2, and the disease it causes was later named COVID-19.[23] According to the Centers for Disease Control and Prevention (CDC), as of June 2022, approximately one out of every five adults who have had COVID-19 still have what is known as "Long COVID,"[24] or also known as "post-COVID" or "Long-haul COVID."[25] Over the past year, more has been learned regarding Long COVID, which includes a wide range of health conditions lasting weeks, months, or even years. Some of the many possible symptoms include postexertional malaise, breathing difficulty, heart palpitations, sleep problems, and depression or anxiety.[25]

Pulmonary Vascular Disease

Pulmonary vascular disease is an umbrella term for any disorder affecting the blood vessels within the lungs. These disorders can lead to cardiovascular problems and interfere greatly with an individual's quality of life.[26] These disorders

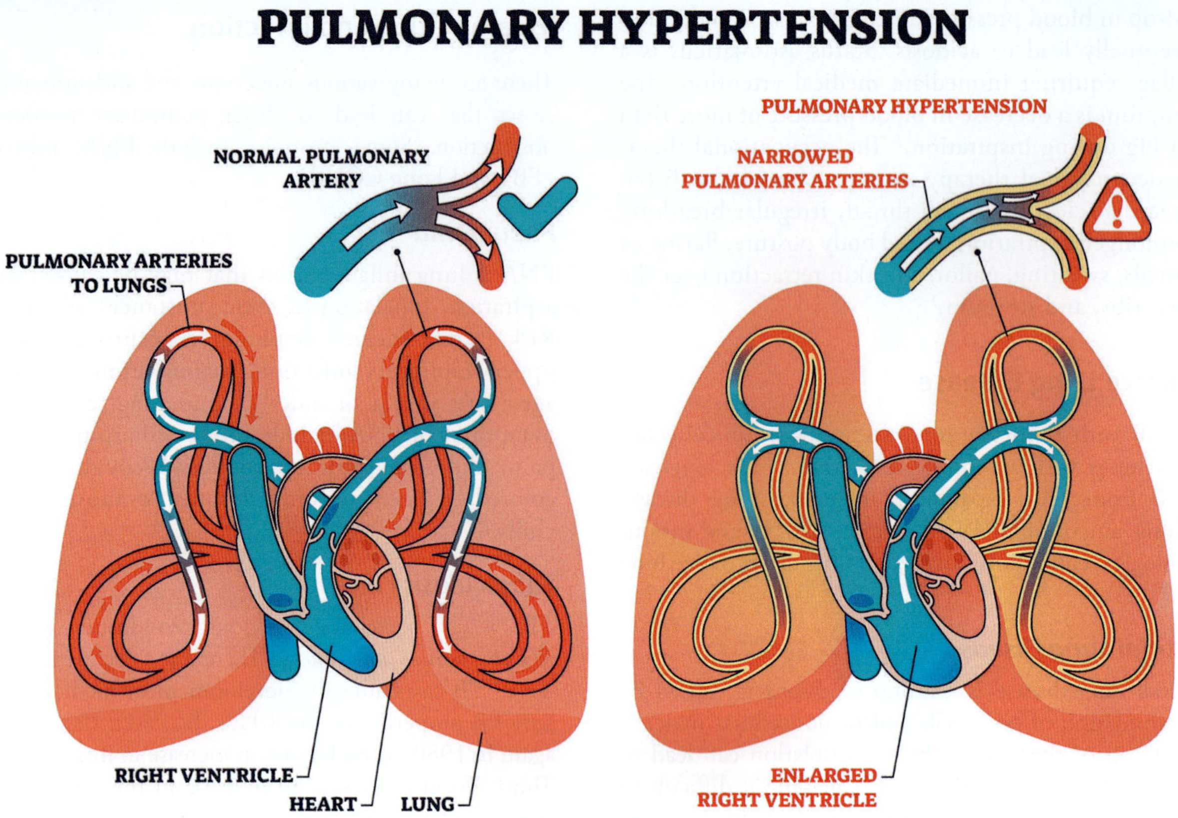

• **Fig. 14.10** Pulmonary hypertension. (From https://iStock.com/VectorMine.)

include pulmonary hypertension (PH), pulmonary vasculitis, and acute PE.[27]

Pulmonary Hypertension

PH is a higher-than-normal blood pressure in your pulmonary arteries.[28] The first symptom is typically shortness of breath while doing normal daily activities and is often the result of an existing heart or lung disease. Other symptoms include dyspnea that worsens over time, cyanosis of the lips and/or skin, dizziness or fainting, and edema in the legs, ankles, or abdominal area. This can be dangerous if the arteries in the lungs narrowed, making the heart work harder to pump blood to the lungs for oxygenation (Fig. 14.10).[28] PH can eventually be fatal without intervention because it can lead to right ventricular hypertrophy and a ripple effect throughout the entire body. It can also lead to eventual cor pulmonale.

There are various types of PH: pulmonary arterial hypertension, PH due to left-sided heart disease, and PH due to lung disease, hypoxia, blockages in the lungs, or other disorders.[28]

Pulmonary Vasculitis

This is a group of severe, progressive diseases characterized by vascular inflammation, resulting in destruction of the lung tissue. The amount of destruction depends on the size of the vessels involved.[29] Although these are rare disorders, an early diagnosis is imperative as it can lead to life-threatening pulmonary bleeding, with subsequent damage to other organs in the body.

Acute Pulmonary Embolism

A PE is a blockage in the vasculature of the lungs by a blood clot or an air bubble (Fig. 14.11). Symptoms include shortness of breath, chest pain, and fainting.[30] When a PE is large, obstructing 60% to 75% of the circulation, acute cor pulmonale can occur.[1] This sudden enlargement of the right ventricle is serious and could result in right-sided heart failure. Symptoms include dyspnea, edema in the legs, liver distention, distention of the veins in the neck, and an elevated hematocrit as the body tries to compensate by producing more erythrocytes.[1]

PE is typically caused by a blood clot that has already formed in one of the deep veins in an extremity called a deep vein thrombosis (DVT).[30] The three major risk factors for DVT include blood stasis from bed rest or obesity, endothelial injury, and hypercoagulable states.[1] Symptoms of DVT include edema and skin redness with associated pain as well as temperature variations on palpation.[1] A test that was once used often was the Homan sign (pain from passive dorsiflexion), but this test has since been considered to be unreliable. An effective indicator to help rule

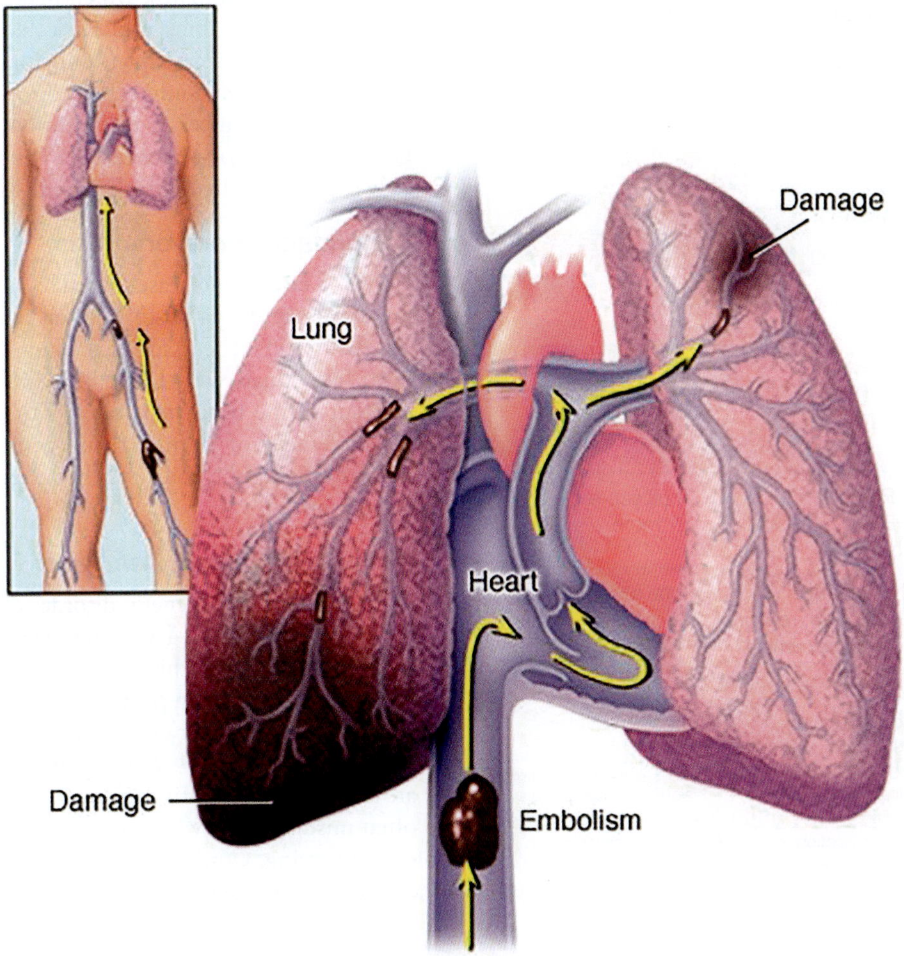

• **Fig. 14.11** Pulmonary embolism. (From https://www.mayoclinic.org/diseases-conditions/pulmonary-embolism/symptoms-causes/syc-20354647, used with permission of Mayo Foundation for Medical Education and Research. All rights reserved.)

out possible PE is the Well's Clinical Decision Rule (see Table 14.1).[1]

Immediate referral to a physician is recommended whenever an individual experiences an abrupt onset of dyspnea, chest pain, shoulder pain with neurologic symptoms, or symptoms of inadequate ventilation.

Neoplasms

There are about 12 different types of neoplastic lung disease (lung cancer). The most prevalent cancer types include small-cell cancers (oat cell carcinoma), squamous cell carcinoma, adenocarcinoma, and large-cell carcinoma.[1] Smoking is the top risk factor, but age (older than 50 years), genetic predisposition, and previous lung disease are also risk factors. Paraneoplastic syndromes occur in about 10% to 20% of individuals with lung cancer.[1] These are believed to be due to the secretion of hormones by the tumor affecting other body organs; these syndromes or symptoms will often mimic neurologic conditions with tremor or ataxia.[1]

Genetic Disorders

Genetic diseases of the lungs are many and varied. Some that might be encountered in clients seen in an occupational therapy setting include cystic fibrosis (CF), lymphangioleiomyomatosis (LAM), and alpha-1 antitrypsin deficiency (AAT deficiency).

Cystic Fibrosis

CF is the most common disease of recessive genetic inheritance in the United States.[1] Both parents must be carriers (Fig. 14.12). In a healthy individual, a channel is developed that allows chloride from salt to pass in and out of cells by a protein called transmembrane conductance regulator (CFTR).[1] People with CF have a defective copy of the gene that helps cells to create that channel. Because

TABLE 14.1 Simplified Well's Criteria to Detect DVT[a]

Criteria	Score
Clinical symptoms of DVT (leg swelling, pain with palpation)	1.0
Other diagnosis less likely than pulmonary embolism	1.0
Heart rate greater than 100 bpm	1.0
Immobilization for 3 or more days or surgery in the past 4 weeks	1.0
History of DVT/PE	1.0
Hemoptysis	1.0
Malignancy	1.0
Screening Clinical Probability Assessment: PE likely; medical consult advised	Total score: 2 or more
Screening Clinical Probability Assessment: PE unlikely; review all other factors then document findings	Total score: 0 or 1

[a]Modified Well's Criteira.
DVT, Deep vein thrombosis; *PE*, pulmonary embolism.
Data from Douma RA. Validity and clinical utility of the simplified Wells rule for assessing clinical probability for the exclusion of pulmonary embolism. *Thromb Haemost*. 2009;101(1):197–200, and Gibson NS. Further validation and simplification of the Wells clinical decision rule in pulmonary embolism. *Thromb Haemost*. 2008;99:229–234.

of this, salt accumulates, which makes the fluids and surrounding mucus thick and sticky, leading to obstructed ducts in the pancreas, liver, and lungs. Individuals with CF were previously only expected to live into their 20s or 30s. Due to advances in intervention for this population, however, those born between the years 2014 and 2018 are now expected to live into their mid-40s.[1]

Lymphangioleiomyomatosis

LAM is a rare lung disease caused by tuberous sclerosis gene mutations, resulting in an unusual type of smooth muscle cell that invades the tissue of the lungs, causing an obstruction. Individuals with LAM have difficulty moving air in and out of the bronchial tubes.[31] There is also sometimes a replacement of normal tissue with cysts or holes, further weakening the ability of the lungs to perform efficient respiration.[31]

Alpha-1 Antitrypsin Deficiency

AAT deficiency is a genetic disorder of autosomal recessive inheritance (see Fig. 14.12); however, it can also be caused by smoking.[32] With this disorder, there is a deficiency in the alpha-1 antitrypsin protein that protects the lungs from destructive illnesses or environmental toxins such as pollution, smoke, or dust.[32] Many people with AAT deficiency are asymptomatic, until they are in their 20s to 50s, and are often misdiagnosed with asthma when they start to experience wheezing. Confirmation of AAT deficiency is done by a blood test or a genetic test.[32]

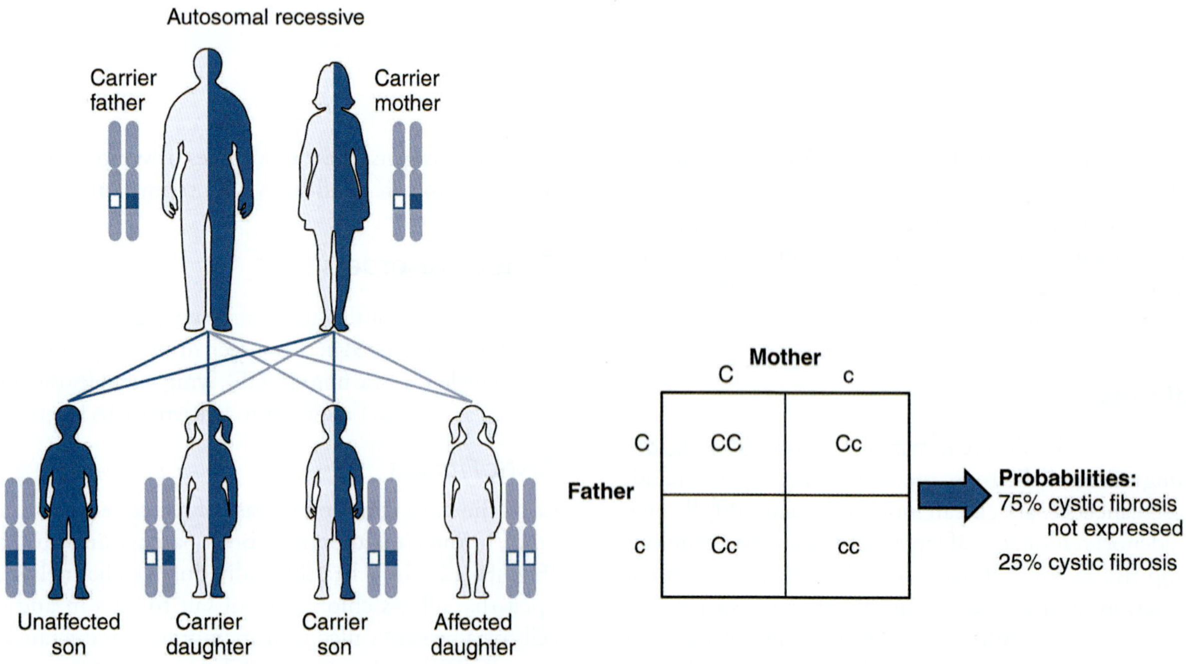

• **Fig. 14.12** Autosomal recessive inheritance. (Courtesy U.S. National Library of Medicine.)

Occupational Lung Disease

Occupational lung diseases include occupational lung cancer, work-related asthma, asbestos mesothelioma, byssinosis (brown lung disease), hypersensitivity PNA, acute respiratory irritation, pneumoconiosis (the dust diseases), and lead poisoning.[1] Home remodeling and certain jobs that involve inhalation of irritants can lead to one of the above occupational lung diseases.

The OT Scope of Practice

Once again, when working as an occupational therapy practitioner (OTP), if a client demonstrates symptoms that are outside of the typical cluster you expect to find with their diagnosis, it is important to report those symptoms to the referring physician. Understanding what would be "normal" and what lies outside that cluster of symptoms expected for that individual's current diagnosis can be the key toward a better understanding of the individual's true condition.

Application—Case Study

CASE EXAMPLE 14.1

A 24-year-old male presented to an outpatient clinic to set up a home exercise program targeting strengthening and activity tolerance after 2 weeks in the acute care setting for severe pneumonia (PNA). No occupational therapy (OT) or physical therapy (PT) services had been ordered to help the client remain active during his hospital stay.

1. **Screen:** During the screening process, the occupational therapist noticed that the client was out of breath, with rapid, shallow breathing and a wheezing sound during inhalation.
2. **Take a Closer Look:** The occupational therapist asked how long this fatigue had been going on, and the client reported that it started as soon as he was able to get out of bed the day prior and was getting worse. The client was worried about going home too soon. The occupational therapist took the client's oxygen saturation level, which was stable at 92% but decreased to 80% after a bout of functional ambulation. She suggested that the client rest and perform pulsed lip breathing.
3. **Determine Flag Status:** Because she was concerned, the occupational therapist determined this to be a potential red flag situation.
4. **Take Action if Needed:** She called the doctor to see if there might have been a reason for the client's current symptoms. The doctor was grateful for the phone call from the occupational therapist and ordered a chest X-ray. Upon discussion with the team, the occupational therapist learned that the physical therapist was also concerned about this client for the same reason.
5. **Document the Findings:** The occupational therapist documented the findings of her examination as well as the phone call to the physician and discussion with the physical therapist.
6. **Take a Second Look:** The X-ray showed a possible atelectasis (a complete or partial collapse of all or a portion of the lung)[33] of the upper lobe of the right lung. The doctor immediately canceled the discharge instructions.
7. **Determine the Flag Status:** This had quickly become a definitive red flag.
8. **Take Action if Needed:** A bronchoscopy was done to remove airway obstructions. The client remained stable in the hospital for several more days, during which time, the occupational therapist saw him at bedside and then in the clinic to gradually improve out-of-bed tolerance. The occupational therapist also met with the physician to request that these individuals be seen sooner for both OT and PT to encourage early mobility and to regain breathing efficiency, strength, and endurance, with the hopes of preventing future occurrences. New policies were implemented at the hospital to ensure that this would be done in the future.

This is a true case. The client had atelectasis, possibly caused by the severe PNA, with a long period of bed rest that was suddenly followed by reentry into the clinical setting to prepare for discharge. The occupational therapist's diplomatic discussions, both with the doctor and other members of the healthcare team, and courage to create change, led to new policies in the hospital ensuring that individuals with pulmonary conditions would be referred to both OT and PT to get out of bed sooner and to gradually be reintroduced to meaningful activity.

References

1. Heick J, Lazaro RT. *Goodman and Snyder's Differential Diagnosis for Physical Therapists: Screening for Referral.* 7th ed. Elsevier; 2023.
2. Menefee W, Jenks J, Mazzasette C, Nguyen K. *20.5: Embryonic Development of the Respiratory System.* Libretexts Med UC Davis; 2023. https://med.libretexts.org/Bookshelves/Anatomy_and_Physiology/Human_Anatomy_(OERI)/20%3A_Respiratory_System/20.05%3A_Embryonic_Development_of_the_Respiratory_System.
3. Rehman S, Bacha D. *Embryology, Pulmonary.* Stats Pearls (Internet), NIH Library of Medicine; 2022. https://www.ncbi.nlm.nih.gov/books/NBK544372/.
4. Kahwar H, Marwaha K. *Surfactant.* Stats Pearls (Internet), NIH Library of Medicine; 2023. https://www.ncbi.nlm.nih.gov/books/NBK546600/.
5. Huff T, Chaudhry R, Arora Y, Mahajan K. *Anatomy, Thorax, Heart Ductus Arteriosus.* Stats Pearls (Internet), NIH Library of Medicine; 2022. https://www.ncbi.nlm.nih.gov/books/NBK470160/.
6. De Gelidi S, Bardill A, Seifnaraghi N, et al. Thoracic shape changes in newborns due to their position. *Sci Rep.* 2021;11:21. https://doi.org/10.1038/s41598-021-83869-8. Article number 4446.
7. Dassios T, Vervenioti A, Dimitriou G. Respiratory muscle function in the newborn: a narrative review. *Pediatric Res.* 2022;91:795–803.
8. Openshaw P, Edwards S, Helms P. Changes in rib cage geometry during childhood. *Thorax.* 1984;39(8):624–627. https://www.ncbi.nlm.nih.gov/pmc/articles/PMC1020518/.
9. Terry PB, Traystman RJ. The clinical significance of collateral ventilation. *Ann Am Thorac Soc.* 2016;13(12):2252–2257. https://doi.org/10.1513/AnnalsATS.201606-448FR.
10. Hislop AA, Wigglesworth JS, Desai R. Alveolar development in the human fetus and infant. *Early Hum Dev.* 1986;13(1):1–11. https://doi.org/10.1016/0378-3782(86)90092-7.

11. Herring MJ, Putney LF, Wyatt G, et al. Growth of alveoli during postnatal development in humans based on stereological estimation. *Am J Physiol Lung Cell Mol Physiol.* 2014; 307(4):L338–L344. https://doi.org/10.1152/ajplung.00094.2014.
12. Biga LM, Bronson S, Dawson S, et al. *22.2 The Lungs. Anatomy & Physiology*. OpenStax, Oregon State University; 2023. https://open.oregonstate.education/aandp/chapter/22-2-the-lungs/.
13. Tomashefski JF, Farver CF. Anatomy and histology of the lung. In: Tomashefski JF, Cagle PT, Farver CF, Fraire AE, eds. *Dail and Hammar's Pulmonary Pathology, Volume I, Nonneoplastic Lung Disease*. 3rd ed. Springer Science; 2008.
14. Klocke RA. *The Mechanisms of Breathing*. Britannica; 2023. https://www.britannica.com/science/human-respiratory-system/The-mechanics-of-breathing.
15. NIH. *How Your Body Controls Breathing*. National Heart Lung and Blood Institute, NIH; 2022. https://www.nhlbi.nih.gov/health/lungs/body-controls-breathing.
16. Al-Ashkar F, Mehra R, Mazzone PJ. Interpreting pulmonary function tests: recognize the pattern, and the diagnosis will follow. *Clevel Clin J Med.* 2003;70(1):866–881. https://internal.medicine.ufl.edu/files/2012/06/5.12.02-How-to-Interpret-Pulmonary-Function-Tests.pdf.
17. Cleveland Clinic. *Peritoneum*. Cleveland Clinic Health Library; 2022. https://my.clevelandclinic.org/health/body/22894-peritoneum.
18. Hoffman M. *Obstructive and Restrictive Lung Disease*. WebMD; 2022. https://www.webmd.com/lung/obstructive-and-restrictive-lung-disease.
19. Cleveland Clinic. *Cor Pulmonale (Right-Sided Heart Failure)*. Cleveland Clinic; 2023. https://my.clevelandclinic.org/health/diseases/24922-cor-pulmonale.
20. Mayo Clinic. *Interstitial Lung Disease Clinic*. Pulmonary Medicine at the Mayo Clinic; 2023. https://www.mayoclinic.org/departments-centers/interstitial-lung-disease-clinic/overview/ovc-20398498.
21. Mayo Clinic. *Sarcoidosis*. The Mayo Clinic; 2023. https://www.mayoclinic.org/diseases-conditions/sarcoidosis/symptoms-causes/syc-20350358.
22. ALS Pathways. *Understanding ALS*. ALS Pathways; 2023. https://www.alspathways.com/als-overview/#about-als.
23. Mayo Clinic. *Coronavirus Disease 2019 (COVID-19)*. Mayo Clinic; 2023. https://www.mayoclinic.org/diseases-conditions/coronavirus/symptoms-causes/syc-20479963.
24. CDC. *Nearly One in Five American Adults Who Have Had COVID-19 still Have "Long COVID."* Centers for Disease Control and Prevention; 2022. https://www.cdc.gov/nchs/pressroom/nchs_press_releases/2022/20220622.htm.
25. CDC. *Long COVID or Post-COVID Conditions*. Centers for Disease Control and Prevention; 2023. https://www.cdc.gov/coronavirus/2019-ncov/long-term-effects/index.html.
26. Brigham and Women's. *Pulmonary Vascular Disease*. Brigham and Women's Hospital; 2023. https://www.brighamandwomens.org/lung-center/diseases-and-conditions/pulmonary-vascular-disease.
27. Bankier AA, Dennie C. Modern diagnosis in the evaluation of pulmonary vascular disease. In: Hodler J, Kubik-Huch RA, von Schulthess GK, eds. *Diseases of the Chest, Breast, Heart and Vessels 2019-2022: Diagnostic and Interventional Imaging [Internet]*. Springer; 2019. https://ncbi.nlm.nih.gov/books/NBK553875/.
28. Cleveland Clinic. *Pulmonary Hypertension (PH)*. Cleveland Clinic; 2023. https://my.clevelandclinic.org/health/diseases/6530-pulmonary-hypertension-ph.
29. Anaev EKh, Baranova A, Belevsky AS. Pulmonary vasculitis: diagnosis and treatment. *Terapevticheskii Arkhiv (Therapeutic Arch J)*. 2018;90(3):99–106. https://doi.org/10.26442/terarkh201890399-106.
30. Mayo Clinic. *Pulmonary Embolism*. Mayo Clinic; 2023. https://www.mayoclinic.org/diseases-conditions/pulmonary-embolism/symptoms-causes/syc-20354647.
31. Cleveland Clinic. *Lymphangioleiomyomatosis (LAM)*. Cleveland Clinic; 2020. https://my.clevelandclinic.org/health/diseases/16022-lymphangioleiomyomatosis-lam.
32. NIH. *Alpha-1 Antitrypsin Deficiency*. National Heart, Lung, and Blood Institute, NIH; 2022. https://www.nhlbi.nih.gov/health/alpha-1-antitrypsin-deficiency.
33. Mayo Clinic. *Atelectasis*. Mayo Clinic; 2023. https://www.mayoclinic.org/diseases-conditions/atelectasis/diagnosis-treatment/drc-20369688.

15

Gastrointestinal Pathophysiology

OBJECTIVES

By the end of this chapter, the reader should be able to:

- Demonstrate a basic understanding of a healthy gastrointestinal system.
- Demonstrate a basic understanding of pathophysiological conditions affecting the gastrointestinal system.
- Explain the pain patterns sometimes associated with the gastrointestinal system.
- Explain some of the palpation techniques used to differentiate an abscess or referred pain.
- Identify possible symptoms associated with various gastrointestinal disorders.
- Explain and/or predict the possible symptoms resulting from the pathophysiology of various gastrointestinal disorders.
- Assess and justify whether a specific gastrointestinal symptom could constitute a yellow or red flag.

The Physiology of Digestion

The gastrointestinal system is made up of the gastrointestinal (GI) tract and the biliary system (liver, pancreas, and gallbladder). The biliary system will be covered in Chapter 16. This chapter covers the GI tract, which consists of a long, convoluted pathway from the mouth, through the esophagus, to the small and large intestines, ending in the anal region (Fig. 15.1).[1]

Healthy Gastrointestinal Physiology

The Mouth

The mouth is the first point of entry for the digestive system, but digestion technically starts before you take a bite of food. Just before the food enters the mouth, salivation takes place.[2] Saliva contains enzymes that mix with the food and begin to break it down for digestion.[3]

The Esophagus

Passive pressure from the tongue during swallowing pushes food down the pharynx and helps regulate movements of the epiglottis. The epiglottis is a flap of cartilage that closes the laryngeal inlet during swallowing so that no food passes into the trachea, which could lead to food in the lungs or aspiration.[4] Swallowing occurs in three phases. The oral phase is voluntary and consists of the passage of food (or bolus) from the oral cavity into the oropharynx. The second stage is involuntary and called the pharyngeal phase, during which the bolus moves from the oropharynx into the esophagus.[5] After the epiglottis moves to block the trachea, a muscle called the upper esophageal sphincter relaxes, allowing food to pass into the esophagus (Fig. 15.2).

The third stage of swallowing is the esophageal phase, when the bolus moves from the esophagus as it pierces the diaphragm, through the lower esophageal sphincter, which opens to allow food to enter the stomach.[5]

The Stomach

The stomach is a hollow muscular container and possibly the most important section of the GI tract. Everything ingested must go through this organ, which is responsible for mechanical digestion, chemical digestion, absorption, and the production of hormones (gastrin, somatostatin, and ghrelin) and regulatory peptides.[6] After the food has been processed, it can be passed into the small intestine.[2]

The Small Intestine

The small intestine begins at the base of the stomach at the duodenum and and is a muscular tube approximately 22 feet long, composed of three segments: the duodenum, jejunum, and ileum. It continues to break down food using enzymes from the pancreas and bile from the liver.[2] Food moves from solid to liquid form after passing through this long tunnel; here, water mixes with the enzymes, bile, and mucus to liquefy the food.

The Pancreas

The pancreas falls within three different systems: the GI system, the biliary system (see Chapter 16), and the endocrine system (see Chapter 18) because it has both endocrine and exocrine functions.[7] As an endocrine gland, the pancreas secretes insulin (the main hormone for sugar metabolism) and other important hormones directly into the bloodstream.[2] For digestion, the pancreas releases peptidases, lipases, nucleases, and amylases.[8] These powerful enzymes help with digestion by breaking down fats, carbohydrates, and proteins.[2]

The Liver and Gallbladder

The liver has many responsibilities, but its primary role in digestion is to take nutrients absorbed in the small intestine and process them. It also secretes bile to help digest various vitamins and fats.[2] The gallbladder acts as the storage unit for bile from the liver. These will both be covered in more detail in Chapter 16.

The Colon (Large Intestine)

The large intestine is a 5- to 6-foot-long muscular tube connecting the small intestine to the rectum.[2,8] Its primary role is to process chyme, or food material that cannot be digested.[9] It begins with the cecum and consists of four parts: the ascending colon, transverse colon, descending colon, and sigmoid colon (Fig. 15.3).[9]

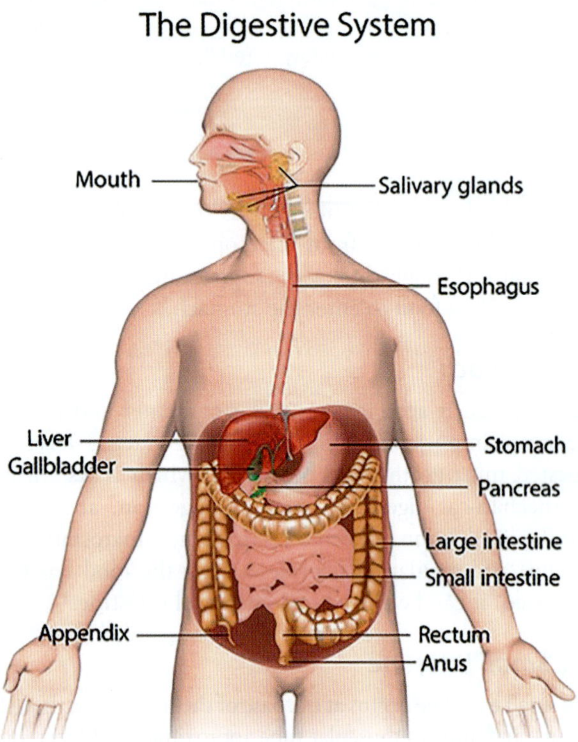

• **Fig. 15.1** The gastrointestinal system. (From https://www.niddk.nih.gov/health-information/digestive-diseases/digestive-system-how-it-works.)

The jobs of the large intestine include separating water and electrolytes from waste material to be absorbed into the system, producing and absorbing vitamins, and forming waste material into feces, which are propelled toward the rectum for eventual elimination.[8]

The Rectum and Anus

The rectum is approximately 8 inches long and connects the colon to the anus. When stool or gas enters this canal and passes toward the anus, a message is sent to the brain to alert the individual.[2] The anus is about 2 inches long with sensors to detect rectal contents. Along with the pelvic floor muscles, an internal sphincter (an involuntary muscle that receives autonomic innervation from the inferior hypogastric plexus) and an external anal sphincter (a voluntary muscle innervated by the pudendal nerve, S2–S4) work to keep the stool from involuntarily leaving the rectum. Our ability to remain continent depends on these nerves and muscles.[2,10,11]

Other Functions of the Gastrointestinal System

About 75% of all cells responsible for immunity are located in the GI tract. In fact, there are more T cells in the epithelial lining of the intestine than in all other bodily tissues combined.[12] There is still much to be learned about the GI system and its innervation (also known as the enteric nervous system). There is a growing field known as psychoneuroimmunology that studies the association between the enteric system, the immune system, and the brain. Many of these studies are performed each year, investigating the association between the GI system and conditions like rheumatoid arthritis and chronic fatigue syndrome.[12]

Gastrointestinal Pathology

There are many different signs and symptoms of possible GI pathophysiology. Early satiety is when the individual is really hungry but becomes full quickly after only a few bites of food.[12] Constipation is when an individual has difficulty eliminating stool. Obstipation is the term for chronic constipation, which is difficult to manage. Diarrhea is described as an abnormal increase in the fluidity and amount of stool. Hydration becomes even more important for these individuals. Fecal incontinence

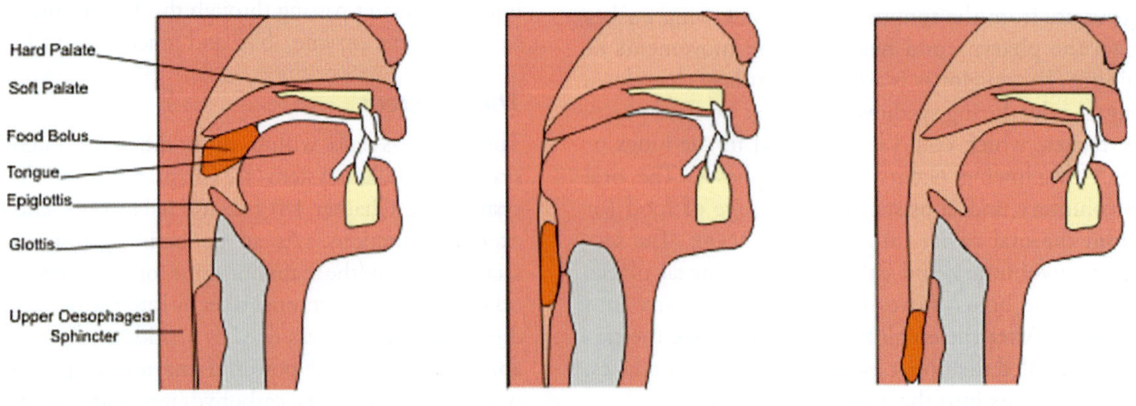

• **Fig. 15.2** Swallowing. (From https://commons.wikimedia.org/wiki/File:Swallow_food.png.)

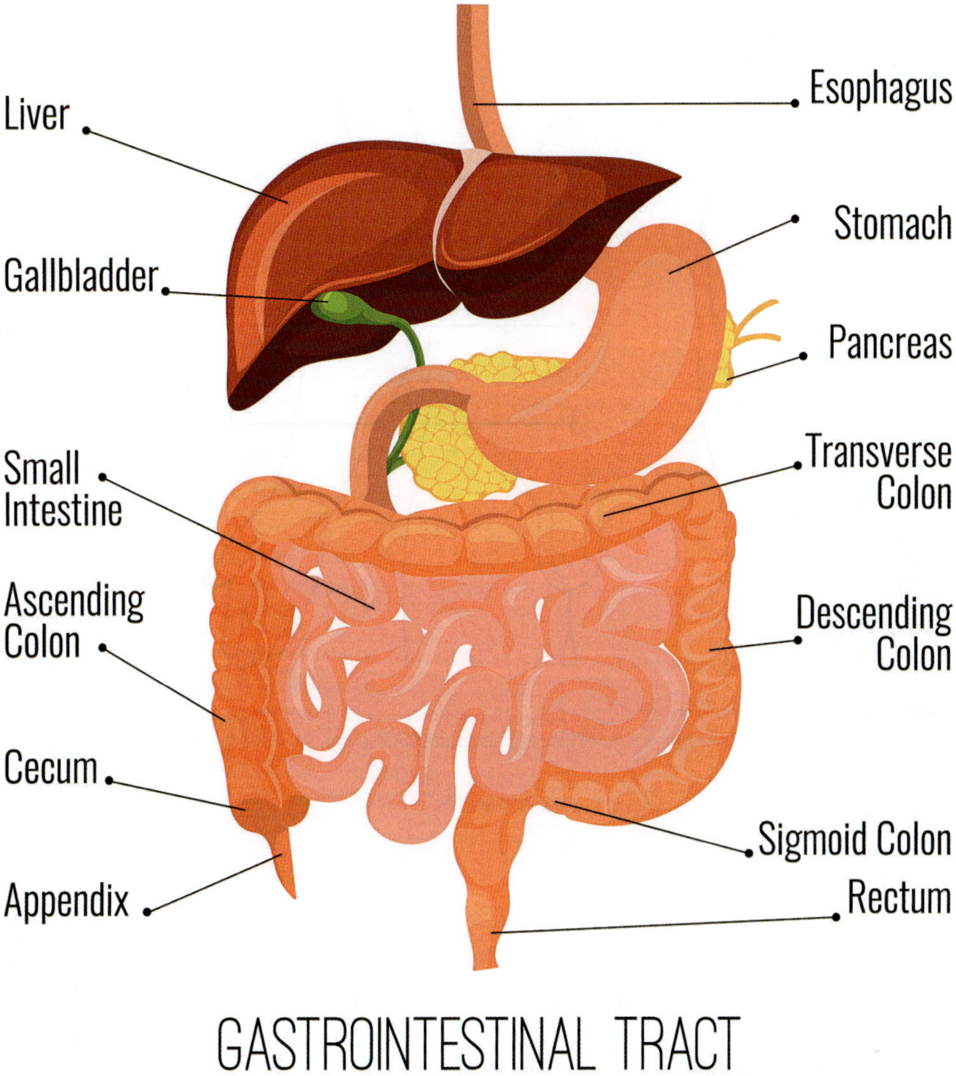

• **Fig. 15.3** Gastrointestinal tract. (From https://www.iStock.com/Godruma.)

is another problem that can be caused by partial obstruction of the rectum, colitis, or even radiation.[12] Other GI symptoms include abdominal pain, dysphagia (difficulty swallowing), psoas abscess, odynophagia (pain with swallowing), and arthralgia (joint pain).

Pain Patterns

GI problems can present with referred pain to the sternum, shoulder, neck, scapula, pelvis, and back.[12] The organs themselves in the abdominal viscera do not perceive pain, but the sensory system is able to inform the body that something is wrong through the sympathetic nervous system. This creates a reflex phenomenon through the peripheral nerves, typically from the same spinal segment, called sympathetic sudomotor changes.[12]

Problems in the epigastric region correspond to the T3–T5 sympathetic nerve distribution with pain coming from the heart, esophagus, stomach, duodenum, gallbladder, or liver and radiating to the ribs, chest, or thoracic spine (mid-back pain) at the T3–T7 levels. Problems in the periumbilical region correspond to the T9–T11 sympathetic nerve distribution, with pain coming from the small intestine, pancreas, and appendix and radiating to the umbilicus and/or low back at around the L3 or L4 level (Fig. 15.4).[12]

An individual might present to occupational therapy with low back pain with or without GI symptoms, but a careful history could reveal that they had a periumbilical pain episode recently that has resolved. Problems in the lower mid-abdominal or hypogastric region correspond to the T10–L2 sympathetic nerve distribution, with pain coming from the large intestines and/or colon (often confused with bladder or uterine pain) and radiating to the pelvis, low back, or sacrum (Fig. 15.5). This referred visceral pain is typically described as deep, aching, burning, sharp, prickling, or knifelike. When referred to other areas, like the shoulder, the location is vague and poorly localized. The areas of referred pain might also have hyperesthesia (increased sensation) or hyperalgesia (excessive sensibility to painful stimuli).[12]

There is sometimes pain over McBurney's point, found one-third of the way between the anterior superior iliac spine (ASIS) and the umbilicus in the lower right quadrant (Fig. 15.6). This pain can be intense when you press on the

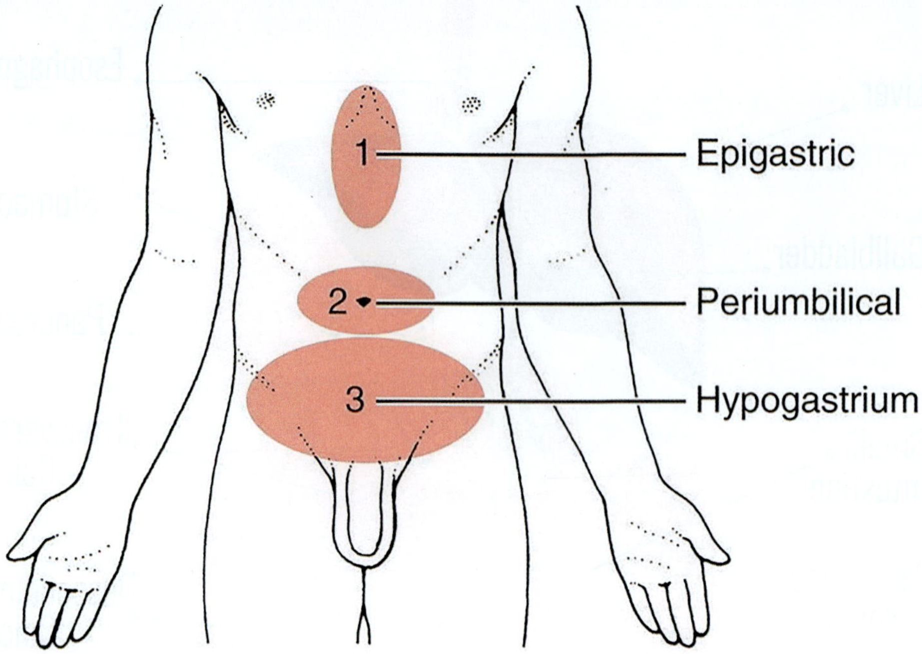

• **Fig. 15.4** Referred gastrointestinal pain patterns—anterior trunk. (From Heick J, Lazaro RT. *Goodman and Snyder's Differential Diagnosis for Physical Therapists: Screening for Referral*. 7th ed. Elsevier; 2023.)

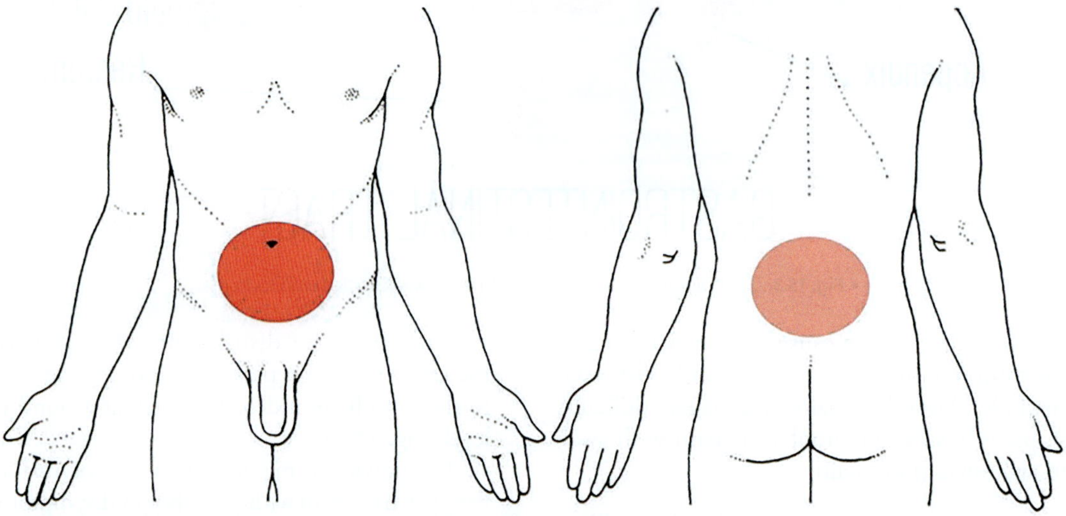

• **Fig. 15.5** Hypogastric pain distribution—anterior and posterior trunk. (From Heick J, Lazaro RT. *Goodman and Snyder's Differential Diagnosis for Physical Therapists: Screening for Referral*. 7th ed. Elsevier; 2023.)

point, but if the pain is worse when you release this pressure (rebound tenderness), this is called a positive Blumberg's sign.

If pain is elicited at McBurney's point when pressure is applied on the opposite side of the body, this is referred to as Rovsing's sign (Fig. 15.7). Either can be indicative of a possible peritonitis or acute appendicitis.[12,13]

Abscess

Obturator or psoas abscess can happen if there is a spread of infection from the GI tract (since these muscles lie behind the GI tract with no protective barrier). Both sides can be involved with general peritonitis (Fig. 15.8).[12]

An antalgic gait (a gait pattern used by a client to avoid a specific pain) might develop with psoas abscess due to a reflex spasm that pulls the leg into internal rotation, resulting in a functional hip flexion contracture. A tender mass can sometimes be palpated in the groin area. The iliopsoas muscle test will result in pain at McBurney's point (Fig. 15.9). The obturator muscle test is performed when trying to rule out appendicitis (Fig. 15.10).[12]

Arthralgia and Joint Inflammation

Many GI conditions have an arthritic component, such as GI infection or inflammatory bowel disease (IBD). The belief is that an antigen crosses the GI mucosa, enters the joint, and an autoimmune response occurs.[12] Enthesitis (inflammation of the entheses, or tendon insertion sites) can occur as well as heel pain with swelling, plantar fasciitis, and enthesopathy (any pathology of the enthesis, typically of the knee, ischial tuberosity, greater trochanter of the femur, or costovertebral and manubriosternal joints).[12] Kehr's sign, or left shoulder pain typically caused by free air in the abdominal cavity, might also be present.[12]

Swallowing and Esophageal Problems

Gastroesophageal reflux disease (GERD) constitutes a group of symptoms caused by the reverse movement of stomach acids and bile into the esophagus (also called acid reflux). Symptoms include chest pain, dysphagia, and a feeling of a lump in the throat. Odynophagia, or pain when swallowing, can be caused by GERD, which may lead to esophagitis.[12] To differentiate between esophagitis and coronary ischemia, upright

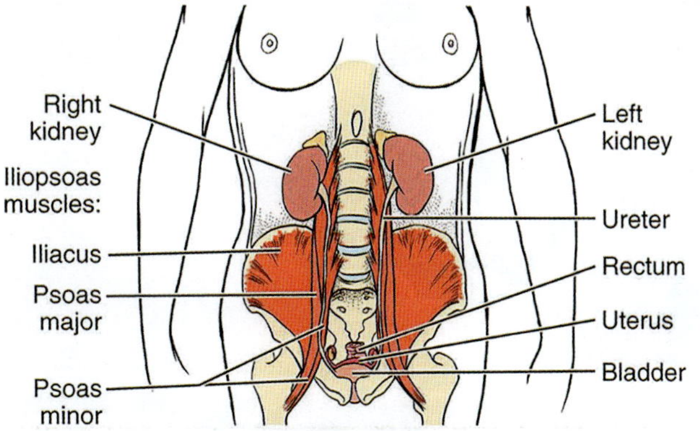

• **Fig. 15.8** Depiction of ilacus and psoas major in relation to the gastrointestinal system. (From Heick J, Lazaro RT. *Goodman and Snyder's Differential Diagnosis for Physical Therapists: Screening for Referral*. 7th ed. Elsevier; 2023.)

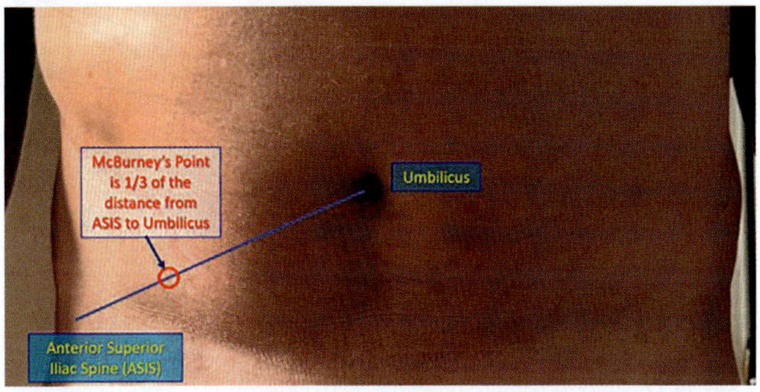

• **Fig. 15.6** McBurney's point.

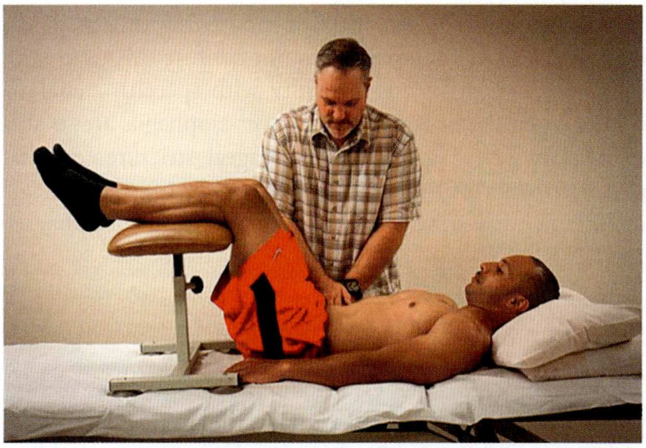

• **Fig. 15.9** The iliopsoas test. (From Heick J, Lazaro RT. *Goodman and Snyder's Differential Diagnosis for Physical Therapists: Screening for Referral*. 7th ed. Elsevier; 2023.)

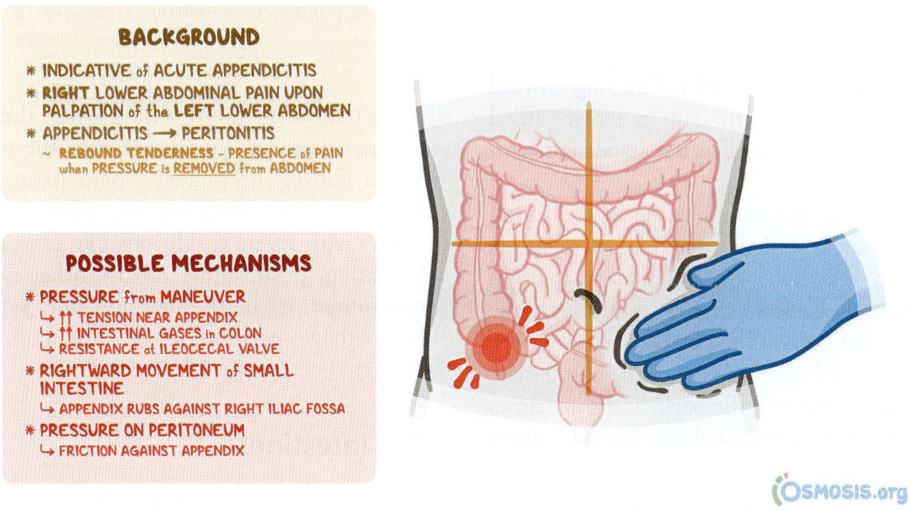

• **Fig. 15.7** Rovsing's sign. (This article was published in Rovsing's Sign, Lily Guo, What Is It, Procedure, Associated Appendicitis, and More, 2021, Copyright Elsevier. https://www.osmosis.org/answers/Rovsing-sign.)

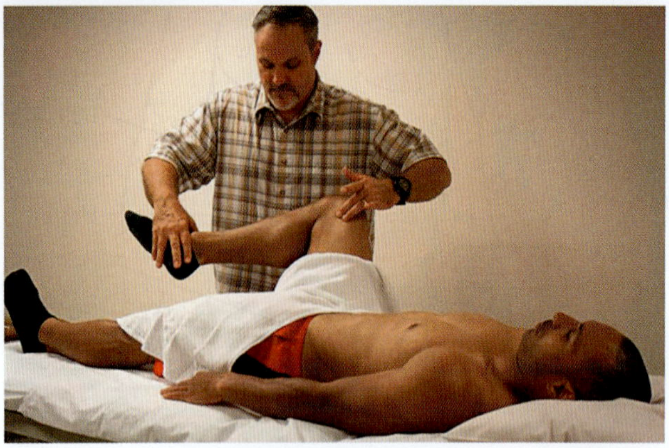

• **Fig. 15.10** The obturator test. (From Heick J, Lazaro RT. *Goodman and Snyder's Differential Diagnosis for Physical Therapists: Screening for Referral*. 7th ed. Elsevier; 2023.)

positioning relieves esophagitis, and supine positioning relieves coronary ischemia. Both conditions require medical referral.[12]

Dysphagia is the sensation of food being caught in the esophagus when swallowing (do not confuse this term with dysphasia, which means difficulty with speech). Achalasia occurs when the muscles of the lower esophagus are unable to relax, which can lead to esophageal stricture (esophageal narrowing). Other problems that can cause dysphagia include peptic esophagitis (inflammation of the esophagus) and GERD.[12]

Stomach and Epigastric Region

When an individual has GI bleeding, it is sometimes accompanied with mid-thoracic back pain. Melena is the presence of large quantities of blood in the stool, giving it a black and tarry appearance.[12] Melenic stool is typically indicative of blood from the upper GI tract. Bright red blood in the stool is typically indicative of blood from the distal colon or rectum, such as from hemorrhoids, rectal fissures, or colorectal carcinoma. Long-standing ulcers can sometimes cause epigastric pain perceived as intense and sharp behind the breastbone with radiation to the back. Epigastric pain that begins at the xiphoid process and radiates up toward the neck might be due to heartburn. This is accompanied by a bitter taste in the mouth and is often associated with GERD.[12]

Peptic ulcers are due to the loss of tissue in the lining of the esophagus, stomach, and duodenum. These ulcers are typically caused by infection with *Helicobacter pylori*, a corkscrew-shaped type of bacteria that bores through the protective layer of the mucosa.[12] The pain comes in waves, will last several minutes, and can radiate into the costal margins, thoracic and lumbar levels of the back, and sometimes the right shoulder. When pain begins about 30–90 minutes after eating, it could be due to gastric ulcers, but when the pain does not begin until about 2–4 hours after eating, it could be due to duodenal or pyloric ulcers. Food will typically not relieve the pain of a gastric ulcer but could relieve the pain of a duodenal ulcer.[12] Duodenal ulcers are typically

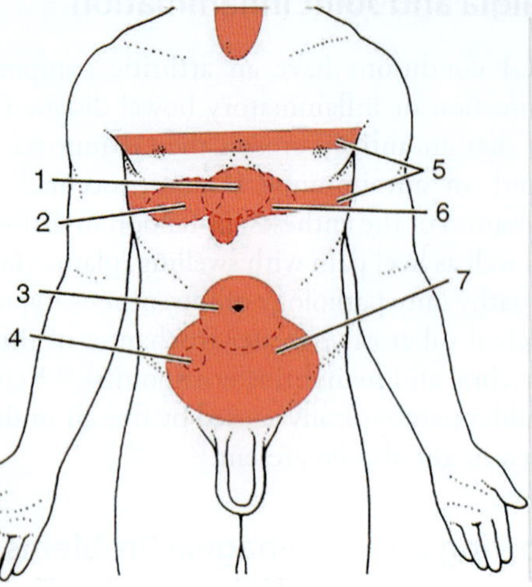

• **Fig. 15.11** Primary gastrointestinal pain patterns. (1) Stomach/duodenum; (2) liver/gallbladder/common bile duct; (3) small intestine; (4) appendix; (5) esophagus; (6) pancreas; and (7) large intestine/colon. (From Heick J, Lazaro RT. *Goodman and Snyder's Differential Diagnosis for Physical Therapists: Screening for Referral*. 7th ed. Elsevier; 2023.)

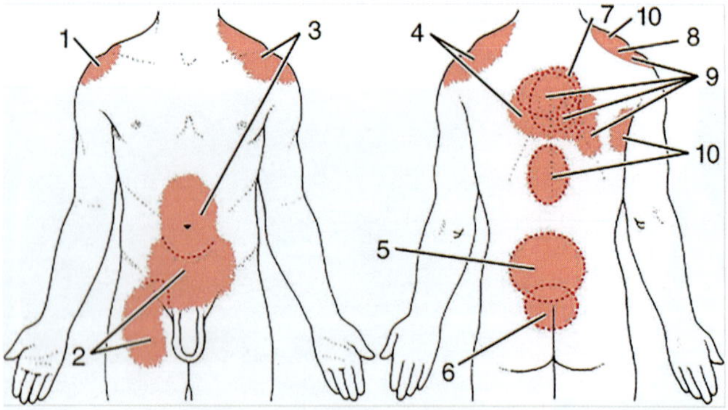

• **Fig. 15.12** Referred gastrointestinal pain patterns. (1) Liver/gallbladder/common bile duct; (2) appendix; (3) pancreas; (4) pancreas; (5) small intestine; (6) colon; (7) esophagus; (8) stomach/duodenum; (9) liver/gallbladder/common bile duct; and (10) stomach/duodenum. (From Heick J, Lazaro RT. *Goodman and Snyder's Differential Diagnosis for Physical Therapists: Screening for Referral*. 7th ed. Elsevier; 2023.)

more painful in the morning when the stomach is empty, and gastric ulcers hurt more with the presence of food. As stated above, the gnawing pain of a duodenal ulcer can be relieved by eating, but the more intense, dull pain that comes with severe conditions like cancer cannot be relieved by eating, positioning, or any other measures. Back pain can sometimes be the first and only symptom of an ulcer, hemorrhage, perforation, or obstruction[12] (Figs. 15.11 and 15.12).

The Intestines

Diverticulosis is a condition that consists of benign pouching or ballooning within the lining of the colon through weakened areas of the mucosal lining. These balloons are called diverticula. Diverticulitis is an infection with inflammation, along with a perforation in one of the diverticula. This can lead to left lower abdominal pain, left pelvic pain, and bloody stools.[12] Appendicitis is an inflammation of the vermiform appendix. It can be very serious, typically requiring surgery. Diseases that can mimic the symptoms of appendicitis include Crohn's disease, perforated duodenal ulcer, gallbladder attacks, right-sided kidney infection, and (in females) ectopic pregnancy or a twisted ovarian cyst. Symptoms typically include pain at McBurney's point, a positive hop test (severe pain when attempting to hop, sometimes used to help determine appendicitis in children), and rebound tenderness (Blumberg's sign).[12]

Irritable bowel syndrome (IBS) is the most common GI disorder in Western society.[12] It is a functional disorder of motility due to abnormal GI smooth muscle contraction with no identifiable abnormality of the bowel. There is visceral pain, constipation or diarrhea, nausea, vomiting, flatulence, foul breath, and bloating, but the disorder rarely progresses and is never fatal. Emotions and stress can aggravate this condition.[12]

IBD is not the same as IBS. There are two types of IBD. The first is ulcerative colitis (UC), an inflammation and ulceration of the inner lining of the large intestine. With this condition, there is often rectal bleeding and diarrhea, with nausea, vomiting, and weight loss. Cancer of the colon is more common among clients with UC than in the general population.[12] The second type is Crohn's disease, an inflammation of the terminal end of the small intestine or ileum.[2] The condition is slow and not as aggressive. There is pain around the umbilicus with some referred pain to the back. There are often symptoms of arthritis and migratory arthralgias.

Colorectal cancer is the third most common cause of death for both males and females in Western society. Mortality can be decreased through a screening process known as fecal occult blood testing.[12]

The Pancreas

Pancreatitis is an inflammation of the pancreas, sometimes resulting in autodigestion of the pancreas by the body's own enzymes.[12] This can be caused by chronic alcoholism, thiazide diuretics, or acetaminophen (i.e., Tylenol).[12] Acute pancreatitis can be self-limiting, but chronic pancreatitis produces recurrent episodes of left upper quadrant pain, with referral to the left lumbar region, mimicking back pain.

Pancreatic carcinoma often produces upper abdominal pain that radiates to the back. This might be the only symptom, so watch for clients with back pain who do not respond to intervention or whose symptoms worsen. Other symptoms of pancreatic cancer might include jaundice, anorexia, light-colored stools, constipation, nausea, vomiting, and weakness. Immediate medical referral is recommended whenever there is a chance of appendicitis, iliopsoas abscess, or retroperitoneal bleeding from a ruptured spleen or ectopic pregnancy.[12] Physician referral is recommended whenever an individual reports that the back pain is relieved after a bowel movement or if the pain seems to be associated with meals, joint involvement, skin irritation, or eye lesions.

Problems affecting the liver and gallbladder will be covered in Chapter 16.

Medications Affecting Gastrointestinal Function

Nonsteroidal anti-inflammatory drugs (NSAIDs) can have negative effects on the entire GI system from the esophagus all the way to the colon. Standard NSAIDs inhibit actions of the two types of cyclooxygenase (COX) enzymes, which are needed to facilitate chemical reactions in the GI tract that promote proper GI function and blood clotting.[12] NSAIDs can also be potent renal vasoconstrictors, leading to lower extremity edema.

A newer type of NSAID called a COX-2 inhibitor (i.e., Celebrex) has been developed to inhibit the effects of only one type of COX and produce less GI irritation. However, these COX-2 inhibitors have been linked to controversial studies regarding risk of cardiovascular problems.[14]

More recent studies have readdressed these safety concerns and continue to be conducted.[14]

The OT Scope of Practice

Once again, when working as an OTP, if a client demonstrates symptoms that are outside of the typical cluster you expect to find with their diagnosis, it is important to report those symptoms to the referring physician.

Application—Case Studies

CASE EXAMPLE 15.1

A 24-year-old female was attending a family reunion. During dinner, she started feeling nauseated. She was talking with her brother, who happens to be an occupational therapist, when she began having sharp pains in her lower right abdominal area. Her brother immediately began investigating further.

1. **Screen:** Her brother asked if she had any other symptoms, and she reported feeling feverish for about 2 days. She had this pain the day before but not with this intensity.
2. **Take a Closer Look:** This was not a clinical setting, but the knowledgeable occupational therapist brought his sister into the house where he could lay her supine and check McBurney's point. There was pain on palpation and definitive rebound tenderness (Blumberg's sign).
3. **Determine Flag Status:** The occupational therapist determined this to be a potential red flag situation. He called 911 for an ambulance pick up, while his sister insisted she was fine.
4. **Take Action if Needed:** The occupational therapist also called his sister's family physician to let him know what was happening. The doctor was grateful for the phone call and ordered an MRI and blood tests upon her arrival at the hospital.
5. **Document the Findings:** This was not a clinical situation, so the occupational therapist was not working at the time and could not document for the record, but he went with his sister to the hospital and made sure to tell the staff the specifics of his sister's condition. This is a great example of how an occupational therapy practitioner (OTP) can be an advocate for a client's situation when talking with other professionals on the medical team.

6. **Take a Second Look:** The MRI showed possible appendicitis, and the sister's bloodwork showed a high white blood cell count, indicating possible infection.
7. **Determine the Flag Status:** This had quickly become a definitive red flag.
8. **Take Action if Needed:** The individual had an emergency appendectomy. The doctor praised the occupational therapist for saving his sister's life. There was nothing further for the brother to do but be there to support his sister.

This is a true case. This author was the occupational therapist's pathology professor three years prior. The occupational therapist called this professor to thank her for the classroom information that helped him save his sister; yet, all the credit goes to this amazing therapist. The sister had appendicitis, and the quick thinking of this OTP was possibly the reason she is alive today.

CASE EXAMPLE 15.2

A 67-year-old male presented to an OTP for assistance with ADLs following a slight right hip flexion contracture from a possible injury.

1. **Screen:** During the occupational therapy screening process, the OTP noticed that the individual had an antalgic gait pattern and a definite lack of full hip extension ROM on the right side. He could not recall any accident or injury leading to this problem. He also reported the pain would be so intense at times, he would feel achy all over and nauseated.
2. **Take a Closer Look:** Concerned this might be a systemic issue, the OTP took the client's temperature and found a low-grade fever of 100.5°F. She asked him to lie on his back with legs elevated on a stool and palpated the area. An area of tenderness, about the size of a golf ball, was palpated in the groin area. There was also severe pain at McBurney's point.
3. **Determine Flag Status:** Because she was concerned, the OTP determined this to be a potential red flag situation.
4. **Take Action if Needed:** She called the client's physician to inform him of the palpable mass, pain at McBurney's point, as well as the low-grade fever. The doctor was grateful for the phone call from the OTP and requested that the OTP send the individual to the ER immediately.
5. **Document the Findings:** The OTP documented the findings of her examination as well as the phone call to the physician.
6. **Take a Second Look:** In the ER, computerized tomography showed an abscess in the right iliopsoas region. The client had an elevated white blood cell count and a high C-reactive protein (this protein is secreted by the liver in response to inflammation).
7. **Determine the Flag Status:** This had quickly become a definitive red flag.
8. **Take Action if Needed:** The client was admitted to the hospital for percutaneous drainage of the abscess and intravenous antibiotics. He made a full recovery and returned to the OTP 2 weeks later for home exercises and ADL and functional mobility education.

This is a true case. The individual had an iliopsoas abscess. The high-level critical thinking skills of the OTP helped to determine the true cause of the client's pain. Although this condition can be difficult to diagnose, the OTP methodically zoomed in on the reason for the client's discomfort and took quick action.

References

1. NIDDK. *Your Digestive System and How It Works.* National Institute of Diabetes and Digestive Kidney Diseases, NIH; 2017. https://www.niddk.nih.gov/health-information/digestive-diseases/digestive-system-how-it-works.
2. Cleveland Clinic. *Digestive System.* Cleveland Clinic; 2024. https://my.clevelandclinic.org/health/body/7041-digestive-system.
3. Vila T, Rizk AM, Sultan AS, Jacra-Rizk MA. The power of saliva: antomicrobial and beyond. *PLOS Pathogens.* 2019;15(11):e1008058. https://doi.org/10.1371/journal.ppat.1008058.
4. Vaskovic J. *Epiglottis.* KenHub. https://www.kenhub.com/en/library/anatomy/epiglottis.
5. Osika A. *Stages of Swallowing (Deglutition).* Ken Hub. https://www.kenhub.com/en/library/anatomy/stages-of-swallowing.
6. Hunt RH, Camilleri M, Crowe SE, et al. The stomach in health and disease. *Recent Br Med J: Adv Clin Pract.* 2015;64:1650–1668. https://doi.org/10.1136/gutjnl-2014-307595.
7. El Sayed SA, Mukherjee S. Physiology, pancreas. In: *StatsPearls (Internet).* National Library of Medicine, NIH; 2023. https://www.ncbi.nlm.nih.gov/books/NBK459261/.
8. Rad A. *Pancreas.* KenHub; 2022. https://www.kenhub.com/en/library/anatomy/the-pancreas.
9. Azzouz LL, Sandeep S, Physiology, large intestine. In: *StatsPearls (Internet).* National Library of Medicine, NIH; 2023. https://www.ncbi.nlm.nih.gov/books/NBK507857/.
10. Pirie E. *External Anal Sphincter.* Ken Hub; 2023. https://www.kenhub.com/en/library/anatomy/external-anal-sphincter.
11. Ahmed A, Arbor TC, Qureshi WA. Anatomy, abdomen and pelvis: anal canal. In: *StatsPearls (Internet).* National Library of Medicine, NIH; 2023. https://www.ncbi.nlm.nih.gov/books/NBK554531/.
12. Heick J, Lazaro RT. *Goodman and Snyder's Differential Diagnosis for Physical Therapists: Screening for Referral.* 7th ed. Elsevier; 2023.
13. Mannarino I. *Rovsing's Sign.* Osmosis from Elsevier. https://www.osmosis.org/answers/Rovsing-sign.
14. El-Malah AA, Gineinah MM, Deb PK, et al. Selective COX-2 inhibitors: road from success to controversy and the quest for repurposing. *Pharmaceuticals.* 2022;15(7):827. https://doi.org/10.3390/ph15070827.

16

Hepatic and Biliary Pathophysiology

OBJECTIVES

By the end of this chapter, the reader should be able to:

- Demonstrate a basic understanding of a healthy liver and biliary system.
- Demonstrate a basic understanding of pathophysiological conditions affecting the hepatic and biliary system.
- Identify possible symptoms associated with various hepatic and biliary disorders.
- Differentiate between the symptoms of viral versus nonviral hepatitis.
- Differentiate between the symptoms of liver versus biliary pathology.
- Explain and/or predict the possible symptoms resulting from the pathophysiology of various liver and/or biliary disorders.
- Assess and justify whether a specific liver and/or biliary symptom could constitute a yellow or red flag.

Physiology of the Hepatic and Biliary System

Beneath the diaphragm, on the right side of the abdominal cavity, there lies a large, cone-shaped organ.[1] This is the liver, consisting of two lobes with eight segments each (Fig. 16.1).

Healthy Hepatic and Biliary Physiology

After the blood in our bodies leaves the stomach and small intestines, it then passes through the liver. The liver contains about a pint of circulating blood at any given time. This blood is filtered of nutrients and certain medications which are then broken down and metabolized.[1] The liver regulates chemical levels and produces bile that carries away waste to the gallbladder and duodenum. This organ is responsible for over 500 vital functions in the human body. The liver is responsible for producing bile, cholesterol, and special proteins. In addition, the liver helps to regulate amino acids, create immune factors, and regulate blood clotting.[1]

The gallbladder is a small, pear-shaped organ located under the liver. It stores the bile that is made in the liver.[2] This bile is made up of cholesterol, bilirubin, and bile salts. It helps to break down and digest fats. There is a series of ducts, called the biliary tract, which carries the bile from the liver to the small intestine.[2]

Hepatic Pathology

Diseases of the liver and gallbladder (like many other body systems) can mimic musculoskeletal pain and impairment.[3] This pain is typically in the regions of the scapula, right shoulder, and upper trapezius with referred shoulder pain. Although this pain might be the only symptom of possible hepatic or biliary problems, there are other occasional symptoms. An individual with a hepatic or biliary problem might have jaundice, which is a yellow discoloration of the skin and sclera of the eyes (Fig. 16.2).[3]

Some individuals with liver problems experience spider angiomas that are branched dilations of the capillaries visible on the skin surface (Fig. 12.7).[3]

Other skin and nail changes include clubbed nails; palmar erythema, or a blotchy redness on the palms of the hands; and/or Terry's nails, which are white and opaque throughout (Fig. 16.3).[3]

Hepatic pathology can also lead to rhabdomyolysis, a serious medical condition that occurs when there is a breakdown of muscle tissue, causing a buildup of creatine phosphokinase levels and severe pain (this can also be a potential complication of long-term statin medications). More symptoms of liver damage include neurologic changes such as confusion, sleep disturbances, muscle tremors, hyperreactive reflexes, and numbness and tingling in the hand and wrist (often misdiagnosed as carpal tunnel syndrome).[3] Asterixis, an inability to maintain wrist

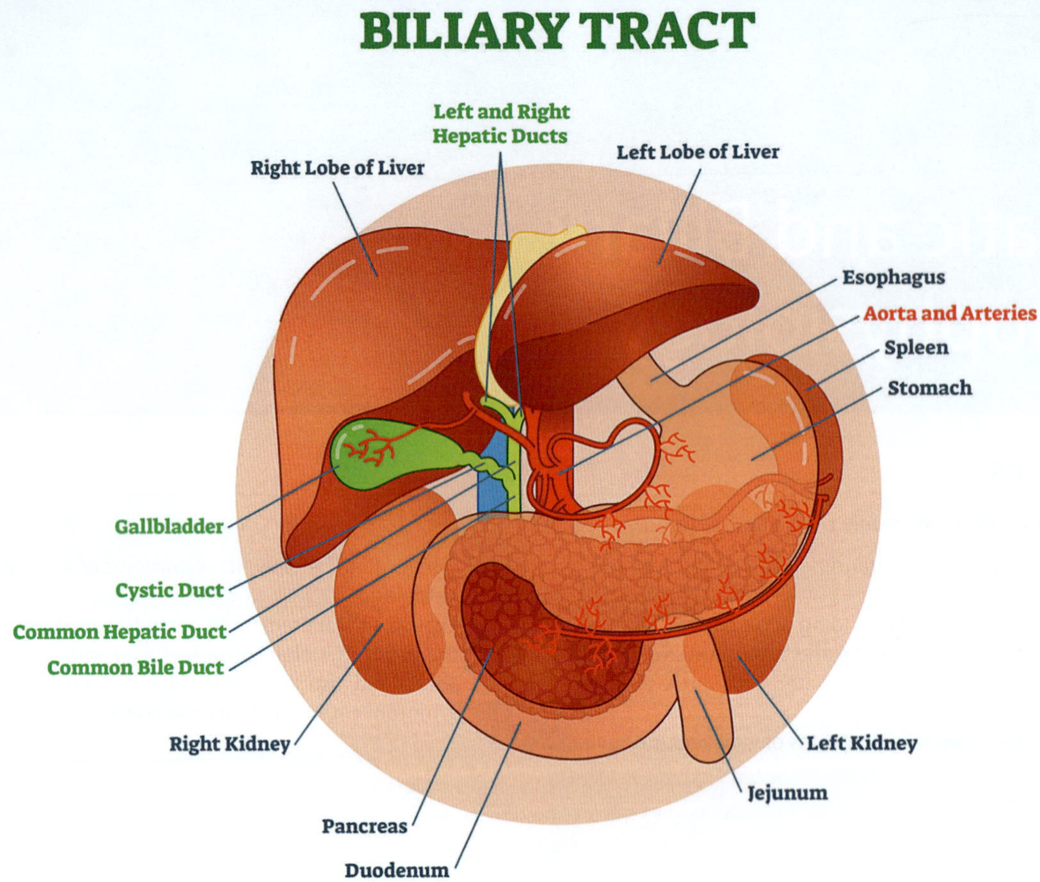

• **Fig. 16.1** The liver and gallbladder. (From https://www.iStock.com/VectorMine.)

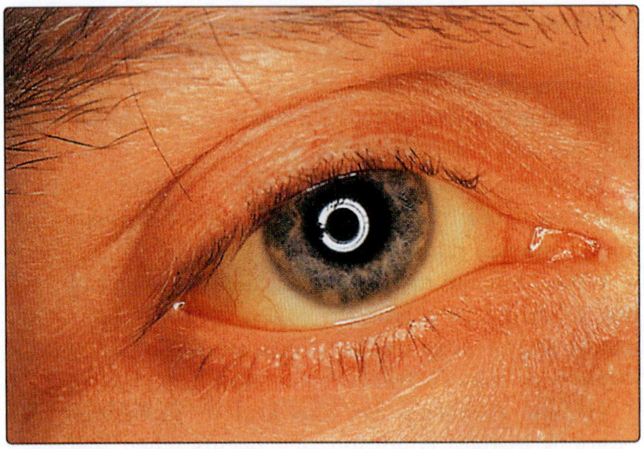

• **Fig. 16.2** Jaundice. (From Srivastava R, et al. *Jaundice in Clinical Biochemistry: An Illustrated Colour Text*. 7th ed. Elsevier; 2024.)

extension without a quick forward flexion of the wrist, also called *flapping tremors*, is also a symptom of hepatic dysfunction (Fig. 16.4).[3]

When a person has bilateral carpal tunnel syndrome, this is possibly due to their line of work, but it might also be due to a systemic condition. The numbness and tingling in the wrist and hand mentioned above will look a lot like carpal tunnel syndrome, and there might even be a positive Tinel sign, or a pins and needles sensation when you lightly tap over the area of the median nerve at an extended wrist (see Fig. 16.5).

Hepatitis

Hepatitis is an inflammation of the liver.[4] This inflammation may be caused by a virus or from alcohol consumption. Hepatitis can also be caused by certain medical conditions,

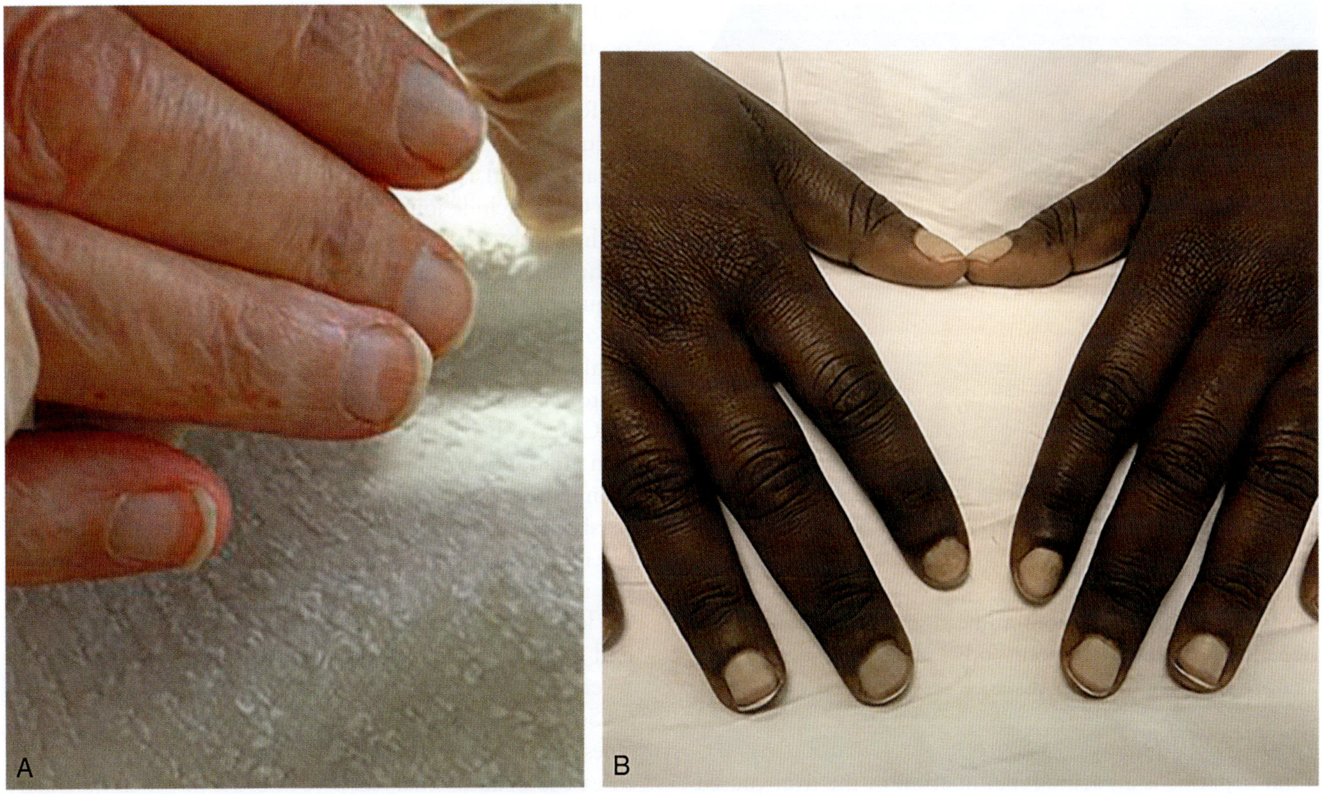

• **Fig. 16.3** Terry's nails. (A, From https://commons.wikimedia.org/wiki/File:Terry%27s_nails.jpg. B, From Meegada S, Verma R. Terry's nails. *Clin Case Rep*. 2020;8(2):404–405.)

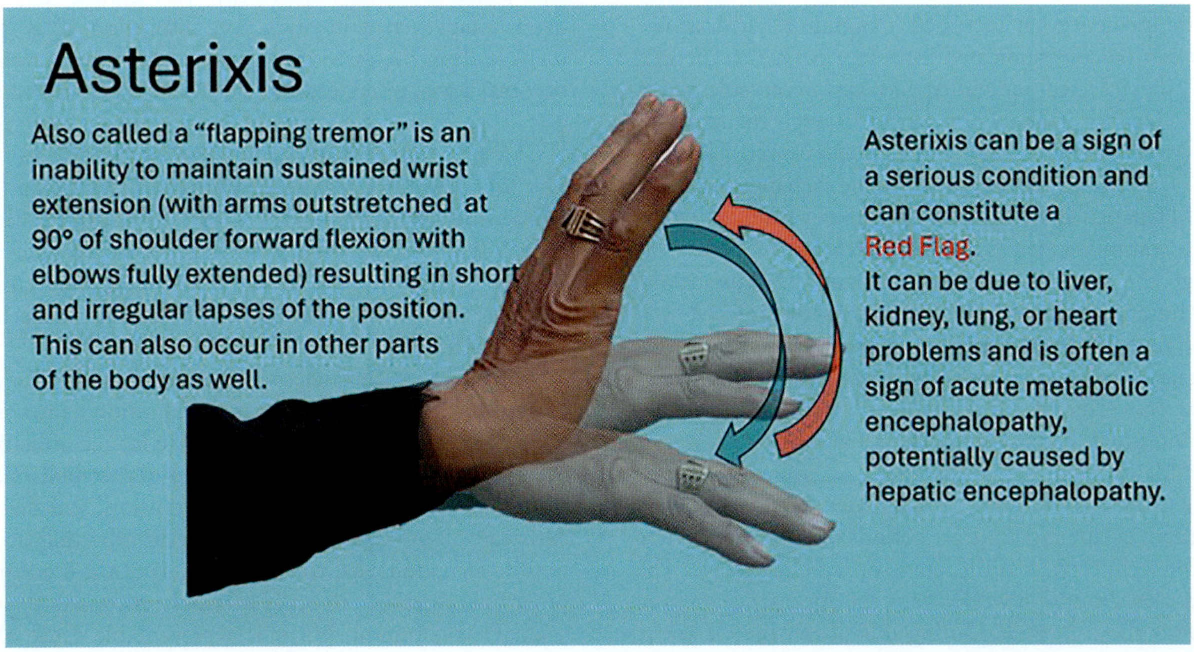

• **Fig. 16.4** Asterixis. (Information from https://www.ncbi.nlm.nih.gov/books/NBK535445/. *Asterixis—StatPearls—NCBI Bookshelf*.)

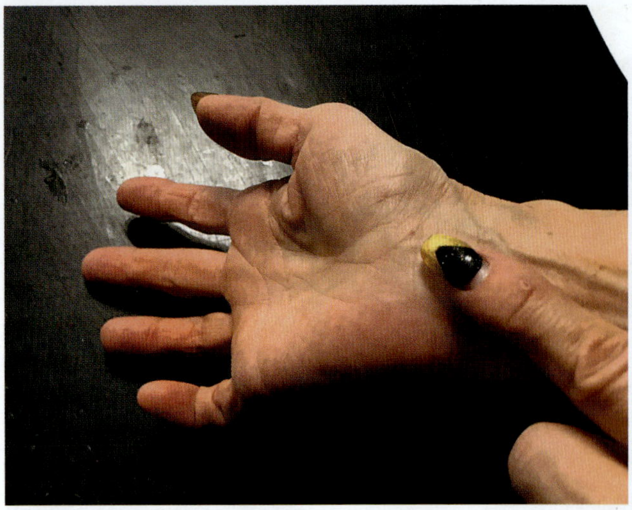

• **Fig. 16.5** Checking for Tinel sign.

medications, or even autoimmune responses. Autoimmune hepatitis happens when your body's antibodies are fighting against your healthy liver tissue.

Viral Hepatitis

Viral hepatitis is an acute inflammation of the liver caused by infectious viruses such as hepatitis A, B, C, D, E, and G viruses. Hepatitis has been difficult to control in our society because not every causative agent has been identified, there is a limited number of drug possibilities to treat the condition, its incidence has increased alongside illicit drug use, and it can be communicated from one person to the next before the infected individual has any observable symptoms.[3] Hepatitis A and E are spread through the fecal-oral route (typically from contaminated food or water). Hepatitis B, C, D, and G are blood-borne and are exchanged via body fluids. Hepatitis B virus (HBV) is a major problem in our society, communicated as a sexually transmitted disease and through the sharing of needles. Hepatitis D virus cannot infect humans unless the HBV is present to coinfect.[3]

The progression of hepatitis occurs in three stages. The first stage is the initial or preicteric stage (lasting 1–3 weeks). During this stage, the individual will typically experience gastrointestinal [GI] symptoms, malaise, fatigue, weight loss, and anorexia, sometimes with an aversion to food with nausea and vomiting. Enlargement of the liver will sometimes occur, and there are periods of intermittent itching. The second phase is the icteric or jaundiced stage. This period lasts about 6–8 weeks, with the appearance of jaundice after about 1 week. During this phase, the GI symptoms begin to go away, and the liver will decrease in size, but post-cervical lymph nodes and spleen become enlarged. The third phase is the recovery period (lasting 3–4 months), during which the person feels better but tires easily.[3] When hepatitis is mild, hospitalization is typically not necessary, especially if the primary causing agent or toxin was known, and has since been removed. Once the causing agent has been removed, it is typically expected that the client's health will improve. When a client has fulminant hepatitis, which occurs suddenly with severe intensity, hospitalization is required because it can be fatal and may spread to others.[3]

Red Flag: Whenever liver problems are suspected by the occupational therapy practitioner (OTP), immediate physician referral is indicated. Other factors that would alert the OTP include joint or muscle pain that is not consistent with the physical findings and the diagnosis of rheumatoid arthritis along with palmar tendinitis.[3] People at high risk of acquiring hepatitis include injection drug users and those who have received prior blood transfusions. Many other systemic problems can occur with HBV and HCV, like rheumatoid arthritis and fibromyalgia.[3]

Chronic hepatitis consists of prolonged liver inflammation after an unresolved viral hepatitis that has lasted longer than 6 months.[5] This condition was once classified as chronic persistent, chronic lobular, or chronic active, but this has recently changed. The classification is now based on etiology, the intensity of inflammation from a histologic perspective, the level of necrosis, and the degree of fibrosis.[5] Inflammation and slight necrosis can be reversible, but fibrosis can only be reversed if the individual does not also have cirrhosis.[5]

Some metabolic disorders can cause chronic hepatitis. These include Wilson disease and hemochromatosis. Wilson disease is an autosomal recessive disorder in which the biliary excretion of copper is impaired. This, in turn, causes copper to build up in the liver and become a toxin, affecting both the liver and neurological system. Hemochromatosis, another autosomal recessive impairment, acts similar to Wilson disease; however, it involves iron absorption. This impairment leads to increased iron in the system which eventually becomes toxic, often leading to arthralgias and arthropathy.[3]

Nonviral Hepatitis

The most common causes of nonviral hepatitis are metabolic-associated fatty liver disease (MAFLD), alcohol-related liver disease (ALD), and drug-induced liver injury (DILI). When the liver becomes inflamed, liver enzymes, aspartate aminotransferase or alanine aminotransferase are typically elevated.[6]

MAFLD was once referred to as nonalcoholic fatty liver disease. Worldwide, it is the most common cause of liver disease. MAFLD is caused by excessive fat accumulation in the liver associated with dysregulation of metabolism and is more likely seen with obesity, hypertension, and diabetes.[6] Although this disease is considered a disorder that does not require any additional comorbidities, it can still occur with other liver diseases and other metabolic disorders.[6]

ALD is common, but it is a preventable cause of liver disease. The primary intervention is a cessation of the consumption of alcohol. DILI is a toxic or drug-induced liver inflammation due to certain medications or illicit drugs.[7] There are more than 1000 medications and herbal supplements that can potentially lead to hepatotoxicity. The most common cause is acetaminophen, but other causes include certain antibiotics, non-steroidal anti-inflammatory drugs, herbal supplements, and cardiac medications.[7]

Cirrhosis of the Liver

Cirrhosis of the liver is a chronic disease with destruction of the liver cells and replacement of damaged connective tissue with fibrous bands. As the liver becomes scarred with these fibrous bands, blood and lymph flow become impaired, leading to hepatic insufficiency. There are many causes of cirrhosis, but alcohol abuse is the most common cause in our country. Problems that can occur as a result of cirrhosis include portal hypertension (elevated pressure in the portal vein, causing blood to back up into the vessels of the esophagus, stomach, and spleen and eventually bypassing the liver altogether through collaterals), ascites (an abnormal amount of fluid in the peritoneal cavity as a result of the back up from the portal vein, with a loss of protein), and esophageal varices (dilated veins of the lower esophagus resulting from the back up from the portal vein).[3]

Hepatic Encephalopathy

Hepatic encephalopathy is a neurologic disorder resulting from a buildup of ammonia (produced from the breakdown of protein) because the liver is no longer able to detoxify this substance.[3] This will lead to the flapping tremors of asterixis and to the numbness and tingling that is often confused with carpal tunnel syndrome. There are four stages of this encephalitis. Stage I, or the prodromal stage, includes subtle symptoms such as a slight tremor, confusion, or disorientation. During stage II, also known as the impending stage, tremors progress to asterixis, and resistance to passive movement is present. Apraxia is best evidenced by having the client draw a circle and a square on each visit and comparing the drawings for progressive deterioration. Stage III, or the stuporous stage, is characterized by marked confusion, muscle rigidity, asterixis, a positive Babinski sign (the toes will spread when stroking the bottom of the foot), and hyperactive deep tendon reflexes. Stage IV, or the comatose stage, is the final stage. During the comatose stage, the client cannot be aroused; there is a positive Babinski sign (stroking the bottom of the foot produces flailing of the toes); no asterixis is present; and there is hepatic fetor, a musty, garlicky smell of the breath.[3,8]

Liver Abscess and Tumors

When bacteria or protozoa inhabit the liver and begin to destroy tissue, producing a cavity in the liver, this is called a liver abscess. This can cause right abdominal pain, right shoulder pain, weight loss, fever, malaise, and chills.[3]

Tumors in the liver can be either benign or malignant. The most common benign tumors are hemangiomas that start in the blood vessels.[9] These typically lead to no symptoms or need for intervention unless they grow into nearby tissues or begin to bleed.[9]

When a malignant tumor begins in the liver, it is called primary liver cancer. The most common type of primary liver cancer in adults is hepatocellular carcinoma.[9] Typically, however, liver cancer is caused by metastasis from another location, for example, the GI tract, esophagus, lung, or breast.[3] This is called secondary liver cancer.

Biliary Pathology

The gallbladder is a small, hollow organ that stores the bile produced by the liver and uses it for digestion.[10] The gallbladder is connected to the cystic duct, which merges with the common hepatic duct to form the common bile duct (Fig. 16.6). Fluids leave the gallbladder through the cystic duct, merge with fluids from the hepatic duct, and then enter the common bile duct, which carries them to the duodenum.

Cholelithiasis

Cholelithiasis is the presence of gallstones, also called calculi. These are hardened masses of material created from the bile.[11] Cholelithiasis can be asymptomatic, but pain and problems will occur when one of these stones leaves the gallbladder and causes an obstruction.[3] This pain is typically right upper abdominal pain that comes and goes in waves; this is called biliary colic. This can lead to other problems like cholecystitis or cholangitis.[3]

Cholecystitis is a blockage or impaction of gallstones in the cystic duct with resulting inflammation and possible infection.[3] There will be steady, severe pain, fever, and nausea.

Cholangitis occurs when the gallstones obstruct an area further down the path in the common bile duct, blocking fluid from both the gallbladder and the liver, and this can lead to jaundice.[3] If the infection travels up the hepatic duct and into the liver, it could be fatal.

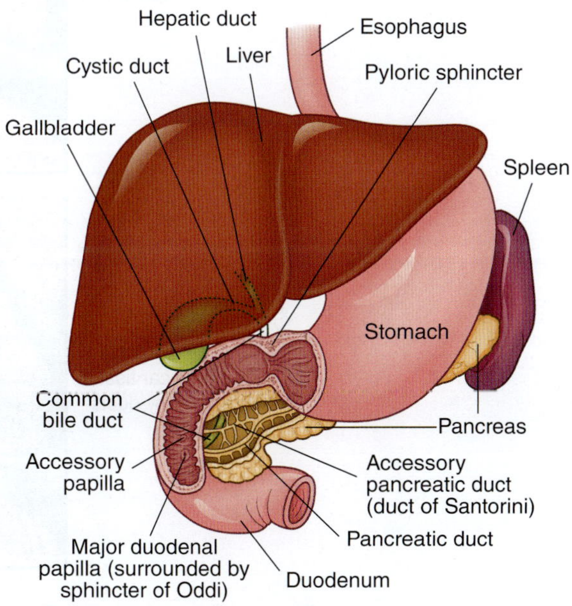

• **Fig. 16.6** Gallbladder. (From McCance KL, et al. *Understanding Pathophysiology*. 8th ed. Elsevier; 2026.)

Signs and symptoms of gallbladder disease are typically a colicky right quadrant pain that occurs after a person has eaten a meal that is high in fat. These symptoms, however, are not the same for everyone, and this pain might not always be in the right upper quadrant pain; it can be a constant pain that is not colicky.[3] There can also be pain in the rectus abdominis over the belly button, indicative of disturbances within the hepatic and biliary systems. This will look like a typical musculoskeletal problem until you ask about the timing of the problem in relation to eating and drinking.[3] If symptoms are worse immediately after eating, then the problem could be cholecystitis. If the problems occur about 1 to 3 hours after eating, it could be gallstones.[3] Another red flag would be musculoskeletal symptoms accompanied by constitutional symptoms (fever, sweats, chills, nausea). These are often the warning signs of a systemic problem.[3]

Primary Biliary Cholangitis

Primary biliary cholangitis was previously called primary biliary cirrhosis. It is a chronic disorder in which the bile ducts slowly deteriorate (Fig. 16.7), interfering with bile secretion.[12] This disorder typically affects females.[12] Although it can be asymptomatic, some individuals experience pruritus (itching), jaundice, GI bleeding, ascites, and

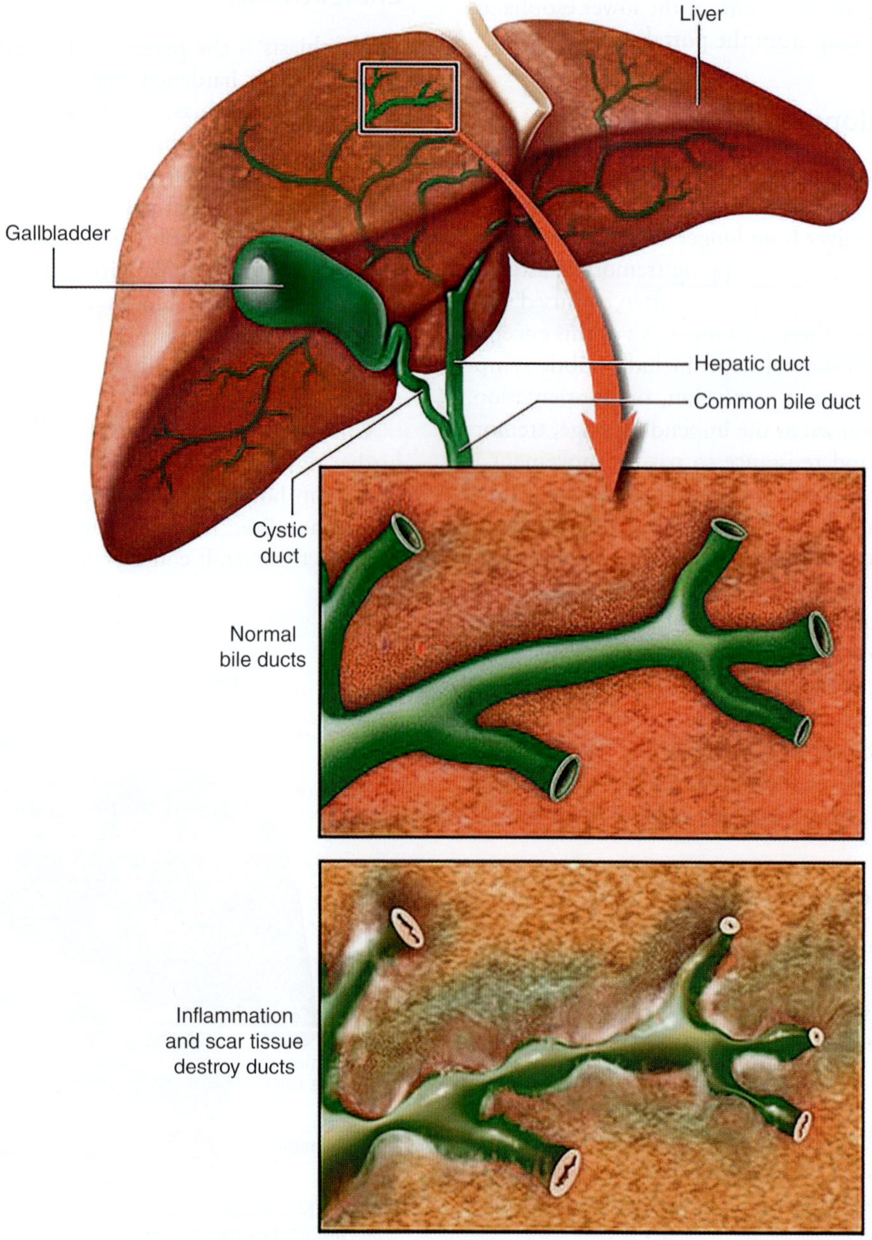

• **Fig. 16.7** Primary biliary cholangitis. (From https://www.mayoclinic.org/diseases-conditions/primary-biliarycholangitis/symptoms-causes/syc-20376874, used with permission of Mayo Foundation for Medical Education and Research. All rights reserved.)

associated autoimmune features like Sjogren syndrome (dry mouth and eyes).

Bile Duct Cancer

Colangiocarcinoma, the second most common form of liver malignancy, is a very serious and sometimes fatal form of cancer.[3]

The OT Scope of Practice

OTPs should be alert to any signs of hepatic or biliary disease in their clients. Some key signs to look for include the development of arthralgias of unknown cause, an apparent bilateral carpal tunnel syndrome, sensory neuropathy, right shoulder or scapular pain of unknown cause, GI symptoms, liver flap, palmar erythema, history of cancer, history of hepatitis, and/or changes in the hue or turgor of the skin.

Application—Case Study

CASE EXAMPLE 16.1

A 68-year-old male presented to an occupational therapy practitioner (OTP) at an outpatient clinic with bilateral carpal tunnel syndrome. The OTP assumed prior to examining the client that he worked in a field that required using repetitive motion of both arms and hands and that would be the reason for the bilateral carpal tunnel. Occam's Razor refers to the premise that the simplest answer is usually the correct answer. When you hear hoofbeats, you think horses before you think zebras, since horses are more common, and therefore, more likely. Although the OTP in this case knew this, she took the time to look a little further.

1. **Screen**: The OTP asked him about his current job duties or hobbies. He was retired and was not doing any labor that required the use of both hands.
2. **Take a Closer Look**: The OTP found that the client had all the signs and symptoms of bilateral carpal tunnel syndrome, including a positive Tinel sign. The OTP again asked the client about hobbies, and he stated that since his wife died, he goes to a local bar every night and "downs about 6 beers and a couple shots of whiskey."
3. **Determine Flag Status**: The OTP determined this to be a potential yellow flag situation.
4. **Take Action if Needed**: The OTP contacted the client's doctor to inform him of the potential for liver problems in this client causing what appeared to be a bilateral carpal tunnel syndrome.
5. **Document the Findings**: The OTP documented this information as well as the phone call with the doctor.
6. **Take a Second Look**: The physician ran blood work and found abnormal liver enzymes. An MRI showed early cirrhosis of the liver.
7. **Determine the Flag Status**: This had quickly become a red flag.
8. **Take Action if Needed**: The client was seen by an expert hepatic team, who were able to encourage the client to stop drinking and to lose weight. They also prescribed some medications to ease his discomfort.

This is a true case. This OTP was able to help the doctors with clues to the client's condition and may have even saved this man's life.

References

1. Hopkins Johns. *Liver: Anatomy and Functions*. John Hopkins Medical Center; 2023. https://www.hopkinsmedicine.org/health/conditions-and-diseases/liver-anatomy-and-functions.
2. Cleveland Clinic. *Gallbladder*. Cleveland Clinic; 2021. https://my.clevelandclinic.org/health/body/21690-gallbladder.
3. Heick J, Lazaro RT. *Goodman and Snyder's Differential Diagnosis for Physical Therapists: Screening for Referral*. 7th ed. Elsevier; 2023.
4. Kahn A. *Hepatitis*. Healthline; 2023. https://www.healthline.com/health/hepatitis.
5. Kumar S. *Overview of Chronic Hepatitis*. Merck Manual; 2022. https://www.merckmanuals.com/professional/hepatic-and-biliary-disorders/hepatitis/overview-of-chronic-hepatitis.
6. Jacob R, Strasser S. Nonviral hepatitis: common causes and their management. *Med Today*. 2022;23(5):25–31. https://medicinetoday.com.au/mt/2022/may/feature-article/nonviral-hepatitis-common-causes-and-their-management.
7. Francis P, Navarro VJ. Drug-induced hepatotoxicity. In: *StatPearls*. National Library of Medicine. National Institutes of Health; 2024. https://www.ncbi.nlm.nih.gov/books/NBK557535/.
8. Marcin J. *Fector Hepaticus*. Healthline; 2018. https://www.healthline.com/health/fetor-hepaticus.
9. ACS. *What Is Liver Cancer?* American Cancer Society; 2023. https://www.cancer.org/cancer/types/liver-cancer/about/what-is-liver-cancer.html.
10. Modric J. *Gallbladder Anatomy and Function*. eHealthStar; 2017. https://www.ehealthstar.com/anatomy/gallbladder.
11. Cleveland Clinic. *Gallstones*. 2022. https://my.clevelandclinic.org/health/diseases/7313-gallstones.
12. Mayo Clinic. *Primary Biliary Cholangitis*. Mayo Clinic; 2023. https://www.mayoclinic.org/diseases-conditions/primary-biliary-cholangitis/symptoms-causes/syc-20376874.

17 Urogenital Pathophysiology

OBJECTIVES

By the end of this chapter, the reader should be able to:

- Demonstrate a basic understanding of healthy urinary and reproductive physiology.
- Demonstrate a basic understanding of pathophysiological conditions affecting the urogenital system.
- Identify possible symptoms associated with various urogenital disorders.
- Differentiate between the symptoms of the upper versus the lower urinary tract.
- Differentiate between the symptoms of the urinary tract versus the reproductive system.
- Explain and/or predict the possible symptoms resulting from the various sexually transmitted infections.
- Assess and justify whether a specific urogenital symptom could constitute a yellow or red flag.

Physiology of the Urogenital System

The urogenital system, also known as the genitourinary system, consists of both the reproductive system and the urinary tract.[1] The components of the urinary tract are the same for both those assigned male at birth (AMAB) and those assigned female at birth (AFAB), but the components of the reproductive system vary between these two groups.[1]

Healthy Urinary Tract Physiology

The urinary system can be divided into two parts: the upper urinary tract and the lower urinary tract.

The Upper Urinary Tract

The upper urinary tract consists of the kidneys and the ureters.[2] The kidneys are bean-shaped organs, located in the peritoneal cavity on either side of the spinal cord at around the level of T11 to L3 (Fig. 17.1).[2] The kidney on the right is typically lower than the one on the left to make room for the liver.

The kidney's primary role is to filter wastes from blood, balancing the body's water and electrolytes. The kidneys filter an estimated 200 quarts of blood per day, eliminating about 2 quarts of fluid in the form of urine.[3] The functional component of the kidney is the renal nephron, which is where the formation of urine takes place (Fig. 17.2).[2]

The kidney's filtration system helps to maintain the acid-base balance in the body and to maintain the balance of electrolytes. The kidneys are able to produce hormones that can stimulate red blood cell production or control calcium metabolism.[4] The kidneys also release renin, an enzyme that helps control blood pressure and balances sodium and potassium in the body.[5]

The rest of the upper urinary tract consists of the ureters. The ureters are the two tubes that carry urine created in the kidneys to the bladder. These tubes travel from the kidneys in the abdominal region to the bladder in the pelvic region (Fig. 17.3).[2]

The Lower Urinary Tract

The lower urinary tract consists of the bladder and the urethra. The bladder is not just a storage site for urine but part of an intricate neural pathway communicating with the autonomic nervous system, the central nervous system, and the somatic nervous system, along with hormonal modulation to alert the body when micturition (or urination) becomes necessary.[6] The body of the bladder consists of smooth muscle called detrusor muscle. This contracts when the body needs to undergo the expulsion of urine.[6]

The urethra is the tube through which urine passes from the bladder to the outside of the body. In individuals who are AMAB, this tube is much longer (about 20 cm in length) than in individuals AFAB (about 3–4 cm in length).[7] For individuals AMAB, this urethra must pass through the prostate and then through the penis, but for individuals AFAB, this tube only goes from the bladder to the front of the outer structures surrounding the vagina, also known as the vulva (Fig. 17.4).[7]

Healthy Reproductive Physiology for AMAB Individuals

Male reproductive organs consist of the testicles (or testes), scrotum, epididymis, vas deferens, prostate, and penis (Fig. 17.5).[8]

The testicles are responsible for sperm production and for making testosterone.[9] The testicles rest in the scrotum, a loose sac of skin, which protects and cools the temperature

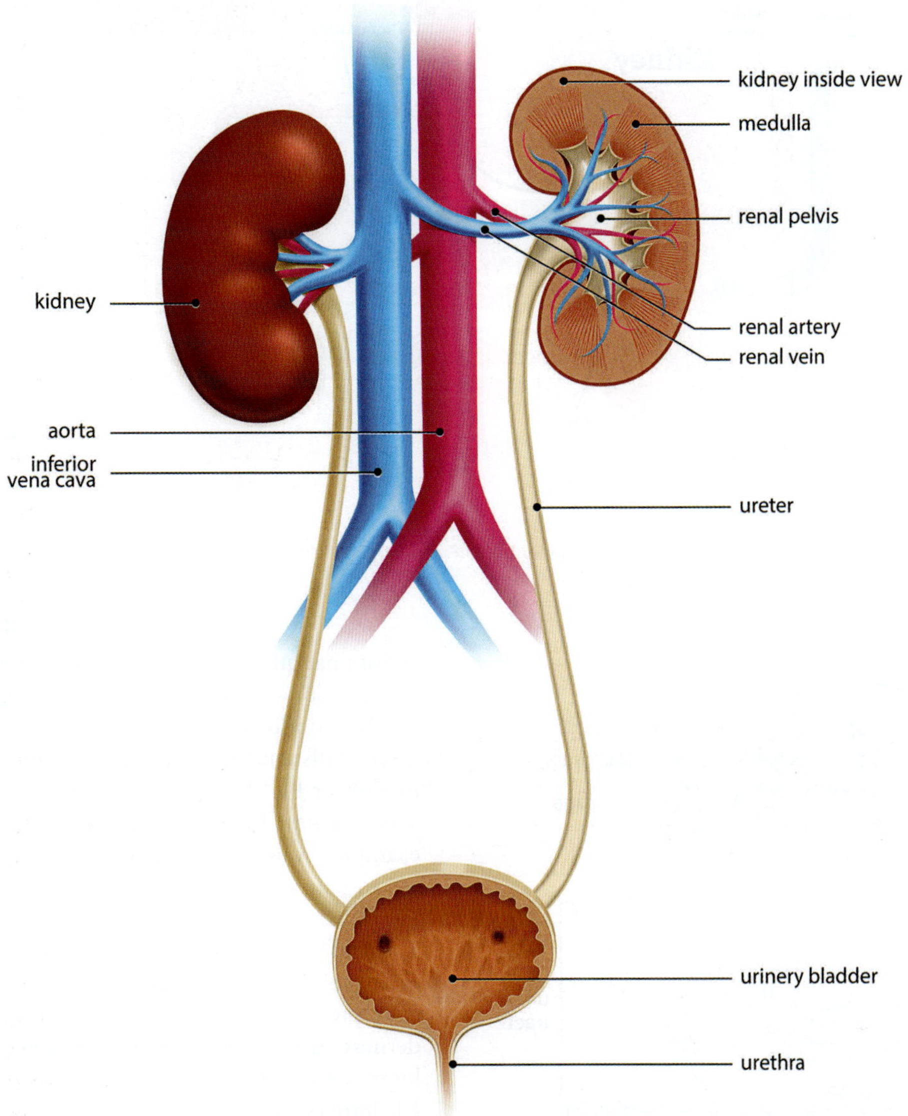

• **Fig. 17.1** The urinary tract. (From https://iStock.com/kocakayaali.)

of the testicles. The epididymis is a coiled tube that rests behind each testicle. It is responsible for storing and transporting the sperm.[9] The vas deferens is a muscular tube that takes the sperm from the epididymis to the urethra. The prostate gland adds extra fluid to the ejaculate to nourish the sperm and allow for smoother passage through the penis upon ejaculation.[9]

Healthy Reproductive Physiology for AFAB Individuals

Female reproductive organs consist of the ovaries, fallopian tubes, uterus, vagina, and vulva (Fig. 17.6).[10]

The ovaries are considered to be the female gonads, which are responsible for gametogenesis, or the development of eggs (also called ova), and the production of sex hormones. Ova leave the ovaries via a process called ovulation and travel from the ovaries to the uterus via tunnels called fallopian tubes.[10] If fertilization takes place, the egg will implant itself into the endometrial lining of the uterus for development, but if fertilization does not take place, this egg will be discharged along with the endometrial lining of the uterus, through the vaginal canal.[10]

Pathophysiology of the Urogenital System

Diseases of the urogenital system (like many other body systems) can mimic musculoskeletal pain and impairment.

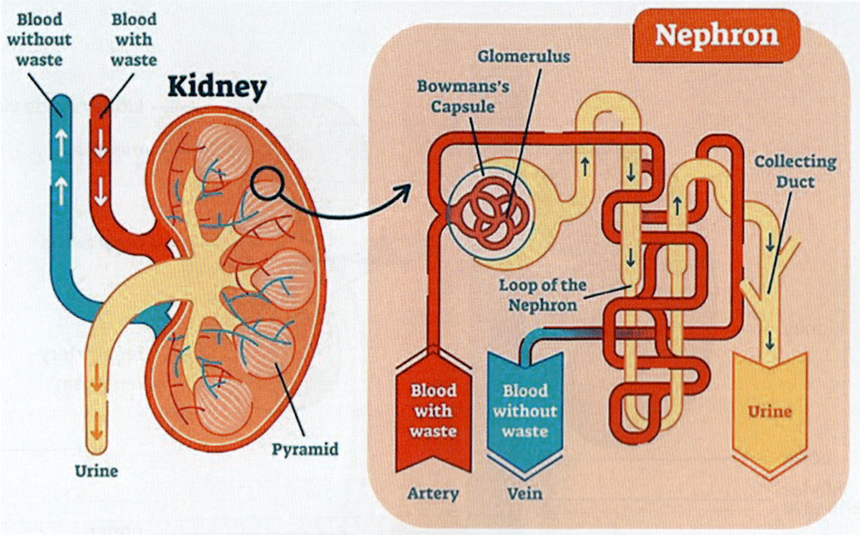

• **Fig. 17.2** The ureters of the upper urinary tract. (From https://biologydictionary.net/urinary-system/.)

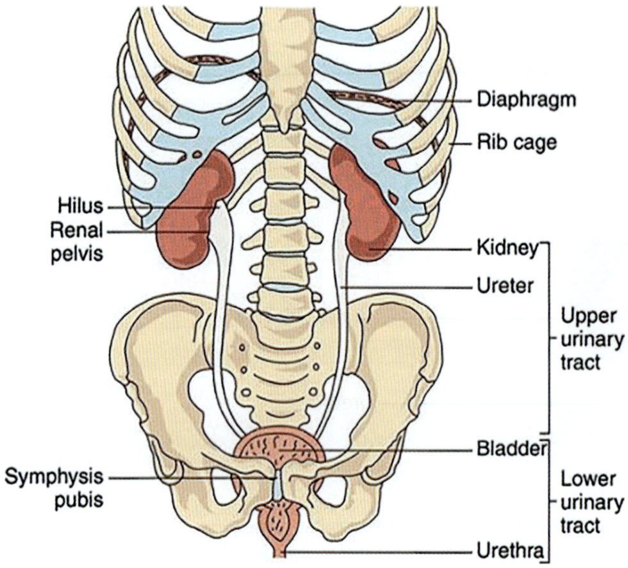

• **Fig. 17.3** The kidney and the renal nephron. (From https://biologydictionary.net/urinary-system/.)

Upper Urinary Tract

Renal pain is not clearly understood, but it is known that both ureteral and renal pain are relayed via sympathetic nerves entering the spinal cord from T10 to L1.[2] This can cause stimulation of cutaneous pain receptors at the same level, resulting in what is called hyperesthesia or skin pain at the T10 to L1 dermatomal distribution. Pain from the kidneys is typically felt in the skin over the subcostal or costovertebral areas of the back.[2]

Pain from a problem with either or both ureters can be felt in the groin or genital areas. With either renal or ureter impairment, pain can occur around the flank and lower abdominal quadrant and can even cause abdominal muscle spasms, along with nausea and vomiting.[2]

One condition seen in the upper urinary tract includes ureteral distention from fluid accumulation due to inflammation or bleeding cysts, resulting in a constant dull and aching pain. There can also be ureteral obstructions, for example, from a stone also called a *calculus*, typically resulting in pain that comes in waves known as *colic*.[2] Stones in the upper urinary tract are relatively common with about 1 out of every 1000 adults treated in the hospital setting each year.[11] An upper urinary tract infection (UTI) typically presents with pain in the flank area, unilateral tenderness in the costovertebral area, with fever, chills, and hypersensitivity over the skin on the back over the T10 to L1 dermatomes.[2]

Sometimes a musculoskeletal injury mimics the symptoms of renal pain. This is called pseudo-renal pain, and it tends to occur secondary to problems in the costovertebral or costotransverse joints, leading to irritation of the costal nerves. This can happen in any of the cervical or thoracic areas but is most common from T10 to T12.[2]

The signs and symptoms of chronic kidney disease are occasionally mistaken for a musculoskeletal disorder. It is important for the occupational therapy practitioner (OTP) to recognize signs and symptoms outside of those typically seen in a musculoskeletal condition.[2] Symptoms of renal impairment include one-sided costovertebral tenderness, ipsilateral shoulder pain, hematuria, dependent edema, decreased urine output, fever, chills, hypertension, and/or weakness.[2]

These symptoms might seem vague and reminiscent of symptoms from other systemic conditions. The key is not for the OTP to diagnose the problem, but to conclude that the problem is more likely systemic, not musculoskeletal, and therefore outside the scope of the OTP to treat. The OTP should, however, document the findings and advocate on

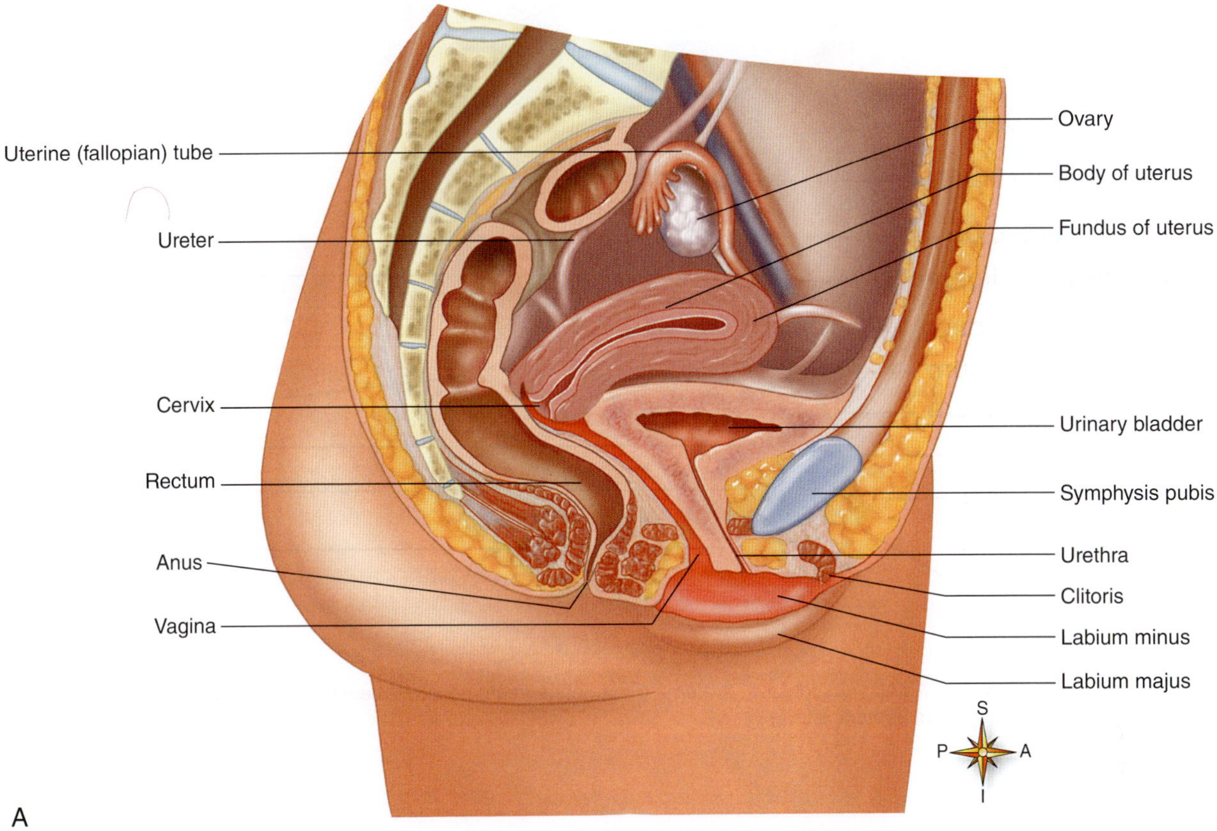

A

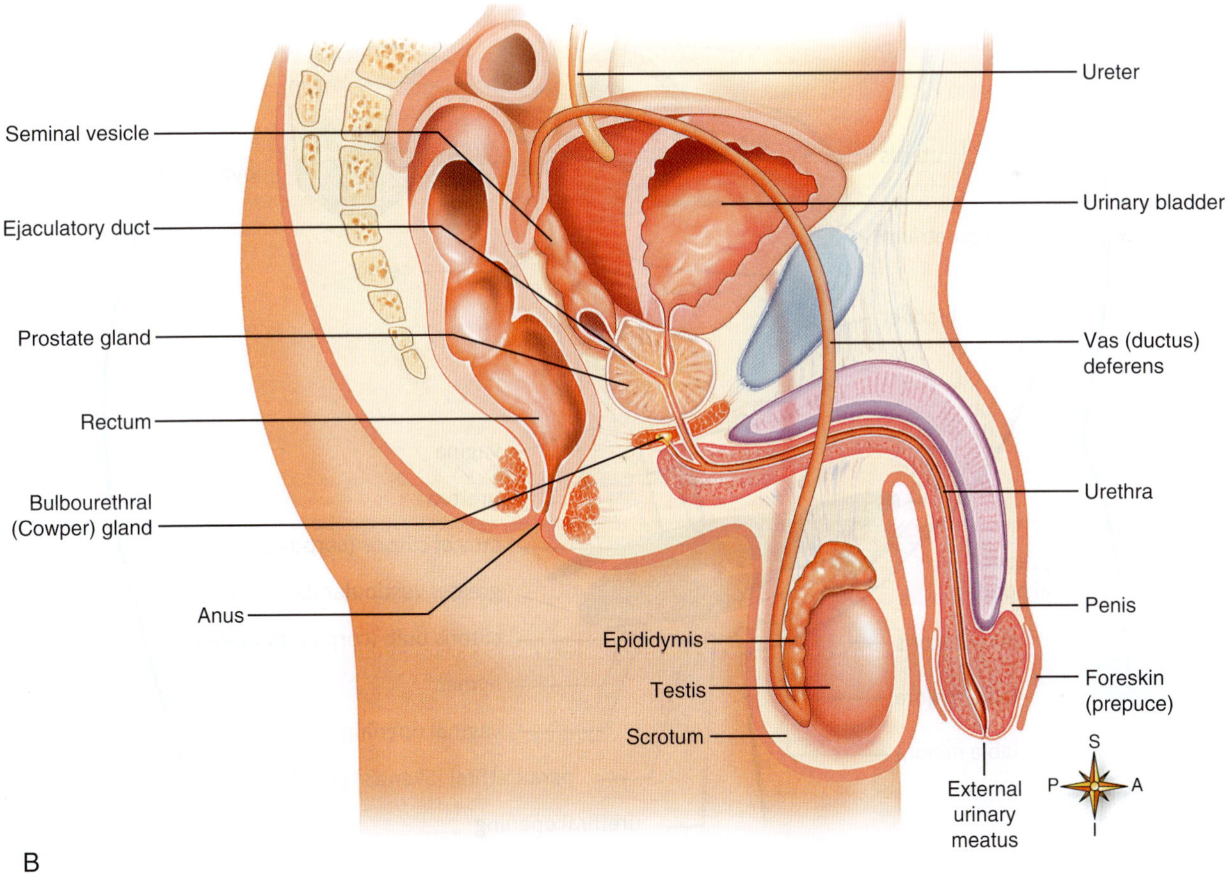

B

• **Fig. 17.4** The AFAB urethra (A) versus the AMAB urethra (B). (From Patton KT, Bell FB, Thompson T, Williamson PL. *The Human Body in Health & Disease*. 8th ed. Elsevier; 2024.)

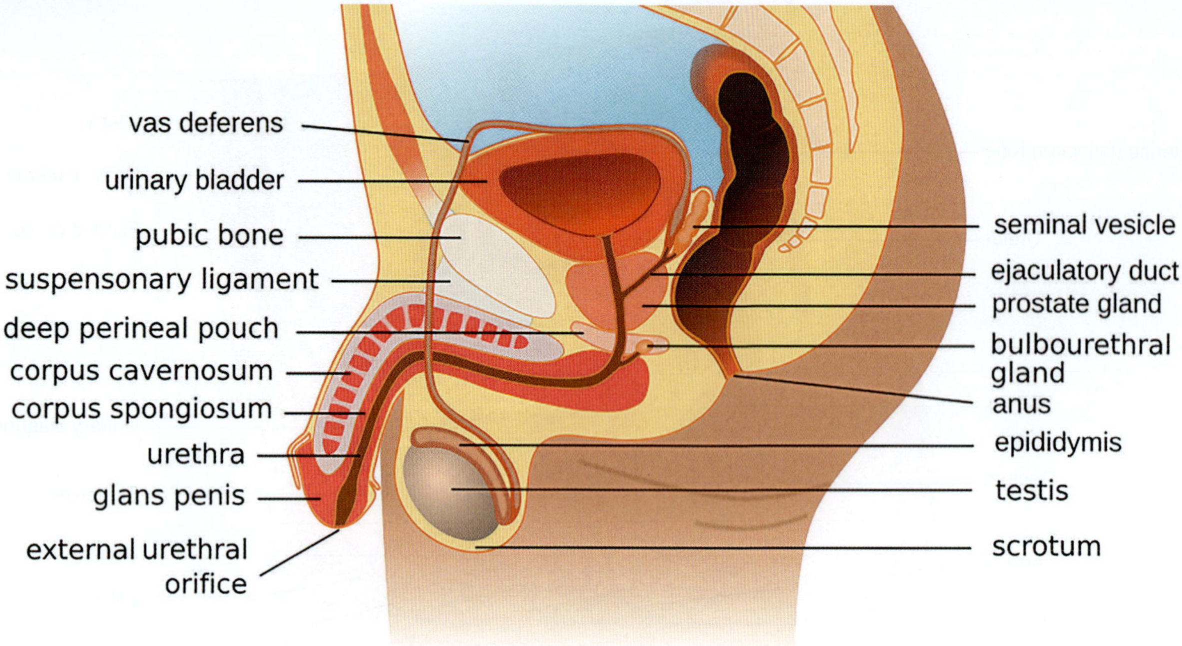

• **Fig. 17.5** The AMAB reproductive system. (From https://commons.wikimedia.org/wiki/File:Human_male_reproductive_system_en.svg.)

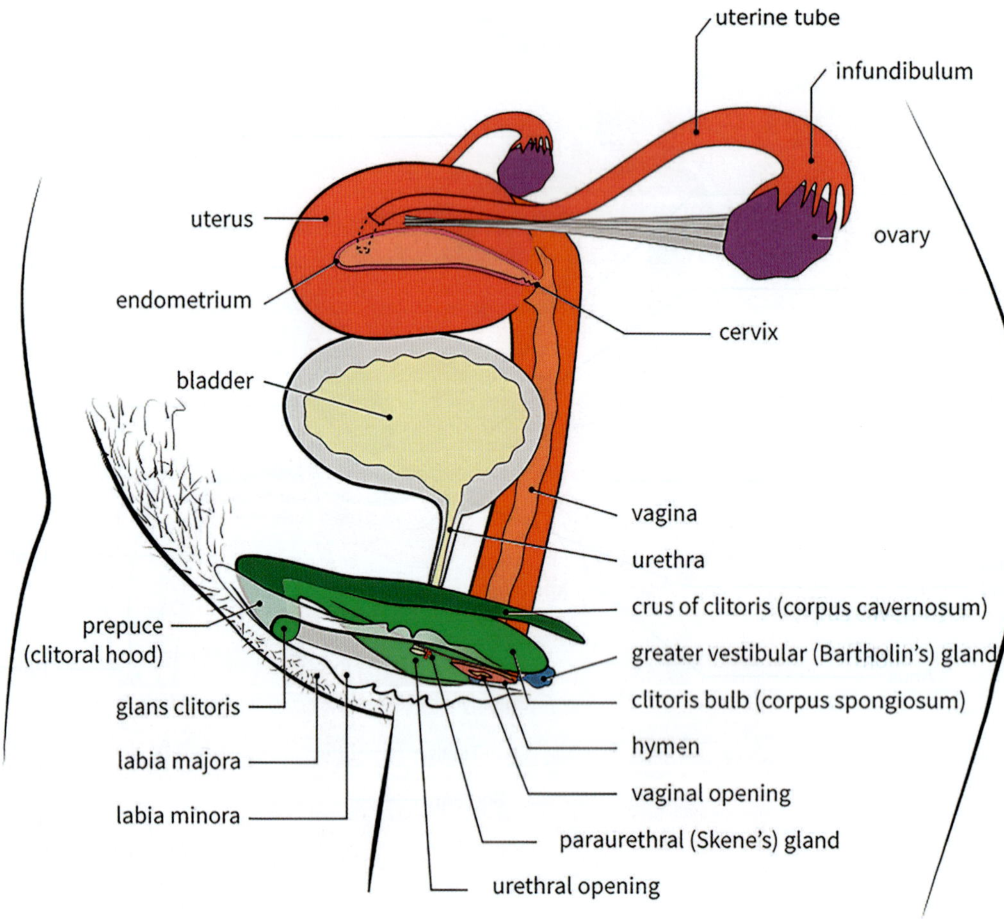

• **Fig. 17.6** The AFAB reproductive system. (From https://commons.wikimedia.org/wiki/File:Female_genital_system_-_3D_view.svg.)

behalf of the client by informing the physician and requesting that further testing be done.

Lower Urinary Tract

Bladder and urethral pain will typically be felt in the lower anterior abdomen or upper pubic (suprapubic) areas. There will occasionally be a sensation of urinary urgency and sometimes pain during urination (dysuria).[2]

A lower UTI typically presents with urinary frequency, low back pain, dysuria, pyuria (pus caused by a high white blood cell count in the urine), bacteriuria (bacteria in the urine), and dyspareunia (painful intercourse).[2] The clinical presentation can be different, however, for elderly adults. These individuals will occasionally have a blunted fever response and might instead exhibit confusion or delirium, lethargy, new onset of incontinence, and/or anorexia.[12]

Although technically a problem with the AMAB reproductive physiology, one common problem in males needs to be mentioned here.[13] Benign prostatic hyperplasia (BPH), also known as an enlarged prostate, is a common health issue in men as they get older. The symptoms include urinary urgency, more frequent need to urinate at night, trouble initiating urination, and inability to fully empty the bladder.[13] This latter problem can lead to a UTI.[13]

Pathology of the Reproductive System

Individuals Born AFAB

There are many pathological conditions that can occur in the female reproductive system. Some of the more common ones include ovarian cysts, endometriosis, and ectopic pregnancy.

Ovarian cysts are fluid-filled sacs that can develop after ovulation. These are typically benign and do not require any intervention, but some can cause pelvic pain, cyst rupture, and blood loss. Those with these complications will typically require medical management.[14]

Endometriosis is a painful condition that occurs when tissue similar to the lining of the uterus grows outside the uterus, often causing pelvic structures and organs to stick to each other.[15] Symptoms include painful menses (periods), pain during sex, pain with urination or bowel movements, excessive bleeding during menses, possible nausea, and fatigue.[15]

An ectopic pregnancy is one in which the egg attaches and grows outside of the endometrial wall of the uterus.[16] These pregnancies typically occur within the fallopian tube. This egg cannot grow normally in this area, and if left alone, it can cause a rupture and be life-threatening. Surgical removal is typically done for these individuals (Fig. 17.7).[16]

Individuals Born AMAB

There are many pathological conditions that can occur with the male reproductive system as well. Some of the more common ones include BPH (mentioned earlier in this chapter) and prostate cancer. Prostate cancer is the second most common type of cancer in men (the first is skin cancer).[17] Early prostate cancer does not typically have any symptoms so frequent screening is important.[18] Individuals born AMAB with more advanced cancer might have difficulty urinating, blood in the urine or semen, difficulty getting an erection, pain in the back or hips, and possible numbness or weakness in the feet or lower extremities.[18]

Sexually Transmitted Infections

Sexually transmitted infections (STIs), formally known as sexually transmitted diseases, are typically bacterial or viral.

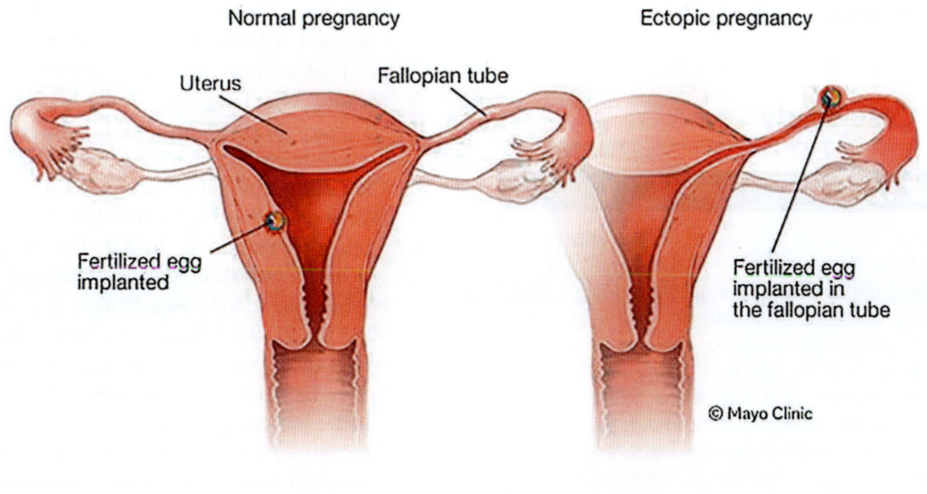

• **Fig. 17.7** Ectopic pregnancy. (From https://www.mayoclinic.org/diseases-conditions/ectopic-pregnancy/symptoms-causes/syc-20372088, used with permission of Mayo Foundation for Medical Education and Research. All rights reserved.)

Bacterial Sexually Transmitted Infections

Some of the more common bacterial infections are chlamydia, gonorrhea, and syphilis.[19] Because these infections are caused by bacteria, they can be treated with antibiotics.[20] Chlamydia is the most frequently reported STI in the United States and is caused by an infection with *Chlamydia trachomatis.*[19] Gonorrhea, caused by *Neisseria gonorrhea,* is a very common STI, especially in people 15 to 24 years of age. Syphilis is caused by the bacterium *Treponema pallidum.* Syphilis is one of the STIs that can cause serious health issues if not treated.[19]

Viral Sexually Transmitted Infections

Some of the more common viral infections are human papillomavirus (HPV), genital herpes, and human immunodeficiency virus (HIV). These infections can be managed with antivirals but not cured by them. HPV is the most common STI.[19] This virus goes away without intervention within 2 years, in most cases, but when it stays longer, it can lead to health problems like cervical cancer in females.[19] Genital herpes is caused by an infection with Herpes simplex virus type 1 or type 2 (HSV-2). This is very common, with almost 12% of the population between the ages of 14 and 49 having HSV-2 infection. Currently, there is no cure, but intervention with antiviral medication can prevent or shorten the length of outbreaks.[19] HIV is the virus responsible for acquired immune deficiency syndrome or AIDS. Although there are new medications to help control the virus, to date, there is no known cure.[21]

The OT Scope of Practice

OTPs should be alert to any signs of possible urogenital impairment in their clients. Clients will often share personal information with their OTP because of the client-therapist trust that develops over time. Continue to actively listen to your clients beyond the initial evaluation. Remember that the OTP should always work within the box (their scope of care) but be able to think outside that box to be a strong client advocate.

Application—Case Study

CASE EXAMPLE 17.1

An 87-year-old woman visited an OTP at her skilled nursing facility. She had been receiving occupational therapy intervention for bathing and dressing, but during today's session, she appeared confused and lethargic.

1. **Screen:** The OTP asked her about her family visit during lunch that day, and the resident clearly could not remember seeing them. She also had difficulty remembering the names of her children. These were new symptoms for this client who was always very coherent and aware of her surroundings, with no prior memory problems.
2. **Take a Closer Look:** The OTP checked the chart and saw a physician's note written earlier that day, reporting that this resident had a "recent onset of dementia." She also saw an entry from one of the nurses saying that the resident was having difficulty urinating.
3. **Determine Flag Status:** Remembering that this female had one of these difficulties the day prior, the OTP was concerned. She determined this to be a potential yellow flag situation.
4. **Take Action if Needed:** The OTP contacted the resident's doctor to inform him of the sudden onset of these symptoms and her concern that something else might be occurring. She informed the physician about the resident's voiding difficulty and asked the physician to order a urinalysis.
5. **Document the Findings:** The OTP documented this information as well as the phone call with the doctor.
6. **Take a Second Look:** The physician immediately ordered bloodwork and a urinalysis.
7. **Determine the Flag Status:** This was still a yellow flag but could escalate to a red flag if the resident's confusion led to injury or a decline in functional status.
8. **Take Action if Needed:** The lab work found a high white blood cell count, and the urinalysis was positive for a UTI with *E. coli* bacteria. Antibiotics were started immediately, and within 48 hours, the patient was no longer confused or lethargic.

This is a true case. This OTP was able to help solve the mystery of the resident's sudden confusion. The doctor asked the OTP, "How did you know?" She answered that she learned it in her OTP program from her professor.

References

1. Santos-Longhurst A. *What Is the Genitourinary System of the Body?* Healthline; 2019. https://www.healthline.com/health/genitourinary-system.
2. Heick J, Lazaro RT. *Goodman and Snyder's Differential Diagnosis for Physical Therapists: Screening for Referral.* 7th ed. Elsevier; 2023.
3. Cleveland Clinic. *Kidney.* Cleveland Clinic; 2023. https://my.clevelandclinic.org/health/body/21824-kidney.
4. NKF. *How Your Kidneys Work.* National Kidney Foundation; 2023. https://www.kidney.org/kidneydisease/howkidneyswrk.
5. Cleveland Clinic. *Renin.* Cleveland Clinic; 2022. https://my.clevelandclinic.org/health/body/22506-renin.
6. Lanzotti NJ, Tariq MA, Bolla SR. Physiology bladder. In: *StatsPearls (Internet).* National Library of Medicine, NIH; 2023. https://www.ncbi.nlm.nih.gov/books/NBK538533/.
7. Cleveland Clinic. *Urethra.* Cleveland Clinic; 2022. https://my.clevelandclinic.org/health/body/23002-urethra.
8. Gurung P, Yetiskul E, Jialal I. Physiology, male reproductive system. In: *StatsPearls (Internet).* National Library of Medicine, NIH; 2023. https://www.ncbi.nlm.nih.gov/books/NBK538429/.
9. WebMD. *The Male Reproductive System.* WebMD; 2022. https://www.webmd.com/sex-relationships/male-reproductive-system.
10. Rosner J, Samardzic T, Sarao MS. Physiology, female reproduction. In: *StatsPearls (Internet).* National Library of Medicine, NIH; 2022. https://www.ncbi.nlm.nih.gov/books/NBK537132/.
11. Cleveland Clinic. *Ureteral Stones.* Cleveland Clinic; 2022. https://my.clevelandclinic.org/health/diseases/16514-ureteral-stones.

12. Rodriguez-Mañas L. Urinary tract infections in the elderly: a review of disease characteristics and current treatment options. *Drugs Context.* 2020;9(2020):4–13. https://doi.org/10.7573/dic.2020-4-13.
13. Mayo Clinic. *Benign Prostatic Hyperplasia (BPH).* Mayo Clinic; 2023. https://www.mayoclinic.org/diseases-conditions/benign-prostatic-hyperplasia/symptoms-causes/syc-20370087.
14. Mobeen S, Apostol R. Ovarian cyst. In: *StatsPearls (Internet).* National Library of Medicine, NIH; 2023. https://www.ncbi.nlm.nih.gov/books/NBK560541/.
15. Mayo Clinic. *Endometriosis.* Mayo Clinic; 2023. https://www.mayoclinic.org/diseases-conditions/endometriosis/symptoms-causes/syc-20354656.
16. Mayo Clinic. *Ectopic Pregnancy.* Mayo Clinic; 2023. https://www.mayoclinic.org/diseases-conditions/ectopic-pregnancy/symptoms-causes/syc-20372088.
17. ACS. *Prostate Cancer.* American Cancer Society; 2023. https://www.cancer.org/cancer/types/prostate-cancer.html.
18. ACS. *Signs and Symptoms of Prostate Cancer.* American Cancer Society; 2023. https://www.cancer.org/cancer/types/prostate-cancer/detection-diagnosis-staging/signs-symptoms.html.
19. CDC. *Sexually Transmitted infections (STIs).* Centers for Disease Control; 2023. https://www.cdc.gov/sti/?CDC_AAref_Val=https://www.cdc.gov/std/default.htm.
20. Cleveland Clinic. *Urinary System.* Cleveland Clinic; 2023. https://my.clevelandclinic.org/health/body/21197-urinary-system.
21. Cleveland Clinic. *HIV & AIDS.* Cleveland Clinic; 2022. https://my.clevelandclinic.org/health/diseases/4251-hiv-aids.

18

Endocrine and Metabolic Pathophysiology

OBJECTIVES

By the end of this chapter, the reader should be able to:

- Demonstrate a basic understanding of healthy endocrine physiology.
- Demonstrate a basic understanding of pathophysiological conditions affecting each endocrine gland.
- Identify possible symptoms associated with various urogenital disorders.
- Differentiate between the symptoms occurring when there are anomalies in the typical amounts of various hormones.
- Demonstrate a basic understanding of healthy metabolic physiology.
- Demonstrate a basic understanding of pathophysiological conditions affecting human metabolism.
- Identify possible symptoms associated with various types of metabolic imbalance.
- Differentiate between the symptoms occurring when there is metabolic acidosis compared to metabolic alkalosis.
- Explain and/or predict the possible symptoms resulting from the various endocrine or metabolic conditions.
- Assess and justify whether a specific metabolic or endocrine symptom could constitute a yellow or red flag.

Physiology and Pathophysiology of the Endocrine System

Glands are groups of cells that together create a substance that is either secreted into a duct or secreted directly into the blood.[1] Glands with ducts are called exocrine glands. These glands secrete substances, such as sweat, into a duct that leads to the epithelial surface. Glands without ducts are called endocrine glands.[1] Endocrine glands create hormones that help maintain a plethora of bodily functions. Hormones are vital chemicals, secreted directly into the bloodstream, that work to coordinate various functions in the body by traveling to other organs and delivering messages for proper function.[2]

The list of endocrine glands and other hormone-secreting organs includes the pituitary gland, hypothalamus, pineal gland, parathyroid glands, thyroid gland, thymus, adrenal glands, pancreas, kidneys, testes, and ovaries (Fig. 18.1).

The Pituitary Gland

The pituitary gland is considered to be the "master" gland of the endocrine system.[3] This gland is located below the hypothalamus. Although it is a small gland about the size of a pea, it releases eight hormones that trigger other glands in the endocrine system to release their hormones.[2] The pituitary gland has two lobes (Fig. 18.2). The anterior lobe of the pituitary creates growth hormone, prolactin (PRL), adrenocorticotropic hormone (ACTH), thyroid-stimulating hormone (TSH), follicle-stimulating hormone (FSH), and luteinizing hormone (LH). The posterior lobe of the pituitary stores and releases antidiuretic hormone (ADH) and oxytocin. Each of these hormones is listed below. For normal hormone levels, see Table 18.1.

Growth Hormone

This hormone is responsible for normal growth in childhood, and it helps to maintain the integrity of human organs throughout the lifespan. This hormone will begin to decrease after the onset of middle age.[4] The current medical community suggests that individuals avoid taking synthetic human growth hormone supplements, as doing so can increase the risk of other medical conditions or complications.[4] Excess growth hormone production during childhood can lead to gigantism, characterized by a marked increase in height. In adulthood, excess growth hormone production can result in acromegaly, a slowly progressive disorder marked by enlargement of the bones in the hands, feet, and face.[5]

Prolactin

This hormone is also known as lactotropin and PRL. It causes lactation, breast development, milk production, and many other bodily functions.[6] Levels of this hormone are

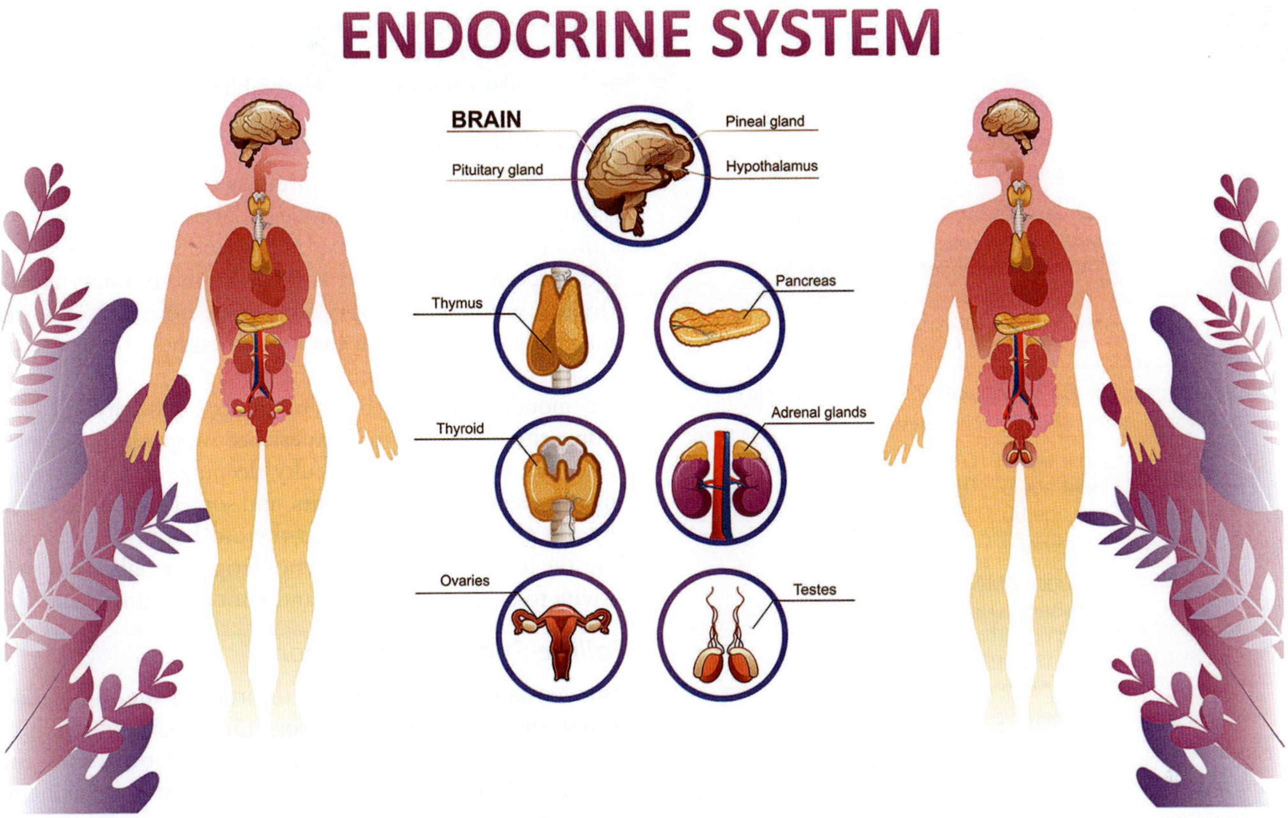

• **Fig. 18.1** Endocrine glands. (From https://www.iStock.com/marrishuanna.)

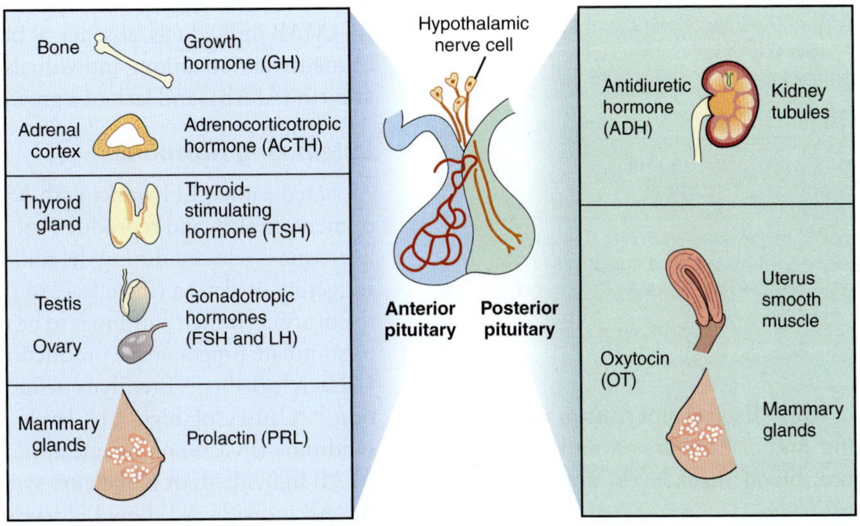

• **Fig. 18.2** The roles of the anterior and posterior pituitary gland. (From Thibodeau GA, Patton KT. *Structure and Function of the Body*. 17th ed. Mosby; 2024.)

typically low in individuals who are not pregnant nor lactating and in people assigned male at birth (AMAB).[6] When these levels get too high, it can cause infertility, irregular periods, amenorrhea (absence of periods), loss of interest in sex, low testosterone levels in males, enlarged breast tissue (gynecomastia), and erectile dysfunction.[6]

Adrenocorticotropic Hormone

This hormone triggers the adrenal glands to produce androgens (sex hormones) and cortisol, often referred to as the "stress hormone."[7] When an individual experiences feelings related to stress, the pituitary secretes ACTH, which then triggers cortisol production.[7] Cortisol works to help regulate

TABLE 18.1 Hormones from the Pituitary Gland

Hormone	Normal Levels
Growth hormone[16]	Adults AMAB: 0.4–10 ng/mL Adults AFAB: 1–14 ng/mL Children: 10–50 ng/mL
Prolactin[6]	AMAB: <20 ng/mL AFAB—not pregnant or breastfeeding: <25 ng/mL AFAB—pregnant or breastfeeding: 80–400 ng/mL
ACTH[7]	7.2–63.3 pg/mL taken in the morning from 7:00 a.m. to 10:00 a.m.
TSH[17]	Under age 18: 0.55–5.31 mU/L Under age 50: 0.5–4.1 mU/L Over age 50: 0.5–4.5 mU/L Over age 70: 0.5–4.5 mU/L
FSH[10]	For adults AMAB Prepuberty: 0–5.0 mIU/mL During puberty: 0.3–10.0 mIU/mL Adults: 1.5–12.4 mIU/mL For adults AFAB Prepuberty: 0–5.0 mIU/mL During puberty: 0.3–10.0 mIU/mL Menstruating: 4.7–21.5 mIU/mL Adults: 1.5–12.4 mIU/mL
LH[11]	AMAB: 1.42–15.4 IU/L AFAB: First 2 weeks of menstrual cycle: 1.3–9 IU/L Preovulation: 6.17–17.2 IU/L Second 2 weeks of menstrual cycle: 1.09–9.2 IU/L Postmenopausal: 19.3–100.6 IU/L
ADH[12]	1–5 pg/mL
Oxytocin[15]	Ovulary peak: 5–10 ng/mL Random: 1.25–5 pg/mL

ACTH, Adrenocorticotropic hormone; *ADH*, antidiuretic hormone; *AFAB*, assigned female at birth; *AMAB*, assigned male at birth; *FSH*, follicle-stimulating hormone; *LH*, luteinizing hormone; *TSH*, thyroid-stimulating hormone.

the body's response to stress. It also helps control the metabolism of fats, proteins, and carbohydrates, and it helps to control blood pressure, blood sugar levels, and the body's inflammatory response.[7]

When ACTH gets too high, it could be because the cortisol levels are too low. This can be due to primary adrenal insufficiency. The most common cause is Addison's disease (a chronic autoimmune condition where the adrenal glands cannot produce enough cortisol).[7] Symptoms would include low blood pressure, weight loss, nausea, weakness, and vomiting.[8] However, when ACTH is abnormally high, like in the case of an adenoma (a benign tumor in the pituitary gland), cortisol will become too high.[7] This is called Cushing disease (not to be confused with Cushing syndrome, which will be discussed later in this chapter). Symptoms of too much cortisol (hypercortisolism) include a round face (moon face), central obesity (buffalo hump), acne, delayed wound healing, and avascular necrosis of the femoral head.[8]

Thyroid-Stimulating Hormone

This hormone is sent by the pituitary to trigger the thyroid gland to make thyroid hormone. If levels of TSH are high, it means that the thyroid level is low, and when thyroid levels are too low, more TSH is made by the pituitary gland. Thyroid hormone is a very important hormone affecting practically every organ in the human body.[9] This hormone helps to control body temperature, weight, muscle strength, and mood. When the body produces excess thyroid hormone, the individual may experience weight loss, irregular heartbeat, nervousness, difficulty sleeping, excessive sweating, frequent bowel movements, and sometimes an enlarged thyroid gland (goiter).[9] When thyroid hormone levels are low, the individual will experience fatigue, weight gain, sensitivity to cold, constipation, and joint and muscle aches.[9]

Follicle-Stimulating Hormone

This hormone works with LH to promote the stimulation of testosterone in boys and estrogen in girls.[10] It is also produced in the pituitary of the developing fetus during the second and third trimesters.[10] Too much FSH in childhood can lead to earlier puberty. Too little or too much FSH due to a problem with the pituitary or hypothalamus is typically due to hypogonadism, which would cause a lack of production of the sex hormones. Symptoms of hypogonadism include an abnormally small penis or undescended testicles in AMAB individuals, absence of breast development or lack of menstruation among individuals who are assigned female at birth (AFAB), and lack of a growth spurt in both groups.[10]

Luteinizing Hormone

As stated earlier, LH works with FSH to aid in sexual development, health, and reproduction. In AFAB individuals, this hormone is released during the middle of the menstrual cycle, triggering ovulation (the release of the egg from the follicle in the ovary).[11] It then continues to be released for about 2 weeks to stimulate progesterone production. In AMAB individuals, LH is released consistently to stimulate testosterone production.[11] Causes of high LH levels include polycystic ovary syndrome (PCOS) or genetic anomalies such as Fragile X in AFAB individuals or Klinefelter syndrome (see Chapter 3) in AMAB individuals.[11] Low LH levels can be due to functional hypothalamic amenorrhea (when menstrual cycles are missed or irregular in relation to excessive exercise) or Kallmann syndrome, a rare condition that can lead to insufficient estrogen or testosterone production.[11]

Antidiuretic Hormone or Vasopressin (Arginine Vasopressin)

ADH is made in the hypothalamus and stored in the posterior pituitary gland.[12] This hormone helps the kidneys to create an osmotic balance (regulating the amount of water stored in the body).[13] When water levels in the body are high, this triggers osmotic sensors and baroreceptors to tell the pituitary to secrete less vasopressin.[12] When an individual is dehydrated (hypovolemia), more ADH will be released from the posterior pituitary.[13] When ADH levels are low, it can be due to decreased production in the hypothalamus or decreased secretion from the pituitary.[12] Regardless of the cause, this can result in a disorder known as diabetes insipidus, in which the individual may experience polyuria (excessive urination), clear urine, fatigue, and polydipsia (extreme thirst). If the body produces too much ADH, this could be secondary to a condition known as the syndrome of inappropriate ADH (SIADH), resulting in symptoms such as headache, nausea, vomiting, and possible coma.[12]

Oxytocin

Oxytocin is stored in the pituitary but made in the hypothalamus. Its primary function is to facilitate childbirth by stimulating the muscles of the uterus to contract, but it also helps to promote positive feelings about the experience.[14] When labor is slow, females are sometimes given oxytocin to speed up the labor. After the baby is born, oxytocin helps move the milk from ducts to the nipple of the breast, and this helps to foster the mother-child bond.[14] In AMAB individuals, oxytocin helps with ejaculation, by connecting to the vas deferens to help propel the sperm forward. Oxytocin also has an effect on the production of testosterone in the testes.[15] Lower than normal oxytocin levels have been linked with autism spectrum disorders and depression. Higher than normal levels of oxytocin have been linked to an overactive uterus in those AFAB and benign prostatic hyperplasia in those AMAB.[15]

The Hypothalamus

The hypothalamus is an area of the brain consisting of various nuclei, located in the center of the brain in an area called the diencephalon, that serves as the primary link between the endocrine system and the nervous system (Fig. 18.3).[18,19] It is like a smart computer (except there is nothing artificial about this intelligence) because it makes predictions and decisions to maintain the body's stable state or homeostasis.[18]

The hypothalamus receives signals from nerve cells in both the brain and the body and responds to these signals in an effort to maintain body temperature, feelings of hunger and thirst, blood pressure, memory, mood, sleep cycle, and sex drive.[18,19] Because the hypothalamus is also part of the central nervous system, it can manage some of these things via direct communication with the autonomic nervous system. This aspect of the hypothalamus will be discussed more in Chapter 20. As part of the endocrine system, however, this region of the brain can also communicate via the release of hormones. The hypothalamus makes two hormones that were already discussed above: vasopressin (ADH) and oxytocin. These two hormones are stored in the posterior pituitary until they are needed, at which time, the hypothalamus signals the pituitary to release the hormone(s) into the system.[18] The hypothalamus also produces growth hormone–releasing hormone, gonadotropin-releasing hormone, corticotropin-releasing hormone (CRH), and thyrotropin-releasing hormone. These signal the release of various hormones from the anterior pituitary in response (Fig. 18.4).[18] The hypothalamus also releases

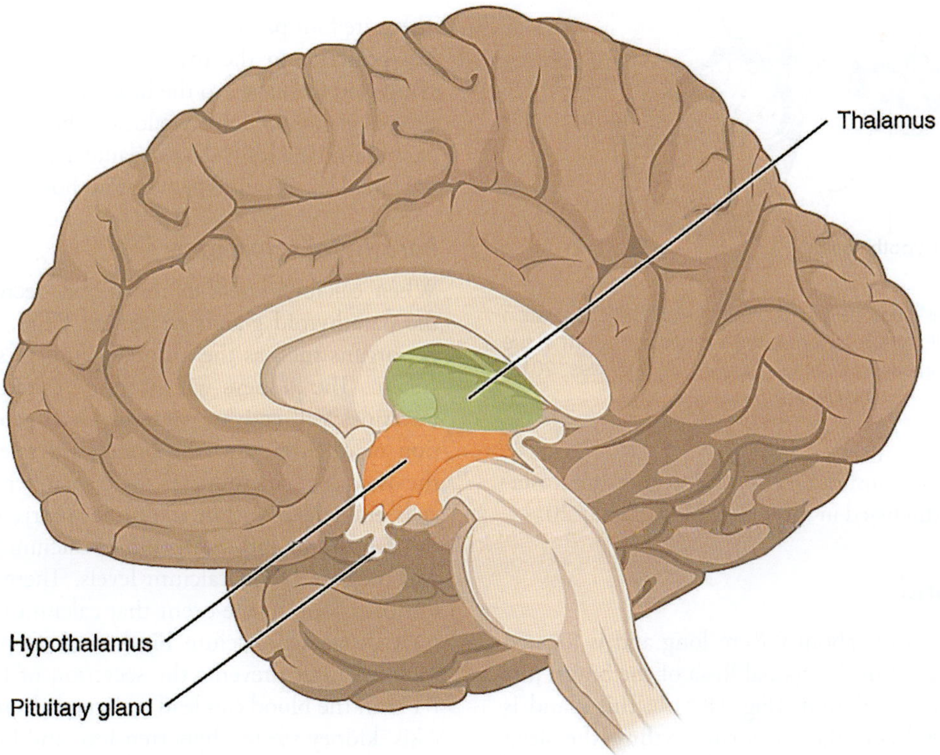

• **Fig. 18.3** The hypothalamus. (From https://www.lecturio.com/concepts/hypothalamus/.)

Hormone from the Hypothalamus	Triggered Pituitary Response
Growth-Releasing Hormone (GH-RH or GHRH)	Release of Human Growth Hormone (hGH or GH), which stimulates the growth of the long bones and larger muscles.
Thyrotropin-Releasing Hormone (TRH)	Release of Thyroid-Stimulating Hormone (TSH), which stimulates the thyroid gland to secrete thyroxine (T4) and triiodothyronine (T3).
Corticotropin-Releasing Hormone (CRH)	Release of Adrenocorticotropic Hormone (ACTH), which stimulates the adrenal glands to release stress hormone (cortisol) as well as regulates the immune response and metabolism.
Dopamine	Inhibits Prolactin synthesis, refines movements, stimulates milk production, and provides pleasure.
Gonadotropin-Releasing Hormone (GnRH)	Release of Follicle-Stimulating Hormone (FSH) and Luteinizing Hormone (LH), which both control the menstrual cycle. In males, FSH controls sperm production, and LH increases testosterone production.
Somatostatin	Inhibits the secretion of many hormones, including Growth Hormone and Thyroid-Stimulating Hormone.

• **Fig. 18.4** The pituitary response from hormones released by the hypothalamus.[18] (Modified from https://my.clevelandclinic.org/health/body/22566-hypothalamus.)

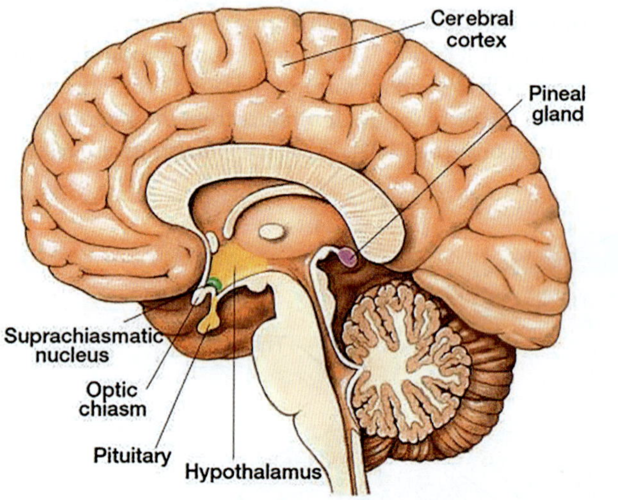

• **Fig. 18.5** The pineal gland. (From Tan D-X, et al. CSF generation by pineal gland results in a robust melatonin circadian rhythm in the third ventricle as an unique light/dark signal. *Med Hypotheses*. 2016; 86:3–9.)

two important neurotransmitters, dopamine and somatostatin, which will be discussed in more detail in Chapter 20.

The Pineal Gland

The pineal gland is only about 0.8 cm long and is located in the posterior region of the cranial fossa of the brain, just inferior to the corpus callosum (Fig. 18.5).[20] This gland is responsible for regulating the circadian rhythm (the sleep and wakefulness cycle). It does this through the secretion of melatonin and 5-methoxytryptophol (5-MTX).[20]

Melatonin

Melatonin is the hormone most responsible for the circadian rhythm. Production of melatonin increases during darkness and decreases when there is light. The light hits the retina, and specialized ganglia (collections of nerve cell bodies) send the impulse to the hypothalamus, and the message is sent to the pineal gland from the hypothalamus via the superior cervical ganglia in the spinal cord.[20] The circadian rhythm is a 24-hour, synchronized cycle that involves mental, physical, and behavioral changes.[21] The pineal gland secretes higher levels of melatonin at night and lower levels during the day.[21] Levels that are too low could cause irregular sleep patterns. This can be caused by shift work, aging, neurodegenerative disorders, or beta-blockers and other medications. Levels that are too high are very rare but can be due to hypogonadism, anorexia nervosa, or polycystic ovarian syndrome.[21]

5-Methoxytryptophol

This hormone is activated by stimulation from radiation, such as sunlight, and is synthesized from serotonin. It performs a dance with melatonin to the tune of the circadian rhythm, with the pineal gland secreting increased levels of 5-MTX during the day.[22] It is for this reason that the blood levels of these two hormones are typically inversely proportional. These are called antagonistic hormones. Because this hormone has antioxidant and immunological modulation properties, it has been considered a possible intervention as an agent against COVID-19.[22]

The Parathyroid Glands

There are four parathyroid glands, located two on either side, just posterior to the thyroid gland (Fig. 18.6).[23] The two glands located closer to the head are called the superior parathyroid glands, and the two located below that are the inferior parathyroid glands.[24] These glands regulate calcium levels in the blood by secreting parathyroid hormone (PTH).

Parathyroid Hormone

When calcium levels in the blood decrease, it stimulates the parathyroid glands to secrete PTH, which affects target organs such as the kidneys, intestines, and the skeletal system. The kidneys will promote calcium resorption, the intestines will activate vitamin D to promote the absorption of calcium, and the bones will release calcium from the osteocystic membranes.[24] (Remember, osteocytes are the cells embedded within the bone matrix that help regulate the deposition and resorption of calcium.) All these actions will increase blood calcium levels. There is also a negative feedback loop in the event that calcium in the blood is too high. Increased calcium binds with G protein, creating a molecule that prevents the secretion of PTH.[23] Too much PTH in the blood can lead to hypercalcemia, with osteoporosis, kidney stones, hypertension, and heart disease.[25] Too little PTH can lead to hypocalcemia with uncontrollable spasms of the face, hands, arms, and feet and a burning or

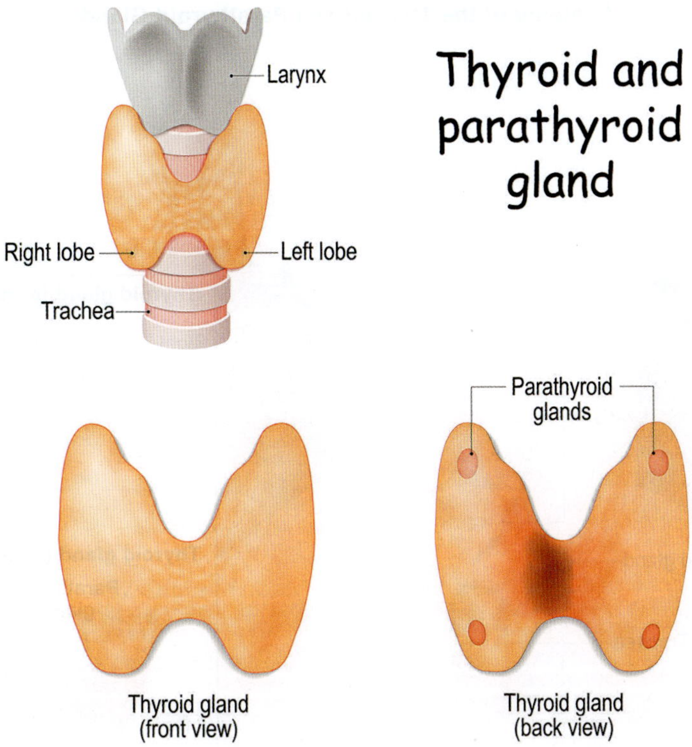

• **Fig. 18.6** The parathyroid glands. (From https://www.iStock.com/ttsz.)

prickling feeling in the hands, feet, and sometimes around the mouth.[26]

The Thyroid Gland

The thyroid gland is a butterfly-shaped organ located in the anterior neck that plays a vital role in metabolism, growth, and the lifelong development of the body (Fig. 18.7).[27] The organ consists of multiple lobules, each containing many small vesicles or sacs that contain thyroid hormone. There are three types of thyroid hormone: tetraiodothyronine or thyroxine (T4), triiodothyronine (T3), and calcitonin. The primary thyroid hormones are T3 and T4, and the thyroid cannot make these if there is not enough iodine in the diet.[27] For normal blood levels of thyroid hormones, see Table 18.2.

As stated above, the process of thyroid hormone secretion requires the work of the hypothalamus to first secrete TRH, triggering the pituitary to release TSH, and this causes the thyroid to secrete more T3 (Fig. 18.4).[28]

Tetraiodothyronine or thyroxine (T4)

This hormone is considered to be an inactive prohormone that requires enzymes from other tissues, such as the kidneys or the liver, to convert the inactive T4 to active T3.[28]

Triiodothyronine (T3)

About 80% of the T3 in the human body is from conversion of T4, but the rest is produced directly by the thyroid gland. This hormone helps to regulate the body's metabolic rate (the rate that food is transformed into energy), heart functions, digestive functions, brain development, bone maintenance, and muscle control.[29] Too much T3 results in weight loss, fast heart rate, irritability, muscle tremors, muscle weakness, sleep problems, and heat sensitivity. Individuals with high thyroid levels over long periods may develop an enlarged thyroid gland or goiter (Fig. 18.8).[9] Too little T3 results in weight gain, slower heart rate, forgetfulness, fatigue, dry skin, hoarse voice, and intolerance to cold.[28] For the comparison between hyperthyroidism and hypothyroidism, see Fig. 18.9.

Calcitonin

This hormone, also secreted by the thyroid gland, plays a role in calcium balance by opposing the role of PTH (the antagonistic hormone), thereby reducing levels of calcium in the blood. It can also act to decrease the resorption of calcium in the kidneys, further reducing blood calcium levels.[30]

The Thymus

The thymus is located posterior to the sternum in the chest, between the apexes of the lungs (Fig. 18.10). This small gland produces white blood cells to help fight infection (T cells and B cells specifically) and produces important hormones, including thymosin and insulin. The thymus also produces some hormones previously discussed, as they are also made in other glands, including growth hormone, PRL, and melatonin.[33] The gland is larger in infants and children, but decreases in size after puberty.

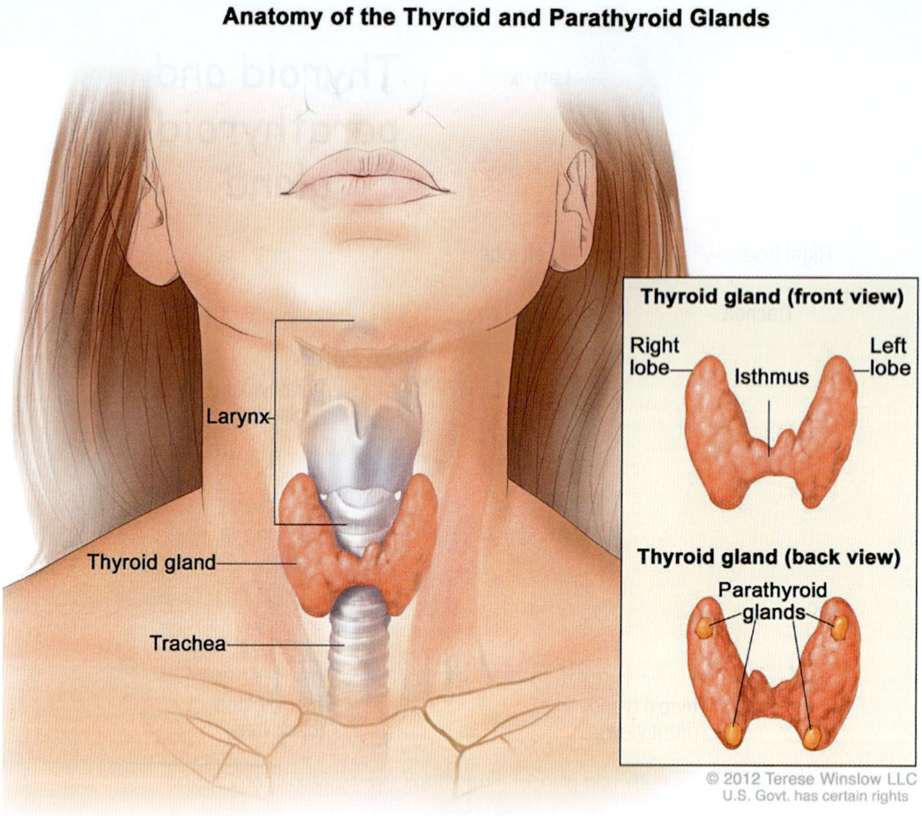

• **Fig. 18.7** The thyroid gland. (From https://www.niddk.nih.gov/health-information/endocrine-diseases/primary-hyperparathyroidism.)

TABLE 18.2 Hormones From the Thyroid Gland

Hormone	Normal Levels
Tetraiodothyronine or thyroxine (T4)[31]	Total levels in adults: 5–12 µg/dL
Triiodothyronine (T3)[29]	Levels are age dependent: Children under age 5: 106–203 ng/dL This gradually declines with age Ages 15–17 years: 71–175 ng/dL Over age 18 years: 79–165 ng/dL
Calcitonin[32]	May vary across laboratories AMAB: 0–7.5 pg/mL AFAB: 0–5.1 pg/mL

AFAB, Assigned female at birth; *AMAB*, assigned male at birth.

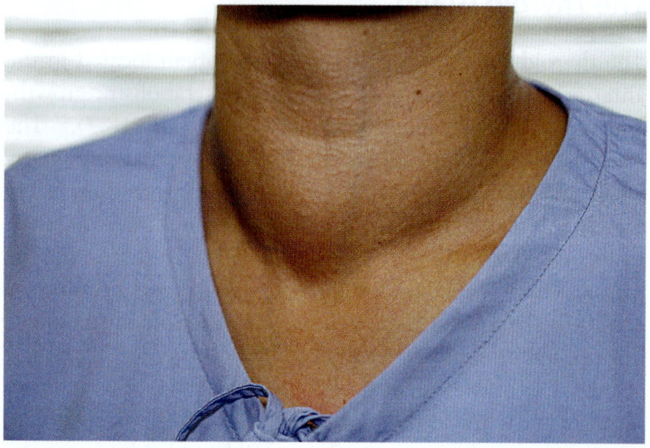

• **Fig. 18.8** Goiter (enlarged thyroid). (From www.istock.com/sasarinpamai.)

Thymosin

Thymosin stimulates T-cell production. These cells mature within the thymus, but they are not yet able to fight infection. Once these cells leave the thymus, thymosin encourages further maturation of the cells, making them powerful agents for the body's immune system.[34] Thymosin "teaches" the T cells to identify cancerous cells, allergens, and pathogens.[33] These cells also "remember" the bacteria and viruses they meet and use that information to give immunity if those pathogens return, but none of this can be done without thymosin.[34] Too much thymosin can result in a runny nose, swollen lymph nodes, and inflammation of the tonsils.

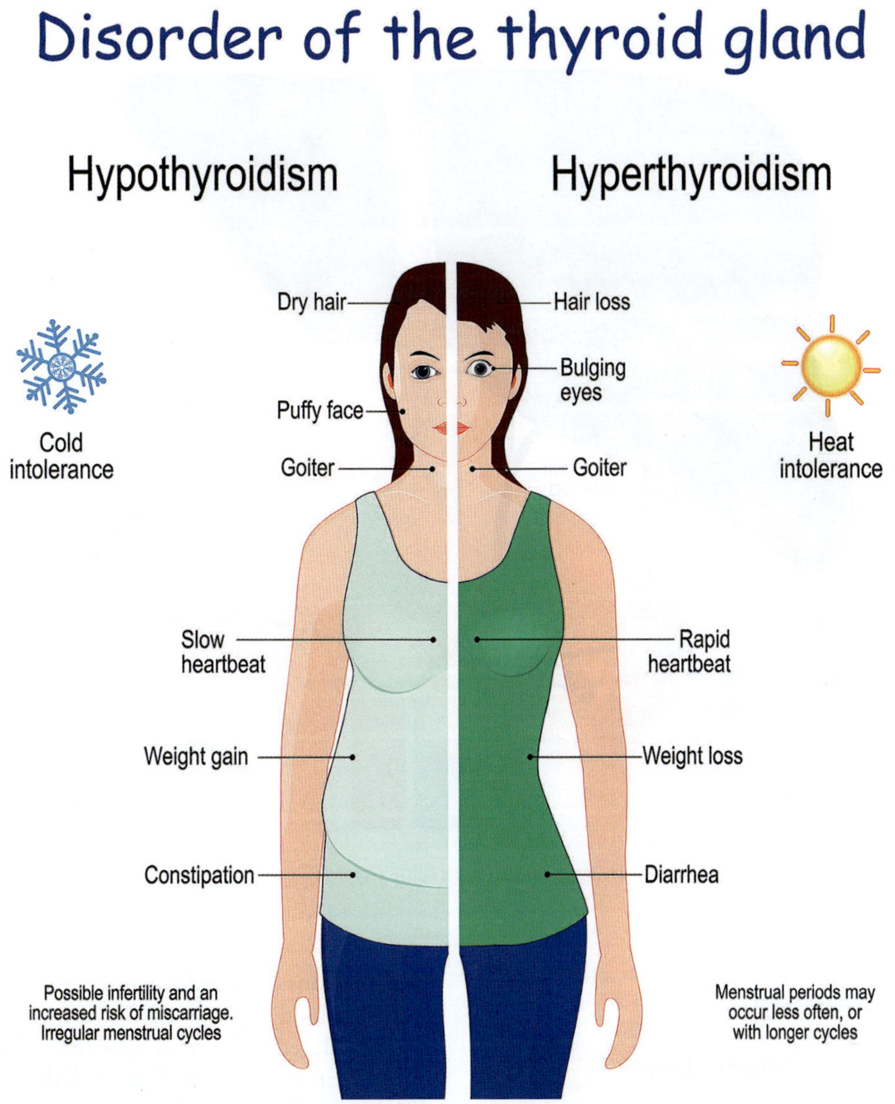

• **Fig. 18.9** Symptoms of hypothyroidism versus hyperthyroidism. (From https://www.iStock.com/ttsz.)

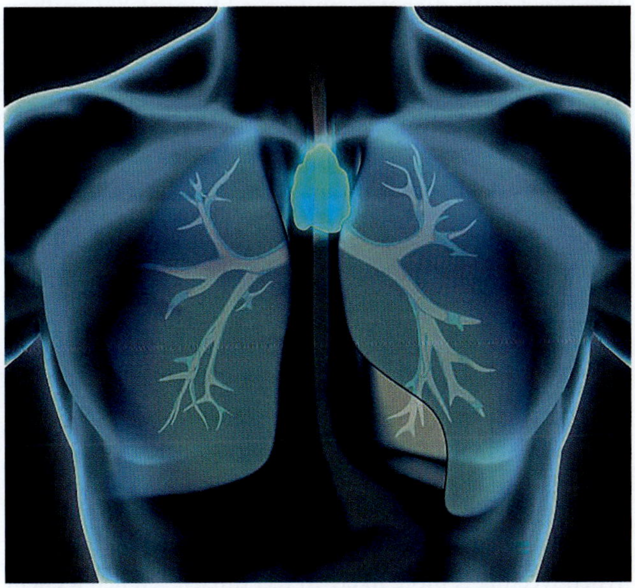

• **Fig. 18.10** The thymus. (From https://www.istockphoto.com/photos/thymus-gland.)

Insulin

Insulin helps to turn food into energy and controls blood sugar levels. Although it is made in the thymus, the primary endocrine gland for insulin is the pancreas. When the body lacks enough insulin, blood sugar rises (hyperglycemia), and diabetes can result. There are various types of diabetic conditions.[35] Gestational diabetes is the type that occurs during pregnancy. *Prediabetes* is when the body cannot use insulin, but blood sugars are not quite high enough to be called Type 2 diabetes. *Type 1 diabetes* happens when the pancreas and thymus cannot make insulin or cannot make enough insulin to control blood sugar levels.[35] *Type 2 diabetes* happens when the pancreas does not produce enough insulin, or the body cannot use the insulin. *Metabolic syndrome* is a group of factors that increase the risk of diabetes, including insulin resistance.[35] More on the symptoms of hyperglycemia and hypoglycemia can be found in the section that follows on the pancreas.

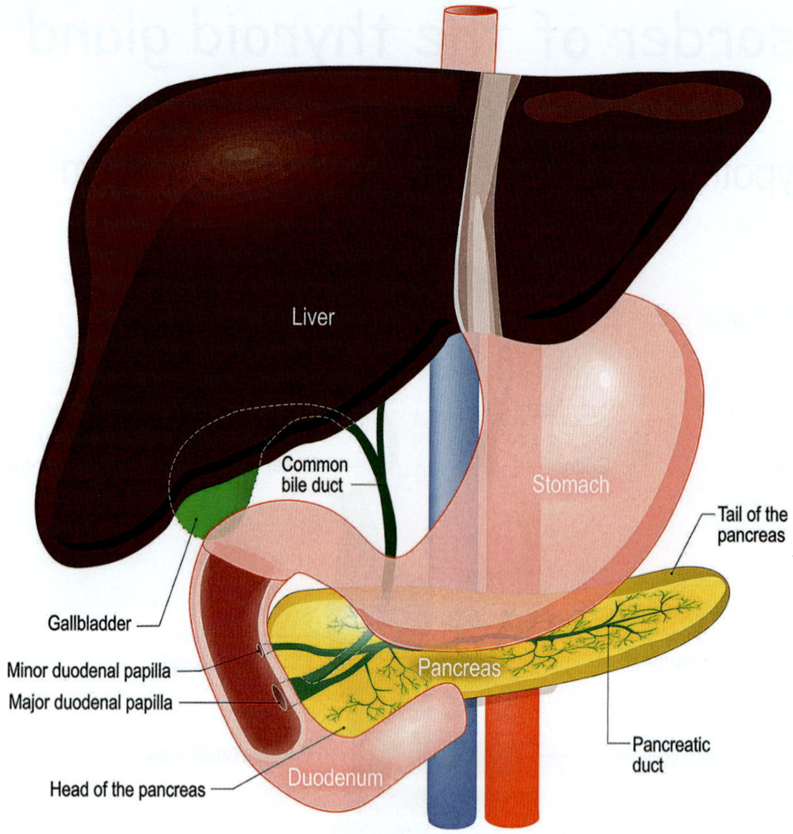

• **Fig. 18.11** The pancreas. (From https://www.iStock.com/ttsz.)

TABLE 18.3 Hormones From the Pancreas

Hormone	Normal Levels
Insulin[36]	60–140 mg/dL
Glucagon[41]	50–100 pg/mL

The Pancreas

Although the pancreas is considered to be a part of the gastrointestinal system, it also secretes hormones, so it is also considered to be an endocrine gland.[35] This organ is located in the posterior aspect of the abdominal cavity, posterior to the stomach, and inferior to the liver (Fig. 18.11). The pancreas acts as both an exocrine gland, producing enzymes that aid in digestion, and an endocrine gland, creating insulin and glucagon, the hormones that control blood sugar.[36] For normal insulin and glucagon levels, see Table 18.3.

Insulin

Although insulin was already mentioned in the discussion of the thymus, it is discussed more here, since the primary insulin-producing gland in the body is the pancreas. The primary job of insulin is to decrease blood sugar levels.[36] During a typical day, there will be slight fluctuations in blood sugar for people without diabetes.[37] When blood sugar goes above 140 mg/dL, an individual is considered to be hyperglycemic. Although blood sugar levels can go high in Type 2 diabetes, they can go even higher in Type 1 diabetes. As of 2021, the Centers for Disease Control and Prevention estimated that 29.7 million people (of all ages) in the United States had been diagnosed with diabetes, and an additional 8.7 million people had undiagnosed diabetes.[38]

When blood sugar goes below 60 mg/dL, an individual is considered to be hypoglycemic.[37] This sometimes happens in response to exercise or to insulin intervention.[40]

It is important for the occupational therapist and occupational therapy assistant (together referred to as occupational therapy practitioners or OTPs) to know the symptoms of hyperglycemia and hypoglycemia, especially in individuals with diabetes (Fig. 18.12).[37] When looking at the table below, it appears that it would be very difficult to know whether a client is hypoglycemic or hyperglycemic. There are ways to differentiate between the two. Talk to your client, and determine when they last took insulin. If it was recent, they are more likely to be hypoglycemic.[40] If the event occurred immediately after or during exercise, it is also more likely to be hypoglycemia.[41] An individual with hypoglycemia is more likely to feel hungry, and an individual with hyperglycemia is more likely to feel thirsty.[40] When a client with diabetes is acting in a way other than usual, and it is

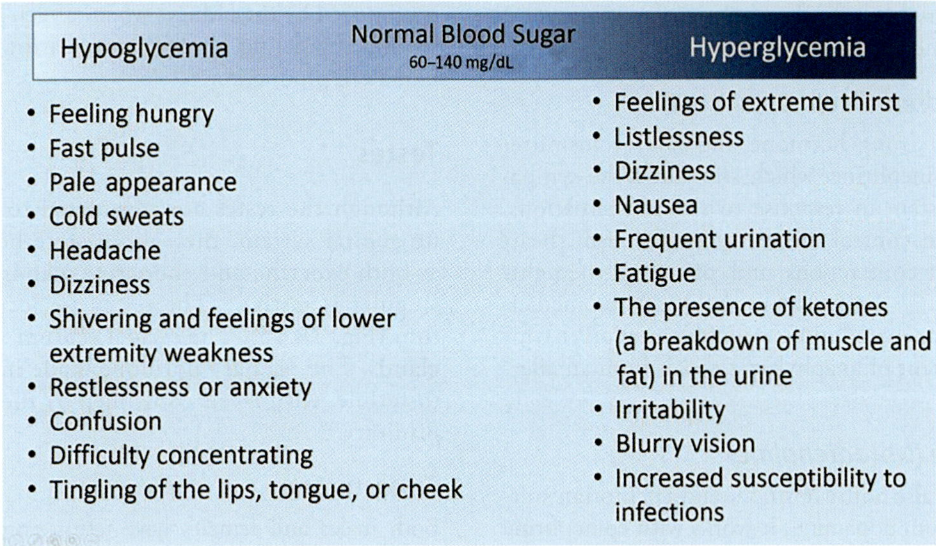

• **Fig. 18.12** Hypoglycemia versus hyperglycemia.

pressing but not urgent, inform the doctor's office immediately, and they can help you determine the best measures to help the client.

Glucagon

The primary job of glucagon is to increase blood sugar levels when needed by triggering the liver to convert the stored glucose (called glycogen) into a more usable form and then secrete it into the bloodstream.[36,42] This hormone is made by the pancreas to prevent blood sugar in the body from dropping too low. More is released during periods of fasting, exercise, a drop in blood sugar, or after protein-rich meals.[42] This hormone works with insulin to create a balanced homeostasis.

The Adrenal Glands

The two adrenal glands (also called suprarenal glands) are small glands located superior to each kidney (Fig. 18.13). The outermost part of each gland is called the adrenal cortex, and the innermost part is called the medulla.[43] There are three separate zones in the adrenal cortex, and each secretes a different hormone: cortisol, aldosterone, and dehydroepiandrosterone along with androgenic hormones. The medulla secretes what is known as the "fight-or-flight" hormones: epinephrine (adrenaline) and norepinephrine.[43]

Cortisol

Cortisol works to control the use of fats, carbohydrates, and proteins in the body. It also decreases inflammation and helps to regulate blood pressure and increase blood sugar.[43] It can also help during times of stress, when more energy is needed due to an emergency situation. The hypothalamus must first release CRH, and this triggers the pituitary to release ACTH, which triggers the adrenal glands to release cortisol.[43]

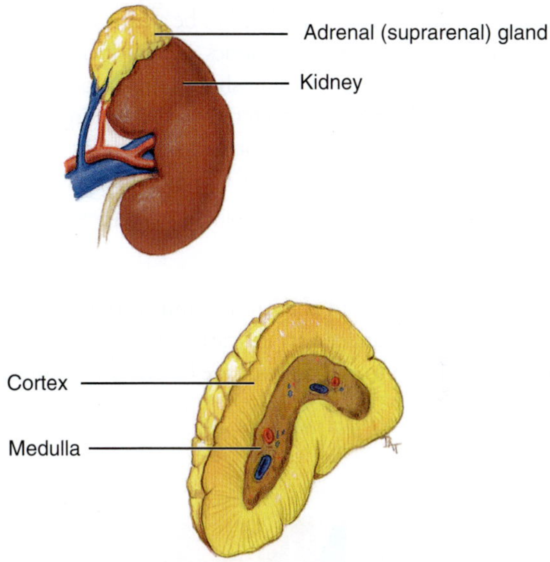

• **Fig. 18.13** The adrenal glands. (From Applegate E. *The Anatomy and Physiology Learning System*. 4th ed. Saunders; 2011.)

Aldosterone

Aldosterone helps to regulate sodium and potassium levels in the blood, and this helps to control blood pressure.[44] It does this by triggering the kidney to favor water and sodium reabsorption and potassium excretion. Aldosterone works to increase water retention and increase blood pressure. It also helps to maintain an acid-base balance.[44]

Dehydroepiandrosterone and Androgenic Hormones

These are weak male hormones that, in individuals AFAB, can be converted into female hormones in the ovaries. They serve as the precursors to the female hormones (estrogens) and the male hormones (androgens).[43]

Epinephrine (Adrenaline)

Epinephrine is a strong hormone and neurotransmitter made from norepinephrine, which stimulates the sympathetic nervous system in response to stressful situations. This hormone can control breathing, metabolism, heart rate, focus, muscle contractions, and, of course, the fight-or-flight response.[43,45] Epinephrine also has some medicinal value, as it can be administered (via an EpiPen) for emergency treatment of anaphylactic shock from an allergic reaction.[43,45,46]

Norepinephrine (Noradrenaline)

Norepinephrine is also both a hormone and a neurotransmitter and is made from dopamine. It works with epinephrine to increase alertness, attention, and arousal by constricting the blood vessels. It also works on the sleep-wake cycle.[47]

Kidneys

Although the kidneys are considered to be a part of the urogenital system, they also secrete hormones, so it is included in this chapter. The kidneys are two bean-shaped organs on either side of the abdominal cavity, just posterior to the floating ribs (Fig. 18.14). In addition to the filtration of bodily fluids performed by the kidneys discussed in Chapter 17, the kidneys also produce vitamin D and secrete a hormone called erythropoietin.[48]

Erythropoietin

This hormone is vital in the production of red blood cells. Red blood cells are necessary to carry oxygen via a protein called hemoglobin to all tissues of the body.[48] Erythropoietin is produced by the kidneys when oxygen levels in the blood are low, by acting on the bone marrow to stimulate red blood cell production.[48]

Testes

Although the testes are considered to be a part of the urogenital system, they also secrete hormones, serving as both exocrine and endocrine glands (plural is testes, singular is testis).[49] The testes are located in the scrotum (Fig. 18.15). The scrotal septum separates the two glands. The primary hormone made in the testes is testosterone, with levels controlled by the LH made in the pituitary.[49]

Testosterone

Both males and females have testosterone (which is made in the ovaries as well as the testes), but it is made in much larger amounts in individuals AMAB. Testosterone production increases during puberty and begins to dip after 30 years of age.[50] This hormone is associated with sex drive and sperm production. This hormone tapers off as males age, and low levels of testosterone in males can lead to a decrease in sex drive, less energy, weight gain, moodiness, hair loss, and osteopenia.[50]

Ovaries

Although the ovaries are considered to be part of the urogenital system, they also serve as endocrine glands. The ovaries are located on either side of the uterus (Fig. 6.2).[51]

The ovaries are responsible for the production of two hormones that play an important role in reproduction and menstruation: estrogen and progesterone.[51]

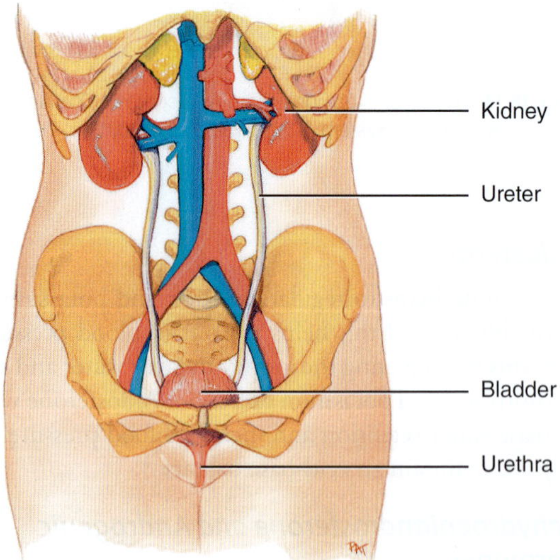

• **Fig. 18.14** The kidneys. (From Applegate E. *The Anatomy and Physiology Learning System*. 4th ed. Saunders; 2011.)

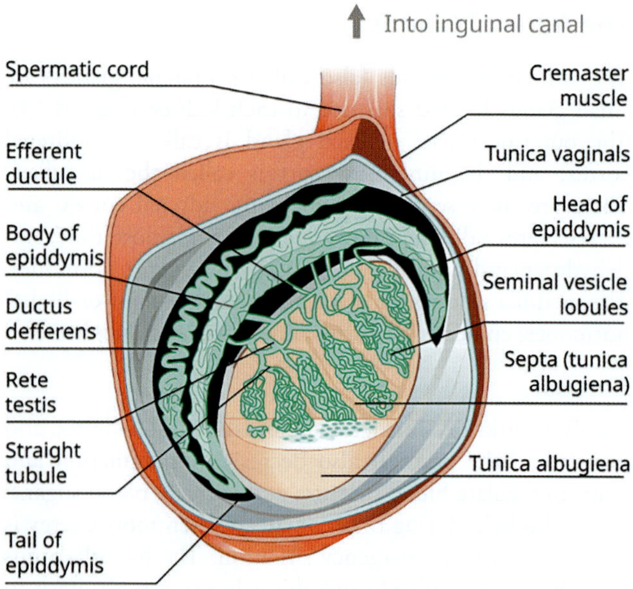

• **Fig. 18.15** The testis. (From Anatomy & Physiology, Connexions Web site. http://cnx.org/content/col11496/1.6/.)

Estrogen

During puberty, the ovaries secrete higher levels of estrogen to help develop primary sex characteristics (those needed for reproduction) and secondary sex characteristics (those that go along with being AFAB, higher voice, or lack of facial hair).[52] This level of estrogen rises and falls along with the menstrual cycle. Estrogen protects the heart by helping to stabilize blood pressure, lowering bad cholesterol (low-density lipoproteins) and increasing good cholesterol (high-density lipoproteins). As individuals AFAB age, the number of egg sacs in the ovaries decreases and so does estrogen production. Estrogen also works to improve muscle mass and bone density.[52]

Progesterone

In individuals AFAB, progesterone helps with menstruation and gives support during the early stages of pregnancy. When conception occurs, progesterone increases to thicken the uterine lining and help sustain the pregnancy.[53]

Antagonistic Hormones

As this chapter has progressed, the reader may have noticed that many of the body's hormones have an antagonistic hormone performing the opposite job. This is necessary for homeostasis. See Table 18.4 for some of the more well-known antagonistic hormones.

Physiology of the Metabolic System

Metabolism is the process whereby the body converts what we eat and drink into energy. Human metabolism is closely tied with endocrine physiology. Many of the previously mentioned hormones directly affect the body's metabolism. For example, hyperthyroidism will increase metabolism, and hypothyroidism will slow metabolism.

The human body performs two metabolic processes: catabolism (breaking down food to release energy) and anabolism (using energy to repair and build cells in the body).[54] Metabolism can also be defined as the sum of all the enzyme-mediated chemical reactions that occur within a cell to provide energy for life.[55] Metabolism is measured in units of energy called kilojoules. A calorie is also a measurement of energy. One calorie is equal to 4.18 kilojoules.[54]

Healthy metabolism affects not only energy creation and utilization but also fluid balance and pH homeostasis.[56]

The Comprehensive Metabolic Panel

A comprehensive metabolic panel is a blood test that measures 14 various substances in the blood to help detect any problems with metabolism. The substances measured in this panel are glucose, calcium, four electrolytes, albumin, total protein, three liver enzymes, bilirubin, blood urea nitrogen (BUN), and creatinine.[56] For estimated normal levels of each of these, see Table 18.5.

Glucose

Glucose is also known as blood sugar. It is a simple carbohydrate (a monosaccharide), with fat and protein, and serves as one of the body's primary sources of energy.[56,57] The thymus and the pancreas help to maintain blood sugar homeostasis. The symptoms of hyperglycemia and hypoglycemia were discussed earlier in this chapter, under the "Insulin" section.

TABLE 18.4 Hormones and Their Antagonists

Homeostasis	Hormone	Antagonistic Hormone
Blood sugar levels	**Insulin** This hormone works to decrease blood sugar levels.	**Glucagon** This hormone works to increase blood sugar levels.
Blood calcium levels	**Parathyroid Hormone** This hormone works to increase blood calcium levels.	**Calcitonin** This hormone works to decrease blood calcium levels.
Growth	**GHRH** This hormone is released by the hypothalamus to increase the secretion of growth hormone in the pituitary.	**Somatostatin** This hormone is released by the hypothalamus, alternatively to GHRH, to decrease the secretion of growth hormone in the pituitary.
Sleep-wake cycle	**Melatonin** This hormone is released by the pineal gland. Production of melatonin increases during the darkness and decreases when there is light, encouraging sleep.	**5-Methoxytryptophol** This hormone is also released by the pineal gland. Production increases when there is light, encouraging wakefulness.

GHRH, Growth hormone–releasing hormone.

TABLE 18.5 Basic Metabolic Panel

Substance	Normal Levels
Glucose[36]	60–140 mg/dL
Calcium[57]	Total: 8.5–10.5 mg/dL Ionized: 4.65–5.2 mg/dL
Sodium (Na^+)[58]	135–145 mEq/L
Potassium (K^+)[60]	3.6–5.2 mmol/L
Bicarbonate (HCO_3^-)[72]	22–26 mEq/L
Chloride[65]	96–106 mmol/L
Albumin[66]	3.4–5.4 g/dL
Total protein[67]	6.0–8.0 g/dL
ALP[69]	40–129 U/L
ALT[69]	7–55 U/L
AST[69]	8–48 U/L
Bilirubin[69]	0.1–1.2 mg/dL
BUN[70]	6–24 mg/dL
Creatinine[71]	Adult males: 0.74–1.35 mg/dL Adult females: 0.59–1.04 mg/dL

ALP, Alkaline phosphatase; *ALT*, alanine transaminase; *AST*, aspartate aminotransferase; *BUN*, blood urea nitrogen.

Calcium

Calcium is a valuable mineral stored in the bones and teeth. Proper levels of calcium in the blood are needed for muscles, nerves, and the heart to function normally.[56] Some of the calcium in the blood is not bound to a protein. This is called free calcium. A total calcium test is a measurement of both the free calcium and the bound calcium. An ionized test only measures the free calcium.[58] The parathyroid gland helps to control the levels of calcium in the blood. The symptoms of hypercalcemia and hypocalcemia can be found earlier in this chapter, under the "Parathyroid Hormone" section.

Electrolytes

Electrolytes are molecules that carry a positive or negative charge. There are four primary electrolytes in the human body needed for proper metabolism: sodium, potassium, bicarbonate, and chloride.[56]

Sodium (Na^+) is a positively charged ion that is necessary for muscle and nerve function. It also helps to maintain fluid balance in the body. Too much sodium (hypernatremia) will lead to water retention and raise blood pressure (with thirst, weakness, swelling in the hands and feet, and insomnia), and too little will do the opposite, lowering blood pressure (with nausea, vomiting, loss of appetite, hallucinations, dizziness, and fatigue).[59]

Potassium (K^+) is also a positively charged ion that is necessary for muscle and nerve function, which works as a counterbalance to sodium, helping to maintain the fluid balance in the body.[60] Hyperkalemia (too much potassium in the body) can cause abdominal pain, nausea, vomiting, and diarrhea, and if the levels are severely high, it can cause arrhythmias, numbness in the hands and feet, and possible damage to the heart, that is, a heart attack.[61] Hypokalemia (too little potassium in the body) can cause constipation, extreme fatigue, muscle weakness and spasms, tingling and numbness, muscle twitches, low blood pressure, excessive thirst, and excessive urination.[62]

Bicarbonate (HCO_3^-), a form of carbon dioxide, is a negatively charged ion that is needed to help maintain the pH balance of our blood. Bicarbonate is a base (alkali), and low levels are an indicator of metabolic acidosis (low pH, or high acidity in the blood). Symptoms of metabolic acidosis are fatigue, weakness, vomiting, loss of appetite, long deep breaths, and fast heart rate.[63] Too much bicarbonate will cause metabolic alkalosis (high pH, or alkalinity in the blood). This risk is higher if a person is dehydrated. Symptoms of metabolic alkalosis include muscle twitching, muscle cramps, spasms, fatigue, confusion, tremors, abnormal heart rate, and seizures (Fig. 18.16).[64]

Chloride (Cl^-) is a negatively charged ion that also helps with muscle and nerve function and helps to maintain the pH balance of the body fluids. A high chloride level can be indicative of dehydration, kidney disease, metabolic acidosis (low blood pH), respiratory alkalosis (too little carbon dioxide in the blood sometimes due to hyperventilation), or Cushing syndrome.[65]

Albumin

This is the primary type of protein in the human body synthesized in the liver and needed for tissue healing.[56] These levels are tested and part of the metabolic panel when the physician suspects liver or kidney malfunction.[66]

Total Protein

This is the sum of different types of protein in the body including albumin and globulins, which are created in the liver.[56] These levels are also tested and part of the metabolic panel when the physician suspects liver or kidney malfunction, with albumin included in this total. This can be tested by evaluating the blood or the urine. High levels of protein in the urine can be indicative of kidney disease.[67] High levels of protein in the blood can be a sign of infection, dehydration, cancer, or liver disease. Low protein levels can occur with malnutrition, congestive heart failure, liver disease, or kidney disease.[67]

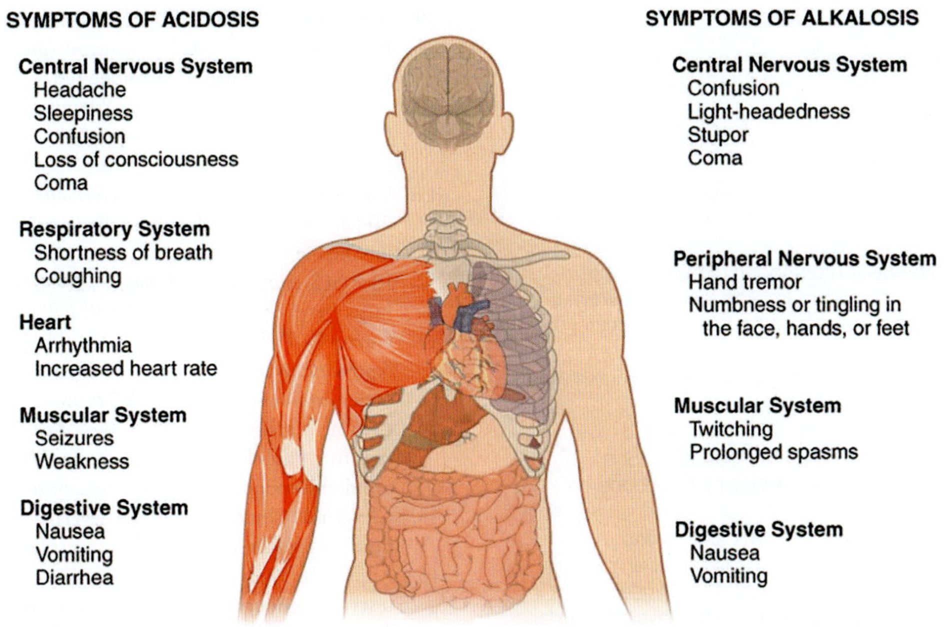

• **Fig. 18.16** Acidosis versus alkalosis. (From https://courses.lumenlearning.com/suny-ap2/chapter/disorders-of-acid-base-balance/.)

Liver Enzymes

There are three main liver enzymes: alkaline phosphatase, alanine transaminase (ALT), and aspartate aminotransferase (AST). There is also gamma-glutamyl transferase and serum bilirubin.[68,69] All of these enzymes can act as catalysts for certain chemical reactions that occur in the body.[56] Liver enzyme testing typically focuses on the levels of ALT and AST.[68] Elevated liver enzymes can be a sign of fatty liver disease, metabolic syndrome (a group of symptoms that increase the risk of heart disease: high blood sugar, high blood pressure, high cholesterol, and high body mass index), hepatitis, cirrhosis, or alchoholism.[68]

Bilirubin

This is a waste product that is left behind after the body breaks down old red blood cells. Most of this is removed from the body by the liver.[56] Higher than normal levels of bilirubin can be an indicator of liver damage or certain types of anemia.[69]

Blood Urea Nitrogen and Creatinine

These are both waste products filtered out of the blood by the kidneys and eliminated via the urinary tract.[56] A BUN test gives information about how the kidneys are working. Ammonia is produced in the liver, and this contains nitrogen that combines with other elements to form urea. This travels from the liver to the kidneys.[70] Healthy kidneys filter waste products such as urea from the blood. When BUN is high, it could indicate a problem in the kidneys.[70] Creatinine is a waste product formed from energy-producing processes in the muscles.[71] The kidneys filter this from the bloodstream, but high levels of creatinine in the blood is also an indicator of possible kidney disease.[71]

The OT Scope of Practice

OTPs should be alert to any signs of endocrine or metabolic problems in their clients. The symptoms of endocrine or metabolic malfunction may not be immediately clear and often resemble those of gastrointestinal, cardiovascular, or other systemic disorders. As stated before in this text, it is not the job of the OTP to make a medical diagnosis. It is, however, the job of the OTP to act as an advocate, sending the client back to the referring physician (when warranted) for bloodwork, urinalysis, and other tests that will possibly provide more information, in an effort to better help the client.

Application—Case Study

CASE EXAMPLE 18.1

A 72-year-old male presented to an OTP at an outpatient clinic with peripheral neuropathy from diabetes. The OTP was working with him to show how to perform skin checks on his feet and to help him with other instrumental activities of daily living.

1. **Screen:** The OTP asked him about his diabetes during the first day working together and made it a point to ask him before each session if he had taken his insulin that day.

2. **Take a Closer Look:** The OTP noticed that the client had an acute tremor in his fingers. The client seemed oblivious to this until the OTP asked him about it. She asked him if he had any other symptoms, and he said that he was feeling very hungry. When she asked if he was thirsty, he said, "No, just hungry."
3. **Determine Flag Status:** The OTP determined this to be a potential yellow flag situation and kept a close eye on the client.
4. **Take Action if Needed:** After about 15 minutes, the client became pale, started mumbling fast, and swaying in his chair. The OTP quickly grabbed a small bottle of orange juice from the clinic refrigerator that she kept specifically for this type of emergency. Within minutes, he was feeling better and thanking the OTP.
5. **Document the Findings:** The OTP phoned the physician to inform them that this happened. She documented this information as well as the phone call with the doctor.
6. **Take a Second Look:** The OTP was able to find someone to give the client a ride to his physician's office (she made sure that he did not drive himself, even though he kept insisting he was fine). The physician ran bloodwork, and adjustments were made to the client's morning dose of insulin.
7. **Determine the Flag Status:** The OTP determined that the situation had quickly escalated to a red flag status.
8. **Take Action if Needed:** The client was cared for immediately by an attentive OTP.

This is a true case. This OTP planned ahead, asking all her clients with diabetes if they had taken their insulin yet that day, keeping orange juice on hand, and really listening to the client's complaints to know that this was an episode of hypoglycemia, possibly saving the client's life.

References

1. Freeman SC, Malik A, Basit H. Physiology, exocrine gland. In: *StatPearls [Internet]*. National Library of Medicine; 2023. https://www.ncbi.nlm.nih.gov/books/NBK542322/.
2. Cleveland Clinic. *Endocrine System*. Cleveland Clinic; 2023. https://my.clevelandclinic.org/health/body/21201-endocrine-system.
3. Hopkins. *Pituitary Gland*. Johns Hopkins Medicine; 2023. https://www.hopkinsmedicine.org/health/conditions-and-diseases/the-pituitary-gland.
4. Mayo Clinic. *Human Growth Hormone (HGH): Does It Slow Aging?* Mayo Clinic Healthy Lifestyle; 2023. https://www.mayoclinic.org/healthy-lifestyle/healthy-aging/in-depth/growth-hormone/art-20045735.
5. Mayo Clinic. *Acromegaly*. Mayo Clinic; 2023. https://www.mayoclinic.org/diseases-conditions/acromegaly/symptoms-causes/syc-20351222.
6. Cleveland Clinic. *Prolactin*. Cleveland Clinic; 2022. https://my.clevelandclinic.org/health/articles/22429-prolactin.
7. Cleveland Clinic. *Adrenocorticotropic Hormone (ACTH)*. Cleveland Clinic; 2022. https://my.clevelandclinic.org/health/articles/23151-adrenocorticotropic-hormone-acth.
8. Allen MJ, Sharma S. Physiology, adrenocorticotropic hormone (ACTH). *StatPearls [Internet]*. National Library of Medicine; 2023. https://www.ncbi.nlm.nih.gov/books/NBK500031/.
9. MedLinePlus. *TSH (Thyroid Stimulating Hormone) Test*. MedLinePlus; 2022. https://medlineplus.gov/lab-tests/tsh-thyroid-stimulating-hormone-test/.
10. Cleveland Clinic. *Follicle-Stimulating Hormone (FSH)*. Cleveland Clinic; 2023. https://my.clevelandclinic.org/health/articles/24638-follicle-stimulating-hormone-fsh.
11. Cleveland Clinic. *Luteinizing Hormone (LH)*. Cleveland Clinic; 2022. https://my.clevelandclinic.org/health/body/22255-luteinizing-hormone.
12. Rice SC. *Antidiuretic Hormone (ADH) Test*. Healthline; 2018. https://www.healthline.com/health/adh.
13. Cuzzo B, Padala SA, Lappin SL. Physiology vasopressin. In: *StatPearls*. National Library of Medicine; 2023. https://www.ncbi.nlm.nih.gov/books/NBK526069/.
14. LeWine HE. *Oxytocin: The Love Hormone*. Harvard Health Publishing; 2023. https://www.health.harvard.edu/mind-and-mood/oxytocin-the-love-hormone.
15. Cleveland Clinic. *Oxytocin*. Cleveland Clinic; 2022. https://my.clevelandclinic.org/health/articles/22618-oxytocin.
16. Appendix: Normal values of metabolic parameters and tests of endocrine function. In: Molina PE, ed. *Endocrine Physiology*. 4th ed. McGraw Hill; 2013. https://accessmedicine.mhmedical.com/content.aspx?bookid=507&sectionid=42540511.
17. Jewel T. *All About Standard TSH Ranges by Age and Life Stage*. Healthline; 2020. https://www.healthline.com/health/tsh-normal-range-by-age.
18. Cleveland Clinic. *Hypothalamus*. Cleveland Clinic; 2022. https://my.clevelandclinic.org/health/body/22566-hypothalamus.
19. Oiseth S, Jones L, Maza E. *Hypothalamus*. LecturiMedical; 2022. https://www.lecturio.com/concepts/hypothalamus/.
20. Ilahi S, Beriwal N, Ilaki TB. Physiology, pineal gland. In: *StatPearls*. National Library of Medicine; 2023. https://www.ncbi.nlm.nih.gov/books/NBK525955/.
21. Cleveland Clinic. *Melatonin*. Cleveland Clinic; 2022. https://my.clevelandclinic.org/health/articles/23411-melatonin.
22. Şehirli AO, Sayıner S. Daylight is critical to preserve 5-methoxytryptophol levels in suspected and confirmed COVID-19 patients. *Med Hypotheses*. 2021;147:110504. https://doi.org/10.1016/j.mehy.2021.110504.
23. UChicago. *Parathyroid Disease*. UChicago Medicine; 2023. https://www.uchicagomedicine.org/conditions-services/endocrinology-metabolic-disorders/parathyroid-disease.
24. Ilahi S, Muco E, Ilaki TB. Anatomy, head and neck, parathyroid. In: *StatPearls*. National Library of Medicine; 2023. https://www.ncbi.nlm.nih.gov/books/NBK537203/.
25. Johns Hopkins. *Hyperparathyroidism*. Johns Hopkins Health; 2023. https://www.hopkinsmedicine.org/health/conditions-and-diseases/hyperparathyroidism.
26. Johns Hopkins. *Hypoparathyroidism*. Johns Hopkins Health; 2023. https://www.hopkinsmedicine.org/health/conditions-and-diseases/hypoparathyroidism.
27. NIH. *How Does the Thyroid Gland Work?* National Library of Medicine: Informed Health; 2018. https://www.ncbi.nlm.nih.gov/books/NBK279388/
28. You and Your Hormones. *Thyroid Gland*. You and Your Hormones, The Society for Endocrinology; 2020. https://www.yourhormones.info/glands/thyroid-gland/.
29. Cleveland Clinic. *T3 (Triiodothyronine Test) Test*. Cleveland Clinic; 2022. https://my.clevelandclinic.org/health/diagnostics/22425-triiodothyronine-t3.

30. You and Your Hormones. *Calcitonin*. You and Your Hormones, The Society for Endocrinology; 2021.
31. Ames H. What to know about T4 levels. *Medical News Today*; 2023. https://www.medicalnewstoday.com/articles/t4-levels.
32. Cleveland Clinic. *Calcitonin*. Cleveland Clinic; 2022. https://my.clevelandclinic.org/health/articles/22330-calcitonin.
33. West M. What is the thymus gland? *Medical News Today*; 2023. https://www.medicalnewstoday.com/articles/thymus.
34. Taylor M. Thymus gland: what to know. *Medical News Today*; 2023. https://www.webmd.com/a-to-z-guides/thymus-gland-what-to-know.
35. Cleveland Clinic. *Insulin*. Cleveland Clinic; 2022. https://my.clevelandclinic.org/health/articles/22601-insulin.
36. Cleveland Clinic. *Pancreas*. Cleveland Clinic; 2022. https://my.clevelandclinic.org/health/body/21743-pancreas.
37. NIH. *Hyperglycemia and Hypoglycemia in Type 2 Diabetes*. National Library of Medicine: Informed Health; 2020. https://www.ncbi.nlm.nih.gov/books/NBK279510/.
38. CDC. *National Diabetes Statistics Report*. The Centers for Disease Control and Prevention; 2021. https://www.cdc.gov/diabetes/data/statistics-report/index.html.
39. Mayo Clinic. *Diabetes*. The Mayo Clinic; 2023. https://www.mayoclinic.org/diseases-conditions/diabetes/symptoms-causes/syc-20371444.
40. Mayo Clinic. *Hypoglycemia*. The Mayo Clinic; 2023. https://www.mayoclinic.org/diseases-conditions/hypoglycemia/symptoms-causes/syc-20373685.
41. Crider C. *Can Exercise Cause Hypoglycemia?* Healthline; 2023. https://www.healthline.com/health/exercise-induced-hypoglycemia.
42. Cleveland Clinic. *Glucagon*. Cleveland Clinic; 2022. https://my.clevelandclinic.org/health/articles/22283-glucagon.
43. Johns Hopkins. *Adrenal Glands. Health*. Johns Hopkins; 2023. https://www.hopkinsmedicine.org/health/conditions-and-diseases/adrenal-glands.
44. Scott JH, Menouar MA, Dunn RJ. Physiology, aldosterone. In: *StatPearls [Internet]*. StatPearls Publishing; 2023. https://www.ncbi.nlm.nih.gov/books/NBK470339/.
45. Charles S. *What Is Epinephrine?* Very Well Health; 2023. https://www.verywellhealth.com/what-is-epinephrine-5078652.
46. Cleveland Clinic. *Epinephrine (Adrenaline)*. Cleveland Clinic; 2022. https://my.clevelandclinic.org/health/articles/22611-epinephrine-adrenaline.
47. Cleveland Clinic. *Norpinephrine (Nordrenaline)*. Cleveland Clinic; 2022. https://my.clevelandclinic.org/health/articles/22610-norepinephrine-noradrenaline.
48. You and Your Hormones. *Hormones. Kidneys*. You and Your Hormones, The Society for Endocrinology; 2019. https://www.yourhormones.info/glands/kidneys/.
49. Tiwana MS, Leslie SW. Anatomy, abdomen and pelvis: testes. In: *StatPearls [Internet]*. StatPearls Publishing; 2023. https://www.ncbi.nlm.nih.gov/books/NBK470201/.
50. Roland J, Robinson D. *What Is Testosterone?* Healthline; 2023. https://www.healthline.com/health/what-is-testosterone.
51. Cleveland Clinic. *Ovaries*. Cleveland Clinic; 2022. https://my.clevelandclinic.org/health/body/22999-ovaries.
52. Cleveland Clinic. *Estrogen: What It Does and 5 Benefits*. Cleveland Clinic; 2022. https://health.clevelandclinic.org/what-does-estrogen-do.
53. Cleveland Clinic. *Progesterone*. Cleveland Clinic; 2022. https://my.clevelandclinic.org/health/body/24562-progesterone.
54. Healthdirect. *Metabolism*. Health Direct: Free Australian Advise You Can Count on; n.d. https://www.healthdirect.gov.au/metabolism.
55. Kornberg H. *Metabolism*. Encyclopedia Britannica; 2023. https://www.britannica.com/science/metabolism.
56. MedLine Plus. *Comprehensive Metabolic Panel (CMP)*. Medline: National Library of Medicine: NIH; 2023. https://medlineplus.gov/lab-tests/comprehensive-metabolic-panel-cmp/.
57. Wright SA. *Everything You Need to Know About Glucose*. Healthline; 2022. https://www.healthline.com/health/glucose.
58. Shital K. *Why Do I Need a Calcium Blood Test?* WebMD; 2023. https://www.webmd.com/a-to-z-guides/do-i-need-a-calcium-blood-test.
59. Case-Lo C. *Blood Sodium Test*. Healthline; 2018. https://www.healthline.com/health/hyponatremia#Outlook.
60. Begum (Reviewer) J. *What Is a Potassium Blood Test?* WebMD; 2021. https://www.webmd.com/a-to-z-guides/potassium-blood-test.
61. Cleveland Clinic. *Hyperkalemia (High Potassium)*. Cleveland Clinic; 2023. https://my.clevelandclinic.org/health/diseases/15184-hyperkalemia-high-blood-potassium.
62. Cleveland Clinic. *Hypokalemia*. Cleveland Clinic; 2022. https://my.clevelandclinic.org/health/diseases/17740-low-potassium-levels-in-your-blood-hypokalemia.
63. NKF. *Metabolic Acidosis*. National Kidney Foundation; 2023. https://www.kidney.org/atoz/content/metabolic-acidosis.
64. Cleveland Clinic. *Metabolic Alkalosis*. Cleveland Clinic; 2021. https://my.clevelandclinic.org/health/diseases/21529-metabolic-alkalosis.
65. Cleveland Clinic. *Chloride Blood Test*. Cleveland Clinic; 2021. https://my.clevelandclinic.org/health/diagnostics/22023-chloride-blood-test.
66. University of Rochester. *Albumin (Blood)*. Health Encyclopedia: University of Rochester; 2023. https://www.urmc.rochester.edu/encyclopedia/content.aspx?contenttypeid=167&contentid=albumin_blood.
67. Eske J. What to know about the protein test and results. *Medical News Today*; 2023. https://www.medicalnewstoday.com/articles/325320.
68. Burgess L. Elevated liver enzymes: everything you need to know. *Medical News Today*; 2023. https://www.medicalnewstoday.com/articles/325838.
69. Mayo Clinic. *Liver Function Tests*. The Mayo Clinic; 2023. https://www.mayoclinic.org/tests-procedures/liver-function-tests/about/pac-20394595.
70. Mayo Clinic. *Blood Urea Nitrogen (BUN) Test*. The Mayo Clinic; 2023. https://www.mayoclinic.org/tests-procedures/blood-urea-nitrogen/about/pac-20384821.
71. Mayo Clinic. *Creatinine Test*. The Mayo Clinic; 2023.
72. Cleveland Clinic. *Arterial Blood Gas (ABG)*. Cleveland Clinic; 2022. https://my.clevelandclinic.org/health/diagnostics/22409-arterial-blood-gas-abg.

19

Environmental Pathogens and Neoplasms

OBJECTIVES

By the end of this chapter, the reader should be able to:

- Identify some of the major environmental pathogens.
- Demonstrate a basic understanding of pathophysiological conditions resulting from environmental pathogens.
- Identify possible symptoms associated with various types of environmental pathogens.
- Differentiate between the symptoms occurring when there is an environmental pathogen versus when there is another physiological condition.
- Explain and/or predict the possible symptoms resulting from exposure to various environmental pathogens.
- List the transmission-based precautions for protection from blood-borne pathogens.
- Differentiate between some of the characteristics of benign versus malignant tumors.
- Assess and justify whether a symptom from an environmental pathogen could constitute a yellow or red flag.

Harmful Agents in the Environment

There are many agents in the environment that can threaten human health. This chapter will cover tobacco use, alcohol, harmful chemicals, radiation, temperature, altitude, malnutrition, bacteria, viruses, eukaryotes (fungus, helminths, protozoa), and parasites. Some of these pathogens can lead to the formation of a tumor or neoplasm. A tumor is a mass of tissue consisting of cells that either closely resemble normal cells (benign) or look different from normal cells (malignant). Neoplasms will also be discussed in this chapter.

Tobacco

The harmful effects of cigarette smoking cannot be overstated. The overall death rate for smokers in the United States is about three times higher than nonsmokers.[1] Cigarette smoking is believed to be responsible for more than 480,000 deaths annually, and it is not just the smoker who is at risk.[1] Smoking during pregnancy can affect the unborn fetus, and nonsmokers exposed to environmental tobacco smoke (ETS) are also at risk.[1]

Smoking

Individuals who smoke have a shortened life expectancy of about 10 years.[1] Smoking is responsible for about 90% of all lung cancer and about 80% of deaths from chronic obstructive pulmonary disease (Fig. 19.1).[2] Females who smoke increase their risk of dying from heart disease by almost 5-fold and from emphysema or bronchitis by more than 12-fold.

Smoking During Pregnancy

According to the Cleveland Clinic, just one cigarette can have serious consequences while pregnant.[3] Smoking while pregnant can lead to stillbirth, miscarriage, or sudden unexpected infant death within the child's first year of life.[3] One cigarette releases toxic chemicals that can lower the levels of oxygen and nutrients carried to the fetus, causing fetal distress, premature birth, asthma, or even cleft lip or palate.[3]

Exposure to Environmental Tobacco Smoke

ETS refers to a nonsmoker's exposure to someone else's tobacco smoke.[4] Breathing in ETS has been called various names like secondhand smoking, involuntary smoking, or passive smoking.[4,5] Many chemicals have been reported in ETS, but nicotine and particulate matter, along with carbon monoxide, have been extensively measured. Inhalable suspended particles in homes with one or more smokers averaged about 20 to 100 μg/m^3 higher than in nonsmoking homes, but the highest concentrations were reported in restaurants and bars, with an average concentration of 35 to 986 μg/m^3.[5] Long-term exposure to this ETS can lead to lung cancer. Biomarkers like cotinine, a byproduct of nicotine, have also been studied (Fig. 19.2).[5]

Alcohol

There is little evidence in the literature that clearly depicts the possible benefits of drinking alcohol versus the risks.[6] Some of the problems with this area of research lie in the clear recall and truthful reporting of an individual's drinking habits. From what is known, any possible benefits of alcohol have not been proven in the literature and cannot be applied to everyone.[6]

The words "drinking responsibly" and "drinking in moderation" are often used. The Mayo Clinic defines *moderation* as one drink per day for females and two drinks per day for males. A *drink* is one of the following: 12 ounces of beer, 5 ounces of wine, and 1.5 ounces of distilled spirits (80 proof). With everything, however, there are pros and cons. The pros (although not proven) of moderate drinking include a decrease in the risk of heart disease, ischemic stroke, and diabetes. The cons of heavy alcohol use include cancer, pancreatitis, heart muscle damage, liver problems, stroke, high blood pressure, accidental injury, or even suicide.[6]

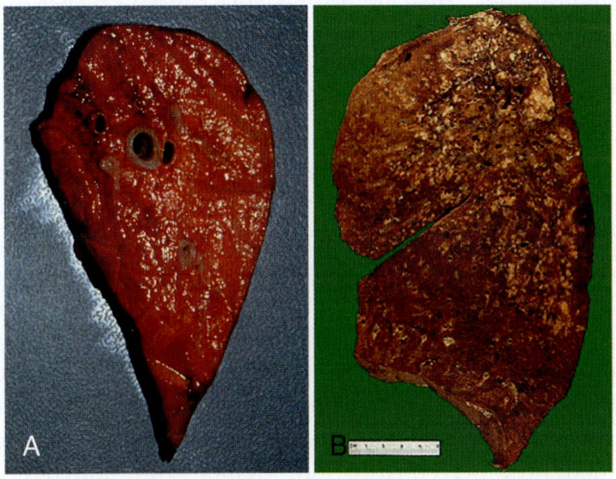

• **Fig. 19.1** The lungs of a nonsmoker compared to a smoker. (From Leonard PC. *Quick & Easy Medical Terminology*. 10th ed. Elsevier; 2024.)

Drinking During Pregnancy

Alcohol has definitive teratogenic properties. A teratogen is any substance that can interfere with the normal development of the unborn embryo or fetus.[7] Alcohol has the ability to pass quickly through the placenta, directly to the developing brain and other organs of the fetus.[7] The term *fetal alcohol spectrum disorder* (FASD) refers to a wide range of possible behavioral, physical, and cognitive disorders resulting from alcohol exposure while in utero.[8] It is estimated somewhere between 1% and 5% of first graders have FASD. The National Health Survey from 2015 to 2018 revealed about 10% of pregnant females reported using alcohol during their pregnancy.[8]

Although heavy drinking during pregnancy puts the unborn child at the greatest risk, even lesser amounts can harm the developing fetus, so it is strongly advised that no alcohol be consumed during the entire pregnancy.[8] FASD constitutes a range of disorders, and each can cause problems with executive functioning and self-regulation; however, the symptoms vary and can be unpredictable. Although most of these children have a normal IQ, FASD is still the most

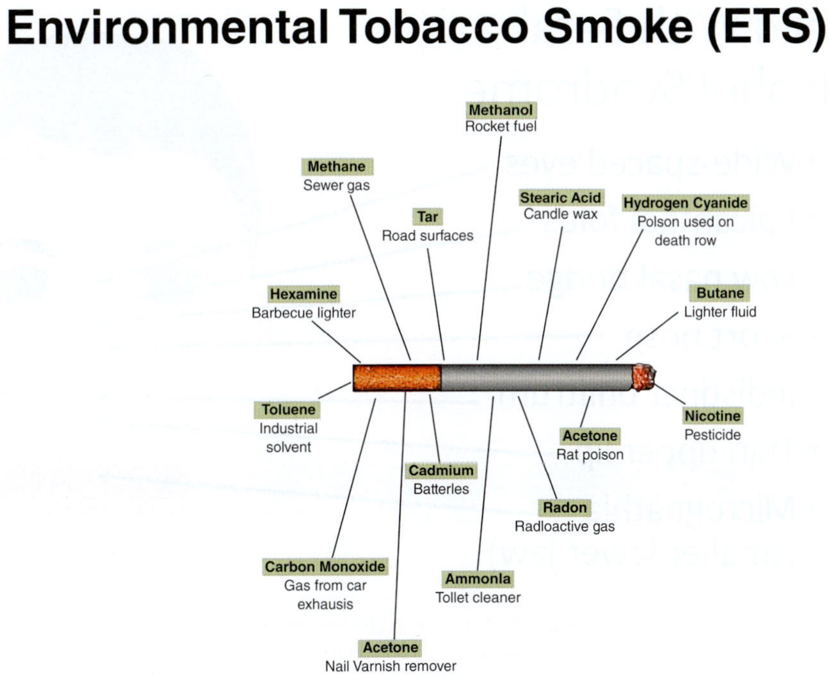

• **Fig. 19.2** Components of ETS. (From Environmental Protection Agency. *Health Effects of Exposure to Secondhand Smoke*. 2010. https://www.epa.gov/smokefree/healtheffects.html.)

common preventable cause of intellectual disability in the world. One of the conditions under the FASD umbrella is fetal alcohol syndrome (FAS). These children often present with characteristic facial features like small eyes, flattened philtrum (the indentation above the upper lip), micrognathia (a small jaw), and microcephaly (a smaller than normal head and forehead) (Fig. 19.3). For more about FASD, see Chapter 3.

Harmful Chemicals

There are many chemicals that can harm us, whether by ingestion, injection, or simple exposure. Those covered in this section include illicit drugs, pharmaceutical medications, and some of the more common environmental chemicals.

Illicit Drugs

The list of illicit (illegal) drugs in the United States is extensive with varying ability to cause harm to human tissues.

Cannabis is the name given to the common hemp plant, which is known to have calming properties, and has recently been used for medicinal purposes.[9] Although a 2024 publication reported that frequent smoking of cannabis might lead to a 25% increased risk of heart attack and a 42% increased risk of stroke,[10] the use of specific cannabinoids (a group of substances that are found in a cannabis plant, like THC and cannabidiol or CBD) has been found to help alleviate symptoms from many disorders, including anxiety, chronic pain, epilepsy, multiple sclerosis, and glaucoma.[11]

Cocaine is a stimulant derived from the coca bush. It causes an increase in heart rate, sweating, and dilation of the pupils. Cocaine can lead to addiction by rewiring pathways in the brain responsible for feelings of reward via the reuptake of serotonin, norepinephrine, and dopamine.[12]

Heroin is a semisynthetic morphine derivative.[9] It is often abused because of its euphoric effects. It is used as a pain reliever in other countries but not in the United States because it can cause decreased breathing, infected heart valves, and even death.[12]

Hallucinogens, like lysergic acid diethylamide (LSD), psilocybin, and peyote, affect sensation, thinking, and self-awareness. They are psychoactive substances that cause anomalies in perception and other emotional changes.[12]

Pharmaceutical Medications

A class of drugs called opioid analgesics has been in the news a great deal over the past 10 years. Opiates are a class of medications prescribed to relieve moderate to severe pain. They work by binding to opioid receptors in the body, which are part of the system that controls pain and addiction.[11] When prescribed by a doctor to be taken for a few days, there is a low risk of addiction, but the longer they are prescribed for, the more likely an individual will begin to develop a dependence on them. Side effects include drowsiness, breathing difficulty, itchy skin, low blood pressure, constipation, tremor, and slowed heart rate.[13]

Hormonal contraceptives are prescribed medications that help prevent pregnancy and control bleeding and pain

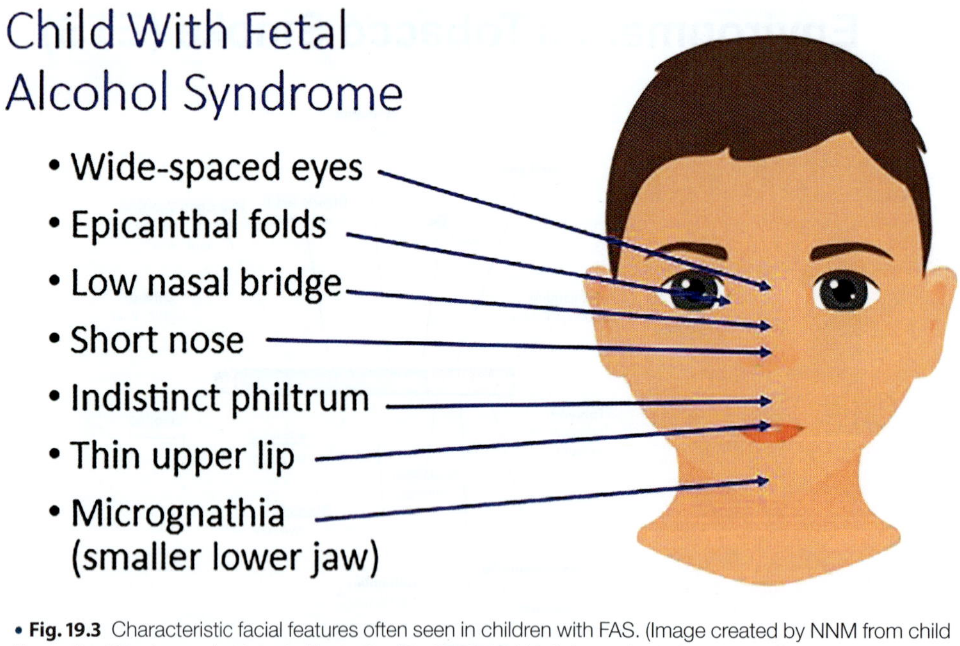

• **Fig. 19.3** Characteristic facial features often seen in children with FAS. (Image created by NNM from child illustration iStock.com/art4stock, Illustration ID: 1362740410; Information is from https://my.clevelandclinic.org/health/diseases/15677-fetal-alcohol-syndrome.)

during menstruation.[14] Certain medications, however, can prevent these oral contraceptives from working, including some antibiotics, antivirals, and seizure medications.[14] Side effects of hormonal contraceptives include acne, bloating, higher than normal blood pressure, fluid retention, headache, mood swings, insomnia, bleeding or spotting between periods, and weight gain.[15]

Environmental Chemicals

Many chemicals in our environment can be harmful to individuals exposed to them. Organic solvents and vapors, agricultural chemicals, and aromatic halogenated hydrocarbons (like polyvinyl chlorides or PVCs), used mainly in industrial settings, can harm the respiratory system or even cause cancer.[16] Exposure to asbestos can lead to mesothelioma (an aggressive, deadly cancer that occurs in the mesothelium, or the thin tissue covering most internal organs).[17] Air pollutants, like particulate matter, sulfur dioxide, nitrogen dioxide, and carbon monoxide, can negatively affect health, as can exposure to certain metals, like mercury, arsenic, or lead.[18,19] Particulate matter can penetrate the lung or bloodstream causing ischemic heart disease or stroke. Sulfur dioxide and nitrogen dioxide (a strong precursor to ozone) can also cause asthma. Carbon monoxide can diffuse across the lung tissue into the bloodstream, making it hard for the cells to bind to oxygen, causing difficulty breathing and flu-like symptoms.[18] Exposure to heavy metals in foods, work environments, or drinking water can lead to mercury, arsenic, or lead attaching to cells and preventing normal functions, which can be life-threatening.[19] Symptoms of heavy metal exposure include abdominal pain, chills, dehydration, diarrhea, nausea, and difficulty breathing (Fig. 19.4).[19]

Radiation

Radiation is energy that consists of subatomic particles moving in electromagnetic waves. It can come from both natural sources (sun, soil, water, air, or the human body itself) and from man-made sources (such as X-ray and MRI machines).[20] Exposure to excessive amounts of radiation can cause damage to the deoxyribonucleic acid (DNA) in cells, lead to illnesses like acute radiation syndrome, and can increase the risk of certain types of cancer and even death.[20,21] Some materials, like lead, can help block certain types of radiation (Fig. 19.5).

The amount of radiation absorbed by an object is typically measured in rads or grays. A rad (the radiation-absorbed dose) is a unit used to measure the amount of radiation absorbed by a person.[22] A gray is the equivalent of 100 rad. These units are often adjusted for the effects of the radiation on the human body. This is called the dose equivalent, "dose equivalent man," or rem.[23] The amount of cellular damage not only depends on the amount of radiation received but also on the rate at which it occurred. More radiation during shorter periods of time can cause more harm.[21] The yearly dose of radiation for the average American is about 0.62 rem or 620 mrem.[24] Doses for typical medical procedures that use radiation can be found in Table 19.1. These doses, and their comparisons to the dose limit for the annual nuclear worker as set by the Nuclear Regulatory Commission (NRC), can be found in Fig. 19.6.

Temperature

It has been commonly believed that normal body temperature is around 98.6°F or 37°C. These numbers originated from a study conducted in the mid-1800s. More recent studies, however, have found normal body temperature to rest between 97.5°F (36.4°C) and 97.9°F (36.6°C), with the range of "normal" anywhere between 97°F and 99°F, dependent upon the person and the circumstances.[25]

Hypothermia, or a body temperature below 95°F (35°C), occurs when the body loses heat faster than it can be produced.[26] This is a medical emergency. Hypothermia is typically due to immersion in cold water or exposure to cold weather for a longer than acceptable period. If this is not rectified, it can lead to complete respiratory or heart failure and eventually death.[26] Symptoms of hypothermia include shivering, slowed or slurred speech, weak pulse, confusion, and eventual ischemia of the tissues.[26]

Hyperthermia is the term given to a group of conditions with a high body temperature of over 100.4°F (38°C). This occurs when the body's heat regulation becomes overwhelmed by external factors in the environment, causing body temperature to rise.[27] This is not the same as a fever, which is due to internal body factors, like infection or drug reactions. Hyperthermia can occur when exercising in hot, humid environments, leading to heat fatigue with excessive sweating, exhaustion, muscle cramps, and headache.[27] Heat exhaustion can lead to heat stroke, which can be life-threatening. Heat stroke is when the body temperature increases from above 103°F to 104°F and can be serious, especially in young children and individuals over 65 years of age.[27] Symptoms of heat stroke include a very fast strong pulse or a very weak pulse, dizziness or confusion, blurred vision, decreased coordination, fainting, seizures, coma, or even death.[27]

Altitude

When at sea level, the human body enjoys a comfortable partial pressure of oxygen (PO_2) with a resultant arterial oxygen saturation (O_2 sat) of about 97% to 100% at rest. At an altitude of 10,000 feet, however, the inspired PO_2 is only about 69% of that at sea level, which can lower the body's O_2 sat levels to as low as 88%.[28] This can result in hypoxic stress, which is dependent upon the rate of ascent and the

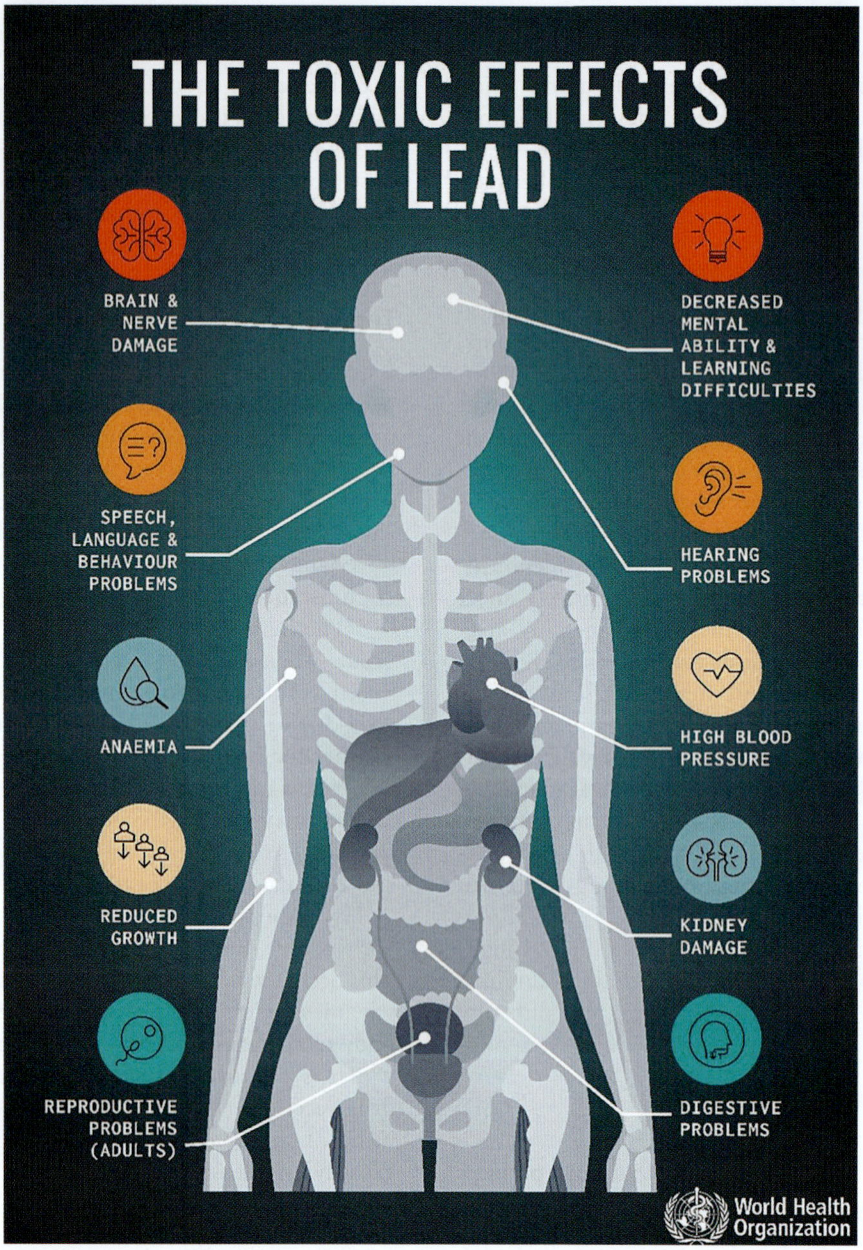

• **Fig. 19.4** Effects of lead exposure. (From https://www.who.int/images/default-source/infographics/chemical-safety/toxic-effects-lead-who-logo.jpg?sfvrsn=ba1a04c1_8.)

duration, with the greatest hypoxemia occurring during sleep. There is also the danger of exposure to colder temperatures, low humidity, increased radiation, and decreased air pressure.[28] The human body can acclimate to this but needs time for this to happen. Altitude illness syndromes can take the form of acute mountain sickness (with headache, dizziness, and fatigue and is self-limiting), high-altitude cerebral edema (with ataxia, confusion, and drowsiness), and high-altitude pulmonary edema (with chest congestion, cough, and dyspnea, and if not treated can lead to bloody sputum, with mandatory descent required).[28]

Diving

Whether an individual is one of the estimated 0.4 to 4 million recreational divers in the United States, or an individual who dives for a living, it is important to know the risks associated with this activity. As stated above, higher altitudes can lead to illnesses caused by a decrease in air pressure.[29] Diving, on the other hand, can lead to illness caused by an increase in pressure on the body due to hydrostatic forces. The deeper the dive, the greater the force (Fig. 19.7).[30]

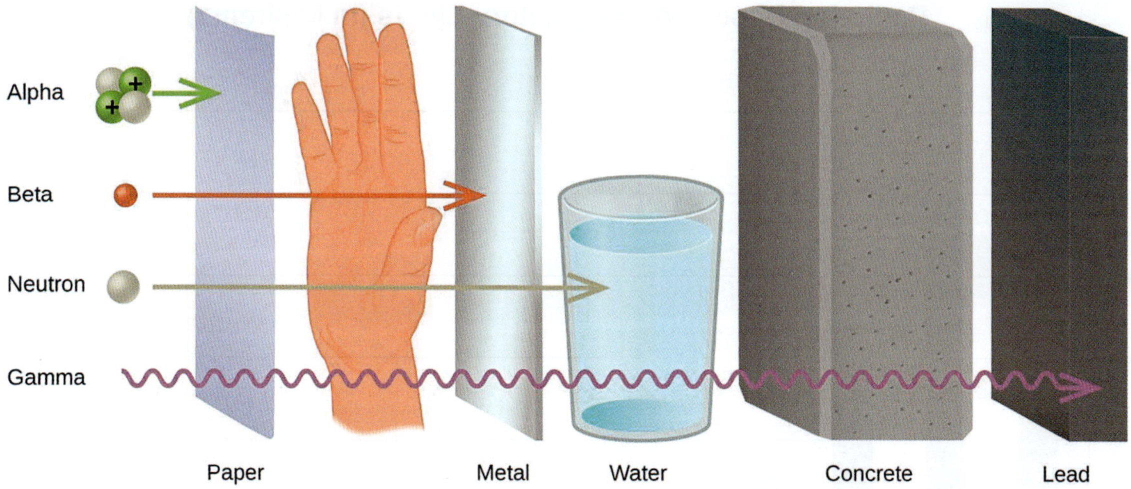

• **Fig. 19.5** Materials that can block the various types of radiation. (From https://openstax.org/books/chemistry-2e/pages/1-introduction.)

TABLE 19.1 The Typical Dose of Radiation From Various Medical Procedures

Procedure	Dose (mrem)
One single exposure of an x-ray:	
• Pelvis	70
• Abdomen	60
• Chest	10
• Dental	1.5
• Hand/foot	0.5
• Mammogram (2 views)	72
• Nuclear medicine	400
CT scans:	
Full body	1000
Chest	700
Head	200

From https://www.nrc.gov/about-nrc/radiation/around-us/doses-daily-lives.html.

When forces on either side of a membrane are not equal, it can result in barotrauma.[29] The most common type of barotrauma in diving is ear and sinus barotrauma, caused by an inability to equalize the pressure in the middle ear, resulting in the eardrum curving into the space. Pulmonary barotrauma is much more severe and occurs when a diver ascends too rapidly, resulting in an overexpansion of the lungs on the ascent.[29,31] This can cause lung tissue to rupture and can enable bubbles to escape, causing a pulmonary embolism (arterial gas embolism) and constitutes a medical emergency. Decompression sickness, or the bends, occurs when collections of excess inert gas, typically nitrogen, saturate the tissues from a quick rate of ascent.[29] Nitrogen narcosis can occur at increased depths over 100 feet, when the partial pressure of nitrogen increases, causing some confusion while diving. This can clear on a controlled ascent.[29]

Malnutrition

To live a healthy life, it is imperative that people receive the right amount of vitamins and nutrients. Malnutrition is a condition that develops when the body does not have the minerals and nutrients necessary for healthy organ function. About one in every hundred children in the United States suffers from chronic malnutrition.[32] Symptoms include easy bruisability, bleeding gums, night blindness, weight loss, thin hair, achy joints, and pale, thick skin. Table 19.2 lists some of the hazards of various vitamin and mineral deficiencies.

Bacteria

Bacteria are microscopic unicellular organisms.[47] There are many various types of bacteria, some of which keep the human body healthy, making up the body's microbiome, and others that can make people ill. Although most bacteria are harmless to humans, some reproduce quickly in the human body, releasing toxins and causing infection. Some of the more common bacteria include *Streptococcus* (causing strep throat), *Staphylococcus* (causing various staph infections), and *Escherichia coli* (causing various *E. coli* infections) (Fig. 19.9).[47] Other bacterial infections include diphtheria, Lyme disease, and pertussis. Some sexually transmitted infections (STIs) that are bacterial in nature include chlamydia, syphilis, and gonorrhea. Because bacteria are living organisms,

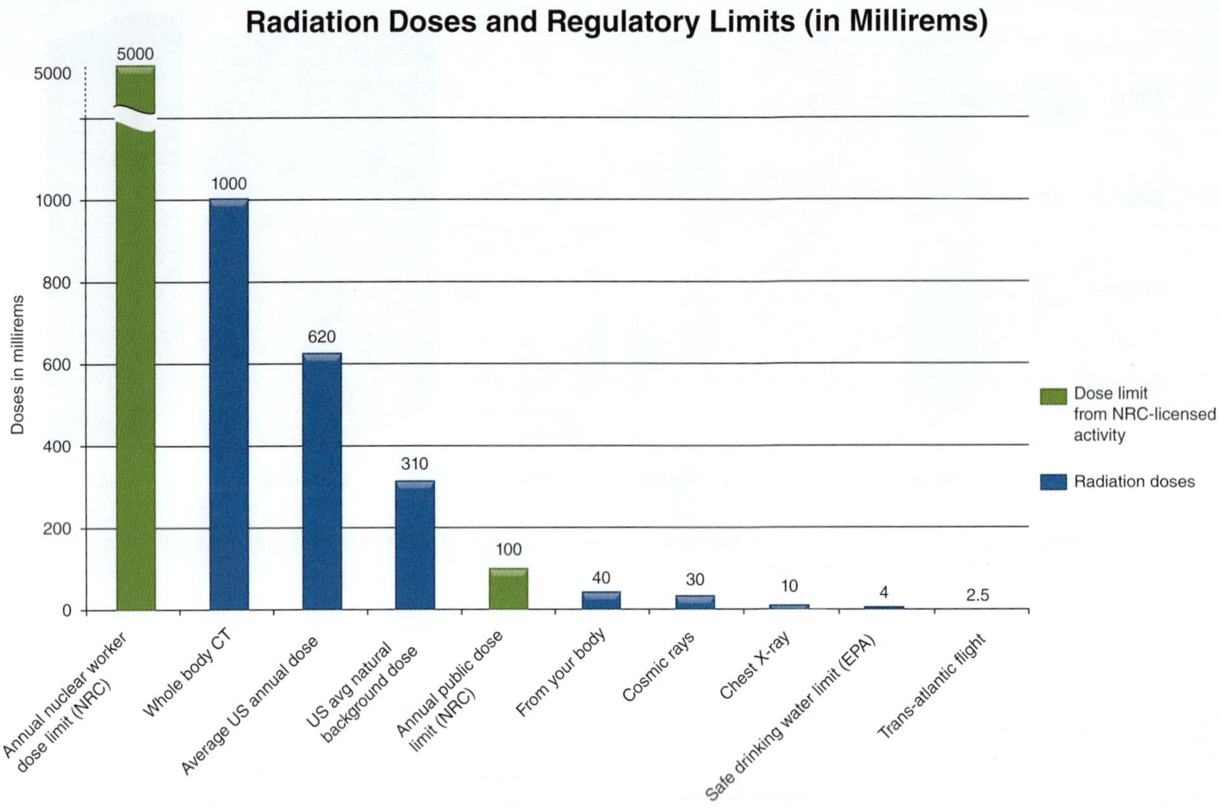

• **Fig. 19.6** Radiation of medical procedures compared to the yearly limits of the typical NRC employee. (From https://www.nrc.gov/about-nrc/radiation/around-us/doses-daily-lives.html.)

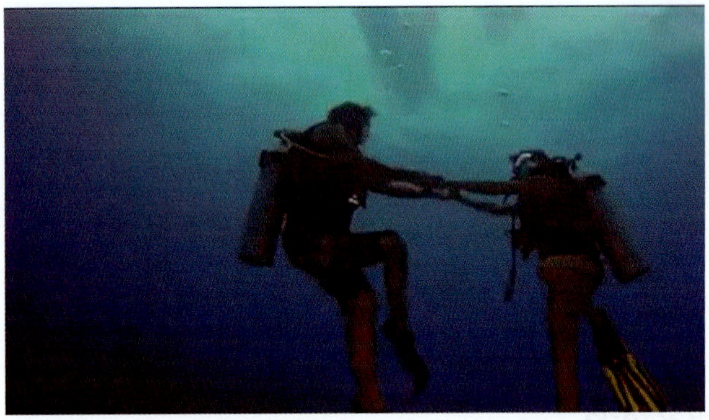

• **Fig. 19.7** The author (N. Michaels) scuba diving with her husband with the boat overhead.

they can live outside a host for various periods of time. The good news is there are antibiotics that can be used to combat most bacteria.[47]

Viruses

Viruses are microscopic particles consisting of genetic material wrapped in a coat of protein.[48] This genetic material consists of either DNA or ribonucleic acid (RNA). It is uncertain whether or not these qualify as living organisms, and they do not live long outside a host. Viruses work by entering a cell and "hijacking" it, releasing their own genetic material and proteins. It then reproduces to hijack more cells.[48] Before releasing proteins, a DNA virus must first change to RNA, where an RNA virus is already available to do so (Table 19.3). Some RNA viruses include the common cold, the mumps, HIV, and COVID-19. Some DNA viruses include Herpes, Epstein-Barr, and human papillomavirus (which has been linked to cervical cancer).

Long COVID-19 and the Need for Occupational Therapy

Long COVID is defined by the Centers for Disease Control and Prevention as a chronic condition occurring after SARS-CoV-2 infection that is present for at least 3 months.[49] Millions of adults in the United States have been affected by long COVID,[49] and this has affected the ability to work and participate in daily activities. OTPs have their expertise in this arena.[50] They are able to customize interventions that enable people to fully participate in life's meaningful activities and are in a unique position to help individuals suffering from the effects of long COVID.[50] A recent article in the *American Journal of Occupational Therapy* written by Kehl-Floberg et al. has stressed the need for OTPs to take the forefront to help maximize function and quality of life for these individuals.[50]

TABLE 19.2 Some of the More Common Nutrients and the Hazards of Malnutrition

Inadequate Nutrient	Name of Resulting Condition(s)	Symptoms
Protein	Hypoproteinemia	Fatigue, weakness, thinning hair, brittle nails, dry skin, and, if severe, can result in liver and kidney problems and even kwashiorkor.[33,34] See Fig. 19.8.
Calcium (Ca^+)	Hypocalcemia	Problems with the teeth, cataracts, muscle aches, osteoporosis, changes in the brain, convulsions, arrhythmias, and possible death.[35]
Sodium (Na^+)	Hyponatremia	Nausea, vomiting, muscle weakness, muscle cramps, confusion, seizures, and coma.[36]
Potassium (K^+)	Hypokalemia	Weakness, fatigue, muscle cramps, constipation, arrhythmias, and heart problems.[37]
Magnesium (Mg^+)	Magnesium deficiency (hypomagnesemia)	Fatigue, appetite loss, nausea, stiffness, weakness, arrhythmias, personality changes, and seizures.[38]
Chloride (Cl^-)	Hypochloremia	Fever, difficulty breathing, confusion, and edema.[39]
Phosphate (P^-)	Hypophosphatemia	Muscle and joint pain, weakness, altered mental state, numbness, and seizures.[40]
Iron	Iron deficiency anemia	Extreme fatigue, weakness, pale skin, chest pain, headache, inflammation of the tongue, poor appetite, and cold hands and feet.[41]
Iodine	Iodine deficiency	Hypothyroidism, choking, enlarged thyroid gland, puffy skin, confusion, hoarseness, and thinning hair. In pregnant females, lack of iodine can cause miscarriage or birth defects.[42]
Zinc	Zinc deficiency	Hypogonadism, emotional lability, impaired taste and smell, immune dysfunction, GI symptoms, complications from infections, and nutritional dwarfism.[43]
Vitamin A	Vitamin A deficiency	Night blindness, increased infections, dry eyes and skin, itchy skin, and dry hair.[44,45]
Vitamin B_1 (thiamine)	Vitamin B_1 deficiency	Fatigue, polyneuropathy, irritability, and cardiac and circulatory problems.[44,45]
Vitamin B_2 (riboflavin)	Vitamin B_2 deficiency	Skin lesions, mouth dryness and cracking, fatigue, and problems with brain function.[44,45]
Vitamin B_3 (niacin)	Vitamin B_3 deficiency	Depression, anxiety, paranoia, scaly dermatitis, and diarrhea.[44,45]
Vitamin B_5 (pantothenic acid)	Vitamin B_5 deficiency	Behavioral changes, seizures, rash, and red tongue.[44,45]
Vitamin B_6 (pyridoxine)	Vitamin B_6 deficiency	CNS problems, irritability, dementia, and depression.[44,45]
Vitamin B_7 (biotin)	Biotin deficiency	This vitamin is bound to proteins. Deficiency can cause hair loss, brittle nails, lethargy, seizures, and hallucinations.[44–46]
Vitamin B_9 (folate or folic acid)	Folic acid deficiency	Cognitive decline, psychosis, vascular dementia, red sore tongue, reduced sense of taste, weight loss, and psychosis. Increased risk of spina bifida in unborn children.[44,45]
Vitamin B_{12} (cobalamin)	Pernicious anemia	Fatigue, paleness, loss of sensation in hands and feet, confusion, and vascular dementia.
Vitamin C	Scurvy	Loss of teeth, bleeding gums, easy bruising, and poor wound healing.[44,45]
Vitamin D	Rickets	Softening of the bones or bone distortion, osteoporosis, and osteomalacia.[44,45]
Vitamin E	Vitamin E deficiency (rare)	Muscle damage, nerve complications, and visual difficulties.[44,45]
Vitamin K	Vitamin K deficiency (rare in adults)	Ineffective blood clotting, osteoporosis, and risk of cardiovascular problems.[44,45]

Key:

Organic Compound	Macrominerals	Trace Minerals	Vitamins

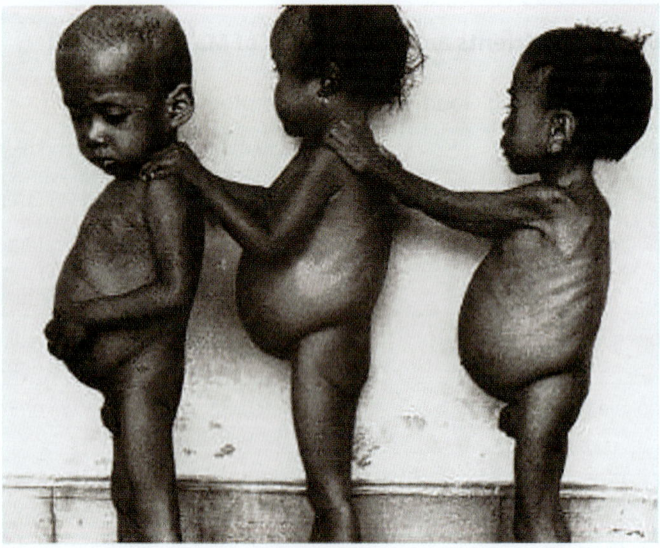

• **Fig. 19.8** Children with Kwashiorkor. (From Mitchell RN, McManus LM. *Pathobiology of Human Disease: A Dynamic Encyclopedia of Disease Mechanisms*. Elsevier; 2014.)

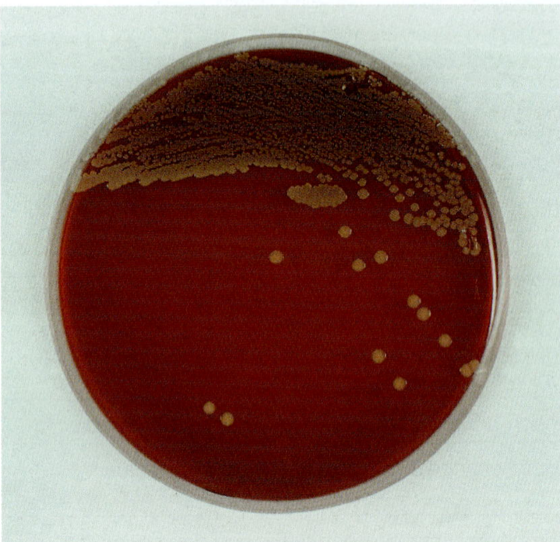

• **Fig. 19.9** Petri dish showing the grape-like clusters of *Staphylococcus*. (From Samaranayake LP. *Essential Microbiology in Dentistry*. ed 4. Churchill Livingstone; 2012.)

Prions

Prions are proteins that can cause the normal proteins located in the brain to behave abnormally.[51] These proteins can infect humans and animals, and some are spread from one to another through infected meat. Although prion diseases are rare in the United States, there is one that is most common called Creutzfeldt-Jakob disease, which can be either inherited or caused by infected tissue during a medical intervention (such as a corneal transplant).[51] It can lead to disability and possible death. Kuru is a disease first identified in the 1950s in New Guinea, caused by ritualistic consumption of prion-infected human brain tissue[51,52] (Fig. 19.10).

TABLE 19.3 Deoxyribonucleic Acid (DNA) Viruses Versus Ribonucleic Acid (RNA) Viruses

DNA Viruses	RNA Viruses
Double-stranded viruses are more common than single-stranded ones	Single-stranded viruses are more common than double-stranded ones
Replicate in the nucleus of the cell	Transcribe and replicate in the cytoplasm of the cell
Must first transcribe DNA into RNA, then synthesize proteins	Can bypass the stage when DNA transcribes into RNA

Eukaryotes (Fungus, Protozoa)

A eukaryotic cell has a cell membrane and organelles such as a nucleus, endoplasmic reticulum, and mitochondria (Fig. 19.11).[53] These cells are different from bacteria because the organelles in eukaryotic cells have membranes, whereas bacteria are prokaryotic cells in which the DNA (or RNA) floats around in the cytoplasm without a membrane.[53] Organisms that have eukaryotic cells include not only plants and animals but also fungi and protozoa.

Fungi

A fungus is made up of cells similar to plant cells, but the cell wall is made of chitin, which is found in insect exoskeletons.[53] Examples of fungal infections include candida (yeast infection) and a type of pneumonia (*Pneumocystis jirovecii*).

Protozoa

Protozoa are microscopic organisms that consist of a single cell. Some have small hairs called cilia to help them move about, and others have a structure that looks like a tail called a flagellum.[53] Infections in humans caused by protozoa include malaria and toxoplasmosis.

Helminths

Helminths are parasites that resemble worms.[54] These are known to infect humans and other animals, and there are three types of worms that can live inside the body: Trematodes (flukes and flatworms), Cestodes (tapeworms), and Nematodes (roundworms, such as hookworms or pinworms).[54] There is also a segmented worm that can live outside the body (ectoparasite), called a leech, which will cling to the skin with a proboscis used to suck blood from the host[55] (Fig. 19.12).

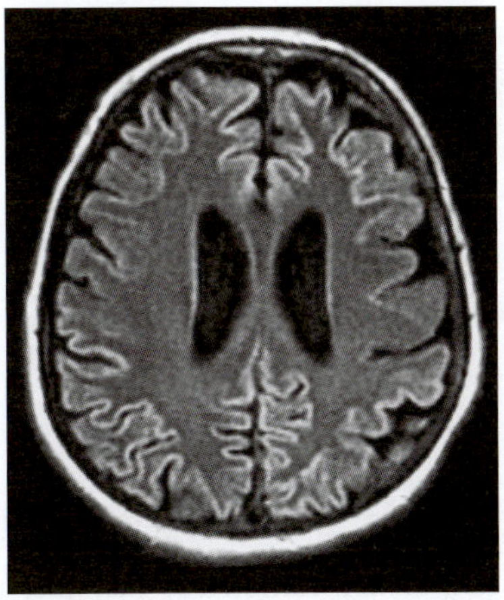

• **Fig. 19.10** Brain magnetic imaging of the brain of an individual with Creutzfeldt-Jakob disease showing cortical diffusion caused by prions. (From Creutzfeldt-Jakob disease, MRI scan #3 Photograph by Science Photo Library—Fine Art America.)

Protection from Contagions

The Centers for Disease Control (CDC) recommends hand washing as the best means of preventing the spread of infection. Standard precautions are to be used for every client and are often based on the nature of the OTP-client interaction. Please see https://www.cdc.gov/infection-control/hcp/basics/standard-precautions.html. The CDC recommends the use of personal protective equipment (PPE) for transmission-based precautions, such as gloves, masks, goggles, and gowns.[56,57] There are three different types of transmission-based precautions: contact precautions, droplet precautions, and airborne precautions. Please see Table 19.4.

Neoplasms

Neoplasms (or tumors) are included in this chapter because they are often caused by environmental factors, like radiation, viruses, or hazardous chemicals. The cause of most types of cancer is yet unknown.

Tumors

The cells in our body go through a life cycle that includes many replications through mitosis, dependent upon the cell

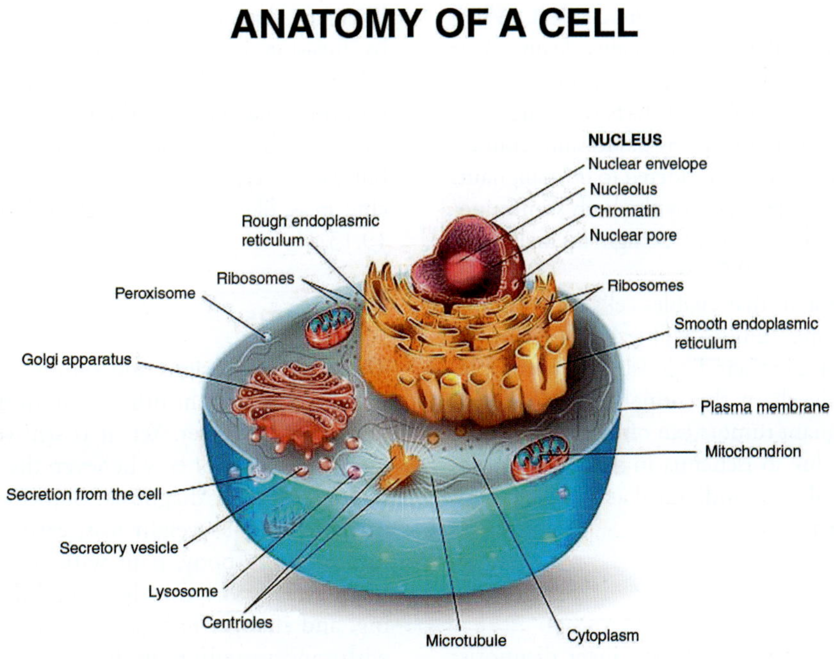

• **Fig. 19.11** The parts of a human cell. (From https://biologydictionary.net/eukaryotic-cell/.)

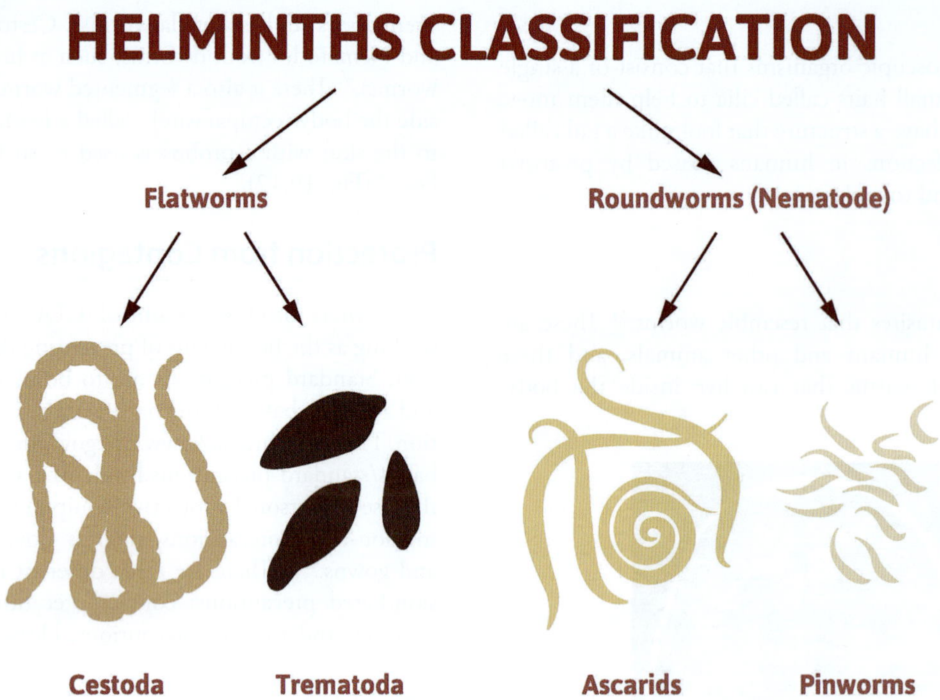

• **Fig. 19.12** Types of helminths. (From https://iStock.com/marochkina.)

type.[58] Typically, the body eliminates old or damaged cells (a process called apoptosis), but there are times when some cells get past these safety measures and begin to replicate. This leads to a collection or mass of cells that can either be benign (noncancerous) or malignant (cancerous).[58]

Benign tumors look a lot like their predecessors and are somewhat organized. They do not invade surrounding tissue and are typically not a medical concern unless they are pressing against a vital organ, nerve, or blood vessel. When the cells of a previously benign tumor change, losing their resemblance to normal cells, they are then considered to be precancerous.[58] As the DNA in the cell starts to change further, the cells then begin to invade nearby tissues and replicate at a faster rate. This tumor is now considered to be malignant. These malignant cells are able to slip by the body's immune/apoptosis system.[58] A comparison of benign to malignant tumors can be found in Table 19.5.

A cytokeratin is a protein that enables cells to withstand mechanical stress.[59] Some tumors will excrete abnormal cytokeratin, which can aid in their diagnosis.[60] For example, checking glycoprotein levels in the urine can help detect prostate cancer.[61] Malignant tumors can often be very painful, especially at night due to ischemia in surrounding tissues.[62] This pain can awaken an individual and make it very difficult to return to sleep.

Terminology

The term *oncology* refers to the study of cancer diagnosis, intervention, and prevention.[63] Typically, the suffix "oma" alone refers to a benign tumor. For example, a *lipoma* is a benign fatty tumor. The suffix "carcinoma" typically refers to a malignant epithelial tumor, and the suffix "sarcoma" refers to a malignant connective tissue tumor. For more terminology, refer to Table 19.6.

How Malignant Tumors Spread

There are three different ways malignant tumors can spread: by invasion into neighboring tissues, by metastasizing to other tissues via the blood or lymphatic system, or by seeding into other parts of the body (typically body cavities).[63] Cancer is able to spread almost anywhere in the human body, but various types of cancer are more likely to spread to specific areas, like the liver, bones, or lungs (Table 19.7 and Fig. 19.13).[64]

Symptoms

There are many signs and symptoms that something may be affecting the health of an individual that could be unrelated to cancer. Yet, it is still very important to contact the practitioner whenever the client's symptoms do not match their diagnosis. Some signs of cancer include extreme fatigue, weight loss, eating difficulty, swelling or lumps in the body, pain with no known cause, fever or night sweats, vision or hearing difficulties, unusual bleeding, and changes in bowel or bladder habits.[65] Individuals with cancer might even develop paraneoplastic syndrome, which is a cluster of disorders that occur when the immune

TABLE 19.4 Transmission-Based Precautions

Transmission-Based Precautions	What to Wear	When to Wear it
Contact Precautions	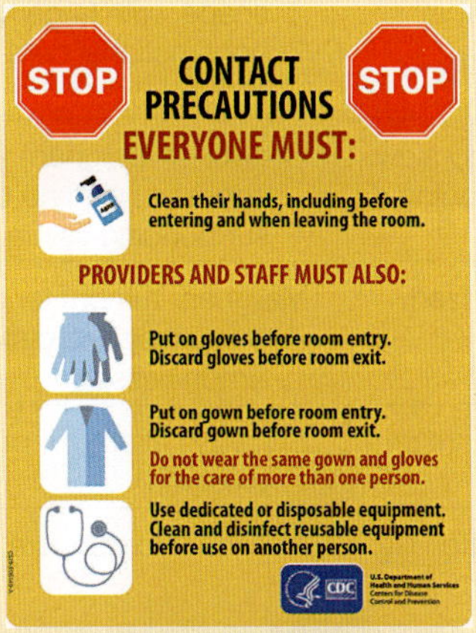	The OTP should use contact precautions whenever there might be contact with bodily fluids on either the client or the surrounding environment.
Droplet Precautions	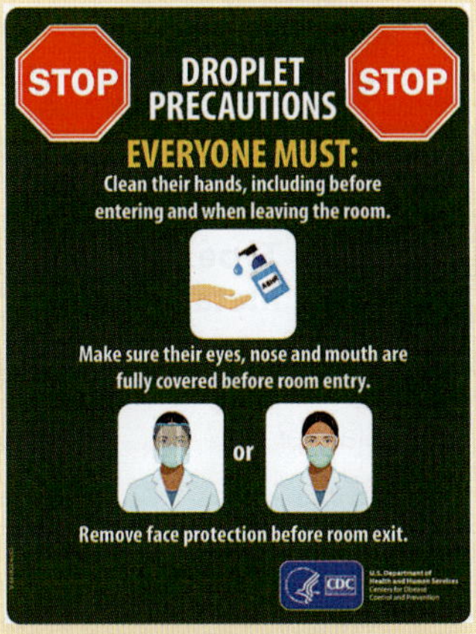	The OTP should use droplet precautions whenever there might be an interaction with a client that requires close contact with respiratory secretions in air droplets. Some pathogens that can spread this way include influenza virus, adenovirus, *B. pertussis*, group A streptococcus, rhinovirus, and *N. meningitides.*
Airborne Precautions	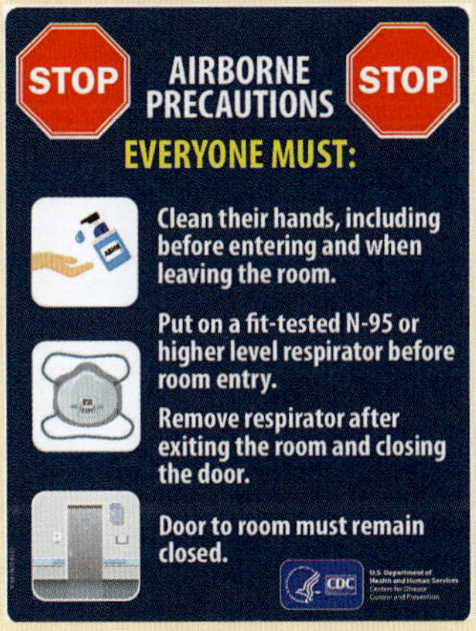	The OTP should use airborne precautions whenever there might be the possibility of infectious transmission through the air. Some pathogens that can spread this way include measles, smallpox, Severe acute respiratory syndrome (SARS), COVID (SARS-CoV2), and Tuberculosis.

Images from https://www.cdc.gov/infection-control/hcp/basics/transmission-based-precautions.html. Text from https://www.cdc.gov/infection-control/hcp/isolation-precautions/precautions.html.

system trying to fight the cancer also mistakenly attacks other bodily organs.[66]

The symptoms of metastatic cancer are many and varied, dependent upon the location and severity. When cancer spreads to the bones, there is severe pain and increased chance of fracture.[64] Cancer in the brain tends to cause dizziness, headache, and seizures. Cancer in the lungs will cause dyspnea and shortness of breath, and cancer in the liver will often

TABLE 19.5 Comparison of Benign Tumors With Malignant Tumors[63]

Typical Characteristics	Benign Tumors	Malignant Tumors
Cells	Benign tumors have cells that are similar to normal cells. They are somewhat differentiated, and mitosis is fairly normal.	Malignant tumors have cells that are varied in size and shape, with large nuclei and many undifferentiated, nonfunctional cells with atypical, increased mitosis.
Growth	Growth of benign tumors is relatively slow, expanding in mass but not spreading, and frequently encapsulated.	Growth of malignant tumors is rapid. The cells are not adhesive, with no capsule, and they can infiltrate surrounding tissue.
Spread	Benign tumors tend to remain localized.	Malignant tumors tend to invade nearby tissues or metastasize to distant sites through blood and lymph vessels.
Systemic effects	Systemic effects of benign tumors are rare.	Systemic effects of malignant tumors are often present.
Threat to life	Benign tumors usually do not threaten life unless they are in critical locations like the brain.	Malignant tumors are often life-threatening.

Adapted from VanMeter KC, Hubert RJ. *Gould's Pathophysiology for the Health Professions*. 7th ed. Elsevier; 2022.

TABLE 19.6 Terminology Associated With Benign and Malignant Tumors

Terminology	Benign Tumors	Malignant Tumors
Suffixes	-oma	-carcinoma -sarcoma
Examples	Chondroma—cartilage Epithelioma—squamous epithelium Adenoma—glandular epithelium	Osteogenic sarcoma—bones Adenocarcinoma—glands Comedocarcinoma—breast

Adapted from VanMeter KC, Hubert RJ. *Gould's Pathophysiology for the Health Professions*. 7th ed. Elsevier; 2022.

TABLE 19.7 Types of Cancer and Primary Sites of Metastasis

Cancer Type	Primary Sites of Metastasis
Bladder	Bone, liver, lung
Breast	Bone, brain, liver, lung
Colon	Liver, lung, peritoneum
Kidney	Adrenal gland, bone, brain, liver, lung
Lung	Adrenal gland, bone, brain, liver, other lung
Melanoma	Bone, brain, liver, lung, skin, muscle
Ovary	Liver, lung, peritoneum
Pancreas	Liver, lung, peritoneum
Prostate	Adrenal gland, bone, liver, lung
Rectal	Liver, lung, peritoneum
Stomach	Liver, lung, peritoneum
Thyroid	Bone, liver, lung
Uterus	Bone, liver, lung, peritoneum, vagina

From NIH. *Metastatic Cancer: When Cancer Spreads*. NIH: National Cancer Institute; 2020. https://www.cancer.gov/types/metastatic-cancer#where-cancer-spreads.

produce jaundice.[64] There are limited ways to stop or control the growth of metastatic cancer, like radiation, surgery, or chemotherapy. Care is typically given throughout the intervention to help relieve pain for the individual and improve their quality of life. This is referred to as palliative care.[64]

The OT Scope of Practice

As stated earlier, there are many signs and symptoms that something may be affecting the health of an individual. OTPs should be alert to any changes in their client's health that cannot be explained by their diagnosis. They should also ask open-ended questions to learn if the individual has been exposed to any environmental agents that could be affecting their health. OTPs do not diagnose; however, thinking outside of the box and communicating observations to the client's physician could be potentially lifesaving.

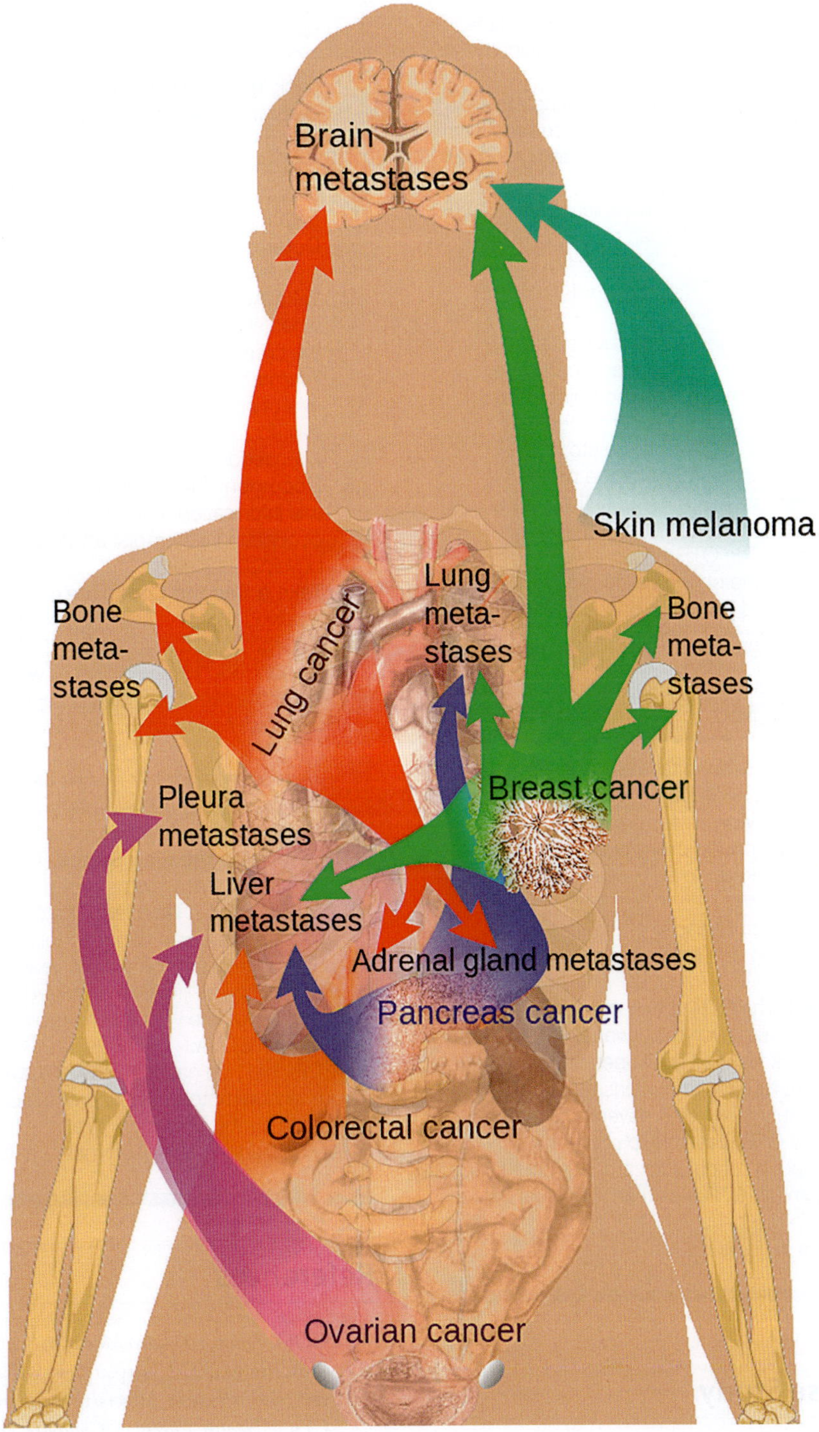

• **Fig. 19.13** The typical pathways for metastatic cancer. (From https://en.wikipedia.org/wiki/Metastasis#/media/File:Metastasis_sites_for_common_cancers.svg.)

Application—Case Study

CASE EXAMPLE 19.1

A 38-year-old female was visited by an occupational therapist (OTR) in home health, to initiate a home exercise program, after an automobile accident left her with multiple fractures. She complained of extreme fatigue and difficulty breathing.

1. **Screen:** The OTR examined the individual thinking maybe there was a possible rib fracture that had been missed in the hospital. When asked how long this had been going on the client responded, "Just today."
2. **Take a Closer Look:** The longer the therapist stayed with the client, the more tired she began to feel. She also thought she smelled gas fumes.
3. **Determine Flag Status:** The OTR determined this to be a potential red flag situation.
4. **Take Action if Needed:** The therapist grabbed the client's walker and helped her outdoors and called her superintendent on her cell phone. The therapist waited outside with the client. The superintendent checked the apartment and found a gas leak in the stove. A neighbor, who was also a close friend of the client, offered to have the client stay with her until the leak was fixed.
5. **Document the Findings:** The OTR documented this information as well as the phone call to the superintendent and followed up with a phone call to the client's physician, which was also documented.
6. **Take a Second Look:** The OTR brought the woman along with one of her neighbors to the ER. She left the woman there with the neighbor to see her next client but returned 2 hours later to check on the client and see what had occurred. The hospital ruled out the presence of any remaining negative effects from the gas inhalation and cleared the woman for discharge. The gas leak had been fixed, and the client was back in her apartment. The client thanked the OTR again for her help that day.
7. **Determine the Flag Status:** Because of the therapist's quick thinking, this situation had quickly gone from a red flag to a green flag.
8. **Take Action if Needed:** The OTR checked again with the superintendent to ensure everything was fixed and thanked him for the quick repairs. The superintendent had also given the client a CO_2 alarm in case this happened again in the future, which it never did.

This is a true case. This OTR was able to prevent a situation that involved an environmental hazard that could have killed the client. Again, an OTR saved an individual's life. The client wrote the therapist a beautiful letter, and her family later sent the OTR flowers in gratitude.

Application—Case Study

CASE EXAMPLE 19.2

A 45-year-old female was seen by an occupational therapy assistant (COTA) in the outpatient setting for exercise after a whiplash injury in an automobile accident.

1. **Screen:** The COTA discussed current pain level with the client while examining her, who had neck pain that was typical for her injury.
2. **Take a Closer Look:** While teaching the client safe methods for functional reaching during ADLs, the client became dizzy and asked to rest. The COTA helped her to lie down on a treatment table and took her vitals, which were normal. After the client began to feel better, the COTA asked an open-ended question: "Other than the neck injury, do you have any additional symptoms?" The client then informed the COTA she had been very tired, losing weight, and that eating became difficult. She also had severe pain at night in her axilla and shoulder, and after awakening with this pain, she had a difficult time getting back to sleep.
3. **Determine Flag Status:** The COTA determined this to be a potential yellow or red flag situation.
4. **Take Action if Needed:** The COTA asked the client when she had her last breast exam or mammogram, and the client said she had not had one "in years." The COTA informed the OTR, who called the physician and informed him of her symptoms. The doctor saw the client the next day, for lab work and to schedule a mammogram, which was performed the next day.
5. **Document the Findings:** The COTA documented this information as well as the conversation with the occupational therapist and the phone call to the physician.
6. **Take a Second Look:** The occupational therapist received a phone call the next day from the doctor asking, "How did you know?" The occupational therapist responded, "How did I know what?" The doctor replied, "That the client had breast cancer." The occupational therapist had to sit down. Her head was spinning. "Wow, I didn't really know, but my COTA noticed symptoms that were unusual for her diagnosis, so we contacted you." The therapist made sure to give a special mention and thank you to her COTA.
7. **Determine the Flag Status:** This had quickly gone from a possible yellow flag to a red flag.
8. **Take Action if Needed:** The client had an immediate mastectomy, with radiation followed by chemotherapy. She returned to the clinic a year later to thank the COTA for saving her life. She admitted that the intervention was brutal, but she was in remission and very grateful to her "angel" COTA.

This is a true case. This COTA was able to analyze the signs and symptoms and communicate this to the OTR, followed by the physician, in a way that helped lead to a diagnosis and intervention that eventually saved a life.

References

1. CDC. *Tobacco-Related Mortality*. Centers for Disease Control and Prevention; 2022. https://www.cdc.gov/tobacco/data_statistics/fact_sheets/health_effects/tobacco_related_mortality/.
2. CDC. *Health Effects of Cigarette Smoking*. Centers for Disease Control and Prevention; 2022. https://www.cdc.gov/tobacco/data_statistics/fact_sheets/health_effects/effects_cig_smoking/index.htm.
3. Clinic Cleveland. *What Happens of You Smoke While Pregnant?* Health Essentials: Cleveland Clinic; 2023. https://health.clevelandclinic.org/smoking-while-pregnant.

4. CCOHS. *Environmental Tobacco Smoke (ETS)*. Canadian Centre for Occupational Health and Safety; 2023. https://www.ccohs.ca/oshanswers/psychosocial/ets/ets_health.html#section-9-hdr.
5. NIH. Institute of Medicine (US) Committee on the Assessment of Asthma and Indoor Air. Exposure to environmental tobacco smoke. In: *Clearing the Air: Asthma and Indoor Air Exposures*. National Academies Press (US); 2000:7. https://www.ncbi.nlm.nih.gov/books/NBK224469/.
6. Clinic Mayo. *Alcohol Use: Weighing Risks and Benefits*. Healthy Lifestyle: Mayo Clinic; 2021. https://www.mayoclinic.org/healthy-lifestyle/nutrition-and-healthy-eating/in-depth/alcohol/art-20044551.
7. Chung DD, Pinson MR, Bhenderu LS, et al. Toxic and teratogen effects of alcohol exposure on fetal development, adolescence, and adulthood. *Int J Mol Sci*. 2021;22(16):8785. https://doi.org/10.3390/ijms22168785.
8. NIH. *Understanding Fetal Alcohol Spectrum Disorders*. NIH: National Institute on Alcohol Abuse and Alcoholism; 2023. https://www.niaaa.nih.gov/publications/brochures-and-fact-sheets/understanding-fetal-alcohol-spectrum-disorders.
9. CIA. Field listing: illicit drugs. In: *The World Fact Book*. CIA; 2015. https://www.cia.gov/the-world-factbook/field/illicit-drugs/.
10. Messina N. *Dangers of Illicit Drugs, Their Effects and Treatment Options*. Addiction Resource; 2022. https://addictionresource.com/drugs/illicit/.
11. Pope C. *Opioids (Narcotic Analgesics)*. Drugs.com; 2023. https://www.drugs.com/drug-class/narcotic-analgesics.html.
12. Drugs.com. *Hormonal Contraceptives*. Drugs.com; 2023. https://www.drugs.com/cg/hormonal-contraceptives.html.
13. Gotter A. *What Are the Side Effects of Birth Control Pills?* Healthline; 2018. https://www.healthline.com/health/birth-control-side-effects.
14. CDC. *Organic Solvents*. Centers for Disease Control and Prevention; 2018. https://www.cdc.gov/niosh/topics/organsolv/default.html.
15. Mayo Clinic. *Mesothelioma*. Mayo Clinic; 2022. https://www.mayoclinic.org/diseases-conditions/mesothelioma/symptoms-causes/syc-20375022.
16. WHO. *Air Quality and Health*. The World Health Organization; 2024. https://www.who.int/teams/environment-climate-change-and-health/air-quality-and-health/health-impacts/types-of-pollutants.
17. Clinic Cleveland. *Heavy Metal Poisoning (Toxicity)*. Cleveland Clinic; 2022. https://my.clevelandclinic.org/health/diseases/23424-heavy-metal-poisoning-toxicity.
18. WHO. *Radiation and Health*. World Health Organization; 2023. https://www.who.int/news-room/questions-and-answers/item/radiation-and-health.
19. CDC. *Radiation and Your Health*. Centers for Disease Control and Prevention; 2021. https://www.cdc.gov/nceh/radiation/health.html.
20. WHO. *Rad (Radiation Absorbed Dose)*. World Health Organization; 2023. https://www.nrc.gov/reading-rm/basic-ref/glossary/rad-radiation-absorbed-dose.html.
21. NRC US. *Measuring Radiation*. United States Nuclear Regulatory Commission; 2020. https://www.nrc.gov/about-nrc/radiation/health-effects/measuring-radiation.html.
22. NRC US. *Doses in Our Daily Lives*. United States Nuclear Regulatory Commission; 2022. https://www.nrc.gov/about-nrc/radiation/around-us/doses-daily-lives.html.
23. Clinic Cleveland. *What is a normal body temperature? Health Essentials*. Cleveland Clinic; 2023. Retrieved January 6, 2024. https://health.clevelandclinic.org/body-temperature-what-is-and-isnt-normal.
24. Mayo Clinic. *Hypothermia*. Mayo Clinic; 2022. https://www.mayoclinic.org/diseases-conditions/hypothermia/symptoms-causes/syc-20352682.
25. Huizen, J. *What Is a Normal Body Temperature? Medical News Today*. 2017. https://www.medicalnewstoday.com/articles/320226.
26. CDC. *High Elevation Travel & Altitude Sickness*. Centers for Disease Control and Prevention, Yellow Book; 2024. https://wwwnc.cdc.gov/travel/yellowbook/2024/environmental-hazards-risks/high-elevation-travel-and-altitude-illness.
27. CDC. *Scuba Diving: Decompression Illness & Other Dive-related Injuring*. Centers for Disease Control and Prevention, Yellow Book; 2024. https://wwwnc.cdc.gov/travel/yellowbook/2024/environmental-hazards-risks/diving.
28. NOAA. *How Does Pressure Change With Ocean Depth?* National Ocean Service; 2023. https://oceanservice.noaa.gov/facts/pressure.html.
29. Scuba Legend. *Scuba Tips: Tips for Ascending Properly*. Scuba Legend; 2023. https://scubalegend.com/scuba-diving/scuba-skills-tips-for-ascending-properly/.
30. Johns Hopkins. Malnutrition. In: *Health*. Johns Hopkins; 2024. https://www.hopkinsmedicine.org/health/conditions-and-diseases/malnutrition.
31. Berry J. What to know about hyproteinemia. *Medical News Today*; 2024. https://www.medicalnewstoday.com/articles/320050#symptoms.
32. Benjamin O, Lappin SL. *Kwashiorkor*. National Institute of Health, National Library of Medicine; 2023. https://www.ncbi.nlm.nih.gov/books/NBK507876/.
33. Barhum L. What happens when calcium levels are low? *Medical News Today*; 2023. https://www.medicalnewstoday.com/articles/321865.
34. Mayo Clinic. *Hyponatremia*. Mayo Clinic; 2022. https://www.mayoclinic.org/diseases-conditions/hyponatremia/symptoms-causes/syc-20373711.
35. Mayo Clinic. *Hypokalemia*. Mayo Clinic; 2022. https://www.mayoclinic.org/symptoms/low-potassium/basics/when-to-see-doctor/sym-20050632.
36. Clinic Cleveland. *Signs You May Have a Magnesium Deficiency*. Cleveland Clinic Health Essentials; 2022. https://health.clevelandclinic.org/feeling-fatigued-could-it-be-magnesium-deficiency-and-if-so-what-to-do-about-it.
37. WebMD. *What Is Hypochloremia?* WebMD; 2023. https://www.webmd.com/a-to-z-guides/what-is-hypochloremia.
38. Cleveland Clinic. *Hypophosphatemia*. Cleveland Clinic; 2022. https://my.clevelandclinic.org/health/diseases/24040-hypophosphatemia.
39. Mayo Clinic. *Iron Deficiency Anemia*. Mayo Clinic; 2022. https://www.mayoclinic.org/diseases-conditions/iron-deficiency-anemia/symptoms-causes/syc-20355034.
40. Clinic Cleveland. *Iodine Deficiency*. Cleveland Clinic; 2022. https://my.clevelandclinic.org/health/diseases/23417-iodine-deficiency.
41. Maxfield L, Shukla S, Crane JS. Zinc deficiency. In: *StatPearls*. National Institute of Health; 2023. https://www.ncbi.nlm.nih.gov/books/NBK493231/.
42. Adkins-Ali C. The ABCs of vitamin deficiency: symptoms you can treat yourself. *University Health News Daily*; 2017. https://universityhealthnews.com/daily/nutrition/the-abcs-of-vitamin-deficiency-symptoms-you-can-treat-yourself/.

43. Lewis R. *What to Know About Vitamin Deficiencies: Symptoms, Signs, and Causes.* Health Grades; 2022. https://www.healthgrades.com/right-care/food-nutrition-and-diet/vitamin-deficiency.
44. WebMD. *Biotin – Uses, Side Effects, and More.* WebMD, 2020. Retrieved January 15, 2024. https://www.webmd.com/vitamins/ai/ingredientmono-313/biotin.
45. Cleveland Clinic. *Bacteria.* Cleveland Clinic; 2022. https://my.clevelandclinic.org/health/articles/24494-bacteria.
46. Crosta P. What to know about viruses. *Medical News Today*; 2023. https://www.medicalnewstoday.com/articles/158179.
47. Johns Hopkins. *Prion Diseases.* Johns Hopkins Medicine: Health; 2024. https://www.hopkinsmedicine.org/health/conditions-and-diseases/prion-diseases.
48. Welsh J. *What Is Kuru?* Very Well Health; 2023. https://www.verywellhealth.com/kuru-7375144.
49. Buckley G. *Eukaryotic Cell.* Biology Dictionary; 2020. https://biologydictionary.net/eukaryotic-cell/.
50. CDC. *Long COVID Basics.* Centers for Disease Control and Prevention; 2024. Long COVID Basics | COVID-19 | CDC 60.
51. Kehl-Floberg K, Pop-Vicas A, Giles, G, Edwards D. The functional consequences of long COVID need to be addressed by occupational therapists. *Am J Occup Ther.* 2023;78:7805205190. 78,7805205190. https://doi.org/10.5014/ajot.2024.05070007.
52. Burch K. *What Are Helminths?* Very Well Health; 2021. https://www.verywellhealth.com/helminths-5207511.
53. Rafferty JP. *Leech.* Encyclopedia Britannica; 2023. https://www.britannica.com/animal/leech.
54. Llor X. *Neoplasm (Tumor).* Yale Medicine; 2024. https://www.yalemedicine.org/conditions/neoplasm.
55. Lee O, Kang H, Yun SJ. Chapter 6 – Urine cytology and urinary biomarkers. In: *Bladder Cancer.* Elsevier; 2018:67–81. https://doi.org/10.1016/B978-0-12-809939-1.00006-0.
56. Barak V, Goike H, Panaretakis KW, Einarsson R. Clinical; utility of cytokeratins and tumor markers. *Clin Biochem.* 2004;37(7):529–540. https://doi.org/10.1016/j.clinbiochem.2004.05.009.
57. Dong M, Lih TM, Chen S, et al. Urinary glycoproteins associated with aggressive prostate cancer. *Theranostics.* 2020;10(26):11892–11907. https://doi.org/10.7150/thno.47066.
58. CDC. *Transmission-Based Precautions.* Centers for Disease Control and Prevention; 2024. http://www.cdc.gov/infection-control/hcp/basics/transmission-based-precautions.html.
59. Jeffers A, Glanz S, Byers AL, Keyhani S. Association of cannabis use with cardiovascular outcomes among US adults. *J Am Heart Assoc.* 2024;13(5):5. https://doi.org/10.1161/JAHA.123.030178.
60. NIH. *Cannabis (marijuana) and cannabinoids*: What you need to know. National Center for Complimentary and Integrative Health; 2019. National Institutes of Health.
61. OSHA. *Worker Protections Against Occupational Exposure to Infectious Diseases.* Occupational Safety and Health Administration. Accessed 2025. https://www.osha.gov/bloodborne-pathogens/worker-protections.
62. Heick J, Lazaro RT. *Goodman and Snyder's Differential Diagnosis for Physical Therapists: Screening for Referral.* 7th ed. Elsevier; 2023.
63. VanMeter KC, Hubert RJ. *Gould's Pathophysiology for the Health Professions.* 7th ed. Elsevier Inc; 2022.
64. NIH. *Metastatic Cancer: When Cancer Spreads.* NIH: National Cancer Institute; 2020. https://www.cancer.gov/types/metastatic-cancer#where-cancer-spreads.
65. ACS. *Signs and Symptoms of Cancer.* American Cancer Society; 2024. https://www.cancer.org/cancer/diagnosis-staging/signs-and-symptoms-of-cancer.html.
66. Clinic Mayo. *Paraneoplastic Syndromes of the Nervous System.* Mayo Clinic; 2022. https://www.mayoclinic.org/diseases-conditions/paraneoplastic-syndromes/symptoms-causes/syc-20355687.

20 Neuromusculoskeletal Pathophysiology

OBJECTIVES

By the end of this chapter, the reader should be able to:

- Demonstrate a basic understanding of the perception of normal sensation.
- Demonstrate a basic understanding of the systemic connection to neuromusculoskeletal pain with a focus on the head, neck, and back.
- Demonstrate a basic understanding of the systemic connection to neuromusculoskeletal pain with a focus on the chest, breast, and ribs.
- Demonstrate a basic understanding of the systemic connection to neuromusculoskeletal pain with a focus on the extremities.
- Identify possible symptoms associated with various types of referred pain.
- Differentiate between the symptoms occurring when there is a neuromusculoskeletal cause versus a systemic cause.
- Assess and justify whether a specific neuromusculoskeletal symptom could constitute a yellow or red flag.

This book has covered some of the many systemic and viscerogenic causes of pain in the nerves, muscles, and bones. This chapter begins with some information about sensation, then goes through various areas of the human body, and lists some of the more common systemic causes of pain.

The Perception of Sensation

The postcentral gyrus is considered to be the primary somatosensory part of the brain's cortex, responsible for sensations related to proprioception, touch, temperature, pressure, and pain (Fig. 20.1).[1]

The part of the brain responsible for vision resides in the occipital lobe,[2] and hearing centers are located mainly in the temporal lobe.[3] Centers for taste appear to be in the insular cortex that separates the frontal and temporal lobes,[4] and smell is processed in both the cerebral cortex and the limbic system.[5] Posture, balance, and equilibrium functions are processed in the cerebellum.[2] Any injury to these areas of the brain can result in problems with these basic sensory functions. Various receptors in the body are responsible for proprioception, interoception, touch, and pain.

Proprioception

Proprioception is the sense of body position. This is the ability to know where a body part is in space without looking. Kinesthetic awareness is the sense of movement. This is the ability to know if a body part is moving and in what direction, without looking.[6] The primary sensory organs for proprioception are stretch receptors called muscle spindles, although other receptors have been mentioned in the literature including low-threshold mechanoreceptors and Golgi tendon organs.[6] This information then travels via afferent nerve fibers up the dorsal column-medial lemniscal pathway[7] of the spinal cord to the postcentral gyrus.[1]

Interoception

Interoception is the sense, interpretation, and regulation of signals from within the body. This is how the brain communicates with internal organs using not only the nervous system but also non-neuronal systems like the endocrine and metabolic systems.[8] Interoceptors, like chemoreceptors, specific mechanoreceptors, and nociceptors (pain receptors), detect various stimuli and change them to electrical signals.[8]

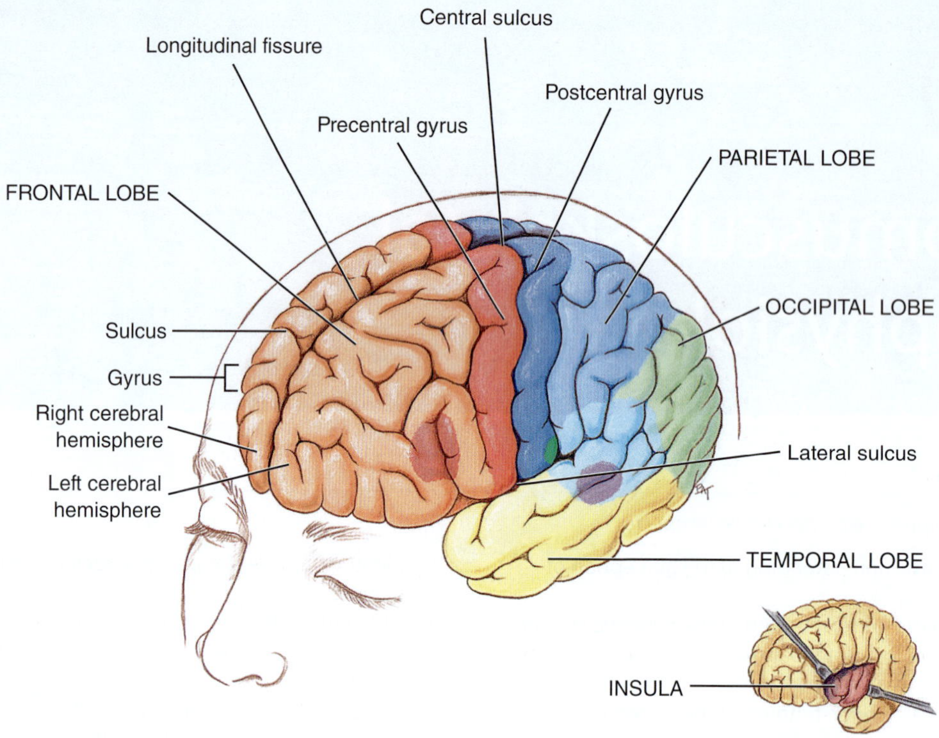

• **Fig. 20.1** Postcentral gyrus in the parietal lobe. (From Applegate E. *The Anatomy and Physiology Learning System*. 4th ed. Saunders; 2011.)

Hormonal or other signals are carried up the ascending neural pathways to the brain. It is believed that this information is then processed in subcortical areas of the brain and moved up to the hypothalamus, insula, postcentral gyrus, and other higher areas for interpretation.[8]

Touch and Pain

Sensations of touch and pain are first perceived by low-threshold mechanoreceptors located in the skin. This information then travels up the spinothalamic tract to the postcentral gyrus of the brain for interpretation.[9] The primary nerve endings in the skin for touch and pain are Merkel cells (which detect fast touch and can determine special differences), Ruffini endings (which respond to slow touch and skin stretch), Meissner corpuscles (which detect the fastest touch but cannot determine special differences), Pacinian corpuscles (which sense high-frequency vibrations but lack special acuity), and the pilosebaceous unit (which produces hair fibers that have mechanoreceptors and help with wound healing).[9] Kraus end bulbs, or bulboid corpuscles, are thought to be thermoreceptors (Fig. 20.2).

Nociceptor nerve endings (which detect pain) protect organisms by causing pain so the individual can avoid a noxious stimulus.[10] Some of the more common mechanical pain receptors are represented in Fig. 20.3.

The rest of this chapter is derived primarily from Chapters 15 through 19 of Ref. 11.

The Systemic Connection to Neuromusculoskeletal Pain

Whenever an individual presents with pain, or any other potential symptoms that could merit occupational therapy (OT) intervention, a thorough screening is needed. This includes a review of the client's history, their symptoms, and their living environment, along with consultation with the interdisciplinary team.[12] When pain is from a neuromusculoskeletal problem, it is typically localized to a part of the body the client can point to. It is generally unilateral, decreases with rest, increases with specific movements, improves with recumbency, and it is often reduced through OT modalities. It is not associated with fever or other systemic symptoms, and it is usually brought on by a specific injury or event.[11] Systemic causes of pain, however, tend to break one or more of these rules.

The Head, Neck, and Back

Although most cases of back and neck pain in adults are due to injuries, physical loading, or age-related degenerative processes,[11] there will be individuals who require imaging or bloodwork to identify the cause of other symptoms that lie outside the typical symptomatology. Occupational therapy practitioners (OTPs) need to not only know how to screen individuals for possible OT intervention but also how to identify signs and

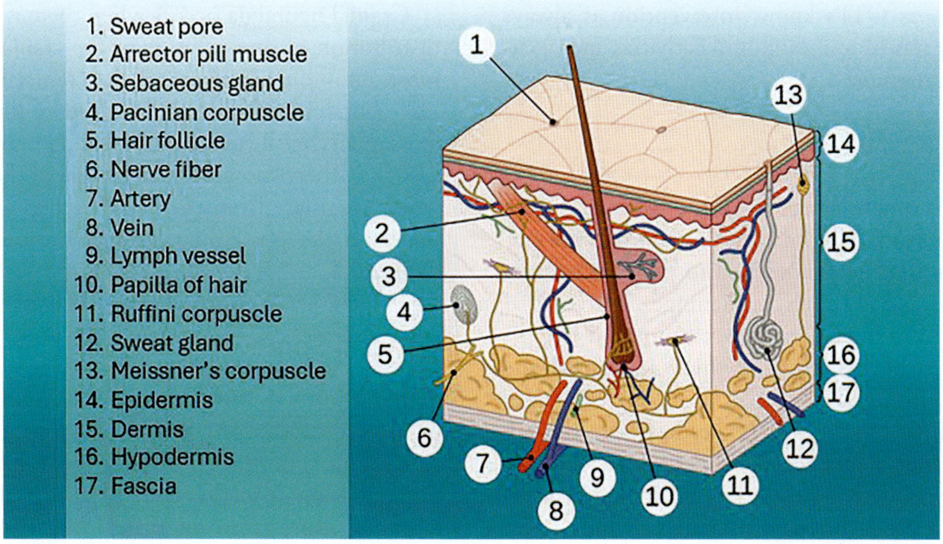

• **Fig. 20.2** Some of the more common receptors of touch. (Image from https://commons.wikimedia.org/wiki/File:Human_skin_anatomy_numbered.svg.)

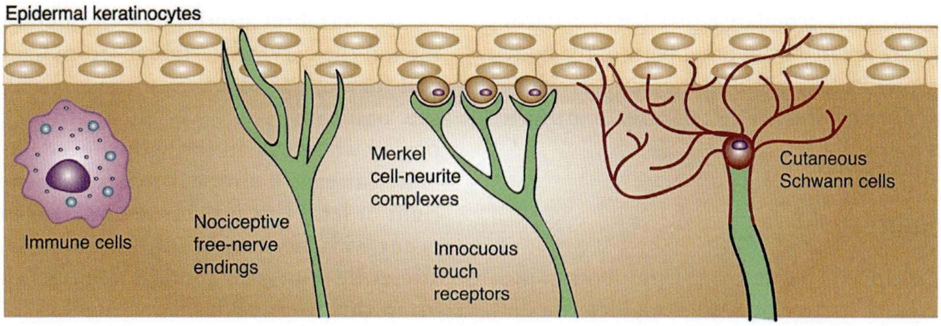

• **Fig. 20.3** Mechanical pain receptors. (From Hill RZ, Bautista DM. Getting in touch with mechanical pain mechanisms. *Trends Neurosci*. 2020;43:311–325.)

symptoms of disorders that fall outside of the cluster of symptoms that are typical for their client's diagnosis. These extraneous symptoms might be signs of a different, or additional, condition. Yet, what happens when the symptoms mimic those of neuromuscular or musculoskeletal pain? This chapter will help work through some of the possibilities.

Past Medical History

There are always important questions to ask the client during screening, such as a past medical history of cancer (even if long ago), back or neck pain that has been ongoing for years, new episodes of serious back or neck pain, gradually increasing pain over a 6-month period, history of any accidents or injury, or a history of other disorders like diabetes, hypertension, or osteoporosis. A recent history of fever or chills is a possible indicator of infection somewhere in the body.[11]

Another clue to better understand the source of the client's pain is the quality of the pain (sharp, dull, throbbing, etc.), what causes the pain to worsen, and what relieves it. The OTP should also ask about the pattern of the pain (if it covers a dermatomal distribution, for example), the duration of the pain (when it started, how long it lasts each time if it tends to fluctuate), and any symptoms (such as if it hurts more after eating, during menses, etc.). The OTP should also ask if the pain is aggravated or relieved by any positions and if it hurts more at night or when awakening in the morning. Pain at night, especially pain that awakens a person after falling asleep, can be a sign of something serious like a tumor or an infection.[11]

Remember, yellow flags signify caution, which are findings that require special attention but not immediate action. Whereas, red flags signify warning, which are findings that require immediate attention.[11]

Yellow flags are often accompanied by psychosocial factors that can either help or hinder rehabilitation progress. The Optimal Screening for Prediction of Referral and Outcome Yellow Flag (OSPRO-YF) tool helps to identify psychosocial factors (fear avoidance, negative mood, and positive affect/coping) in individuals with musculoskeletal pain.[13] Of course, as OTPs know, intervention is always dependent upon a return to meaningful activities and occupation-based intervention.

Head

Because there are no pain receptors in the brain itself, the brain does not feel pain. Pain from elements inside the cranium (intracranial disorders) is related to pressure on cranial nerves, sinuses, blood vessels, or meninges. Extracranial headache pain is from outside of the cranium and is typically considered to be benign. The third edition of the *International Classification of Headache Disorders* divides headaches into three parts: primary headache, secondary headache, and cranial neuralgias.[14] Primary headaches are not caused by any underlying disorder and include cluster headaches, tension headaches, and migraines, which affect different areas of the head and face (Fig. 20.4).

Secondary headaches are caused by an underlying disorder or injury and include headaches due to dehydration, concussion, hormonal imbalance, eye strain, stress, or tension. Cranial neuralgias are due to cranial nerve pain.[11,15] OTPs are most likely to see clients with secondary headaches or cervicogenic headaches that are referred from other parts of the body to the head.[11] Examples include neck injuries such as whiplash or postural strain, intervertebral disc disease, or arthritis in the cervical facet joints.[14]

Cranial Nerve Pain

Most of the body's peripheral nerves come from roots in the spinal cord. The cranial nerves, however, originate in the brain and go directly to various parts of the body. There are 12 cranial nerves, and their points of origin can be seen in Fig. 20.5.

Cranial neuralgia occurs when there is severe pain in the distribution of one or more of the cranial nerves. The two most common neuralgias of the cranial nerves are trigeminal neuralgia (affecting cranial nerve five or CN V) and glossopharyngeal neuralgia (affecting cranial nerve nine or CN IX). There can also be neuralgia of the occipital nerves, which originate from the spinal nerves at C2 and C3 and travel up the posterior aspect of the neck and scalp (see Table 20.1).

Cervical Spine

Either a joint dysfunction, like a shoulder impingement or facet dysfunction, or a medical problem, like a fracture, tumor, or infection, can cause cervical pain without radiation into the arm. If pain is referred, however, it could come from an infection, cancer, or other systemic condition like a cardiac, pulmonary, or abdominal disorder. This radiation can occur with any cervical myelopathy and can be accompanied by coordination problems, weakness, bowel or bladder problems, or sexual dysfunction.[11]

The vertebral arteries pass through the transverse foramen of the cervical vertebrae (from C6 to C2) (Fig. 20.6) and then merge together at the levels of the pons to form the basilar artery.[20] Vertebral artery syndrome is suspected whenever an individual needs to turn their whole body instead of simply the head and neck when looking right or left. This is because dizziness and nystagmus will occur with neck motions, like combined extension and lateral flexion. The cervical spine is often affected early on in the progression of rheumatoid arthritis, with deep aching pain in the occipital and temporal regions of the head, sometimes referred to the face from C2 nerve root irritation.[11]

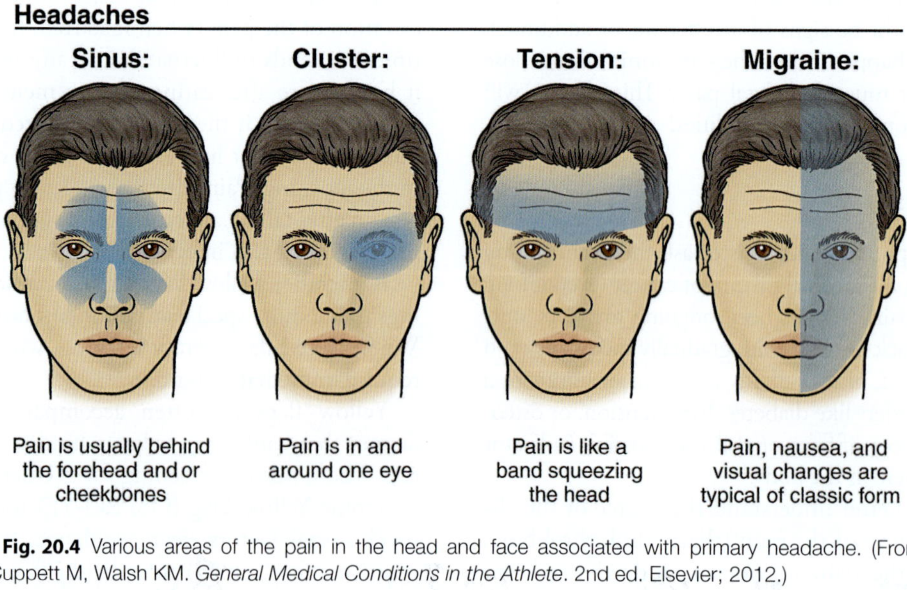

• **Fig. 20.4** Various areas of the pain in the head and face associated with primary headache. (From Cuppett M, Walsh KM. *General Medical Conditions in the Athlete*. 2nd ed. Elsevier; 2012.)

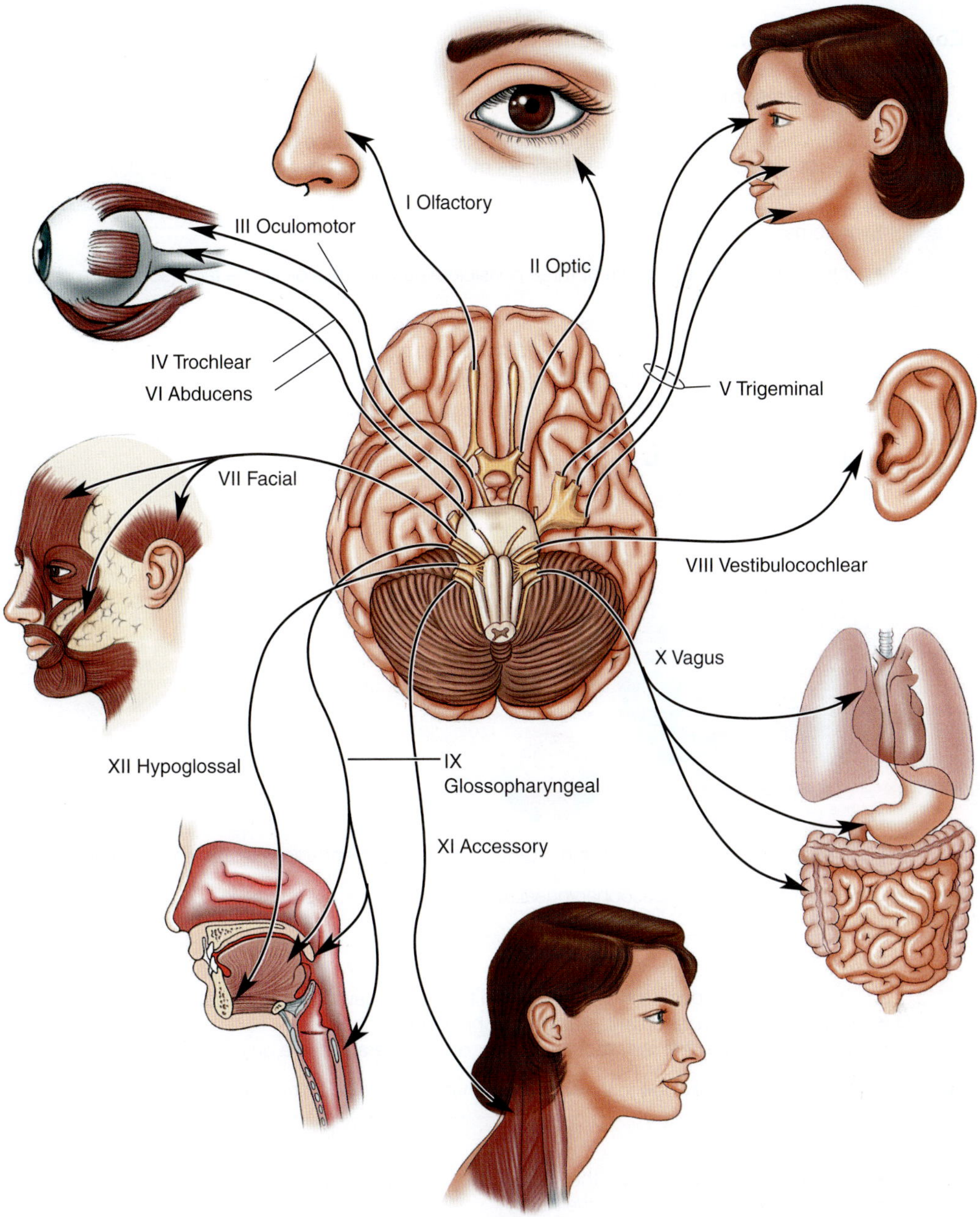

• **Fig. 20.5** The origins of the 12 cranial nerves and their functions. (From Barbara Herlihy, *The Human Body in Health and Illness*. 8th ed. Elsevier; 2026.)

Thoracic Spine

Pain in the thoracic spine is typically from musculoskeletal causes, such as muscle strain, vertebral or rib fracture, spinal stenosis, costotransverse and costovertebral joint dysfunction, intervertebral disc herniation, and mechanical problems in the cervical spine referring pain to the thoracic spine. If pain is of a systemic origin, it is typically accompanied by constitutional symptoms (fever, fatigue, malaise, etc.).[11] Because these additional symptoms often develop after the initial onset of back pain, the individual might think it is something new and not mention it to the OTP. Careful observation and open-ended questions help the OTP to facilitate this discussion.[11]

Lumbar Spine

It is estimated that around 80% of adults will experience acute low back pain (LBP) at some point in their lives. When this pain is persistent and limits activity, it constitutes a yellow flag and requires a second look.[11] The Centers for Disease Control and Prevention (CDC) reported that 39% of adults in the United States were experiencing LBP in 2019.[21] This was most common in white females over the age of 65 whose income fell below the federal poverty level. Only 28.4% of people between the ages of 18 and 29 reported LBP in 2019, but this gradually increased in the older population groups, with 45.6% of individuals over the age of 65 reporting LBP.[21]

TABLE 20.1 Most Common Types of Cranial Nerve Pain

Disorder	Clinical Presentation
Trigeminal (CN V) neuralgia (also called tic douloureux)[16,17]	Cause: This is thought to result from a disruption in the function of the nerve due to contact between the nerve and a nearby blood vessel. It occurs most often in individuals over the age of 50 and is more common in women than in men. Symptoms: • Intense pain in one or more of three possible areas on the side of the face (see image below), lasting days, weeks, or months • Pain that feels like stabbing or electric shock in the cheek or jaw • This pain is only felt when awake and not during sleep • Periods of relief between episodes • Anxiety between episodes 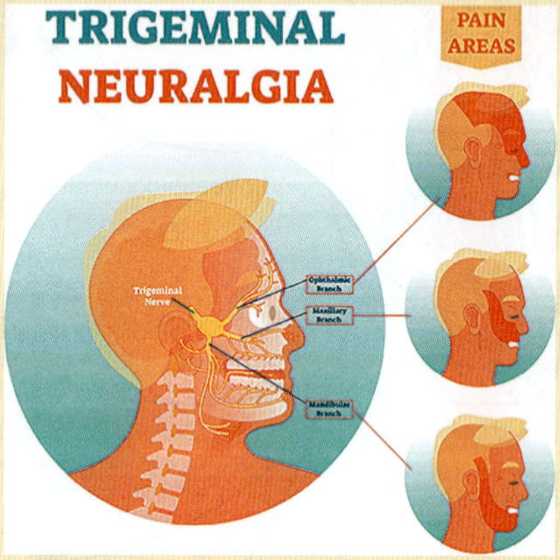 From https://www.hopkinsmedicine.org/health/conditions-and-diseases/trigeminal-neuralgia
Glossopharyngeal (CN IX) neuralgia[18]	Cause: Irritation of the glossopharyngeal nerve resulting from compression by a blood vessel, a tumor, or an infection. Symptoms: • Severe pain that occurs in brief attacks in the mouth, jaw, tongue, throat, tonsils, and/or ear • This pain is sharp, shooting, stabbing, aching, and/or burning • Intense episodes that last about a minute, often several times a day
Occipital neuralgia[19]	Cause: This is typically due to injury or inflammation of the occipital nerves (see image below). Symptoms: • Aching or burning pain from the base of the head up through the scalp • Pain on one or both sides of the head • Pain behind the eyes • Numbness • Light sensitivity • Pain with neck movements 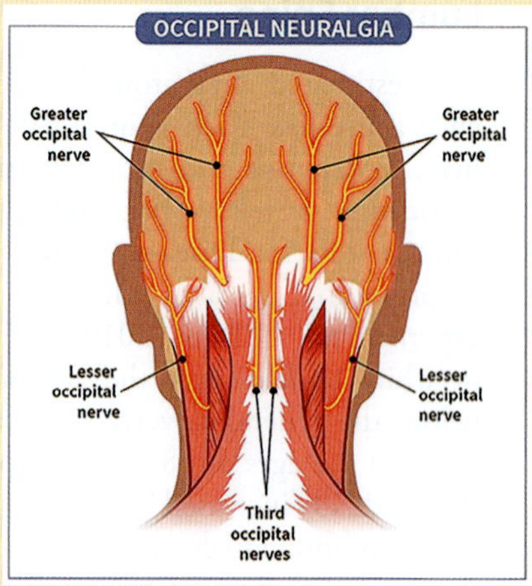

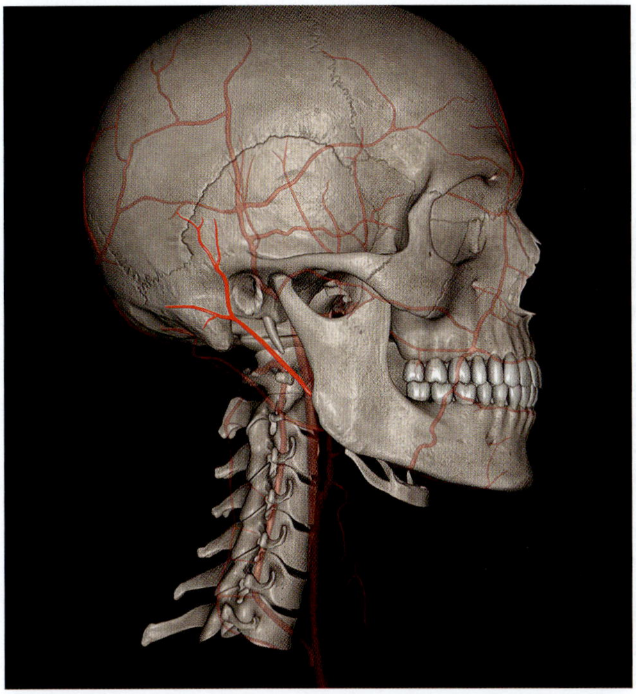

• **Fig. 20.6** The vertebral arteries. (From iStock.com/benote.)

Systemic causes of LBP can be due to problems in the pelvic and abdominal viscera that are referred to the back directly from the organ structures, but this pain could also be produced by irritation of the posterior abdominal wall by blood, inflammation, pus, or leaking enzymes, causing the pain to arise directly from irritation in the anterior structures of the back.[11]

Spinal Cord Injuries

Although the topic of spinal cord injury (SCI) is typically covered in a neurology course, it will be briefly mentioned here. A spinal cord injury may result from trauma or other causes, such as a tumor. This injury can be complete or incomplete. If either type of SCI is suspected, it is always a **red flag**. Although it is likely that this diagnosis would be made prior to the initial OT visit, it is important for the occupational therapist and/or the occupational therapy assistant to know signs and symptoms of a SCI and what to expect at various levels of spinal cord involvement. Fig. 20.7 lists the levels of spinal cord injury and the movements affected.

Sacrum

Often, sacroiliac (SI) pain is due to trauma causing inflammation and a condition called sacroilitis. This condition can affect one or both SI joints (Fig. 20.8).[22]

When there is no trauma, and no pain associated with tests that diagnose facet joint injury in the spine, the SI pain could be from more serious pathology, such as one of the spondyloarthropathies (i.e., ankylosing spondylitis and various types of arthritis, including psoriatic arthritis and arthritis with chronic inflammatory bowel disease).[11]

An individual with spondyloarthropathy will often have pain occurring in the second half of the night, with stiffness that improves with activity. As with most systemic causes of pain, there are often constitutional signs and symptoms (such as fever, skin lesions, anorexia, fatigue, and weight loss). When these are seen in any individual, it constitutes a red flag, with immediate referral to the physician[11] (Table 20.2). The sacrum will be discussed again later in this chapter.

Some of the more common red flags that could be associated with systemic problems can be found in Table 20.3.

The Chest, Breast, and Ribs

There will be times when a client with an injury with resultant pain in the chest will come to an OT clinic for improved functional mobility and participation in occupations (such as with an athletic injury or after a mastectomy). During therapy, however, when new pain develops in this area, it constitutes a definitive red flag. It is important to remember that OTPs must work within their scope of practice and, therefore, should not attempt to make a medical diagnosis. Still, they have to know when to treat and when to refer the client back to the physician or to the emergency room. OTPs have to work inside the box but be able to think outside the box.

Chest

Screening a client with chest pain requires questions geared toward medical history involving cardiac problems and cancer. As stated in the previous chapter, hearing hoof beats, OTPs need to think of horses (the more common animal) as opposed to zebras. In this case, a heart attack and breast cancer are zebras, but both are still deadly, and risk factors must be identified. Obviously, if the client has crushing chest pain, 911 should be called immediately. It is better to contact the paramedics and not need them than it is to not contact them and have a crisis on your hands. It is always better to err on the side of caution, especially when it comes to chest pain.

Cardiac Symptoms

Risk factors for cardiac-associated symptoms include advanced age, menopause in females, family history of high blood pressure (hypertension), tobacco use, family history of heart disease, and high cholesterol. The clinical presentation of the client will provide a great deal of information. Heart rate can help to determine if there is reduced cardiac output. In this case, the rate of the heart will quicken (tachycardia). If there is myocardial ischemia or trauma, the heart rate will slow (bradycardia). Always ask about associated signs and symptoms, like nausea or dizziness, and see if light pressure over the area increases or decreases the pain. Watch for pain that feels crushing or searing and spreads to the back, neck, or jaw. This could be a sign of a heart attack.[14] Signs of possible pericarditis (or inflammation of the lining around the heart) include sudden stabbing pain in the center or left side of the chest that occurs quickly, often increasing when

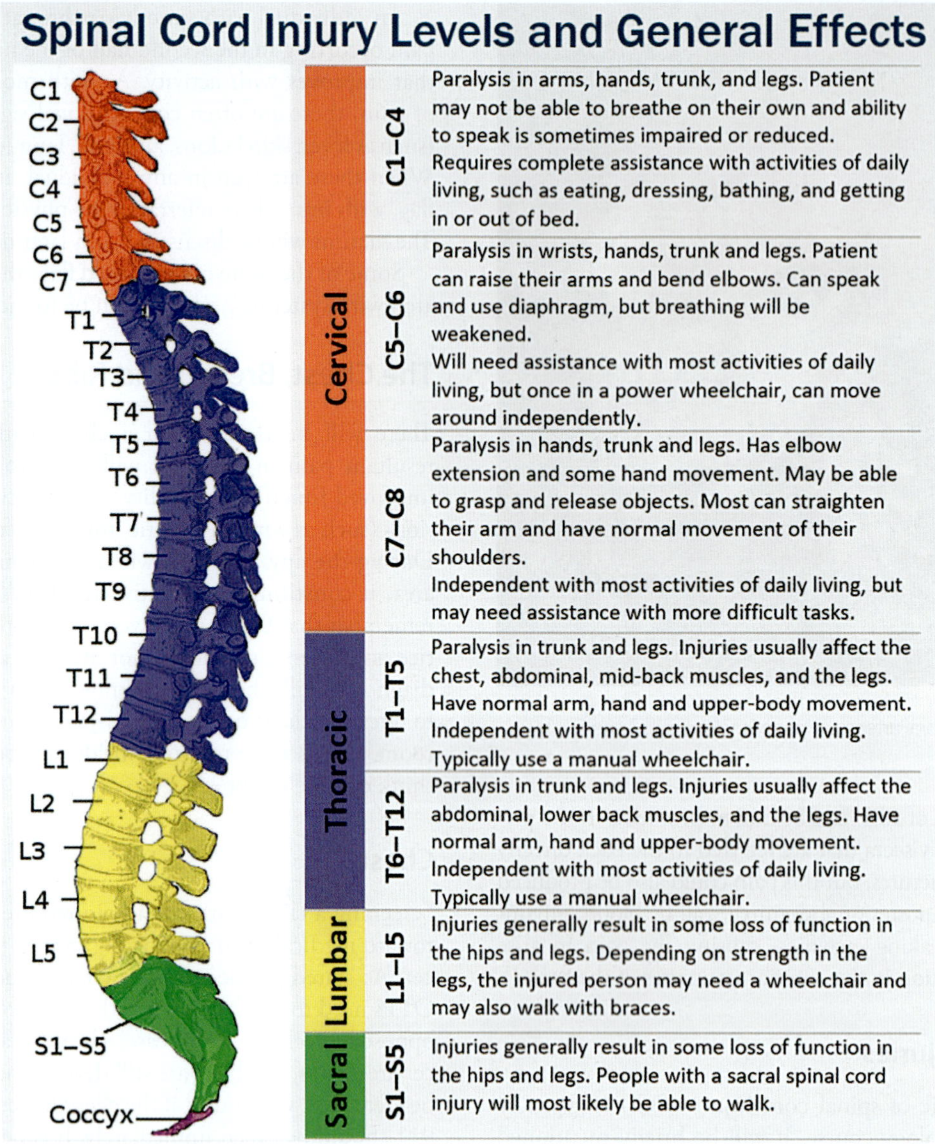

• **Fig. 20.7** Levels of spinal cord injury. (From https://www.pngkit.com/view/u2w7w7i1e6i1y3q8_spinal-cord-injury-levels/.)

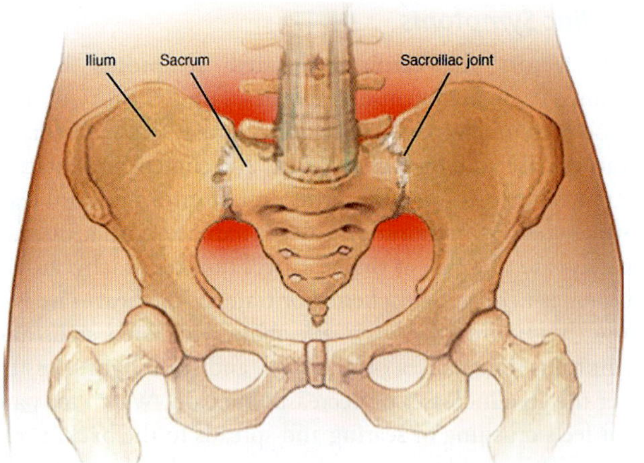

• **Fig. 20.8** The sacroiliac joints. (From https://www.mayoclinic.org/diseases-conditions/sacroiliitis/symptoms-causes/syc-20350747, used with permission of Mayo Foundation for Medical Education and Research. All rights reserved.)

lying down, and sometimes accompanied by weakness and fever.[28] Angina pectoris is chest pain caused by a reduction in blood flow to the heart.[29] It is relatively common and typically treated with nitroglycerin.[30]

Whatever the cause, chest pain always constitutes a red flag and is a medical emergency, requiring an immediate call to 911.[28] Although it is estimated that over 50% of all chest pain has a noncardiac basis, it is always best to err on the side of caution.[11] While it may feel embarrassing to send someone to the emergency room for a noncardiac condition, it would be far more troubling to face the consequences of delayed action during a true cardiac event.

Breast

Sometimes, breast pain is the primary complaint, but typically, this will occur in conjunction with shoulder, neck, or back pain.[11] Performing a breast examination is not within the scope of occupational therapy intervention,[31] but

TABLE 20.2 Potential Systemic Causes of Neck and Back Pain

Potential Cause	Cervical	Thoracic	Lumbosacral
Cancer	• Metastatic lesions (leukemia, Hodgkin disease) • Cervical bone tumors • Cervical cord tumors • Lung cancer; Pancoast tumor • Esophageal cancer • Thyroid cancer	• Mediastinal tumors • Metastatic extension • Pancreatic cancer • Breast cancer • Multiple myeloma	• Primary bone tumors • Neurogenic tumors (sacrum) • Metastatic lesions • Prostate cancer • Testicular cancer • Pancreatic cancer • Colorectal cancer • Multiple myeloma • Lymphoma
Cardiovascular	• Angina • MI • Aortic aneurysm • Occipital migraine • Cervical artery ischemia or dissection • Arteritis	• Angina • Myocardial infarction • Aortic aneurysm • Occipital migraine • Cervical artery ischemia or dissection • Arteritis	• Abdominal aortic aneurysm • Endocarditis • Myocarditis • Peripheral vascular: ◦ Postoperative bleeding from anterior spine surgery
Pulmonary	• Lung cancer; Pancoast tumor • Tracheobronchial irritation • Chronic bronchitis • Pneumothorax • Pleuritis involving the diaphragm	• Respiratory or lung infection • Empyema • Chronic bronchitis • Pleurisy • Pneumothorax • Pneumonia	• COPD[23]
Renal/urologic	• Renal parenchymal disease (muscle cramps and headache)[24]	• Acute pyelonephritis • Kidney disease	• Acute pyelonephritis • Perinephritic abscess • Nephrolithiasis • Ureteral colic (kidney stones) • Urinary tract infection • Dialysis (first-use syndrome) • Renal tumors

GI	• Esophagitis
	• Esophageal cancer
		• Esophagitis (severe)
		• Esophageal spasm
		• Peptic ulcer
		• Acute cholecystitis
		• Biliary colic
		• Pancreatic disease
			• Small intestine:
			  ◦ Obstruction (neoplasm)
			  ◦ Irritable bowel syndrome
			  ◦ Crohn's disease
			• Colon:
			  ◦ Diverticular disease
			• Pancreatic disease
			• Appendicitis

Gynecologic	• Diaphragmatic endometriosis[11] • Pregnancy[12]	• Diaphragmatic endometriosis[25] • Pregnancy[26] • Thoracic endometriosis[27]	• Cancer • Retroversion of the uterus • Uterine fibroids • Ovarian cysts • Endometriosis • PID • Incest/sexual assault • Rectocele, cystocele • Uterine prolapse • Normal pregnancy • Multiparity
Infection	• Vertebral osteomyelitis • Meningitis • Lyme disease • Retropharyngeal abscess; epidural abscess (post-steroid injection)	• Vertebral osteomyelitis • Herpes zoster • HIV • Epidural abscess	• Vertebral osteomyelitis • Herpes zoster • Spinal tuberculosis • Candidiasis (yeast) • Psoas abscess • HIV

(Continued)

TABLE 20.2 Potential Systemic Causes of Neck and Back Pain—cont'd

Potential Cause	Cervical	Thoracic	Lumbosacral
Other	• Osteoporosis • Fibromyalgia • Psychogenic (non-organic causes) • Fracture • Rheumatoid: o RA and atlantoaxial subluxation o Psoriatic arthritis o Polymyalgia rheumatica • Ankylosing spondylitis • Viral myalgia • Cervical lymphadenitis • Thyroid disease	• Osteoporosis • Fibromyalgia • Psychogenic (non-organic) • Acromegaly • Cushing syndrome • Fracture	• Osteoporosis • Fibromyalgia • Psychogenic (non-organic) • Fracture • Cushing syndrome • Type III hypersensitivity disorder (back/flank pain) • Post-regional anesthesia • Ankylosing spondylitis

COPD, Chronic obstructive pulmonary disease; *MI*, myocardial infarction; *PID*, pelvic inflammatory disease; *RA*, rheumatoid arthritis; *HIV*, human immunodeficiency virus; *GI*, gastrointestinal.

Derived primarily from Heick J, Lazaro RT. *Goodman and Snyder's Differential Diagnosis for Physical Therapists: Screening for Referral*. 7th ed. Elsevier; 2023.

TABLE 20.3 Common Red Flags Associated With Systemic Causes of Neck and Back Pain

Some of the More Common Red Flags Associated with Systemic Causes of Neck and Back Pain
• Age less than 20 years or over 50 years (malignancy)/ over 70 years (fracture)
• Previous history of cancer
• Constitutional symptoms (e.g., fever, chills, unexplained weight loss)
• Failure to improve with conservative care (usually over 4–6 weeks)
• Recent urinary tract infection, blood in urine (or stools), difficulty with urination
• History of injection drug use
• Immunocompromised condition (e.g., prolonged use of corticosteroids, transplant recipient, autoimmune diseases)
• Pain is not relieved by rest or recumbency
• Severe, constant nighttime pain
• Progressive neurologic deficit; saddle anesthesia; urinary or fecal incontinence
• Back pain accompanied by abdominal, pelvic, or hip pain
• History of falls or trauma (screen for fracture, osteoporosis, domestic violence, alcohol use)
• Significant morning stiffness with limitation in all spinal movements (ankylosing spondylitis or other inflammatory disorder)
• Skin rash (inflammatory disorder [e.g., Crohn's disease, ankylosing spondylitis])

From Heick J, Lazaro RT. *Goodman and Snyder's Differential Diagnosis for Physical Therapists: Screening for Referral*. 7th ed. Elsevier; 2023.

TABLE 20.4 Clinical Signs and Symptoms Associated With Breast Cancer

Some of the More Common Signs and Symptoms Associated With Breast Cancer
• Nontender (painless), firm, or hard lump
• Unusual discharge from nipple
• Skin or nipple retraction dimpling; erosion, retraction, itching of nipple
• Redness or skin rash over the breast or nipple
• Generalized hardness, enlargement, shrinking, or distortion of the breast or nipple
• Unusual prominence of veins over the breast
• Enlarged rubbery lymph nodes
• Axillary mass
• Swelling of arm
• Bone or back pain
• Weight loss

From Heick J, Lazaro RT. *Goodman and Snyder's Differential Diagnosis for Physical Therapists: Screening for Referral*. 7th ed. Elsevier; 2023.

referring the client back to the physician is something that the OTP should do, just to rule out the possibility of any unknown lumps or lesions that could be cancerous. This can also be true for male clients. The most common site of cancer in females is the breast.[11] For clinical signs of possible breast cancer, see Table 20.4.

Although rare, if a client complains of itching, redness, and flaking of the skin around the nipple, it could be Paget disease, a form of ductal cancer[11] (Fig. 20.9).

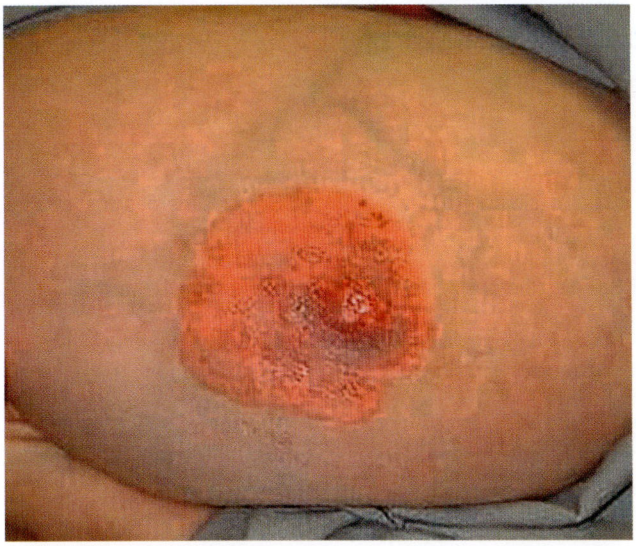

• **Fig. 20.9** Paget disease of the breast. (Courtesy Lily Chu, National Naval Medical Center, Bethesda. https://en.wikipedia.org/wiki/Paget%27s_disease_of_the_breast#/media/File:Paget_Disese_of_the_Nipple.jpg.)

Not all breast problems are life-threatening. Mastodynia is caused by irritation of the upper dorsal intercostal nerve and presents as unilateral breast pain typically during the menstrual cycle. Mastitis is inflammation of the breast tissue and is often associated with breastfeeding. Breast cysts (small fluid-filled sacs) are common in females, and there may be only one or many. These are typically asymptomatic, but when there is pain, physicians might drain the fluid to decrease the symptoms.[32] Gynecomastia is the overdevelopment of breast tissue in men or boys and is typically benign.[33] It is often caused by hormonal changes but can also be caused by various medications like antibiotics, antidepressants, chemotherapy, or prostate cancer medications or by certain illicit drugs like marijuana or heroin.[33]

Ribs

As stated earlier, its estimated that over 50% of all chest pain is noncardiac, but only 20% to 25% of what remains is musculoskeletal.[11] Problems in the cervical spine can refer to pain in the ribs, and musculoskeletal disorders, like muscle exertion, myofascial trigger points, osteomyelitis, and costochondritis, can lead to pain in the chest and arms. This pain can be differentiated from angina pectoris because it can last for seconds or hours and is not relieved with nitroglycerin.[11]

It is possible to differentiate some musculoskeletal syndromes from those of possible visceral-related causes, especially heart attacks.[11]

Conditions like costochondritis, Tietze syndrome, xiphoid hypersensitivity, and slipping rib syndrome are described in the following subsections.

Costochondritis

Costochondritis refers to pain without swelling in the cartilage that connects the ribs to the sternum (costochondral joints). This disorder can occur at any time over the lifespan, but it is most common in individuals over 40 years of age.[11] The individual will complain of sharp pain along the edges of the sternum, typically near the second through fifth costochondral joints. This pain will sometimes radiate into the arm or back and is often confused with a heart attack. The difference is that with a heart attack, the pain is not along the edges of the sternum but in the center of the chest.[11] In addition, the typical symptoms of a cardiac or pulmonary condition such as nausea, vomiting, dyspnea, and diaphoresis will not typically be seen with costochondritis.[11] Still, it is not within the scope of OT to make this determination. Whatever the cause, chest pain always constitutes a red flag and is a medical emergency, requiring an immediate call to 911.[28]

Tietze Syndrome

Tietze syndrome refers to inflammation and pain with swelling in the area of the costochondral joints. It is often confused with costochondritis, but these two disorders are not identical. This disorder can occur any time over the lifespan, but it is most common in individuals under 40 years of age. The individual will complain of chest pain along the edges of the sternum, typically near the second and third costochondral joints. There will be swelling, tenderness on palpation, and a feeling of warmth, with possible skin coloration.

Xyphodynia

This is a general term that refers to pain and/or sensitivity at the xyphoid process and/or the xiphisternal joint. This pain can increase with movement or overeating and is often associated with nausea.[34] Because the pain is central in the chest, it might present like a heart attack, but with xyphodynia, gentle palpation over the xyphoid process will increase the pain, sometimes accompanied by nausea and radiation into the back and the arms.[34]

Slipping Rib Syndrome

Slipping rib syndrome occurs when there is abnormal movement of a false rib (rib 8–10), leading to impingement of one of the intercostal nerves. There is hypermobility of the false rib costal cartilages (the anterior end), causing the rib to slip under the rib located superior to it.[35]

This causes pain from the lower chest to the upper abdominal region.[35] This pain increases when the individual side bends to the affected side.[11] This condition can occur at any age but is most common in middle-aged females.[35]

For a list of potential systemic and neuromuscular causes of chest, breast, and rib pain, see Table 20.5.

The Neck, Chest, and Abdomen

Whenever an individual is referred to occupational therapy for a musculoskeletal condition, it is important to not only evaluate the joint in question but also the area above and below the joint.[11]

Pain in the shoulder can be referred from other areas of the body such as the pulmonary, renal, or gynecological systems. Problems like heart disease, peptic ulcers, or even

TABLE 20.5 Potential Systemic and Neuromuscular Causes of Chest, Breast, and Rib Pain

Possible Cause	Chest	Breast	Ribs
Systemic	Cancer • Mediastinal tumors Cardiac • Myocardial ischemia (unstable angina) • Myocardial infarct • Cardiomyopathy • Myocarditis • Pericarditis • Dissecting aortic aneurysm • Aortic aneurysm • Aortic stenosis or regurgitation • Mitral valve prolapse • Tachycardia Pleuropulmonary • Asthma/COPD • Pulmonary embolism • Pneumothorax • Pulmonary hypertension • Cor pulmonale • Pneumonia with pleurisy or pleuritis • Mediastinitis Epigastric/upper GI • Esophagitis • Esophageal spasm • Reflux or other motility disorder • Hiatal hernia • Upper GI ulcer • Cholecystitis • Pancreatitis Hematologic • Anemia • Polycythemia • Sickle cell crisis Other • Rheumatic disease (sternoclavicular joint) • Infection (sepsis): sternoclavicular joint (injection drug use) • Anxiety, panic attack • Vertebroplasty (possible pulmonary embolism) • Cocaine use • Anabolic steroids • Collagen vascular disorder with pleuritis or pericarditis • Fibromyalgia • Hyperthyroidism • Dialysis (first-use syndrome) • Type III hypersensitivity reaction • Herpes zoster (shingles) • Psychogenic	Infection • Mastitis (lactating females) • Abscess • Shingles (herpes zoster) Cancer • Malignant tumor • Inflammatory carcinoma of the breast Inflammation • Pleuritis GI • GERD Other • Acute fat necrosis (after trauma) • Lymph disease • PMS, menstrual, or hormonal influence (including early pregnancy) Paget disease • Benign tumor, cyst, calcific change • Medication (e.g., some hormone, cardiovascular, psychiatric drugs) • Anxiety	Infection • Shingles (herpes zoster) Gastrointestinal • Gallbladder disease (at the level of the tenth rib) Cancer • Cancer that has metastasized to the bone Other • Pleurisy • Osteoporosis

TABLE 20.5 Potential Systemic and Neuromuscular Causes of Chest, Breast, and Rib Pain—cont'd

Possible Cause	Chest	Breast	Ribs
Neuromuscular	Neurologic • Nerve root compression • Intercostal neuritis • Dorsal nerve root irritation • TOS • Thoracic disc disease Other • Postoperative pain • Tietze syndrome • Costochondritis, sternochondritis • Sternoclavicular joint strain • Hypersensitive xiphoid, xyphodynia • Slipping rib syndrome • TrPs • Myalgia • Cervical spine disorder, arthritis	Neurologic • Mastodynia (mammary neuralgia) • Cervical radiculopathy • TOS Injury • Trauma (including motor vehicle accident, assault, breast biopsy, heavy breasts, or surgery) • Rib fracture, costochondral • Dislocation, chest contusion Inflammation • Costochondritis Other • Pectoral myalgia or other conditions affecting the pectoralis muscles • TrPs • Breast implants, augmentation, reduction • Scar tissue • Connective tissue disorders	Neurologic • TOS Injury • Trauma (e.g., bruise, fracture) Inflammation • Costochondritis Other • Slipping rib syndrome • Tietze syndrome • TrPs

GERD, Gastroesophageal reflux disease; *GI*, gastrointestinal; *PMS*, premenstrual syndrome; *TOS*, thoracic outlet syndrome; *TrPs*, trigger points.
Adapted from Heick J, Lazaro RT. *Goodman and Snyder's Differential Diagnosis for Physical Therapists: Screening for Referral*. 7th ed. Elsevier; 2023.

ectopic pregnancy can refer pain to the shoulder. Knowing what questions to ask and actively listening to the client can help make a more accurate determination.[11] See Table 20.6 for potential systemic and neuromuscular causes of neck, chest, back, and abdominal pain.

The Shoulder and Upper Extremity

A thorough review of past medical history can help to determine the cause of an individual's discomfort, but it could also save a life. For example, when a client has a history of any type of cancer, it could constitute a red flag. Lung cancer and breast cancer are the most common types of cancer that can metastasize to the shoulder.[11] The next part of a good screening is the clinical presentation. There are many types of visceral conditions that manifest as shoulder pain. See Table 20.7 for a list of factors to keep in mind when a client presents with shoulder pain of unknown cause.

The forearm and wrist are also common areas of the body where individuals experience pain. Some of this pain is musculoskeletal in origin, but this pain can also be caused by systemic problems. Carpal tunnel syndrome, for example, is caused by an impingement of the median nerve as it passes through the carpal tunnel in the wrist.[11] This can cause intense burning pain that radiates into the hand and up the arm to the elbow and beyond. It is typically a musculoskeletal problem, but when it presents as bilateral, and the client reports similar symptoms in the feet, it may be caused by liver dysfunction that causes a buildup in serum ammonia and urea levels, leading to peripheral nerve impairment. When the OTP suspects this, some questions need to be asked of the client. Ask if there is a history of liver disease, look for medications that are hepatotoxic or signs of possible alcoholism, and ask questions like, "How many acetaminophen (Tylenol) do you take each day?" Also look at the client for signs of yellowing (jaundice) in the whites of their eyes; spider angiomas; palmer erythema; changes in the nail beds; and liver flap (asterixis).[11]

The Sacrum, Sacroiliac, and Pelvis

The most common piece of information linking sacroiliac (SI) joint or pelvic pain to a musculoskeletal reason is a memorable physical event, such as a fall or a misstep off a curb.[11] When pain occurs without a history of accident, injury, or assault, it may mean there is a systemic cause for the pain.[11]

The Sacrum and the Sacroiliac Joints

SI joint pain is typically unilateral and centered over the area of the posterior superior iliac spine, with tenderness on palpation over the same area.[11] This pain will sometimes radiate down the posterior-lateral thigh and beyond to the knee and

TABLE 20.6 Potential Systemic and Neuromuscular Causes of Neck, Chest, Back, and Abdominal Pain

Possible Cause	Neck	Chest, Trunk, or Back	Abdomen
Systemic	Cancer • Metastasis (leukemia, Hodgkin lymphoma) • Cervical cord tumor • Bone tumor Cardiovascular/vascular • TOS Pulmonary • Primary tuberculosis Other • Cervical central cord lesion • Trauma: cervical fracture or ligamentous instability; whiplash	Cancer • Metastasis to nodes in axilla or mediastinum • Metastasis to lungs from: o Bone o Breast o Kidney o Colorectal o Pancreas o Uterus • Bone metastasis to thoracic spine: o Breast o Lung o Thyroid o Breast cancer o Lung cancer Cardiovascular/vascular • Angina/MI • Acute coronary syndrome • ICU s/p CABG • Pacemaker (complications) • Bacterial endocarditis • Pericarditis • Thoracic aortic aneurysm • Empyema and lung abscess • Collagen vascular disease Pulmonary • Pulmonary embolism • Pulmonary tuberculosis • Spontaneous pneumothorax • Pancoast tumor • Pneumonia Gastrointestinal/hepatic • Hiatal hernia Infection • Septic arthritis • Necrotizing fasciitis • Mononucleosis • Osteomyelitis/transverse myelitis • Syphilis/gonorrhea • Herpes zoster (shingles) • Pneumonia • Cellulitis (skin anywhere on neck, chest, arm, hand) Other • Mastodynia (breast) • Diabetic adhesive capsulitis • Sickle cell disease • Hemophilia	Cancer • Pancreatic cancer • Spinal metastases • Kidney • Testicle • Prostate Cardiovascular/vascular • Dissecting aortic aneurysm Renal/urologic • Kidney stones • Obstruction, inflammation, or infection of upper urinary tract Gastrointestinal/hepatic • Peptic/duodenal ulcer (perforated) • Ruptured spleen • Liver disease • Gallbladder disease • Pancreatic disease Infection • Subphrenic abscess Gynecologic • Ectopic pregnancy (rupture) • Endometriosis (cyst(s)) Other • Diaphragmatic hernia • Anterior spinal surgery (postoperative hemorrhage)

TABLE 20.6 Potential Systemic and Neuromuscular Causes of Neck, Chest, Back, and Abdominal Pain—cont'd

Possible Cause	Neck	Chest, Trunk, or Back	Abdomen
Neuromuscular	Neurologic • Nerve root compression • Intercostal neuritis • Dorsal nerve root irritation • TOS • Cervical disc disease Other • Postoperative pain • Sternoclavicular joint strain • Myalgia • Cervical spine disorder, arthritis	Neurologic • Mastodynia (mammary neuralgia) • Cervical radiculopathy • TOS Injury • Trauma (including motor vehicle accident, assault, breast biopsy, heavy breasts, or surgery) • Rib fracture, costochondral • Dislocation, chest contusion Inflammation • Costochondritis • Tietze syndrome Other • Conditions affecting the pectoralis muscles • Congenital conditions affecting the skeletal system • Breast implants, augmentation, reduction • Scar tissue • Connective tissue disorders • Pectoral myalgia or other conditions affecting the pectoralis muscles	Neurologic • Nerve root compression • Intercostal neuritis Injury • Trauma (e.g., bruise, fracture) • Rectus abdominalis strain Other • Muscle strain during pregnancy • Overexertion (i.e., repetitive sit-ups)

CABG, Coronary artery bypass grafting; *MI*, myocardial infarction; *TOS*, thoracic outlet syndrome; *TrPs*, trigger points.
Adapted from Heick J, Lazaro RT. *Goodman and Snyder's Differential Diagnosis for Physical Therapists: Screening for Referral*. 7th ed. Elsevier; 2023.

TABLE 20.7 Potential Systemic Causes of Shoulder Pain

Possible Cause	Right Shoulder	Left Shoulder
Gastrointestinal	Lateral border of the scapula • Peptic ulcer	Left shoulder (Kehr sign) • Internal bleeding • Spleen (trauma, rupture) Postoperative laparoscopy
Cardiac	Right shoulder radiating down the arm • Myocardial ischemia	Left pectoral region • Myocardial Ischemia Left shoulder between the scapula • Thoracic aortic aneurysm
Hepatic and biliary	Right shoulder between the scapula and subscapular area • Acute cholecystitis Right shoulder and right upper trapezius • Gallbladder problems Right shoulder and right subscapular area • Liver disease (hepatitis, cirrhosis, metastatic tumor, abscess)	Left shoulder • Pancreas Left shoulder and left upper trapezius • Infectious mononucleosis (hepatomegaly, splenomegaly)
Pulmonary	Ipsilateral shoulder; upper trapezius • Pulmonary problems • Pleurisy • Pneumothorax • Pancoast tumor • Pneumonia	Ipsilateral shoulder; upper trapezius • Pulmonary problems • Pleurisy • Pneumothorax • Pancoast tumor • Pneumonia
Kidney	Ipsilateral shoulder • Kidney problems	Ipsilateral shoulder • Kidney problems
Gynecological	Ipsilateral shoulder, dependent upon location of the lesion(s) • Gynecologic problems • Endometriosis	Ipsilateral shoulder • Gynecologic problems • Endometriosis • Ectopic pregnancy

Adapted from Heick J, Lazaro RT. *Goodman and Snyder's Differential Diagnosis for Physical Therapists: Screening for Referral*. 7th ed. Elsevier; 2023.

ankle and to the buttocks but rarely above the L5 level of the back. This occurs without paresthesia to the leg. Symptoms outside of this cluster could be signs of a more systemic cause.[11] See Table 20.8 for some of the red flags associated with possible systemic causes of pain in this region.

The Pelvis

The most common causes of pelvic pain are musculoskeletal and neuromuscular, followed by gynecologic and infectious, but there can also be vascular, neoplastic, and GI disorders.[11] Some potential gynecologic causes include ectopic pregnancy, prolapsed uterus, or endometriosis. Other causes include pelvic inflammatory disease, peripheral vascular disease, pelvic congestion syndrome, cancer, gastrointestinal disorders (like irritable bowel syndrome), iliopsoas abscess, urogenital causes, and appendicitis, to name a few.[11]

The key is to conduct a thorough client history that includes family history and risk factor assessment. This is followed by an evaluation of the client's pain pattern, looking for any potential red or yellow flags. Asking additional questions as they present themselves is good practice, and always ask the client if there are any other associated signs and symptoms.[11] They may have other aches or pains that they did not feel were important to tell you because they seem unrelated. For example, a client might have pelvic pain and also unreported shoulder pain (Kehr sign), or they may have an increase in vaginal discharge along with their pelvic pain.[11] Asking the right open-ended questions will provide the OTP with more information and enable a more accurate depiction of the client's condition. Informing the physician of the findings will aid the doctor to make a correct diagnosis. It is not only good practice but also an excellent way to serve as your client's advocate.

Once this information is known, gentle palpation of the painful area can give the OTP more clues. For example, the iliacus and psoas muscles blend together at around the level of the inguinal ligament to make up the lateral portion of the femoral triangle floor.[36] Due to the proximity of the GI system, this is an area where infected abscesses can occur. The way to palpate for this possibility can be found in Chapter 15. The iliopsoas muscle test will result in pain at McBurney's point (Fig. 15.9).

For possible signs and symptoms of sacral, SI, and pelvic pain, see Table 20.9.

TABLE 20.8 Red Flags Associated With Pain in the SI Region

Screening Criteria	Red Flags
History	• SI/sacral pain without a history of trauma or overuse (rule out assault, anal intercourse) • Previous history of cancer • Previous history of GI disease (ulcerative colitis, Crohn's disease, irritable bowel syndrome) • Previous history of infection (skin, genitourinary tract, heart, septic sacroiliitis)
Risk factors	• Osteoporosis • Sexually transmitted infection or other organ system infection • Intravenous drug abuse • Long-term use of antibiotics (colitis)
Clinical presentation	• Insidious onset/unknown cause • Lack of objective findings • Anterior pelvic, suprapubic, or low abdominal pain at the same level as the sacrum
Associated signs and symptoms	• Pain relieved by passing gas or having a bowel movement • Presence of GI, gynecologic, or urologic signs and symptoms • Fever (septic sacroiliitis); other constitutional symptoms

GI, Gastrointestinal; *SI*, sacroiliac.
From Heick J, Lazaro RT. *Goodman and Snyder's Differential Diagnosis for Physical Therapists: Screening for Referral*. 7th ed. Elsevier; 2023.

The Gluteal Region, Hip, Groin, Thigh, and Leg

The causes of pain in the gluteal area, hip, groin, thigh, and leg, that are systemic in origin, are many and varied. Pain in this region can result from vascular conditions (like abdominal aortic aneurysm or arterial insufficiency), gastrointestinal disease, cancer, infectious disorders, reproductive conditions, or even a combination of these.[11] This pain can be referred to the gluteal and groin areas and down the thigh to the lower leg from the kidneys, scrotum, abdomen, or peritoneal area,[11] which can make screening for OT intervention a challenge.

The process of screening for occupational therapy services entails watching for yellow (caution) or red (warning) flags to direct critical decision-making.[11] OTPs need to ask questions related to significant risk factors, suspicious clinical presentation, past medical history, or associated signs and symptoms. Watching for facial expressions and body language is always important.[11] Pulling together identifiable clusters of signs and symptoms and informing the physician can make the OTP an excellent advocate for their client.

See Table 20.10 for a list of factors to keep in mind when a client presents with gluteal, hip, groin, thigh, and leg pain of unknown or suspicious origin.

See Table 20.11 for a list of various symptoms in neurologic and vascular disorders that can cause leg pain.

TABLE 20.9 Potential Systemic and Neuromuscular Causes of Sacral, SI, and Pelvic Pain

Possible Cause	The Sacrum and SI Joints	The Pelvis
Systemic	Infectious/inflammatory conditions • Vertebral osteomyelitis • Endocarditis • Tuberculosis (uncommon) Spondyloarthropathy • Ankylosing spondylitis • Reactive arthritis • Psoriatic arthritis • IBD (arthritis associated with IBD) Spondylogenic conditions • Fractures (traumatic, insufficiency, pathologic), metabolic bone disease • Osteoporosis (insufficiency fractures) • Paget disease • Osteodystrophy • Osteoarthritis Gynecologic conditions • Reproductive cancers • Uterine fibroids • Ovarian cysts • Endometriosis • PID • Incest/sexual assault • Rectocele, cystocele • Uterine prolapse • Normal pregnancy; multiparity (more than one pregnancy) Gastrointestinal • Ulcerative colitis • Colon cancer • IBS • Crohn's disease (regional enteritis) Cancer • Primary tumors (rare: giant cell, chondrosarcoma, chondroma, synovial villoadenomas, schwannoma, neurofibroma, ependymomas, ganglineuromas) • Metastatic lesions (history of cancer) • Prostate • Lung • Thyroid • Colorectal • Breast • Gastrointestinal • Multiple myeloma • Kidney Other • Fibromyalgia	Gynecologic • Pregnancy (including ectopic, ruptured, or unruptured) • Uterovaginal, urethral, and/or rectal prolapse (rare) • Vulvodynia • Dysmenorrhea • Endometriosis • Premenstrual tension syndrome • Uterine or cervical tumors, fibroids, adhesions, polyps, stenosis • Ovarian cysts, varicosities, torsion, ovulation; any ovarian anomaly • Intrauterine contraceptive device • Adnexal torsion (ovaries, fallopian tubes twisted) (rare) • Spontaneous, therapeutic, or incomplete abortion; postabortion syndrome Infection/inflammation • Septic arthritis; reactive arthritis • Ankylosing spondylitis • Crohn's disease • Acute or chronic appendicitis • Herpes zoster • Osteomyelitis • PID • Sexually transmitted infection • Postpartum infection • Psoas abscess (abdominal or pelvic infectious process) • Osteitis pubis • Shingles (herpes zoster) Vascular disorders • Arterial occlusion; ischemia • Abdominal angina • Abdominal aneurysm • Pelvic congestion • Varicosities or pelvic thrombophlebitis Cancer • Reproductive • Urologic Gastrointestinal disorders • IBD • Crohn's disease • Ulcerative colitis • IBS • Diverticular disease • Constipation (common in older adults) • Neoplasm • Hernia • Bowel obstruction • Abdominal migraine Urogenital • Chronic urinary tract infection • Detrusor-sphincter dyssynergia (bladder spasm) • Interstitial cystitis/painful bladder syndrome • Radiation cystitis • Acute pyelonephritis • Kidney stones (ureteric calculus, urolithiasis) • Chronic nonbacterial prostatitis, prostatodynia, prostate cancer • Chronic orchalgia • Urethral strictures

(Continued)

TABLE 20.9 Potential Systemic and Neuromuscular Causes of Sacral, SI, and Pelvic Pain—cont'd

Possible Cause	The Sacrum and SI Joints	The Pelvis
Neuromuscular/ musculoskeletal/ soft tissue	Neurologic • Nerve root compression (mimics SI joint pain) Joint related • Degenerative joint disease • Discogenic disease (mimics SI joint pain) • Zygapophyseal joint pain (mimics SI joint pain) • Lumbar spine fusion or hip arthrodesis • Enthesis (tendon insertion)/ ligamentous sprain Musculoskeletal • Bone harvesting for grafts (may cause secondary instability) Myofascial or kinetic chain imbalance Myofascial syndromes (mimics SI joint pain) Pelvic floor muscle spasm/myalgia Injury • Trauma (motor vehicle accidents, sexual assault, etc.) Idiopathic (unknown)	Other • Psychogenic; somatization disorder; depression • Sleep disorders • Surgery (abdominal/laparoscopic, tubal, pelvic) • Fibromyalgia • Autonomic nervous system impairment • Paget disease • Lead or mercury toxicity • Substance abuse (cocaine) • Sickle cell anemia Chronic visceral pain syndrome Neurologic • Nerve entrapment (surgical scar in lower abdomen) • Incomplete spinal cord lesion; neoplasia of spinal cord or sacral nerve • Multiple sclerosis • Pudendal neuralgia • Complex regional pain syndrome Joint related • Hip, SI joint, low back, sacral, or coccyx impairment • Total hip arthroplasty (polyethylene wear debris) • Spondylolysis • Pubic strain/sprain/separation (pubis symphysis) • Discogenic lesions (herniation) • Scoliosis Musculoskeletal • Muscle impairment (hamstrings, abdominals, rectus femoris, piriformis, adductor muscles, pelvic floor muscles, pelvic girdle, iliopsoas, quadratus lumborum) • Stress reaction/fracture • Vertebral compression fracture (lumbar spine) • Coccygodynia • Osteoporosis Pelvic floor dysfunctions • Overactive PFM syndrome • Levator ani syndrome • Tension myalgia Injury • Trauma (surgery, labor and delivery, motor vehicle accidents, sexual assault, etc.) • Adhesions Idiopathic (unknown) • Vaginismus • Anismus • Somatization disorders • Abdominal wall myofascial pain, TrPs • Postural alignment issues • Hernia (obturator, sciatic, inguinal, femoral, umbilical)

IBD, Irritable bowel disease; *IBS*, irritable bowel syndrome; *PID*, pelvic inflammatory disease; *PFM*, pelvic floor muscle; *SI*, sacroiliac; *TrPs*, trigger points.
Adapted from Heick J, Lazaro RT. *Goodman and Snyder's Differential Diagnosis for Physical Therapists: Screening for Referral*. 7th ed. Elsevier; 2023.

Neurological Disorders That Can Mimic Musculoskeletal Conditions

Various systemic disorders affecting the neurological system can sometimes mimic musculoskeletal conditions. A few of the more common conditions seen by OTPs can be found in Table 20.12.

Myopathies That Can Mimic Neuromusculoskeletal Injury

Various muscles disorders, known as myopathies, can sometimes mimic neurological or skeletal conditions. A few of the more common conditions seen by OTPs can be found in Table 20.13.

TABLE 20.10 Potential Systemic and Neuromuscular Causes of Gluteal, Hip, Groin, Thigh, and Leg Pain

Possible Cause	Gluteal and Hip Region	Groin and Thigh	Knee and Leg (Specifically Sciatica)
Systemic	Gluteal specific • Sciatica from tumor, infection, endometriosis • Sacroiliitis (pyogenic infection, reactive arthritis, spondyloarthritis) • Neoplasm (primary or regional metastases via lymph nodes) • Osteoid osteoma of the upper femur • Osteomyelitis of the upper femur • Septic arthritis (hip, SI) • Abscess from aseptic necrosis, Crohn's disease, or other retroperitoneal infection; anorectal abscess • Sacral neuralgia from genital herpes • Ischemia (e.g., claudication from PVD, peripheral arterial aneurysm) Cancer • Lumbar or sacral cord tumor • Bone tumor • Pancreatic cancer • Spinal metastases • Kidney • Testicle • Prostate • Osteoid osteoma • Chondrosarcoma • Giant cell tumor • Ewing sarcoma Vascular • Arterial insufficiency • Abdominal aortic aneurysm • Avascular necrosis Urogenital • Kidney (renal) impairment; kidney stones • Testicular cancer Infectious/inflammatory conditions • Abdominal or peritoneal inflammation • Ankylosing spondylitis • Appendicitis • Ischial rectal abscess • Crohn's disease; ulcerative colitis • Diverticulitis	Cancer • Spinal cord tumor • Osteoid osteoma • Hodgkin disease/lymphoma • Leukemia • Testicular • Prostate • Soft tissue mass • Metastasis to the nodes located in the groin Fluid in peritoneal cavity • Ascites (cirrhosis) • Congestive heart failure • Cancer • Hyperaldosteronism Hemophilia • GI bleeding Gynecologic conditions • Cancer (uterine/ovarian masses) • Uterine fibroids • Ovarian cyst • Endometriosis (causing pubalgia) • Ectopic pregnancy (not common) • Sexually transmitted infection • PID Infection • Intra-abdominal or intraperitoneal infection Urologic • Prostate impairment such as prostatitis, BPH, or prostate cancer • Epididymitis; testicular torsion • Urethritis/urinary tract infection • Upper urinary tract problems affecting the kidneys or ureters (inflammation, infection, obstruction) • Hydrocele/varicocele GI • Diverticulitis • Inflammatory bowel disease Other • Osteoporosis • Seronegative spondyloarthropathy • Abdominal aortic aneurysm, peripheral arterial aneurysm	Cancer • Bone cancer • Previous history of cancer (metastases) Metabolic • History of diabetes mellitus • Peripheral neuropathy Vascular • Atherosclerosis • Vascular claudication Peritoneal problems • Presence of intraabdominal or peritoneal inflammatory disease (abscess) • Crohn's disease • PID • Diverticulitis • Endometriosis of the sciatic nerve Other • Tobacco use • Radiation therapy (delayed effects; rare) • Recent spinal surgery, especially with instrumentation • Hypermobility syndromes such as Ehlers-Danlos syndrome • Restless leg syndrome

(Continued)

TABLE 20.10 Potential Systemic and Neuromuscular Causes of Gluteal, Hip, Groin, Thigh, and Leg Pain—cont'd

Possible Cause	Gluteal and Hip Region	Groin and Thigh	Knee and Leg (Specifically Sciatica)
	• Osteomyelitis (upper femur) • PID • Reactive arthritis • Inflammatory arthritis, RA, SLE, seronegative arthropathy, gout) • Septic hip or SI arthritis • Septic hip bursitis • Tuberculosis Metabolic disorders • Osteomalacia, osteoporosis • Gaucher disease • Paget disease • Ochronosis • Hemochromatosis • Diabetes mellitus (associated with neuropathy) Other • Sickle cell crisis • Hemophilia • Ectopic pregnancy • Femoral artery catheterization	Thigh specific • Retroperitoneal or intraabdominal tumor or abscess • Kidney stones (nephrolithiasis, ureteral or renal colic) • Peripheral neuropathy (bilateral, symmetric) • Diabetes mellitus • Neoplasm • Chronic alcohol use • Thrombosis (femoral artery, great saphenous vein) • Bone tumor (primary or metastases) • Bone fracture associated with long-term bisphosphonates (rare; under investigation)	
Neuromuscular	Gluteal specific • Sciatica (nerve compression from surrounding soft tissues; piriformis syndrome) • Posterior facet joint dysfunction • Hip joint disease • Disc disease (thoracic or lumbar) • SI joint dysfunction • Bursitis (psoas, gluteal, ischial, trochanteric) • Hamstring strain • Myofascial syndromes • Spondylolisthesis • Direct trauma • Fracture (sacrum, ilium, pubic ramus) Neurologic • Nerve root compression • Intercostal neuritis • Dorsal nerve root irritation • Lumbar spine problems (especially spondylosis, stenosis, disc), SI joint, sacral, or knee pathology • FAI • Peripheral nerve injury or entrapment; meralgia paresthetica	Neurologic • Nerve compression or entrapment (ilioinguinal, obturator nerves) Musculoskeletal • Musculotendinous strain (adductors, hamstrings, iliopsoas, abdominals, tensor fascia lata, gluteus medius) • Internal oblique avulsion Nerve compression or entrapment (ilioinguinal, obturator nerves) • Stress reaction, stress fracture, avulsion fracture, or complete bone fracture (femoral neck, pubic ramus) • Bursitis (iliopectineal) • Subluxation, dislocation, dysplasia • Labral tear with or without femoroacetabular impingement • SI joint impairment • Lumbar spine impairment (spinal stenosis, disc disease) • Myofascial dysfunction Thoracic disc disease (lower thoracic spine) Other • Pubalgia • Osteitis pubis • Apophysitis (young athletes)	Neurologic • Nerve root compression • Neurogenic claudication Musculoskeletal • Fibromyalgia • Leg length discrepancy • Congenital hip dysplasia; hip or knee subluxation or dislocation • Degenerative disc disease • Piriformis syndrome • Spinal stenosis Injury • Previous low back injury or trauma; direct fall on knee or twisted ankle; gunshot wound • Decubitus ulcer Other • Pregnancy • Work- or occupation-related posture or repetitive movement disorders Knee specific • Musculotendinous strains (e.g., adductor, abductor, quadriceps) • Total knee arthroplasty Torn knee ligaments (ACL, PCL) and/or meniscus Ankle specific • Sprained ankle

Musculoskeletal
- Osteoarthritis
- Synovitis
- Femoral, inguinal, or sports hernia/athletic pubalgia
- Bursitis (trochanteric, iliopectineal, iliopsoas, ischial)
- Fasciitis, myofascial pain
- Muscle impairment (weakness, loss of flexibility, abnormal tone/strain/tear/avulsion); snapping hip syndrome
- Tendinopathy (tendinitis, tendinosis)
- Piriformis syndrome
- Stress reaction/fracture
- Occult fracture of the femoral neck
- Total hip arthroplasty
- Implant loosening
- Bone loss; subsidence
- Acetabular labral or cartilage lesion
- Developmental hip dysplasia; hip dislocation
- Legg-Calvé-Perthes disease
- SCFE

Vascular
- Intraoperative blood vessel injury
- Avascular necrosis of the femoral head
- Osteitis pubis (pubic pain radiates to anterior hip)

Other
- Postoperative pain
- Infection
- Osteitis pubis (pubic pain radiates to anterior hip)

- Trauma (physical, sexual, birth)
- Sports, inguinal, or femoral hernia
- Hip joint impairment
- Avascular necrosis (osteonecrosis)
- Total hip arthroplasty (loosening, infection, bone loss, subsidence)
- SCFE
- Legg-Calvé-Perthes disease
- Arthritis, arthrosis

Thigh specific
- Musculotendinous strains (e.g., adductor, abductor, quadriceps)
- Iliopectineal bursitis (anterior and medial thigh pain); trochanteric bursitis/greater trochanteric pain syndrome (lateral thigh)
- Peripheral neuropathy (unilateral, asymmetric)
- Contusions (collisions with balls, hockey pucks, the ground, other athletes)
- Nerve compression (e.g., meralgia paresthetica from compression of the LFCN, sciatic nerve, obturator nerve)
- Myositis ossificans (injury with contusion and hematoma formation)
- Femoral shaft or subtrochanteric stress reaction or fracture; insufficiency fracture/stress reaction
- Hip disease (osteoarthritis, labral tear)
- Total hip arthroplasty (loose component, polyethylene wear debris, undersized/oversized femoral stem, periosteal irritation)
- SI joint dysfunction
- Upper lumbar spine dysfunction; spondylolisthesis, herniated disc, previous surgery

ACL, Anterior cruciate ligament; *BPH*, benign prostatic hypertrophy; *FAI*, femoroacetabular Impingement; *GI*, gastrointestinal; *LFCN*, lateral femoral cutaneous nerve; *PCL*, posterior cruciate ligament; *PID*, pelvic inflammatory disease; *PVD*, peripheral vascular disease; *RA*, rheumatoid arthritis; *SCFE*, slipped capital femoral epiphysis; *SI*, sacroiliac; *SLE*, systemic lupus erythematosus.
Adapted from Heick J, Lazaro FT. *Goodman and Snyder's Differential Diagnosis for Physical Therapists: Screening for Referral*. 7th ed. Elsevier; 2023.

TABLE 20.11 Potential Neurologic and Vascular Disorders That Can Cause Leg Pain

Disorder	Clinical Presentation
Vascular claudication	Cause: Atherosclerosis in the peripheral arteries Age of onset: • Typically begins in people over age 40 Symptoms: • Pain is usually bilateral • No burning or dysesthesia • Decreased or absent pulses • Change in color and skin of the feet • Normal DTRs may be absent in people older than 60 • Sciatica possible (ischemia) • Pain is consistent in all spinal positions; brought on by physical exertion (e.g., walking, positive van Gelderen bicycle test); increased by climbing stairs or walking uphill (increased metabolic demand) • Relieved promptly by standing still, sitting down, or resting (1–5 min)
Neurogenic claudication	Cause: Can be caused by neoplasm or abscess, disc protrusion, osteophyte formation, or ligamentous thickening Age of onset: • Typically begins in people over age 40 Symptoms: • Pain is usually bilateral but may be unilateral • Burning and dysesthesia in the back, buttocks, and/or legs • Normal pulses • Good skin nutrition • Depressed or absent ankle jerks • Positive pain on SLR • Sciatica • Positive "shopping cart" sign (leaning forward on supportive surface; unable to straighten up because of painful symptoms) • Pain is usually in the low back, buttocks, thighs, calves, feet • Pain is increased in spinal extension, with walking; increased by walking downhill (increased lumbar lordosis) • It is less painful when walking uphill • Pain is decreased by sitting, lying down, bending forward, or flexion exercises (may persist for hours)
Peripheral neuropathy	Cause: More than 100 causes: diabetes; medication; accident; nerve compression; metal toxicity; nutritional deficiency; diseases such as RA, SLE, AIDS; cancer; hypothyroidism; alcoholism Age of onset: • Age of onset varies Symptoms: • Pain, aching, and numbness of feet (and hands) • Motor, sensory, and autonomic changes: burning, prickling, or tingling may be present; extreme sensitivity to touch (or numbness); weakness, falling (foot drop), muscle atrophy; infection, ulcers, gangrene • Feet and hands in stocking-glove pattern • Relieved by pain medication and relaxation techniques; treatment of underlying cause
Restless leg syndrome	Cause: Cause unknown; may be a sleep disorder, arterial disorder, or dysautonomic disorder of the autonomic nervous system; may occur with dehydration or as a side effect of many medications and possibly caffeine, pregnancy, or iron deficiency Age of onset: • Age of onset varies Symptoms: • Crawling, creeping sensation in legs; involuntary • Involuntary contractions of calf muscles, occurring especially at night • Pain or other symptoms can be mild to severe, lasting seconds, minutes, or hours • Sleep disturbance • Paresthesia of the feet, calves, and legs Factors that can decrease symptoms: eliminate caffeine; increase iron intake, movement, walking, moderate exercise; medication; stretching; maintain hydration; heat or cold

DTR, Deep tendon reflexes; *RA*, rheumatoid arthritis; *SLE*, systemic lupus erythematosus; *SLR*, straight leg raise.

From Heick J, Lazaro RT. *Goodman and Snyder's Differential Diagnosis for Physical Therapists: Screening for Referral*. 7th ed. Elsevier; 2023.

TABLE 20.12 Potential Neurologic Disorders That Can Mimic Musculoskeletal Conditions

Disorder	Clinical Presentation
Multiple sclerosis (MS)	Cause: An autoimmune disorder, with an unknown cause, characterized by inflammation and demyelination of neurons in the central nervous system (CNS) Typical Age of Onset: Around ages 20 to 50 Symptoms: • Impaired vision, typically in one eye • Vertigo • Fatigue • Paresthesia • Bowel or bladder dysfunction • Muscle weakness • Spasticity • Ataxia (lack of coordination, resulting in slurred speech, stumbling and wide gait, trouble with fine motor tasks, and problems with eye movements) • Babinski sign (a reflex tested by stroking the bottom of the foot, noted as positive when the toes abduct, indicating potential CNS involvement)
Guillain-Barré syndrome (GBS)	Cause: An acquired autoimmune disorder, with an unknown cause but typically occurring after an infection or a stressful event. It is characterized by inflammation and demyelination of neurons in the peripheral nervous system (PNS). Typical Age of Onset: All age groups can be affected. Symptoms: • A sudden onset of paralysis • Hyporeflexia • Paresthesia • Muscle weakness • Pain • Oculomotor dysfunction • Ataxia
Lyme disease	Cause: Although this disorder is from the bite of a deer tick carrying a bacterium called *Borrelia* burgdorferi, because of the neurological conditions that can occur with this disorder, it is included here. Typical Age of Onset: Almost any age Symptoms: • Erythema migrans ("bull's eye" rash) around the area of the tick bite • Flu-like symptoms • Arthritis will later begin to appear along with neurologic signs and symptoms such as stiff neck, severe headache, meningitis, Bell's palsy radiculopathy, numbness, memory loss, and loss of motor coordination.
Amyotrophic lateral sclerosis (Lou Gehrig's disease)[37,38]	Cause: This is a neurodegenerative condition with an unknown cause. It targets both motor neurons, in the central nervous system (upper motor neurons) and in the peripheral nervous system (lower motor neurons). It is a fatal disorder with quick progression of signs and symptoms. Typical Age of Onset: Around ages 55 to 75 Symptoms: • Muscle stiffness • Hyperreflexia • Difficulty breathing • Limited endurance • Muscle weakness • Atrophy • Respiratory failure

(Continued)

TABLE 20.12 Potential Neurologic Disorders That Can Mimic Musculoskeletal Conditions—cont'd

Disorder	Clinical Presentation
Cerebrovascular accident (CVA or stroke)[39]	Cause: CVA is a term used to describe the disruption in the flow of blood to the brain. There are two types of CVAs, one type is caused by a blockage in a blood vessel (ischemic) and the other type is caused by a rupture in a blood vessel (hemorrhagic). A CVA or stroke typically produces symptoms on one side of the body. Typical Age of Onset: CVAs typically occur in older adults but can occur at any age. Symptoms: • Sudden weakness or paralysis on one side of the body • Sudden headache with nausea or vomiting • Possible facial droop on one side • Blurry, double, worsening, or darkened vision • Difficulty with functional mobility • Dizziness • Loss of sitting and/or standing balance • Decrease in gross motor and fine motor coordination • Speech deficits—difficulty speaking or understanding speech
Cerebral palsy (CP)[40,41]	Cause: This is a group of conditions affecting movement, motor control, balance, and posture. It occurs when there is damage to the developing brain. Typical Age of Onset: The brain damage that can lead to a diagnosis of CP can occur in utero (most common), during birth, or from an injury after birth. Symptoms (can vary): • Exaggerated reflexes • Dystonia, ranging from hypotonicity to spasticity • Choreoathetoid (involuntary) twitching or writhing movements • Difficulty swallowing • Difficulty with functional mobility • Difficulty with fine motor skills (thus affecting developmental milestones) • Eye movement imbalance • Ataxia Types: • **Spastic cerebral palsy** with stiff muscles and sometimes choreoathetoid movements. This can be in the form of *spastic hemiplegia*, affecting either the right or left half of the body, *spastic diplegia*, affecting the legs more than the arms, and *spastic quadriplegia*, affecting all four extremities. • **Dyskinetic cerebral palsy** with involuntary and uncomfortable jerky movement of the arms, legs, or face. • **Ataxic cerebral palsy** with deficits related to depth perception and balance. • There can also be **Mixed types**.
Disorders affecting cognition	Cognitive disorders like Parkinson's disease and Alzheimer's disease are covered in Chapter 22.

From Heick J, Lazaro RT. *Goodman and Snyder's Differential Diagnosis for Physical Therapists: Screening for Referral*. 7th ed. Elsevier; 2023.

TABLE 20.13 **Potential Disorders of the Muscle Fibers That Can Mimic Musculoskeletal Injury**

Disorder	Clinical Presentation
Muscular dystrophy (MD)[42]	Cause: This is a group of conditions that cause progressive loss of muscle mass with resultant weakness, caused by gene mutations that interfere with the production of the proteins that form heathy muscle. There are different types of MD, but the most common are Duchenne and Becker.
	Duchenne MD Typical Age of Onset: Symptoms typically appear in early childhood. This is more common in boys, but girls can be carriers.
	Symptoms: • Frequent falls • Difficulty with changing positions, specifically from a supine or sitting position. Child might need to use their hands to push on the quadriceps muscles to assist in standing (Gower's sign) • Difficulty with gross motor movements (running, ambulating) • Prominent calf muscles • Delays in growth • Learning disabilities
	Becker MD Typical Age of Onset: Symptoms typically appear in the teens but might not occur until the mid-twenties.
	Symptoms: While similar to those of Duchene symptoms tend to be less severe and progress at a slower rate.
Rhabdomyolysis	Cause: This condition is potentially fatal and a definitive **red flag** situation. It occurs when myoglobin and other components of muscle fibers are released into the blood stream because of damage to the muscle cells. This cellular damage can result from trauma, severe burns, overexertion, liver impairment, alcohol abuse, various illicit drugs, high doses of medications metabolized in the liver (such as acetaminophen, diuretics, or statins), and, more recently, Long COVID-19.
	Typical Age of Onset: More likely to occur in adults
	Symptoms: • Muscle aches, cramps, and soreness • Respiratory difficulties • Liver and renal involvement • Reddish-brown urine • Decrease in urine output • Fever • Fatigue • Nausea and vomiting • Confusion
Dermatomyositis[43]	Cause: This is a type of polymyositis, meaning it is an inflammation that affects muscles and one or more systems, in this case, the integumentary system (the skin). This disorder is a serious illness that can become fatal.
	Typical Age of Onset: This typically begins when children are between the ages of 5 and 15 or when adults are between the ages of 40 and 60.
	Symptoms: • Muscle weakness • Muscle degeneration • Rashes on the skin (typically around the eyelids, scalp, neck, and shoulders) • Difficulty breathing • Difficulty changing positions: from lying to sitting, from sitting to standing • Trouble with climbing stairs • Bumps on the knees and elbows • Joint pain • Rough cuticles and visible blood vessels around the folds of fingernails

From Heick J, Lazaro RT. *Goodman and Snyder's Differential Diagnosis for Physical Therapists: Screening for Referral*. 7th ed. Elsevier; 2023.

The OT Scope of Practice

Knowledge of the possible conditions that can refer pain to a region is one of the keys to quick and accurate screening.[11] Remember, OTPs do not diagnose. They work within their scope of practice as designated by the American Occupational Therapy Association (AOTA) and their state licensing board.[44] OTPs must work inside of the box but be able to think outside of the box when screening clients for possible intervention. Collecting information and relaying it to the physician for further workup is one of the most beneficial actions OTPs can take for their clients.

Some tools are available to aid the occupational therapy team in the screening process. Many can be found in the Quality toolkit on the AOTA website.[45] There are also screening tools developed in the physical therapy community that could be useful for OTPs as well, including the OSPRO for Musculoskeletal Pain Conditions (OSPRO) and the OSPRO: Review of System (OSPRO-ROS).[46] The OSPRO-YF adds the psychosocial domains to look more closely at various domains (negative mood domain, fear-avoidance domain, and positive affect and coping).[47]

Application—Case Study

CASE EXAMPLE 20.1

A 68-year-old female was referred to an OT practitioner (OTP) in an outpatient setting with left shoulder pain of unknown origin. The client reported that it may have started while lifting groceries or maybe that is when she first noticed the pain. She was uncertain.

1. **Screen:** The client seemed a little lethargic and tired. Picking up on this, the OTP asked her pertinent questions about her overall health.
2. **Take a Closer Look:** The client reported feeling tired and having lost weight recently without trying. So, the OTP began to ask more questions related to medical history, including medications and past illnesses. The client reported that she underwent a partial mastectomy 6 years ago in her left breast. This information was not in the chart the OTP had been given.
3. **Determine Flag Status:** The OTP determined this to be a potential red flag situation.
4. **Take Action if Needed:** The OTP contacted the client's doctor to inform him of her concerns. The doctor ordered a breast examination and mammogram for the client.
5. **Document the Findings:** The OTP documented this information as well as the phone call with the doctor.
6. **Take a Second Look:** On breast examination, the physician found a quarter-sized lump on the left side in the area of the past partial mastectomy. Mammogram confirmed the tumor.
7. **Determine the Flag Status:** This was a definitive red flag.
8. **Take Action if Needed:** The client was operated on that week for a full mastectomy and lymph node removal. She returned to the OTP 6 months later with flowers and a thank you for saving her life.

This is a true case. Knowing the questions to ask and the potential reasons for systemic pain can be a great asset for an OTP. Once again, an OTP was a hero in someone's life.

CASE EXAMPLE 20.2

A 75-year-old male inpatient, recovering after removal of a ruptured spleen due to an automobile accident, presents with left shoulder pain consistent with Kehr sign.

1. **Screen:** The OTP saw the client at bedside. He was sitting up in bed with good color and seemed in good spirits but complained of shoulder discomfort that "hurts even more than the incision site from the spleen surgery."
2. **Take a Closer Look:** The OTP lightly palpated the shoulder which elicited the pain over the insertion of the supraspinatus tendon. When palpating the area of the spleen, she was unable to elicit a similar response in the shoulder.
3. **Determine Flag Status:** The OTP determined this to be an interesting situation but followed the palpation with some questions related to the client's past medical history. She learned that the client had undergone surgical repair of the left rotator cuff 5 years earlier due to a torn supraspinatus tendon. Because palpation at the site of the spleen did not elicit pain, the OTP believed that this did not fit the cluster of identifiable signs and symptoms typically seen with Kehr sign.
4. **Take Action if Needed:** The OTP contacted the client's doctor to inform him that the client did not exhibit the Kehr sign but did have symptoms more in line with a new tear to his rotator cuff.
5. **Document the Findings:** The OTP documented this information as well as the interaction with the doctor.
6. **Take a Second Look:** The physician referred the client to the orthopedic physician, who determined that there was indeed a tear to the rotator cuff that probably occurred during the car accident and went undetected because of the urgency of the splenectomy.
7. **Determine the Flag Status:** This had quickly become a yellow flag, as it was not life-threatening, but it was a red flag for the client who was in severe pain.
8. **Take Action if Needed:** The client was again seen in surgery for rotator cuff repair and returned to the OTP 2 days later. He thanked the OTP for being "the only observant individual in the hospital."

This is a true case. This OTP was able to help the doctors with clues to the client's condition and helped to redirect the course of his rehabilitation with a much better outcome.

References

1. Diguiseppi J, Tadi P. Neuroanatomy, postcentral gyrus. In: *StatPearls*. NIH; 2023. https://www.ncbi.nlm.nih.gov/books/NBK549825/.
2. Johns Hopkins. *Brain Anatomy and How the Brain Works*. Johns Hopkins; 2024. https://www.hopkinsmedicine.org/health/conditions-and-diseases/anatomy-of-the-brain.
3. Stiepan, D. *Mayo Clinic: How Hearing Affects Your Brain Health*. Mayo Clinic; 2022. https://newsnetwork.mayoclinic.org/discussion/mayo-clinic-minute-how-hearing-affects-your-brain-health/.
4. D'Angelo, S. The sweet spot: research locates taste center in the brain. *Cornell Chronicle*; 2019. https://news.cornell.edu/stories/2019/03/sweet-spot-research-locates-taste-center-brain.
5. Physiopedia. *Olfactory Cortex*. Physiopedia; 2024. https://www.physio-pedia.com/Olfactory_Cortex.
6. Macefield VG, Knellwolf TP. Functional properties of human muscle spindles. *J Neurophysiol*. 2018;120(2):452–467. https://doi.org/10.1152/jn.00071.2018.

7. TeachMe Anatomy. *The Ascending Tracts*. TeachMe Anatomy; 2024. https://teachmeanatomy.info/neuroanatomy/pathways/ascending-tracts-sensory/.
8. Chen WG, Schloesser D, Arensdorf AM, et al. The merging science of interoception: sensing, integrating, interpreting, and regulating signals within the self. *Trends Neurosci*. 2021;44(1):3–16. https://doi.org/10.1016/j.tins.2020.10.007.
9. Whitehead A, Grider MH. Neuroanatomy, touch receptor. In: *StatPearls*. NIH; 2023. https://www.ncbi.nlm.nih.gov/books/NBK547731/.
10. Pinho-Ribeiro FA, Verri WA, Chiu IM. Nociceptor sensory neuron-immune interactions in pain and inflammation. *Trends Immunology*. 2016;38(1):5–19. https://doi.org/10.1016/j.it.2016.10.001.
11. Heick J, Lazaro RT. *Goodman and Snyder's Differential Diagnosis for Physical Therapists: Screening for Referral*. 7th ed. Elsevier; 2023.
12. AOTA. Occupational Therapy Practice Framework: Domain and Process, 4th ed. *Am J Occup Ther*. 2020; 74(Suppl.2):7412410010p1–7412410010p87. https://doi.org/10.5014/ajot.2020.74S2001.
13. Butera KA, George SZ, Lentz TA. Psychometric evaluation of the Optimal Screening for Prediction of Referral and Outcome Yellow Flag (OSPRO-YF) tool: factor structure, reliability, and validity. *J Pain*. 2020;21(5–6):557–569. https://doi.org/10.1016/j.jpain.2019.09.003.
14. IHS. *International Classification of Headache Disorders*. 3rd ed. The International Headache Society; 2018. https://ichd-3.org/.
15. Babale C. Different types of headaches and when to see a doctor. *eMediHealth*. 2023. https://www.emedihealth.com/nervous-system/migraine-headache/treat-headache.
16. Vaskovic J. *Vertebral Artery*. Ken Hub; 2023. https://www.kenhub.com/en/library/anatomy/vertebral-artery.
17. Lucas JW, Conner EM, Bose J. *Back, Lower Limb, and Upper Limb Pain Among U.S. Adults, 2019*. Centers for Disease Control and Prevention: National Center for Health Statistics; 2021:415. https://www.cdc.gov/nchs/products/databriefs/db415.htm#section_2.
18. Mayo Clinic. *Sacroilitis*. Mayo Clinic; 2023. https://www.mayoclinic.org/diseases-conditions/sacroiliitis/symptoms-causes/syc-20350747.
19. Bordoni B, Marelli F, Morabito B, et al. Low back pain and gastroesophageal reflux in patients with COPD: the disease in the breath. *Int J Chronic Obstr Pulmonary Dis*. 2018;13:325–334. https://doi.org/10.2147/COPD.S150401.
20. Yetman D. Overview of renal parenchymal disease. *Healthline*. 2024. https://www.healthline.com/health/kidney-disease/renal-parenchymal-disease.
21. Huizen J. What to know about diaphragmatic endometriosis. *Med N Today*. 2023. https://www.medicalnewstoday.com/articles/321412.
22. Kesikburun, et al.Güzelküçük S, Fidan U, et al. Musculoskeletal pain and symptoms in pregnancy: a descriptive study. *Therapeutic Adv Musculoskelet Dis*. 2018;10(12):229–234. https://doi.org/10.1177/1759720X18812449.
23. Dorwart L. Thoracic endometriosis. *VeryWellHealth*. 2023. https://www.verywellhealth.com/thoracic-endometriosis-7484050.
24. AHA. *Signs and Symptoms of Pericarditis*. American Heart Association; 2021. https://www.heart.org/en/health-topics/pericarditis/symptoms-and-diagnosis-of-pericarditis.
25. Mayo Clinic. *Breast Cysts. Angina*. 2022. https://www.mayoclinic.org/diseases-conditions/angina/symptoms-causes/syc-20369373.
26. Hambrecht R, Berra K, Calfas KJ. Managing your angina symptoms with nitroglycerin: what about exercise? *Circulation*; 2013; 127(22):e642–e654. https://doi.org/10.1161/CIRCULATIONAHA.113.000821.
27. AOTA. Occupational Therapy Scope of Practice. America Occupational Therapy Association. *Am J Occup Ther*. 2021;75(Supplement 3):7513410020. https://doi.org/10.5014/ajot.2021.75S3005.
28. Mayo Clinic. *Breast Cysts*. Mayo Clinic; 2024. https://www.mayoclinic.org/diseases-conditions/breast-cysts/symptoms-causes/syc-20370284.
29. Johns Hopkins. *Gynecomastia*. Johns Hopkins Health; 2024. https://www.hopkinsmedicine.org/health/conditions-and-diseases/gynecomastia.
30. Clevland Clinic. *Tietze Syndrome*. Cleveland Clinic, 2022. https://my.clevelandclinic.org/health/diseases/23565-tietze-syndrome.
31. Noor N, Amgalan A, Vij N. Treatment and management of xiphoidalgia. *Orthopedic Rev*. 2022;14(3):37070. https://doi.org/10.52965/001c.37070.
32. Physiopedia. *Slipping Rib Syndrome*. Physiopedia; 2024. https://www.physio-pedia.com/Slipping_Rib_Syndrome.
33. Basinger H, Hogg JP. Anatomy, abdomen and pelvis: femoral triangle. In: *StatsPearls*. *National Institute of Health*; 2023. https://www.ncbi.nlm.nih.gov/books/NBK541140/.
34. AOTA. *Quality Toolkit*. American Occupational Therapy Association; 2024. https://www.aota.org/practice/practice-essentials/quality/quality-toolkit.
35. George SZ, Beneciuk JM, Lentz TA, et al. Optimal Screening for Prediction of Referral and Outcome (OSPRO) for musculoskeletal pain conditions: results from the validation cohort. *J Orthopedic Sports Phys Ther*. 2018;48(6):460–475. https://www.jospt.org/doi/10.2519/jospt.2018.7811.
36. Razmjou Hh, Palinkas V, Robarts S, Kennedy D. Psychometric properties of the OSPRO-YF screening tool in patients with shoulder pathology. *Physiother Can*. 2021;73(1):26–36. https://doi.org/10.3138/ptc-2019-0046.
37. Johns Hopkins. *Health. What Is Trigeminal Neuralgia?* Johns Hopkins; 2025. https://www.hopkinsmedicine.org/health/conditions-and-diseases/trigeminal-neuralgia.
38. Mayo Clinic. *Trigeminal Neuralgia*. Johns Hopkins; 2023. https://www.mayoclinic.org/diseases-conditions/trigeminal-neuralgia/symptoms-causes/syc-20353344.
39. Cleveland Clinic. *Glossopharyngeal Neuralgia (GPN)*. Cleveland Clinic; 2024. https://my.clevelandclinic.org/health/diseases/15799-glossopharyngeal-neuralgia-gpn.
40. Marks, H, Ellis, RR. *Occipital Neuralgia: What Is It?* Web MD, 2024. https://www.webmd.com/migraines-headaches/occipital-neuralgia-symptoms-causes-treatments
41. Cleveland Clinic. *Amyotrophic Lateral Sclerosis (ALD)*. Cleveland Clinic; 2024. https://my.clevelandclinic.org/health/diseases/16729-amyotrophic-lateral-sclerosis-als.
42. Yang X, Ji Y, Wang W, et al. *Amyotrophic Lateral Sclerosis: Molecular Mechanisms, Biomarkers, and Therapeutic Strategies*. NIH: National Library of Medicine; 2021. https://pmc.ncbi.nlm.nih.gov/articles/PMC8300638/.
43. Ellis ME. Cerebrovascular accident. *Healthline*. 2018 https://www.healthline.com/health/cerebrovascular-accident#types.

44. Mayo Clinic. *Cerebral Palsy*. Mayo Clinic; 2023. https://www.mayoclinic.org/diseases-conditions/cerebral-palsy/symptoms-causes/syc-20353999.
45. NIH. *What Are the Types of Cerebral Palsy?* NIH: Eunice Kenedy Shriver National Institute of Child Health and Human Development; 2021. https://www.nichd.nih.gov/health/topics/cerebral-palsy/conditioninfo/types.
46. Mayo Clinic. *Muscular Dystrophy*. Mayo Clinic; 2022. https://www.mayoclinic.org/diseases-conditions/muscular-dystrophy/symptoms-causes/syc-20375388.
47. Cleveland Clinic. *Dermatomyositis*. Cleveland Clinic; 2022. https://my.clevelandclinic.org/health/diseases/15701-dermatomyositis.

SECTION III

Pathophysiology Affecting Cognition

Introduction to Section III

This section contains two chapters: Chapters 21 and 22.

Chapter 21 discusses cognition from both historical and theoretical perspectives. Awareness of where the field began and the path it has taken can help those studying cognitive pathophysiology appreciate where scientists currently stand in their understanding of this complex topic. It is ironic that the very processes of thinking and reasoning are both difficult to relate to and yet essential for understanding how we think. Metacognition, or "thinking about thinking," has long eluded scientists. Occupational therapy practitioners (OTPs) address cognitive issues regularly in their client interactions, which is one of the many factors that set occupational therapy apart from other healthcare services. However, the theories behind cognition are many and varied. Reading this chapter will, hopefully, help the reader synthesize the information and form their own interpretation of what may be the best approach.

Chapter 22 discussed types of pathophysiology that could affect cognitive ability. This chapter starts with a neurological overview of the cognitive centers of the brain and then covers neurocognitive disorders. The distinction between delirium and dementia is explored, along with various pathological conditions that can contribute to their development. Traumatic brain injury and adult attention-deficit hyperactivity disorder are also covered. The chapter also briefly discusses medications and cognition.

OTPs are uniquely positioned to address not only physical impairments but also cognitive deficits. Therefore, these authors believe Section III is a particularly important part of this textbook.

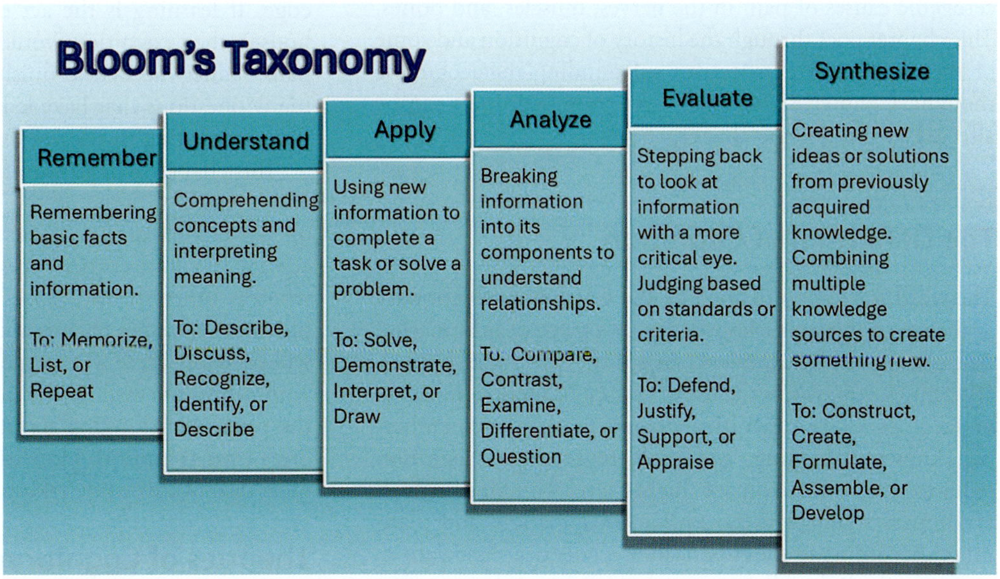

Bloom's Taxonomy. (Courtesy Natalie Norman Michaels. Data https://www.simplypsychology.org/blooms-taxonomy.html.)

21 Cognition: Theoretical Constructs and Historical Overview

OBJECTIVES

By the end of this chapter, the reader should be able to:

- Explain some of the earlier theories used to explain cognitive thought.
- Demonstrate a basic understanding of the way cognitive thought affects everyday choices.
- Compare and contrast theories from various periods of time, such as earlier Herbartian thought with the theories of Behaviorism.
- Justify the need for a systematic approach for clinical decision-making when screening individuals for possible occupational therapy intervention.

Understanding Cognition

This book has covered some of the many systemic and viscerogenic causes of pain in the nerves, muscles, and bones. This chapter goes through the history of cognition and some of the theoretical perspectives surrounding metacognitive thought. Chapter 22 will then cover how cognition can be affected by physiologic change.

The Definition of Cognition

The word *learning* is defined by the Cambridge Dictionary as the act of obtaining knowledge or a piece of information that is acquired by experience or study.[1] This same dictionary defines *cognition* as the use of conscious mental processes or faculties.[2] These faculties include thinking, remembering, knowing, judging, and problem solving.[3] Cognition requires the utilization of higher-level thinking, which encompasses language, perception, imagination, and planning.[3] According to the American Psychological Association, cognition includes all forms of knowledge and awareness, including the acts of perceiving, conceiving, remembering, imagining, judging, reasoning, and problem solving.[4] While learning involves experiences and changes that lead to the acquisition of knowledge, cognition consists of the tools required to incorporate, create, and maintain this knowledge. If learning is the act of building something (e.g., a house), then cognition would be the tools (e.g., a hammer, nails, ladder) needed to finish the project. This brings forth many questions that have led to several theoretical perspectives attempting to address this.

This chapter will go through various theories of learning and cognition. Some of the theoretical perspectives developed over the years have focused solely on an individual's perception of various experiences in order for learning to occur, whereas other theories focus more on the cognitive complexities utilized to change and create knowledge. The reader will probably agree with some of these concepts and disagree with others but will be the ultimate judge! *Metacognition* is the process of thinking about one's own thought processes: one's own cognition. Hopefully, the reader will be doing a great deal of this while taking in the content of this chapter.

Theories of Cognition

Looking at the history of theoretical development should provide an understanding of the trends in thinking over

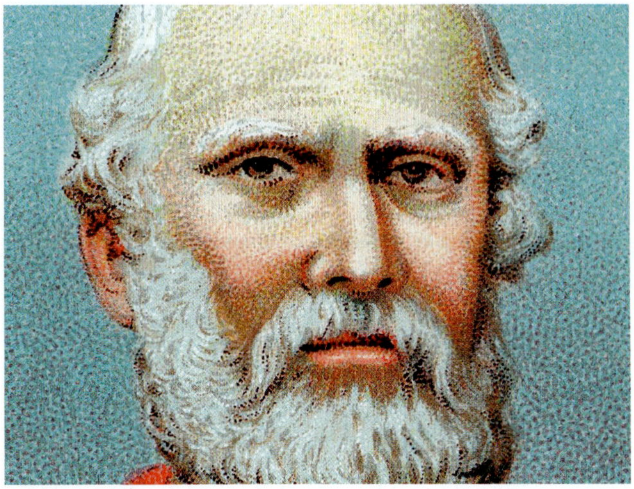

• **Fig. 21.1** Plato. (© Photos.com/Thinkstock.)

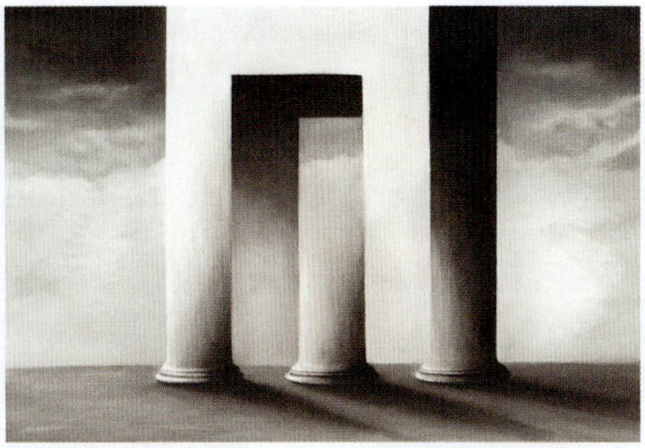

• **Fig. 21.2** Ambiguous figure as an example of perception. (From https://www.iStock.com/francescoch.)

time. Much like the prediction of the path of a hurricane, individuals cannot understand where they are and where they are going without having some knowledge of where they have been. So, the historical context becomes important. The field of learning and cognition is not stagnant, but ever changing and growing along with our knowledge and understanding.

400 Before Common Era (BCE) to the 1800s

The study of learning and cognition dates back thousands of years. It began on a more philosophical note but then changed course in the 1800s when theorists began to ponder the ideas of natural selection and behaviorism. These new ideas made some theorists change the way they perceived learning and cognition from a philosophical perspective to a more psychological one. This historical overview begins with some of the pre-19th-century philosophers.

Plato

One of the most famous of the earlier theoretical perspectives regarding learning and cognition was written by Plato around 400 BCE (Fig. 21.1).[5]

In his work entitled "Allegory of the Cave," which is included in his book *Republic*, Plato suggested that we can only learn from the information that we have taken in with our senses, and that we incorporate this information based on how it is perceived by our minds.[6] He tells a tale about a dialogue between Socrates and Glaucon in which they discussed prisoners who had been residing in a cave since birth. The prisoners are strapped down so all they can see are shadows of their captors. They have never seen anything during their entire lives except for these shadows (Fig. 21.2).

They have never seen each other, the sun, the grass, the animals, or any other human being, except in shadow. In Plato's writing, Socrates asks whether these people believe that the shadows are not just representative images, but actual beings. He suggests that, to these prisoners, all they know is the shadow, so the truth would be nothing more than these shadows. To them, a person looks like a shadow and nothing more. Until they are allowed to sense the world from different perspectives, they will continue to believe (or perceive) that what they have sensed (all they have been shown) is the absolute truth.[6]

When a person has limited information but believes that they know something in its entirety, they may be more likely to make a mistake. The idea behind the allegory of the cave is rooted in sensation and perception. *Sensation* is defined in Britannica as any conscious and concrete experience resulting from the stimulation of a sensory nerve, organ, or area of the brain.[7] *Perception* is the process of translating and organizing various sensory stimulation into a structured experience.[8] Fig. 21.2 depicts an ambiguous figure which becomes more precise as the viewing distance is increased. This is a good example of perception.

If sensation is akin to ingredients in our cupboard, then perception is what we create from those ingredients. The early writings of Plato help us to better understand that to learn, we take in sensations from our environment, and from that, we create our perception. There is no question that the early writings of Plato have influenced many of the learning theories we utilize today.

Tabula Rasa

In the late 1600s, a British philosopher and medical researcher named John Locke (1632–1704) coined the term *tabula rasa,* or "clean tablet" (Fig. 21.3).

Locke, known by many as the "Father of Classical Liberalism," believed that the human mind at birth has no rules for processing information, but as new information is added, the rules of learning are eventually created though one's perception of that incoming information.[9,10] Many philosophers, including Aristotle, believed that the mind was a tabula rasa (smooth or erased slate). Locke, who is believed by some to be one of the greatest philosophers in Europe at the end of the 17th century, wrote the *Essay Concerning Human Understanding* in 1690, where he

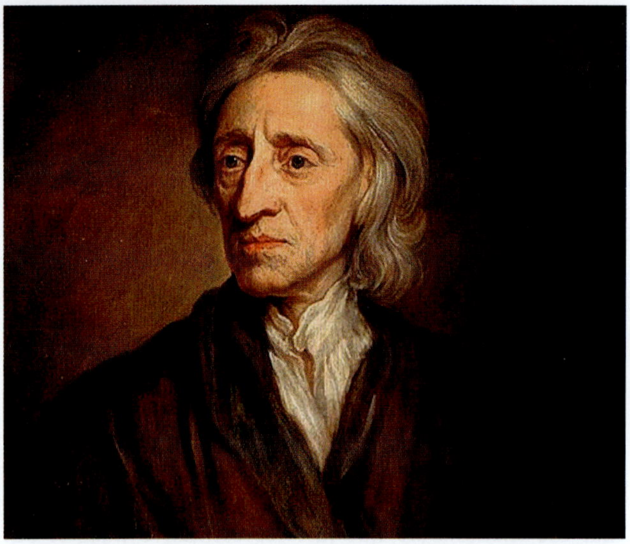

• **Fig. 21.3** John Locke. (From http://www.johnlocke.net/john-locke-maturity-1689-1704/.)

argued that humans have no innate knowledge and that all ideas come from experience.[10]

John Locke's ideas became known as *empiricism*, whereby knowledge comes from experience and people learn the truth about reality from these experiences.[11] This was radical thinking for this time, especially in England. A civil war had just taken place, engulfed by conflicts between the King and Parliament, as well as public unrest regarding differences in religious beliefs.[12] Locke opposed authoritarianism and believed humans should use reason to search for truth rather than accept the opinions of others.

Nature Versus Nurture

At the heart of many theories of learning and cognition is the nature versus nurture controversy.[13] This controversy dates back to Plato's own internal conflict (suggested in his writings) between whether intellect is inherited (*Nature*) or achieved through life experiences (*Nurture*). This debate continues today and is enhanced as we study the human genome and developmental neurobiology, asking whether cognitive ability is gained through genetics, through experience, or through a combination of both.[13] A famous example of this controversy can be seen in Box 21.1.

19th Century and Beyond

The 1800s brought a tide of change as the desire for empirical evidence and scientific study regarding the human mind became more widely recognized. Researchers were hoping for more objective evidence to help explain the workings of the human mind and began to lean away from the more philosophical perspectives of the past regarding learning and cognition.

Herbartian Thought

In the early 1800s, a German philosopher named Johann Friedrich Herbart (1776–1841) was developing a new philosophy on human learning.[15] Herbart was interested in quantitative relationships among ideas and believed researchers could apply complex mathematical equations to describe interactions that occur among ideas in the human mind (Fig. 21.6).

Herbart believed that we have a collection of ideas in the human mind. Some of these ideas oppose each other. This opposition can weaken a new, original idea below the needed threshold for expression. This new idea will stay below the threshold of awareness until a similar idea causes the original one to gain strength, and this will occur at a speed proportionate to the degree of similarity between the two ideas.[15]

• BOX 21.1 The Wild Boy of Aveyron[14] (Language Acquisition: Is It Nature or Nurture?)

It was the year 1800 when he was found on the outskirts of the town of Saint Sernin, France, in the providence of Aveyron; he was a young boy who appeared to have been surviving in the wild all his life. His skin was scarred, and he stood about 4½ feet tall. He was estimated to be about 12 years of age, and the people who found him gave him the name, Victor. Victor was dirty, frightened, and unable to speak. "We'll clean him up and get him into a school, and he will be fine," or so the community thought. Yet no matter how hard they tried, this young boy was unable to learn to communicate through speech (Fig. 21.4). A young man named Jean-Marc-Gaspard Itard decided to give it a try (Fig. 21.5). He worked tirelessly with Victor, believing that the boy's inability to speak might not stem from genetics (Nature) but simply stem from his isolation and his lack of experience (Nurture).

If this was the case, then simply teaching the boy to talk would be the solution. Itard used many conditioning, behavior modification, and modeling techniques when working with Victor. After about 5 years, Victor had made great gains, demonstrating ability to read and write simple sentences, understanding the names of many objects, demonstrating emotion, expressing desires, and obeying commands, but he still could not learn to speak.

Because of both his successes and failures with Victor, Itard's work not only taught the psychological community different teaching strategies (strategies that were way ahead of their time), but it also made researchers more aware of the complexities of human learning. Is some of our ability actually genetic? Could it be that Victor was autistic before he went missing, and Itard's strategies actually allowed Victor to connect with a caring individual?

Do we learn language through socialization (Nurture), or are we born with an innate ability to speak (Nature)? Could it be a combination of both? Does language have a critical period that was simply missed for Victor? This question continued to be asked throughout the 20th century by Skinner, Chomsky, and others and still continues today.

(Continued)

• BOX 21.1 The Wild Boy of Aveyron[14] (Language Acquisition: Is It Nature or Nurture?)—cont'd

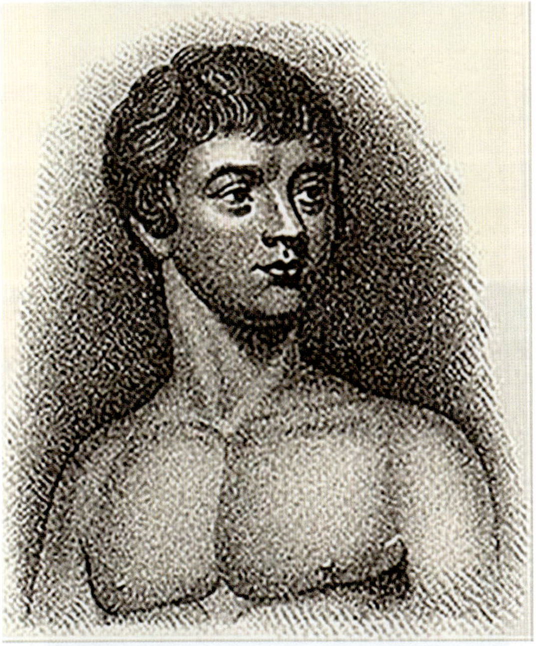

• **Fig. 21.4** Victor of Aveyron. (From https://en.wikipedia.org/wiki/Victor_of_Aveyron.)

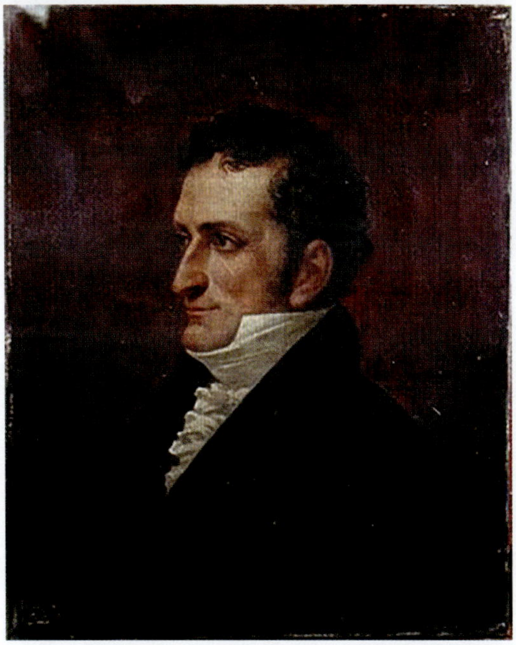

• **Fig. 21.5** Jean-Marc-Gaspard Itard. (From https://commons.wikimedia.org/wiki/File:Jean_marc_gaspard_itard_1775_hi.jpg.)

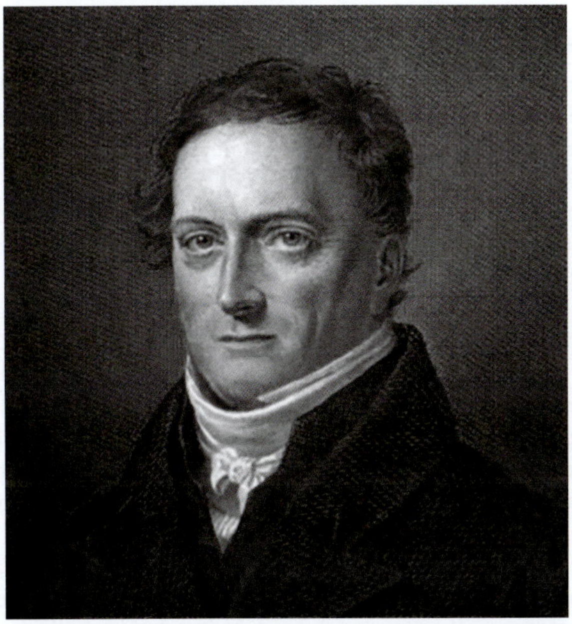

• **Fig. 21.6** Johann Friedrich Herbart. (From "Die großen Deutschen im Bilde" (1936) by Michael Schönitzer.)

According to Herbart's theory, no idea can rise into awareness, unless other ideas are there to help it along. As the original idea rises back into awareness, similar ideas will cling to it, and this cluster of ideas in the human mind make up what Herbart called the *Apperceptive Mass*.[15] The idea is that when teaching students, you can facilitate learning by presenting related ideas with which the student is already familiar. Although not everyone agreed with Herbart's philosophy, his ideas helped build the bridge between the more abstract, philosophical perspectives on human learning to a more concrete, studied psychological forum. His ideas also encouraged Fechner and other early experimentalists to apply mathematics to the psyche.[15]

Natural Selection

Do human beings, as a group, develop and change over the centuries? Charles Darwin brought intrigue to the field when he developed his theory of *Natural Selection* in 1838. Seven years prior, in 1831, Darwin went on a voyage aboard the British HMS Beagle employed as a naturalist to survey the coastline of South America.[16] During this trip through Brazil, Argentina, Chile, and the Galápagos, he collected samples of plants, animals, fossils, and rocks.[16] It was from these samples that his theory began to form (Fig. 21.7).

Darwin actually kept his idea to himself at first, knowing that there may be disagreement from society, until he studied a paper by a naturalist named Alfred Russell Wallace, who had developed a similar idea. The two decided to publish their theory together in 1858 (20 years later).[17] This theory is sometimes called *adaptive evolution*. The idea is that all animals, including humans, will survive and become stronger if they possess certain traits that make survival

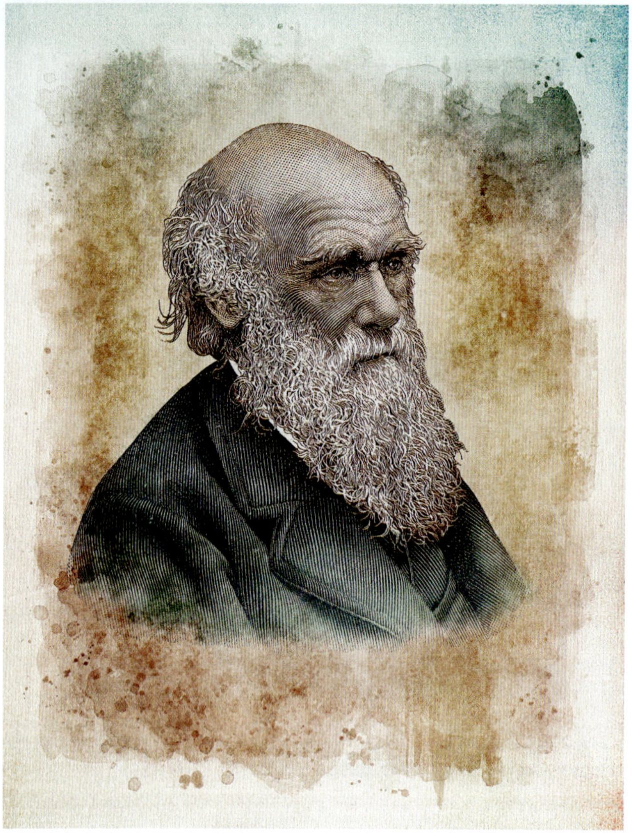

• **Fig. 21.7** Charles Darwin. (From https://iStock.com/Grafissimo.)

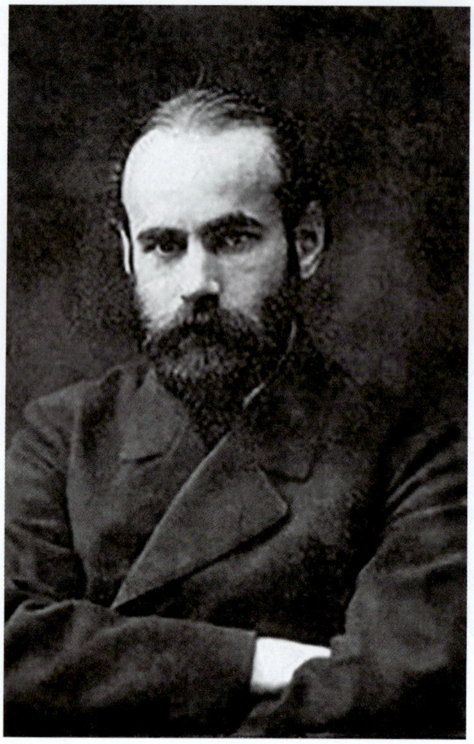

• **Fig. 21.8** Max Wertheimer. (From https://commons.wikimedia.org/wiki/File:Max_Werheimer_(1880-1943).jpg.)

more possible in a given situation. Because these animals are more likely to survive, they are also more likely to reproduce and pass their genes on to future generations. Nature has, therefore, "selected" these traits for the perpetuation of the species. In 1859, Darwin published his book *On the Origin of Species*.[18]

Animal Studies and Behaviorism

One of the major ways we learn is through the observation of animals. Edward Lee Thorndike documented his animal studies in his book *Animal Intelligence: Experimental Studies*, published in 1911.[19] Wolfgang Kohler wrote *The Mentality of Apes* in 1917,[20] and Ivan Pavlov wrote *Conditioned Reflexes* based on his study of dogs in 1927.[21] This marked the beginning of the behaviorist movement. Behaviorism, a term used by John Watson in 1913, is typically defined as a descriptive, objective approach to the study of learning based on the observed behavior in animals and in humans.[22] *Behaviorism* is based on the premise that we make associations with events around us (the stimuli), which cause us to behave in different ways (the responses). While Pavlov and Watson discussed classical conditioning in which the animal receives a stimulus and responds accordingly, Skinner used rats to demonstrate operant conditioning in which the animal makes a choice to act prior to receiving the reinforcement.[23]

Gestalt Theory

Not everyone agreed with the theoretical ideas that stemmed from the behaviorist paradigm. Some of the German theorists at that time believed that the behaviorists focused too much on the collection and analysis of data from the bottom up, without the appreciation of the entire process as a whole. These theorists proposed Gestalt theory. The word *Gestalt* is a German term that refers to an object, concept, or thing made up of many various parts that, when taken together, becomes more than the sum of its parts.[24] *Gestalt Theory* is a school of thought that seeks to understand how the human brain perceives life experiences. This theory was originally proposed by Max Wertheimer, when he wrote "Experimental Studies of the Perception of Movement" in 1912, and other supporters followed (Fig. 21.8).

Wertheimer believed that people tend to organize data and interpret it through grouping. As a result of these mental shortcuts, he came to the conclusion that an individual's perception of the whole is different from the sum of the components.[25] The idea is that the structures of the brain have various properties that are different than the simple sum of their parts.[25] An example when applying this to perception could be letters and words. Letters are just letters, until they come together to form a word, and these words string together into sentences for humans to then interpret as having meaning.[25]

Cognitive Development

Jean Piaget (1896–1980) is believed by many to be the father of *Cognitive Developmental Theory*. He is most famous for his systematic study of cognitive development in children.[26]

Piaget was a Swiss theoretician who began his career as a zoologist but became more interested in psychology as his career progressed. He was inspired by speakers like Carl Jung and Eugen Bleuler.[26] Piaget observed that when children learn, they seem to be creating their own version of reality, gaining mental growth by integrating simpler concepts into more complex concepts at each stage of cognitive change or development (Fig. 21.9).[26]

Piaget was not just interested in how people behave in a given situation, but in how they think and change over time. He concluded that there were four primary stages of cognitive development: the sensorimotor states (from birth to 18 months of age) with object permanence, the preoperational stage (from age 2 to 7 years) with symbolic thought, the concrete operational stage (from age 7 to 11 years) with logical thought, and the formal operational stage (from adolescence to adulthood) with scientific reasoning.

Piaget was not the only developmental theorist who focused on the cognitive realm; for example, James Fowler explained a list of stages for the cognitive development of faith,[27] Lawrence Kohlberg found that there are six developmental stages of moral reasoning,[28] and Carol Gilligan wrote about the stages of moral reasoning and the ethics of care for females.[29]

Contextual Theories

Although Piaget's theories had a high impact on the field of cognitive psychology, some theorists did not agree with his stage theory. They believed that instead of cognitive development occurring in stages, it is more of a continuous process.[30] Some also believed that Piaget's theory failed to take into consideration the *role of situational factors* (the role of the environment, social factors, and contextual factors of learning and behavior).[31] For example, would it be harder to learn in a cold room or in a stark environment? They also wondered if the social processes that occur among and around us affect our ability to learn. These were the issues addressed by Bronfenbrenner and Vygotsky.

Urie Bronfenbrenner was born in Moscow in 1917. He taught at Cornell University for over 50 years and developed his *Bioecological Theory* in 1979.[32] This theory explains the interactions of the many influences that surround and affect the developing person. In Bronfenbrenner's theory, the central focus of learning is the individual person. Over time, he modified his theory adding more of a focus on developmental processes (Fig. 21.10).[33]

Lev Vygotsky was born in Orsha, Russia in 1895.[34] Although he died young from tuberculosis at the age of 37, he was still very influential in the field of cognitive psychology. He developed his *Sociocultural Theory* in the 1930s, but it was not known outside of Russia until well after his death

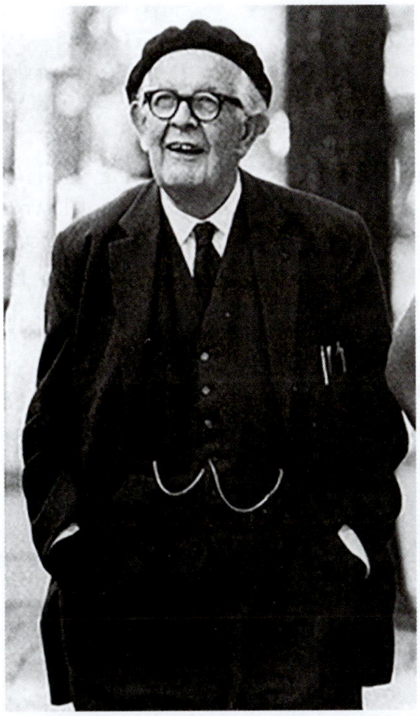

• **Fig. 21.9** Jean Piaget. (From https://commons.wikimedia.org/wiki/File:Jean_Piaget_in_Ann_Arbor.png.)

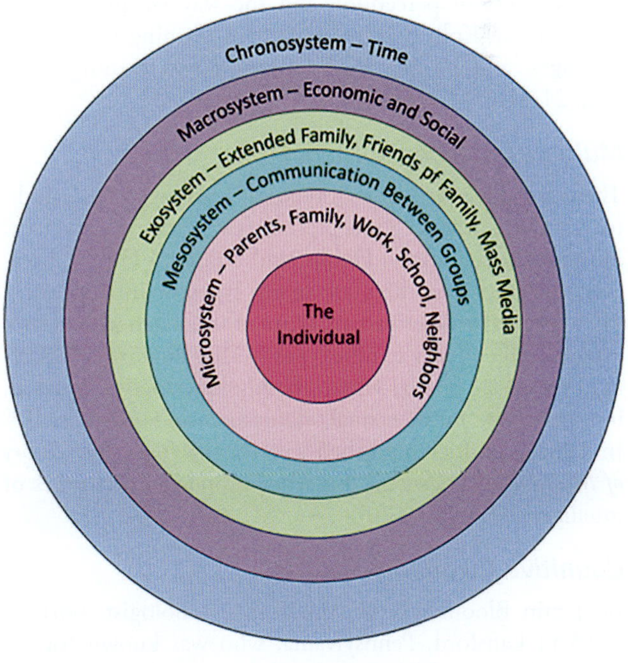

• **Fig. 21.10** Bronfenbrenner's bioecological model, created by Joel Gibbs. (Information from https://www.simplypsychology.org/bronfenbrenner.html.)

in the 1970s.[35] His theory contends that cognitive growth is a collaborative process, very much dependent upon an individual's social, cultural, and historical processes. In Vygotsky's theory, the central focus of learning consists of the social processes the individual experiences.[36]

Information Processing Theories

Encoding, storage, and retrieval might sound like terms from a computer course, but this is the basic premise of the *Information Processing Approach* used to describe human learning and cognition.[37] An individual first receives input (or a stimulus), which is described and stored in the individual's memory to be retrieved when needed. In this model, *sensory memory* holds information perceived through the senses, and although most are ignored, some grab the mind's attention, and those are stored in short-term memory.[37] *Short-term memory* is not meant to be maintained for an extended period of time. However, some important information from short-term memory is encoded and stored into long-term memory. *Working memory* is a type of short-term memory. It pulls components together in an effort to work through and carry out a specific task. *Long-term memory* requires methods to store this information, such as repetition, relating information to other experiences, or breaking it up into chunks.[37]

Learning Style Theory

The focus of learning style theory is that people tend to process information differently based upon their learned and/or inherent traits. There are many different learning style models. In 1975, Rita and Kenneth Dunn defined learning styles as the way in which individuals take in and retain information or skills.[38] In 1984, David Kolb added the elements of perception and the way we process this information. Kolb depicted a cycle of learning that occurs in stages, and he described four different learning styles (Fig. 21.11).[39]

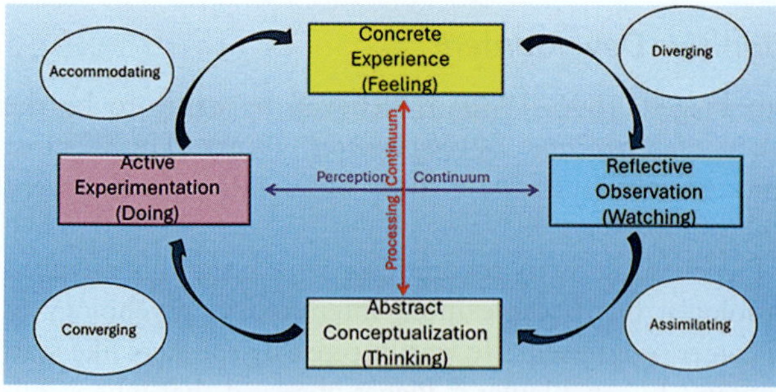

• **Fig. 21.11** Kolb's four learning styles. (Information from https://www.simplypsychology.org/learning-kolb.html.)

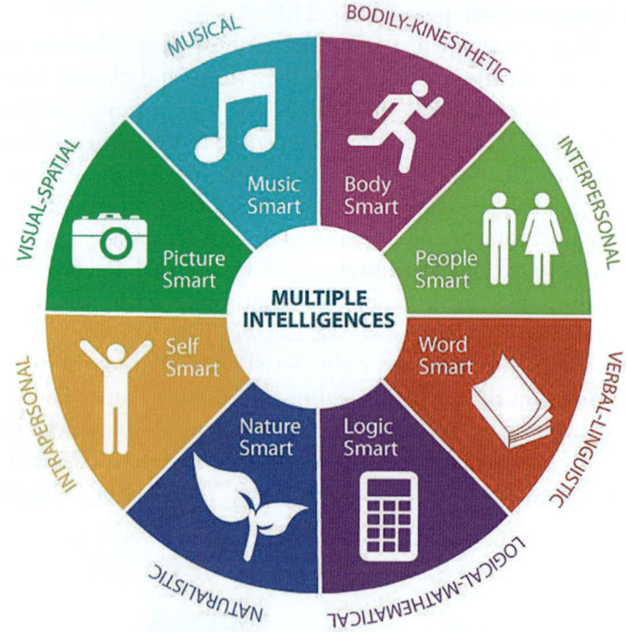

• **Fig. 21.12** Gardner's multiple intelligences. (From Wikipedia Creative Commons. https://en.wikipedia.org/wiki/Theory_of_multiple_intelligences.)

Multiple Intelligence Theory

There are some well-known types of learning: visual, auditory, and kinesthetic. Some professors at Harvard University, Howard Gardner, John Hobbs, and Elizabeth Hobbs, however, believed that there are many types of intelligence.[40] They originally described six types of intelligence that later expanded the theory to nine types (verbal-linguistic, logical-mathematical, spatial-visual, bodily-kinesthetic, musical, interpersonal, intrapersonal, naturalist, and existential).[40] In 1983, Gardner published *Frames of Mind: The Theory of Multiple Intelligences*. This work proposes eight types of intelligence (Fig. 21.12).[41]

Cognitive Taxonomy Theory

Benjamin Bloom was an American psychologist, born in 1913 in Lansford, Pennsylvania, who was known for his optimistic view of education and the impact of education to make human potential possible.[42] He initially focused his research on educational settings and other learning environments as well as mastery learning. He later became known for his hierarchical classification of learning objectives. Although he proposed three psychological domains required for any task (cognitive, affective, and psychomotor), he is best known for his cognitive taxonomy of learning objectives (Fig. 21.13).[42]

Combining Theories

There are many theoretical perspectives discussed in this chapter. The trick is to look at each with an open mind and choose the best for each individual situation encountered.[43] Using an *Eclectic Approach*, or an approach that combines and integrates what is felt by the individual to be the optimal choice from each theory, can help develop a comprehensive and more personalized treatment approach.[43]

Cognitive Disorders

This chapter covered the theoretical perspectives of cognition. Although the profession has learned a great deal about cognition over the years, there is still so much to learn,

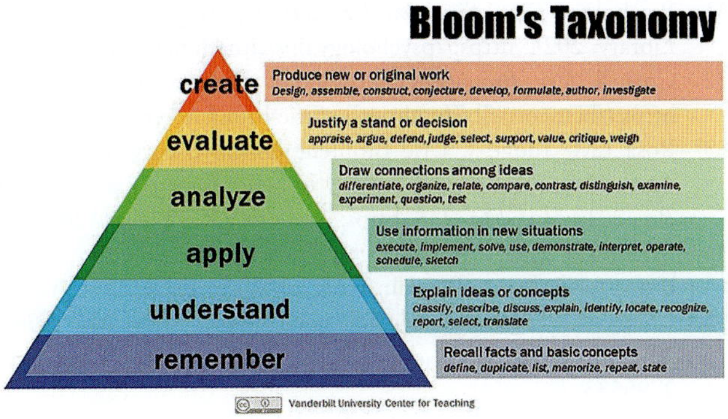

• **Fig. 21.13** Bloom's revised taxonomy. (Used with permission from AdvancED: The Institute for the Advancement of Higher Education, Vanderbilt University. https://www.newworldencyclopedia.org/entry/File:Bloom%27s_Revised_Taxonomy.jpg.)

especially as researchers uncover more information about the human brain and conditions that can affect cognitive ability. Chapter 22 will cover some of the pathophysiological conditions that can affect an individual's cognition.

The OT Scope of Practice

A thorough understanding of cognitive and metacognitive processes, and the ability to teach clients how to apply those concepts, is in part what separates occupational therapy practitioners (OTPs) from other healthcare professions.[44] Helping clients to think through difficult scenarios after an injury, illness, or during a disease process is one of the many jobs of an OTP.[45] Helping collect important information and relaying it to the physician could help the doctor to determine the cause of cognitive decline. Some occupational therapy screening tools are available for use with our clients. Many can be found in the quality toolkit on the AOTA website.[46]

Application—Occupational Therapy Screening Using Bloom's Taxonomy

COGNITIVE STEPS FOR INFORMATION PROCESSING AND PROGRAM SYNTHESIS IN OT SCREENING USING BLOOM'S TAXONOMY

I. Collect the information (data)—**Knowledge**
   A. What do you know about the individual already?
   B. What do you need to know?
   C. What questions should you ask to find out?
II. Consolidate or chunk the information—**Remember**
   A. What is important?
   B. What is not important?
III. Understand the information—**Comprehension (Understanding)**
   A. How does the information affect the client's function?
   B. How does it affect the client's self-efficacy?
   C. How does it affect the client's goals for meaningful activity?
IV. Integrate the information—**Application**
   A. Integrate the information into what you already know from your courses and from your past experiences.
   B. Apply this information
V. Analyze the information—**Analysis**
   A. Categorize the information
   B. Compare and contrast
   C. Look for red and yellow flags
   D. Consult with the medical team
VI. Step back and make a decision of appraisal—**Evaluation**
   A. Make an assessment: treatment or referral back to the physician
   B. Use your information to defend/justify your stance
   C. Implement the treatment or referral plan and test your hypothesis
   D. Make conclusions based upon your outcomes
VII. Synthesizing an idea and a plan—**Synthesis**
   A. Organize your information
   B. Create your hypothesis
   C. Develop a plan for treatment intervention
   D. Document your plan
   E. Revise the plan as needed by the client
VIII. Go back to the other stages as needed for occupational therapy decision-making and as the client's needs change.

References

1. Cambridge University Press. *Learning*. Cambridge Dictionary. Cambridge University Press. https://dictionary.cambridge.org/dictionary/english/learning.
2. Cambridge University Press. *Cognition*. Cambridge Dictionary. Cambridge University Press. https://dictionary.cambridge.org/dictionary/english/cognition.
3. Cherry K. Cognition in psychology: how people think and what's involved in this process. *Very Well Mind*. 2023. https://www.verywellmind.com/what-is-cognition-2794982.
4. APA. *Cognition and the Brain*. American Psychological Association; 2024. https://www.apa.org/topics/cognition-brain.
5. History. *Plato*. History.com; 2023. https://www.history.com/topics/ancient-greece/plato.
6. Plato, Lee D, Lane M, et al. *Republic (Penguin Classics). (4th Century B.C.). Independently*. New Edition: Penguin Classics; 2007.
7. Britannica. *Sensation: Neurology and Psychology*. Encyclopedia Britannica; 2011. https://www.britannica.com/topic/sensation.
8. Britannica. *Perception: Neurology and Psychology*. Encyclopedia Britannica; 2011. https://www.britannica.com/search?query=perception.
9. Famous. *John Locke Biography*. The Famous People. https://www.thefamouspeople.com/profiles/john-locke-134.php.
10. Merriam-Webster. *Tabula rasa*. Merriam-Webster Dictionary; 2021. https://www.merriam-webster.com/dictionary/tabula%20rasa.
11. Maden J. *John Locke's Empiricism: Why We Are All Tabula Rasa (Blank Slates)*. Philosophy Break; 2021. https://philosophybreak.com/articles/john-lockes-empiricism-why-we-are-all-tabula-rasas-blank-slates/.
12. Stanford. *John Locke*. Stanford Encyclopedia of Philosophy; 2022. https://plato.stanford.edu/entries/locke/#LimiHumaUnde.
13. Stiles J. Chapter 1 – Brain development and the nature versus nurture debate. *Prog Brain Res*. 2011;189:3–22. https://doi.org/10.1016/B978-0-444-53884-0.00015-4.

14. Itard JMG, Humphrey G, Humphrey M. *The Wild Boy of Aveyron (L'efant Sauvage)*. English/French Edition. Prentice-Hall; 1962.
15. Stanford Encyclopedia of Philosophy. *Johann Friedrich Herbart.* Stanford Encyclopedia of Philosophy; 2015. https://plato.stanford.edu/entries/johann-herbart/.
16. National Geographic. *Charles Darwin.* National Geographic. https://education.nationalgeographic.org/resource/charles-darwin/.
17. Britannica. *Alfred Russel Wallace.* Encyclopedia Britannica; 2024. https://www.britannica.com/biography/Alfred-Russel-Wallace.
18. Darwin Online. *On Origin of the Species, 1859.* Darwin Online. John Murray. https://darwin-online.org.uk/content/frameset?itemID=F373&viewtype=text&pageseq=1.
19. Thorndike EL. *Animal Intelligence: Experimental Studies.* Macmillan Press; 1911. https://doi.org/10.5962/bhl.title.55072.
20. Köhler W. The mentality of apes, 1917. In: Dennis W, ed. *Readings in the History of Psychology.* Appleton-Century-Crofts; 1948:497–505. https://doi.org/10.1037/11304-054.
21. Pavlov IP. *Conditioned Reflexes: An Investigation of the Physiological Activity of the Cerebral Cortex.* Oxford Univ. Press; 1927.
22. Malone JC. Did John B. Watson really "found" behaviorism? *Behav Anal Pract.* 2014;37(1):1–12. https://doi.org/10.1007 2Fs40614-014-0004-3.
23. Mcleod S, Guy-Evans O. Operant conditioning: what it is, how it works, and examples. *Simply Psychol.* 2024. https://www.simplypsychology.org/operant-conditioning.html.
24. Merriam-Webster. *Gestalt.* Merriam-Webster Dictionary; 2023. https://www.merriam-webster.com/dictionary/gestalt.
25. Mcleod S, Guy-Evans O. What is gestalt psychology? Theory, principles, & examples. *Simply Psychol.* 2023. https://www.simplypsychology.org/what-is-gestalt-psychology.html.
26. Britannica. *Jean Piaget.* Encyclopedia Britannica. 2024. https://www.britannica.com/biography/Jean-Piaget.
27. Armstrong T. *The Sages of Faith According to James W. Fowler.* American Institute for Learning and Human Development; 2020. https://www.institute4learning.com/2020/06/12/the-stages-of-faith-according-to-james-w-fowler/.
28. Mcleod S, Guy-Evans O. Kohlberg's stages of moral development. *Simply Psychol.* 2024. https://www.simplypsychology.org/kohlberg.html.
29. Britannica. *Carol Gilligan: American Psychologist.* Encyclopedia Britannica; 2024. https://www.britannica.com/biography/Carol-Gilligan.
30. Mcleod S, Guy-Evans O. Piaget's theory and stages of cognitive development. *Simply Psychol.* 2024. https://www.simplypsychology.org/piaget.html#Critical-Evaluation.
31. Psychology Tips. *Situational Factors. Psychology Tips.* Manuals Library; 2024. https://psychology.tips/situational-factors/.
32. Cornell. *Urie Bronfenbrenner.* Cornell Human Ecology. 2024. https://bctr.cornell.edu/about-us/urie-bronfenbrenner.
33. Rosa EM, Tudge J. Urie Bronfenbrenner's theory of development: its evolution from ecology to bioecology. *J Family Theory Rev.* 2013;5(4):243–258. https://doi.org/10.1111/jftr.12022.
34. Britannica. *L.S. Vygotsky: Soviet Psychologist.* Britannica; 2024. https://www.britannica.com/biography/Jean-Piaget.
35. Cherry K. Lev Vygotsky's life and theories. *Very Well Mind.* 2023. https://www.verywellmind.com/lev-vygotsky-biography-2795533.
36. Kurt S. Lev Vygotsky – sociocultural theory of cognitive development. *Framew Theories.* 2020 . https://educationaltechnology.net/lev-vygotsky-sociocultural-theory-of-cognitive-development/.
37. Bouchrika I. *What Is Information Processing Theory? Stages, Models & Limitations.* Research.com; 2024. https://research.com/education/what-is-information-processing-theory.
38. Dunn R, Dunn K. Learning styles, teaching styles. *NASSP Bull.* 1975; 59(393):37–49. https://doi.org/10.1177/019263657505939308.
39. Mcleod S, Guy-Evans O. Kolb's learning styles and experiential learning cycle. *Simply Psychol.* 2024. https://www.simplypsychology.org/learning-kolb.html.
40. NIU. *Howard Gardner's Theory of Multiple Intelligences.* Norther Illinois University, Center for Innovative Teaching and Learning; 2024. https://www.niu.edu/citl/resources/guides/instructional-guide/gardners-theory-of-multiple-intelligences.shtml.
41. Gardner H. *Frames of Mind: The Theory of Multiple Intelligences.* Basic Books; 1983.
42. New World. *Benjamin Bloom.* New World Encyclopedia; 2023. https://www.newworldencyclopedia.org/entry/Benjamin_Bloom.
43. Andriy. *Eclectic Approach Psychology: A Versatile Al Effective Method. Psychology Tips.* Manuals Library; 2024. https://psychology.tips/eclectic-approach-psychology/#google_vignette.
44. Lee SS, Powell NJ, Esdaile S. A functional model of cognitive rehabilitation in occupational therapy. *Can J Occup Ther.* 2001; 68(1):41–50. https://doi.org/10.1177/000841740106800105.
45. AOTA. Occupational therapy practice framework: domain and process, 4th Ed. *Am J Occup Ther.* 2020;74(suppl_2): 7412410010p1–7412410010p87. https://doi.org/10.5014/ajot.2020.74S2001.
46. AOTA. *Quality Toolkit.* American Occupational Therapy Association; 2024. https://www.aota.org/practice/practice-essentials/quality/quality-toolkit.

22

Cognitive Pathophysiology

OBJECTIVES

By the end of this chapter, the reader should be able to:

- Demonstrate a basic understanding of the neurology behind normal cognitive functioning.
- Identify possible symptoms associated with various types of delirium, mild cognitive impairment, and dementia.
- Differentiate between the symptoms of delirium versus dementia.
- Explain and/or predict the possible symptoms resulting from a diagnosis of adult attention-deficit/hyperactivity disorder.
- Assess and justify whether a symptom from a cognitive impairment could constitute a yellow or red flag.

The Human Brain and Cognition

This book has covered some of the many systemic and viscerogenic causes of pathology leading to movement and sensory disorders. This chapter goes through cognition and how it can be affected by physiologic change. The parts of the brain responsible for higher levels of cognition are thought to be in the very front of the brain in an area called the prefrontal cortex or PFC.[1] This part of the brain is responsible for planning, decision-making, the modulation of social behavior, and the prediction of consequences of behavior (or executive functions). Cognitive control has been defined as the process of employing these executive functions to guide behavior to achieve a specific goal.[2] Functional magnetic resonance imaging (MRI) has located parts of the dorsal-lateral prefrontal cortex, the anterior cingulate cortex (near the anterior part of the corpus callosum), and the parietal cortex as comprising a complex cognitive control network.[2] The part of the frontal cortex near the eyes, called the orbitofrontal cortex, codes information and helps control impulses, and the ventromedial part of the PFC is responsible for reward processing and the visceral responses to emotions.[1] How neurodevelopment leads to cognitive change is not fully understood,[2] but studies using functional MRI have helped to map various areas of the brain for memory, language, and other aspects of cognition (Figs. 22.1 and 22.2).

Neurocognitive Disorders

Neurocognitive disorders are often divided into one of three types: *mild cognitive impairment, delirium*, and *dementia*. *The Diagnostic and Statistical Manual of Mental Disorders, Fifth Edition (DSM-5)* has classified six key domains of cognition to help determine the severity of a neurocognitive disorder (Fig. 22.3).[3] All six areas of cognition can be addressed by occupational therapy (OT) intervention.

The term *mild cognitive impairment* is often used for individuals with confusion or difficulty concentrating. It is forgetfulness that is more than what is typically expected from normal aging and can be due to early dementia or simple reactions to medication or other physiologic changes.[4] The terms *delirium* and *dementia*, however, are often confused with one another.

Delirium

Delirium can come on quickly, over hours or days. It is an altered state of consciousness that is often accompanied by confusion, lethargy, and feelings of disorientation. Delirium is a symptom, not a disorder.[5] It can be a result of a situation such as bladder infection or recent COVID-19 with a respirator or breathing tube (COVID-19 delirium). It can be hypoactive with drowsiness or lethargy, often seen in ICU patients, or it can be hyperactive with agitation and restlessness.[5]

Dementia

Dementia is a blanket term for a group of symptoms that affect cognition, memory, and social abilities. Dementia typically comes on gradually over the course of months or years. Symptoms include memory loss, difficulty forming

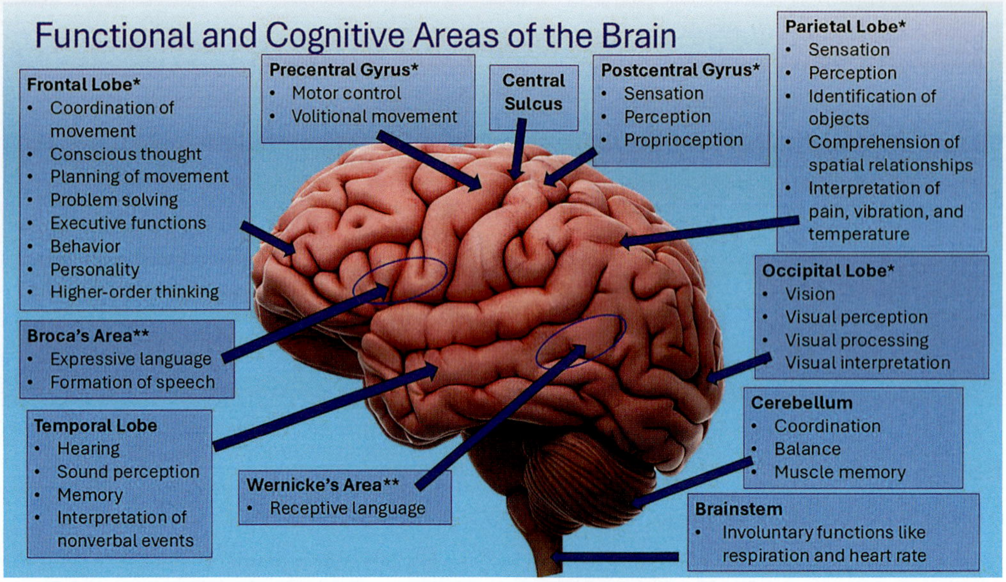

• **Fig. 22.1** The functional and cognitive areas of the brain. (Image from iStock.com/3dMediaSphere, Brain Illustration: ID 484757150; Data from *Cleveland Clinic. *Cerebral Cortex*. 2022. https://my.clevelandclinic.org/health/articles/23073-cerebral-cortex; and **Guy-Evans O. *Wernicke's Area: Location and Function*. Simply Psychology; 2023. https://www.simplypsychology.org/wernickes-area.html.)

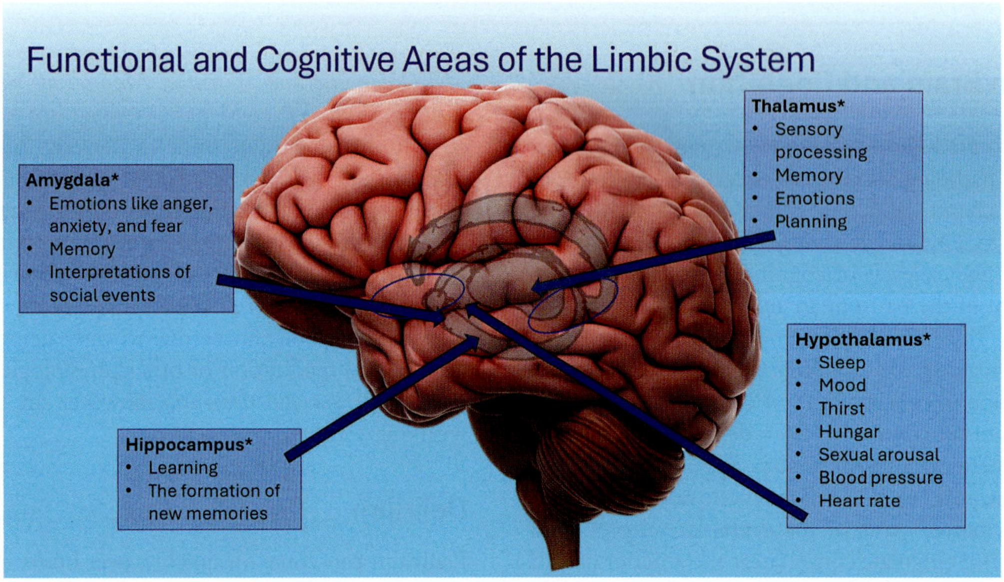

• **Fig. 22.2** The functional and cognitive areas of the limbic system. (Image from iStock.com/3dMediaSphere, Brain Illustration: ID 484757150; Data from Cleveland Clinic. *Brain*. 2025. https://my.clevelandclinic.org/health/body/limbic-system.)

or remembering words, poor coordination of movements, confusion, personality changes, and depression.[6] The most common cause of dementia is Alzheimer's disease, but there are other causes, such as Parkinson's disease or Lewy body dementia, with symptoms varying based on the cause.[6] Unlike delirium, dementia is caused by damage or loss of nerve cells in the brain and a loss of the connections between neurons. Some medications have side effects that can mimic dementia, and lack of certain vitamins can have a similar effect, but these will appear to be closer to delirium, as the symptoms can be resolved after the true cause is found (Table 22.1).[6]

Alzheimer's Disease

Most cases of dementia in the United States are due to Alzheimer's disease which affects more than 5 million Americans.[7] Alzheimer's is a type of dementia accounting for 60% to 80% of cases,[4] and it ranks as the fifth leading cause of death worldwide, affecting approximately 45 million people.[8] About 70% of the individuals diagnosed with Alzheimer's disease are 75 years of age or older.[9] Alzheimer's disease is believed to be caused by an accumulation of amyloid beta

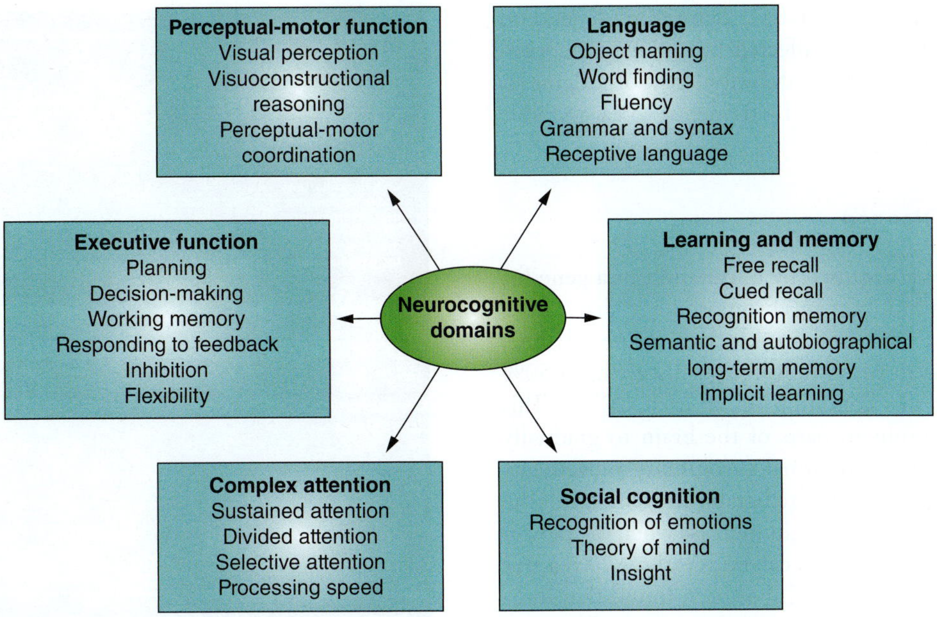

• **Fig. 22.3** The six domains of neurocognitive function. (From Sachdev PS, Blacker D, Blazer DG, Ganguli M, Jeste DV, Paulsen JS, Petersen RC. Classifying neurocognitive disorders: the DSM-5 approach. *Nat Rev Neurol*. 2014;10:634–642.)

TABLE 22.1 A Comparison of Delirium Versus Dementia

Characterstic	Delirium	Dementia
Timing[a]	Acute onset	Chronic, gradual, and progressive
Symptoms[a]	Difficulty paying attention, problems with cognition, and an altered level of consciousness	Loss of previously learned knowledge
Cause[a]	Can be caused by illnesses, dehydration, and/or something in the environment	Typically due to a chronic condition such as a vascular blockage, Alzheimer's, Parkinson's, or Lewy body dementia
Prognosis[b]	The cognitive deficit comes and goes. Can be reversible if treated early	Chronic and progressive. There is a steady loss of the ability to think and reason.
Relationship[a]	People with delirium have a greater chance of developing dementia over time.	People with dementia are more prone to episodes of delirium.

[a]From Fong TG, Inouya SK. The inter-relationship between delirium and dementia: the importance of delirium prevention. *Nat Views Neurol*. 2022;18:579–596.
[b]From Cleveland Clinic. *Delirium*. Cleveland Clinic; 2023. https://my.clevelandclinic.org/health/diseases/15252-delirium.

protein (Aβ) in the brain. The accumulation of these proteins leads to the formation of oligomers (low-weight protein molecules), which can penetrate the cell membranes, leading to cellular dysfunction and even cell death.[8] These oligomers can also recombine into fibrils or chains and form amyloid plaques in the brain. Symptoms of Alzheimer's disease include emotional fluctuations, sleep disorders, cognitive decline, and behavioral changes. As the disorder progresses, it can lead to multiorgan failure and even brain death.[8]

Frontotemporal Dementia

Frontotemporal dementia is a term that encompasses a number of disorders that affect the frontal and temporal lobes of the brain, thereby affecting personality, language, and behavior. These disorders account for approximately 10% to 20% of all dementia cases.[10] With this type of dementia, the affected parts of the brain begin to atrophy (or shrink). This disorder is sometimes misdiagnosed as Alzheimer's disease, but frontotemporal dementia tends to occur at a younger age (ages 40–65).[9] Symptoms depend on the part of the brain that is affected but include inappropriate social behavior, lack of inhibition, lack of judgment, loss of empathy, overeating, and a tendency to eat inedible objects (also known as pica).[10,11]

Huntington's Disease

Huntington's disease is caused by a mutation in a gene for a protein called huntingtin in chromosome 4 that causes many repeats of the DNA building blocks cytosine, adenine, and guanine. A parent with Huntington's disease has a 50% chance of passing this condition on to each child.[12] This disorder causes neurons in parts of the brain to gradually break down, leading to abnormal involuntary movements called chorea (irregular and unpredictable movements of the extremities and face), which might increase when the person is upset or nervous. Age of onset can be as early as 20 years or as late as 60 years and beyond. It has been found that individuals with a young onset of symptoms will typically have a faster functional decline than those with a later onset of symptoms.[13] Some physical symptoms may include slurred speech, trouble swallowing, problems eating, and difficulty walking.[12] Eventually, cognitive problems will occur, starting with problems prioritizing activities, learning new skills, or putting thoughts into words.[12]

Lewy Body Dementia

This type of dementia is caused by abnormal accumulations of a protein called alpha-synuclein (aSyn) in the brain.[14] These deposits are called Lewy bodies, and they affect two neurotransmitters in the brain: acetylcholine (affecting learning and memory) and dopamine (affecting cognition, behavior, movement, motivation, and sleep). This leads to problems with thinking, movement, mood, and behavior.[14] This disorder affects more than a million individuals in the United States aged 50 and over. Some of the cognitive symptoms include visual hallucinations; unpredictable changes in attention, concentration, and wakefulness; and severe loss of thinking abilities. Unlike Alzheimer's disease, problems with memory typically arise later in the progression of the disorder.[14] Although Lewy body dementia is evident when Lewy bodies appear in the cortex and mood centers of the brain, Parkinson's disease (which is covered next) occurs when Lewy bodies appear in the brainstem and movement control centers of the brain (Fig. 22.4).[15]

Parkinson's Disease

The prevalence of Parkinson's disease has doubled over the past 25 years.[16] A 2022 study by the Parkinson's Foundation reported that nearly 90,000 people are diagnosed with Parkinson's disease each year in the United States.[17] This is a

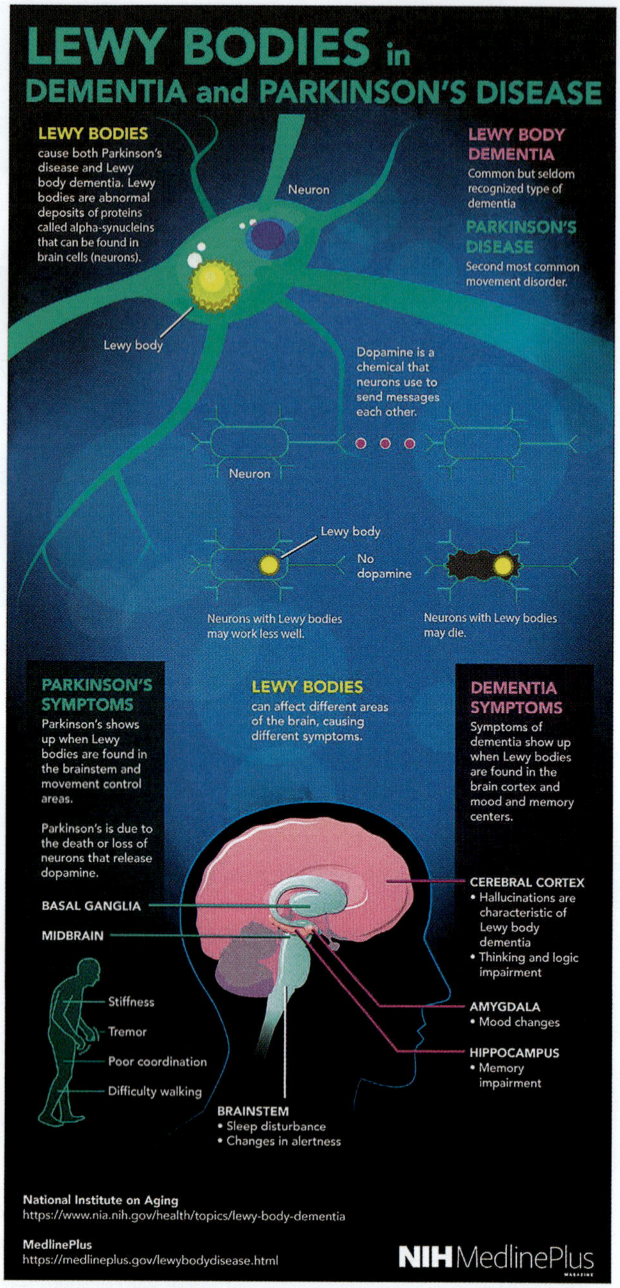

• **Fig. 22.4** Parkinson's disease versus Lewy body dementia. (From https://magazine.medlineplus.gov/multimedia/lewy-bodies-dementia.)

neurodegenerative disorder caused by problems with the dopaminergic (dopamine-producing) neurons in the midbrain, specifically in a basal ganglia structure known as the substantia nigra (Fig. 22.5).[18]

Lewy bodies, consisting of abnormal accumulations of aSyn, are found in the neurons of the substantia nigra in people with this disorder. The motor problems that accompany this disorder typically begin to occur after about 60% to 80% of the neurons in the substantia nigra have become involved.[18] Symptoms of Parkinson's disease include

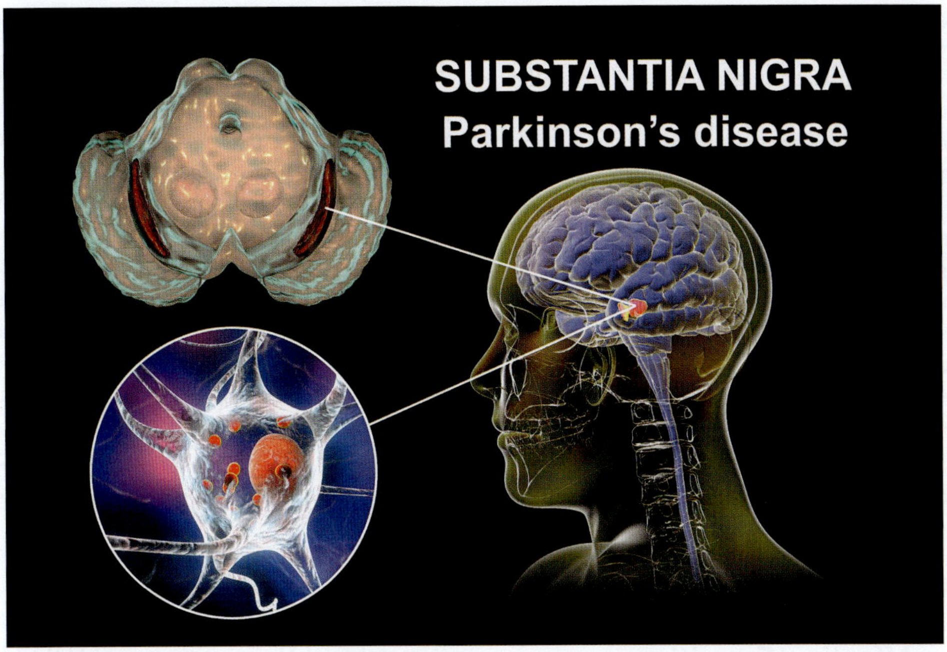

• **Fig. 22.5** The pars compacta of the substantia nigra. (From https://istock.com/Dr_Microbe.)

depression, anxiety, hallucinations, cognitive decline, a tremor mainly at rest and specifically in the hands (called a pill-rolling tremor), slow movement (also called bradykinesia or hyperkinesia), stiffness (rigidity), and problems with posture and gait.[18]

Vascular Dementia

The term *vascular dementia* is a blanket term for cognitive decline caused by impaired blood flow to the brain.[19] This can result from any condition that can damage blood vessels and interfere with circulation, like cerebral vascular accident (stroke). Risk factors for this include diabetes, high cholesterol, high blood pressure, and smoking. Symptoms will depend on the area of the brain that is involved and include confusion, slowed thinking, difficulty organizing thoughts or actions, memory deficits, depression, and unsteady gait.[19]

Traumatic Brain Injury

The term *traumatic brain injury* (TBI) covers injuries that range from a quick blow to the head to an injury with brain penetration.[20] It has been estimated that about 1.7 million people in the United States suffer from some form of TBI,[20] and recent research has linked TBI to neurodegenerative disorders and dementia.[21,22] It is estimated that about 2% of the population in the United States lives with some sort of long-term disability as a result of a prior TBI.[22] Some of this is the result of chronic traumatic encephalopathy, a type of posttraumatic dementia.[21] More studies are currently underway to better understand this phenomenon.[21]

Adult Attention-Deficit/Hyperactivity Disorder

It is estimated that about 2.5% of adults have adult attention-deficit hyperactivity disorder (ADHD).[23] Because the executive functions related to attention and memory are affected, this disorder is categorized as a neurocognitive disorder, so it is listed here in this chapter. Adult ADHD includes a group of persistent problems such as hyperactivity, difficulty paying attention, and impulsivity.[24] This can lead to unstable relationships, inability to perform well at work, and low self-esteem.[24] ADHD has been found to be associated with deficits across various neurocognitive domains, including working memory, planning/organization, reaction time variability, intelligence/achievement, and vigilance.[25] An estimated 8.4% of children are diagnosed with ADHD, and two-thirds of these children will continue to have ADHD as adults.[23] Parts of the brain thought to be involved in individuals with ADHD are the prefrontal cortex, the basal ganglia, limbic system, and reticular activating system.

Significant associations have also been found between an ADHD diagnosis and changes in the superior temporal gyrus; fronto-basal cortex (orbital region, located above the eyes); portions of the frontal lobes; superior longitudinal fasciculus; and cortico-limbic areas, including the prefrontal cortices, hippocampus, and amygdala (Fig. 22.6).[26]

Childhood Neurocognitive Disorders

An estimated four million children in the United States suffer from chronic illnesses including cancer, diabetes, and sickle cell anemia. Major advances in treatment as well as early detection of these disorders have increased the lifespan of these children; however, there are still long-term effects of these illnesses and of the interventions used to treat them. One of the primary long-term effects is impaired cognitive function.[27]

Congenital conditions affecting childhood neurodevelopmental outcomes related to cognition include congenital heart disease and hypoventilation syndrome.[28,29] There are many congenital disorders of the brain and spinal cord that can affect cognition, including but not limited to agenesis of the corpus callosum (partial or complete absence), encephalocele (a rare defect of the neural tube causing a skull groove between the forehead and nose, often accompanied by other brain malformations), and microcephaly (a condition in which the skull is abnormally small due to arrested brain development).[30]

Other Systems Affecting Cognition

This textbook has gone through various systems in the human body, outlining some of the more common disorders that fall within each system. Many of these disorders can cause dementia-like symptoms. Those most often cited in the literature as having this potential effect include endocrine disorders, metabolic disorders, autoimmune disorders, and cancer.[31] There is also a strong association between systemic inflammation and cognitive deficits; levels of inflammation tend to increase as we age.[32] Stress and certain medications can also cause dementia-like symptoms.[33,34]

Medications and Cognition

One dangerous group of medications that can affect cognition is those that block acetylcholine (anticholinergic medications).[34] These medications include tolterodine (for urinary incontinence), certain antidepressants, antipsychotics (e.g., Haldol can cause symptoms that mimic Parkinson's disease), some antivertigo medications, and certain antiparkinsonian medications.[34] Effects of anticholinergic medications include confusion, memory loss, and delirium. Benzodiazepines, like Ativan, Xanax, or Restoril, can also cause dementia-like symptoms when used long term or when mixed with other nonprescribed substances. Corticosteroids, like prednisone, can also cause cognitive changes. Opioid pain medications, chemotherapy drugs, and statins (for cholesterol management) can all cause episodes of confusion.[34]

The OT Scope of Practice

Remember, OT practitioners (OTPs) do not diagnose, but they do need to be able to determine the occupational implications of how a client's condition might impact their everyday life. OTPs work within their scope of practice as designated by the American Occupational Therapy Association (AOTA) and their state licensing board.[35] There are many assessment tools available to aid the OTP in the screening process with respect to cognitive deficit. Many can be found in the Quality toolkit on the AOTA website, under the cognition tab.[36] Table 22.2 provides a quick overview of some of the more common conditions seen by OTPs.

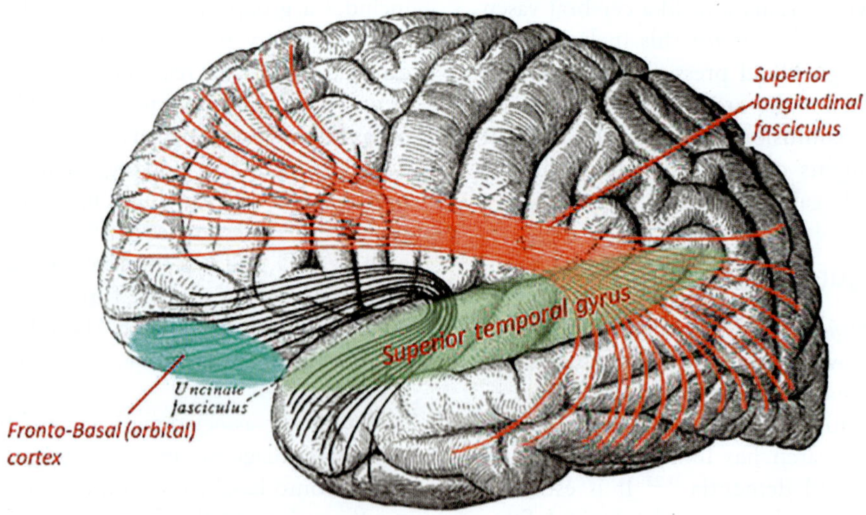

• **Fig. 22.6** Areas of the brain involved with attention-deficit/hyperactivity disorder. (Modified from https://commons.wikimedia.org/w/index.php?curid=30367821.)

TABLE 22.2 Some of the Neurocognitive Conditions Often Seen by OTPs

Condition	Symptoms that could affect occupational performance	Some possible occupational therapy interventions
Delerium	• Comes on suddenly over hours or days • Altered state of consciousness • Confusion, lethargy, disorientation	• Behavioral adaptations such as reassurance, reorientation, and cognitive stimulation[37] • Environmental adaptations such as providing a comfortable setting to promote sleep or mobility[37] • Activities of daily living (ADL) exercises, instrumental activities of daily living (IADL) exercises, and exercises to help regain cognitive function[38]
Dementia	• Comes on gradually over a period of months or years • Affects cognition, memory, and social abilities • May have movement disorders, personality changes, and depression	• Instruction in compensatory strategies[39] • Instruction in environmental strategies[39] • Family education[39] • Promotion of meaningful activities like recreational activities or animal therapy[40] • Verbal and cognitive activities[40] • Agitation management[40]
Alzheimer's disease	• Most common type of dementia in the United States • Believed to be caused by an accumulation of amyloid beta protein (Aβ) in the brain • Can have emotional fluctuations, sleep disorders, cognitive decline, and behavioral changes	• Individual and/or group cognition exercises[41] • Multisensory stimulation intervention[41] • Coordination exercises to music[41] • Imagery and improvisation[41] • Reminiscence therapy[41] • Family education[41]
Lewy body dementia	• A type of dementia • Believed to be caused by abnormal accumulations of a protein called alpha-synuclein (aSyn) or Lewy bodies in the brain • Can have problems with thinking, hallucinations, movement, mood, and behavior	• Skill building through task-oriented motor practice (STOMP)[42] • Repetitive blocked practice[42]
Parkinson's disease	• A neurodegenerative disorder caused by problems with the dopaminergic neurons in the substantia nigra of the midbrain • Depression, anxiety, hallucinations, cognitive decline, and tremor at rest • Festination (strong hesitation like the feet are stuck to the floor) of gait, masked facies (rigid facial expressions), and rigidity of the trunk and extremities	• Client-centered approaches to enhance meaningful occupations including ADLs and IADLs[43] • Cognition exercises[43] • Gross motor, fine motor, and coordination exercises[43] • Non-immersive virtual reality[43] • Use of assistive technology[43] • Timing activities and activities to music[41,43] • Family education[39]

Application—Case Study

CASE EXAMPLE 22.1

A 75-year-old female presents with a diagnosis of sudden-onset Parkinson's disease. She was referred by her physician for balance exercises and improved functional ambulation. The occupational therapist was immediately concerned about the diagnosis because Parkinson's disease does not typically come on "suddenly."

1. **Screen:** The client appeared to have all the signs and symptoms of Parkinson's disease from the rigidity to the pill-rolling tremor. The OTR asked her family how long the client had these symptoms. They said that she was walking fine just 2 days prior.
2. **Take a Closer Look:** The therapist looked at the chart and found that this client had started taking Haldol 2 days prior, right when the symptoms began.
3. **Determine Flag Status:** The therapist felt that this could be a red flag, as a continuation of symptoms could result in a dramatic decline of health for this client.
4. **Take Action if Needed:** The OTR contacted the client's doctor and asked if the client could be taken off the Haldol to see if this was the reason for her symptoms. The doctor said no that this would not be possible as the client was having psychotic episodes, and the Haldol was needed.
5. **Document the Findings:** The OTR documented this information.

6. **Take a Second Look:** The therapist looked up the typical dosage of Haldol based on the weight of the client. This particular client was a small female weighing about 98 pounds. The dosage she was taking was for a heavier person. Armed with this information, the therapist called the physician again and this time asked that the client's dosage of Haldol be decreased by 50%. She explained this lowered dose might be sufficient to control her symptoms while possibly alleviating any side effects. The doctor agreed. After another 48 hours on a lower dose, the client's Parkinson-like symptoms had completely subsided. The lower dosage was also sufficient to control the client's psychotic episodes.
7. **Determine the Flag Status:** Thanks to the quick thinking of the OTR the situation progressed rapidly from a red flag to a yellow flag, and eventually to a green flag within a matter of days.
8. **Take Action if Needed:** The client was again seen in the therapy clinic one more time and was ambulating and talking with none of the prior symptoms. Her family thanked the therapist, calling her a miracle worker!

This is a true case. This therapist was able to help the doctor to prescribe the right amount of medication for the client's weight, alleviating the side effects of the medication, possibly saving the client's life.

References

1. Martin EI, Ressler KJ, Binder E, Nemeroff CB. The neurobiology of anxiety disorders: brain imaging, genetics, and psychoneuroendocrinology. *Psychiatr Clin North Am*. 2009;32(3):549–575. https://doi.org/10.1016/j.psc.2009.05.004.
2. Breukelaar IA, Antees C, Grieve SM, et al. Cognitive control network anatomy correlates with neurocognitive behavior: a longitudinal study. *Hum Brain Mapp*. 2016;38(2):631–643. https://doi.org/10.1002/hbm.23401.
3. Sachdev PS, Blacker D, Blazer DG, et al. Classifying neurocognitive disorders: the DSM-5 approach. *Nat Rev Neurol.* 2014;10:634–642. https://doi.org/10.1038/nrneurol.2014.181.
4. Fifiled K. *Dementia vs. Alzheimer's: Which Is It?* AARP; 2020. https://www.aarp.org/health/conditions-treatments/info-2018/difference-between-dementia-alzheimers.html.
5. Seunghee E. *Delirium*. Johns Hopkins Medicine; 2024. https://www.hopkinsmedicine.org/health/conditions-and-diseases/delirium.
6. Mayo Clinic. *Dementia*. Mayo Clinic; 2024. https://www.mayoclinic.org/diseases-conditions/dementia/symptoms-causes/syc-20352013.
7. Psychology Today. Neurocognitive disorders (mild and major). *Psychol Today*. 2019. https://www.psychologytoday.com/us/conditions/neurocognitive-disorders-mild-and-major.
8. Ma C, Hong F, Yang S. Amyloidosis in Alzheimer's disease: pathogeny, etiology, and related therapeutic directions. *Molecules*. 2022;27(4):1210. https://doi.org/10.3390/molecules27041210.
9. Clinic Mayo. *Alzheimer's Disease*. Mayo Clinic; 2024. https://www.mayoclinic.org/diseases-conditions/alzheimers-disease/symptoms-causes/syc-20350447.
10. Clinic Mayo. *Frontotemporal Dementia*. Mayo Clinic; 2023. https://www.mayoclinic.org/diseases-conditions/frontotemporal-dementia/symptoms-causes/syc-20354737.
11. Cleveland Clinic. *Pica*. Cleveland Clinic; 2022. https://my.clevelandclinic.org/health/diseases/22944-pica.
12. NIH. *Huntington's Disease*. National Institute of Neurological Disorders and Stroke; 2024. https://www.ninds.nih.gov/health-information/disorders/huntingtons-disease.
13. Kwa L, Larson D, Yeh C, Bega D. Influence of age of onset on Huntington's disease phenotype. *TOHM*. 2020;10:21. https://doi.org/10.5334/tohm.536.
14. NIH. *What Is Lewy Body Dementia? Causes, Symptoms, and Treatments*. National Institute of Neurological Disorders and Stroke; 2024. https://www.nia.nih.gov/health/lewy-body-dementia/what-lewy-body-dementia-causes-symptoms-and-treatments.
15. NIH. Lew bodies dementia. *NIH Medline Plus Magazine*. 2019. https://magazine.medlineplus.gov/multimedia/lewy-bodies-dementia.
16. WHO. *Parkinson's Disease*, World Health Organization; 2023. https://www.who.int/news-room/fact-sheets/detail/parkinson-disease.
17. Parkinson's Foundation. *Prevalence & Incidence*. Par Foundation; 2024. https://www.parkinson.org/understanding-parkinsons/statistics/prevalence-incidence.
18. Parkinson's Foundation. *What Is Parkinson's?* Parkinson's Foundation; 2024. https://www.parkinson.org/understanding-parkinsons/what-is-parkinsons.
19. Mayo Clinic. *Vascular Dementia*. Mayo Clinic; 2021. https://www.mayoclinic.org/diseases-conditions/vascular-dementia/symptoms-causes/syc-20378793.
20. Georges A, Das JM. Traumatic brain injury. In: *StatPearls*. NIH, National Center for Biotechnology Information; 2023. https://www.ncbi.nlm.nih.gov/books/NBK459300/.
21. Graham NSN, Sharp DJ. Dementia after traumatic brain injury. *Br Med J*. 2023;383:2065. https://doi.org/10.1136/bmj.p2065.
22. Shively S, Scher AI, Perl DP, Diaz-Arrastia R. Dementia resulting from traumatic brain injury: what is the pathology? *JAMA. Arch Neurol*. 2012;69(10):1245–1251. https://doi.org/10.1001/archneurol.2011.3747.
23. Gharibian, E. *What Is ADHD? An Overview of the Causes and Signs of ADHD*. Verdugo Psychological Associates; 2023. https://verdugopsych.com/what-is-adhd-an-overview-of-the-causes-and-signs-of-adhd/.
24. Clinic Mayo. *Adult Attention Deficit/Hyperactivity Disorder (ADHD)*. Mayo Clinic; 2023. https://www.mayoclinic.org/diseases-conditions/adult-adhd/symptoms-causes/syc-20350878.
25. Pievsky MA, McGrath RE. The neurocognitive profile of attention-deficit/hyperactivity disorder: a review of meta-analyses. *Arch Clin Neuropsychol*. 2018;33(2):143–157. https://doi.org/10.1093/arclin/acx055.
26. Gehricke JG, Kruggel F, thampipop T, et al. The brain anatomy of attention-deficit/hyperactivity disorder in young adults – a magnetic resonance imaging study. *PLOS One*. 2017;12(4):e0175433. https://doi.org/10.1371/journal.pone.0175433.
27. Compas BE, Jaser SS, Reeslund K. et al. Neurocognitive deficits in children with chronic health conditions. *Am Psychologist*, 2017;72(4):326–338. https://doi.org/10.1037/amp0000042.
28. Ortinau CM, Smyser CD, Arthur L, et al. Optimizing neurodevelopmental outcomes in neonates with congenital heart disease. *Pediatrics*. 2022;150(Supplement 2):e2022056415L. https://doi.org/10.1542/peds.2022-056415L.
29. Charnay AJ, Antisdel-Lomaglio JE, Zelko FA, et al. Congenital central hypoventilation syndrome: Neurocognition already reduced in preschool-aged children. *Chest*. 2016;149(3):809–815. https://doi.org/10.1378/chest.15-0402.
30. NIH. *Birth Disorders of the Brain and Spinal Cord*. National Institute of Neurological Disorders and Stroke; 2024.

https://www.ninds.nih.gov/health-information/disorders/birth-disorders-brain-and-spinal-cord.

31. Morlano JR, Kelley BJ. Chapter 4: Dementia and systemic disorders. In: Lewis SL, ed. *Neurological Disorders due to Systemic Disease*. Wiley; 2013. https://doi.org/10.1002/9781118414019.ch4.
32. Lin T, Liu GA, Perez E, et al. Systemic inflammation mediates age-related cognitive deficits. *Front Aging Neurosci*. 2018;10:236. https://doi.org/10.3389/fnagi.2018.00236.
33. McEwen BS. Neurobiological and systemic effects of chronic stress. *Chronic Stress*. 2017;1. https://doi.org/10.1177/2470547017692328.
34. Ellison JM. *Medications That Can Mimic Dementia*. Alzheimer's Disease Research; 2023. https://www.brightfocus.org/alzheimers/article/is-it-something-im-taking-medications-that-can-mimic-dementia.
35. AOTA. *Practice Essentials: Occupational Therapy Scope of Practice*. American Occupational Therapy Association; 2024. https://www.aota.org/practice/practice-essentials/scope-of-practice.
36. AOTA. *Quality: Quality Toolkit*. American Occupational Therapy Association; 2024. https://www.aota.org/practice/practice-essentials/quality/quality-toolkit.
37. Pozzi C, Tatzer VC, Alvarez EA, Lanzoni A, Graff MJL. The applicability and feasibility of occupationl therapy in delirium care. *Eur Geriatr Med*. 2020;11:209–216. https://doi.org/10.1007/s41999-020-00308-z.
38. Zhao J, Fan K, Zheng S, Xie G, Niu X, Pang J, Zhang H, Wu X, Qu J. Effect of occupational therapy on the occurrence of delirium in critically ill patients: a systematic review and meta-analysis. *Front Neurol*. 2024;15:1391993. https://doi.org/10.3389/fneur.2024.1391993.
39. Pimouguet, C, Le Goff M, Wittwer J, Dartigues J, Helmer C. Benefits of occupational therapy in dementia patients: findings from a real-worlld observational study. *J Alzheimer Dis*. 2017;56:509–517. https://doi.org/10.3233/JAD-160820.
40. Uceda-Portillo C, Aranda-Valero S, Moruno-Miralles P. Occupational therapy interventions to improve the quality of life of older adults with dementia living in nursing homes: a systematic review. *Healthcare*. 2024;12:896. https://doi.org/10.3390/healthcare12090896.
41. Smallfield, S, Metzger L, Green M, Henley L, Rhodus EK. Practice guidelines—Occupational therapy practice guidelines for adults living with Alzheimer's disease and related neurocognitive disorders. *Am J Occup Ther*. 2024;78 https://doi.org/10.5014/ajot.2024.078101.7801397010.
42. Ciro CA, Hershey LA, Garrison D. Enhanced task-oriented training in a person with dementia with Lewy bodies. *AJOT*. 2013;67(5):556–563. https://doi.org/10.5014/ajot.2013.008227.
43. Oliveira GM, Basílio SAR, Omura KM, Kovic M, Larsen AE, Cardoso MM, Corrêa VAC. Mapping of practices and approaches of occupational therapists in Parkinson's disease: a scoping review. *Cad Bras Ter Ocup*. 2024;32:e3349. https://doi.org/10.1590/2526-8910.ctoAR256833492.

SECTION IV

Pathophysiology Affecting Mental Health

Introduction to Section IV

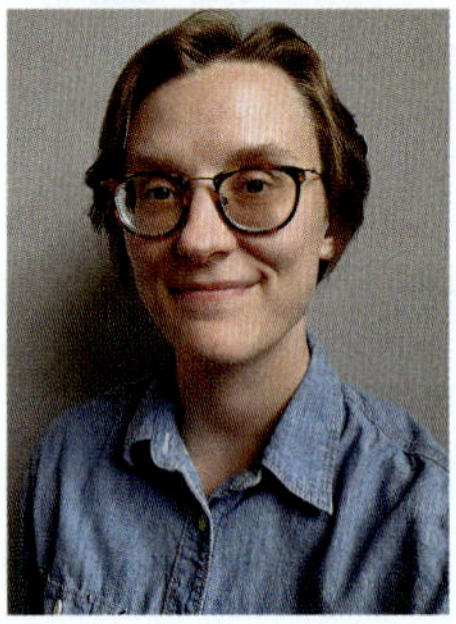

Section IV focuses on the pathophysiological conditions affecting mental health with application to occupational therapy (OT). As occupational therapy practitioners (OTPs), the holistic scope of practice extends beyond the physical to include mental, emotional, and social health and well-being, as these areas impact an individual's participation in meaningful occupations.

We are fortunate to have Dr. Katy Schmidt, OTD, Assistant Professor in the School of OT at Belmont University, and alumna of the Johns Hopkins Mental Health Occupational Therapy Fellowship, as a guest writer for Section IV. Although many graduate occupational therapy programs have a separate mental health course, Dr. Schmidt and the authors of this text found it imperative to introduce mental health–related topics and disorders within the context of pathophysiology to understand how physical and mental health are interrelated, distinguish adaptive versus maladaptive behaviors, and contribute to combating mental health stigma.

There are seven chapters in this section. Chapter 23 begins by differentiating moods and emotions and identifying their physiological factors, then explains the classification of mood disorders, and ends with depressive and bipolar disorders with related signs, symptoms, and etiology. Chapter 24 distinguishes fight-or-flight responses from diagnosable anxiety disorders. Chapter 25 outlines personality theories followed by a brief overview of 10 personality disorders. Chapter 26 reviews the brain and associated "thinking" skills before exploring types of psychotic symptoms, schizophrenia, and schizoaffective disorder. Chapter 27 presents the physiological control centers for eating behaviors in addition to the four types of eating disorders and their commonly associated behaviors and symptoms. Chapter 28 defines trauma, traumatic events, and the physiological response to threats as well as introduces posttraumatic stress disorder and its pathophysiology, symptoms, and physiological factors. Lastly, Chapter 29 begins by detailing the reward system of the brain and how this pathophysiology can negatively translate into the development of a substance use disorder.

Each of the mental health chapters in Section IV includes definitions of important terms, concepts, or related areas of the brain; an overview of various disorders with associated signs, symptoms, behaviors, and contributing factors; and concludes with a section describing the scope of OT practice, including summary tables, OT-specific interventions, and case studies for clinical application.

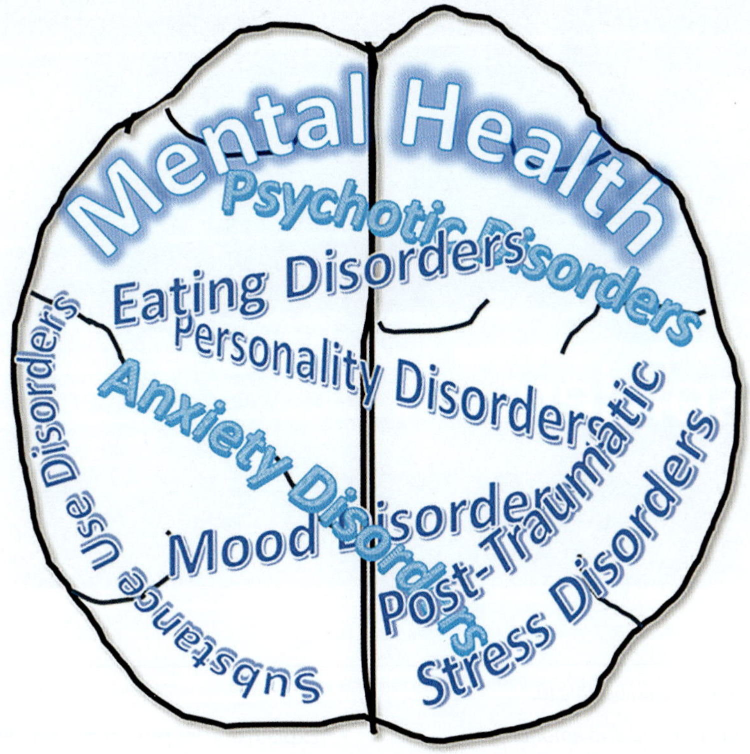

(Courtesy Natalie Norman Michaels and Katy Schmidt.)

23 Mood Disorders

KATY SCHMIDT

OBJECTIVES

By the end of this chapter, the reader should be able to:

- Compare and contrast the terms *mood* and *emotion*, examining their definitions, duration, triggers, physiological processes, and impact on behavior.
- Identify possible symptoms associated with various types of mood disorders.
- Differentiate between depressive disorders and bipolar disorders.
- Explain and/or predict the possible symptoms resulting from a diagnosis of major depressive disorder.
- Assess and justify whether a symptom from a mood disorder could constitute a yellow or red flag.

Healthy Mood

The term *mood* refers to the tendency of an individual's disposition to respond emotionally in a specific way that can last for hours or even weeks.[1] Mood is different from emotions. *Emotions* typically require a specific event or object that has caused the emotions, whereas moods are simply feelings that have no apparent cause.[1]

Mood

Mood has been defined by the National Institute of Mental Health as a persistent internal emotional state that can impact an individual's behavior.[2] Healthy individuals are typically aware of their current mood and can identify related feelings of happiness, sadness, anger, anxiety, or calmness.[3] Mood may change, depending on environment, psychological factors, or behavior. However, mood typically endures longer than emotion.[3] An individual's mood can greatly affect their participation in everyday life activities.

Emotions and Mood

Emotions typically contribute to mood and last a shorter duration than mood. Emotion is the subjective experience of psychological and physiological reactions to stimuli. Emotions are often automatic responses that are not initiated purposefully but are typically due to a response from some sort of stimulus.[4] These emotions may be managed through intentional behaviors and are highly influenced by culture and social learning. Emotions may be experienced as positive (such as joy or love) or negative (such as anger, sadness, or fear).[4]

Multiple physiological factors may contribute to emotion. The reticular formation of cells in the brainstem first receives sensory information. Next, the limbic system processes the information and controls endocrine and autonomic nervous system responses (such as the hormonal processes causing a fight-or-flight response to danger).[4] Finally, the frontal lobe of the cerebral cortex is primarily responsible for the psychological experience of emotion, including awareness, thoughts, beliefs, motivation, and consequent behavior (Fig. 23.1).[4]

The physiologic factors that contribute to mood are more complex since there is typically no underlying sensory information, as seen with emotions. For example, it has long been believed that a chemical imbalance in the brain causes depression, but this does not begin to cover the complexity of the disorder.[5] Depression can be caused by genetic vulnerability, faulty mood regulation at the brain level, and stressful life events. Some recent studies found that the hippocampus is smaller in size in those who are depressed when compared to those who are not.[5]

Disturbances in mood are referred to as mood disorders.[1]

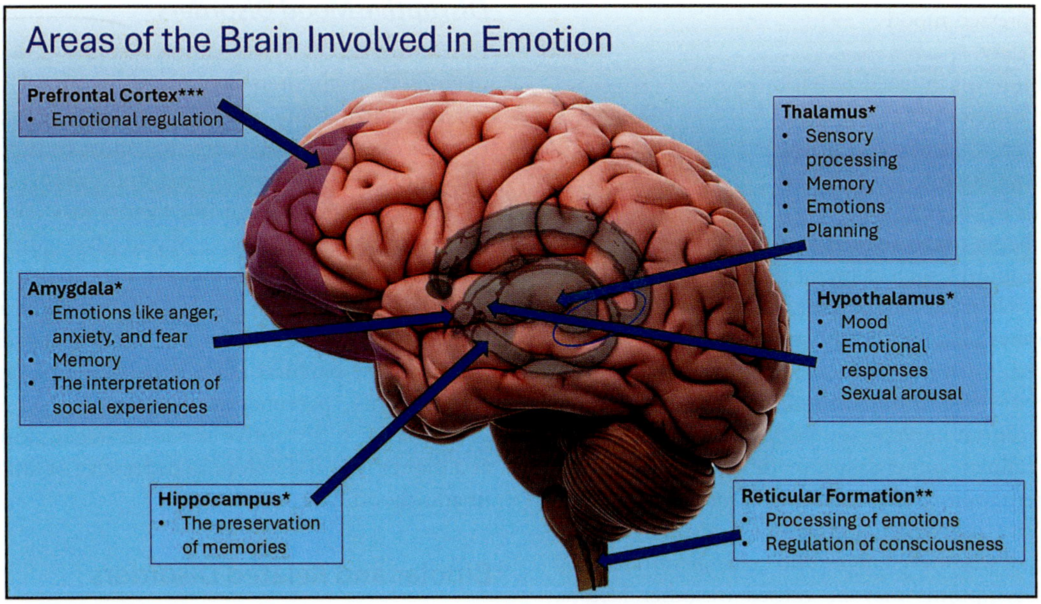

• **Fig. 23.1** Areas of the brain involved in emotion. (From 3dMediSphere/iStock photo 484757150. Information from *https://my.clevelandclinic.org/health/body/limbic-system, **https://www.physio-pedia.com/Reticular_Formation, ***https://pubmed.ncbi.nlm.nih.gov/28616997/.)

Mood Disorders

When a mood disturbance creates impairment in daily functioning, it may be diagnosed as a mood disorder. *The Diagnostic and Statistical Manual of Mental Disorders, Fifth Edition* has listed most of the mood disorders under one of two categories: depressive disorders or bipolar and related disorders.[6]

Depressive Disorders

Depressive disorders are characterized by sad, empty, or irritable mood resulting in an impairment of daily function. The diagnostic criteria for each specific depressive disorder are based on duration, timing, or causative factors.[6]

Major Depressive Disorder

Major depressive disorder is the most commonly recognized depressive disorder, characterized by long and persistent episodes of extreme sadness.[6,7]

This disorder is characterized by the presence of five or more of the following symptoms for at least 2 weeks, causing clinically significant distress or impairment in social or occupational function:

- Depressed mood
- Diminished interest or pleasure in activities
- Increase or decrease in weight or appetite
- Insomnia or hypersomnia
- Psychomotor agitation or retardation
- Fatigue
- Feelings of worthlessness or guilt
- Diminished ability to think, concentrate, or make decisions
- Thoughts of death or suicide

Multiple factors may contribute to the development of major depressive disorder. Physiological risk factors include a family history of depression. First-degree family members of individuals with major depressive disorder have a two to four times higher risk than that of the general population.[6] Heritability is estimated to be approximately 40%. Females may experience an increased risk for depressive disorders during certain reproductive life stages, including the premenstrual, postpartum, and perimenopause phases. Environmental risk factors include adverse childhood experiences, low income, limited education, racism, discrimination, stressful life events, and interpersonal trauma. Neuroticism is a temperamental risk factor. Individuals with high levels of neuroticism are more likely to experience a depressive episode in response to stressful life events.[6]

Persistent Depressive Disorder

Persistent depressive disorder is similar to major depressive disorder, but symptoms continue for at least 2 years in adults or 1 year in children. The etiology of persistent depressive disorder is similar to that of major depressive disorder.[6,7]

Premenstrual Dysphoric Disorder

Premenstrual dysphoric disorder is characterized by the presence of five or more of the following symptoms during the final week before the onset of menses, causing clinically significant distress or impairment in social or occupational function[6]:

- Marked mood lability or mood swings
- Marked irritability or anger

- Marked depressed mood
- Marked anxiety
- Decreased interest in usual activities
- Difficulty concentrating
- Fatigue
- Change in appetite
- Insomnia or hypersomnia
- A sense of being overwhelmed or out of control
- Physical symptoms such as breast tenderness or swelling, joint or muscle pain, bloating, or weight gain

The pathophysiology of premenstrual dysphoric disorder is understudied, with research emerging in recent years.[6] This disorder may be attributed to multiple factors, including abnormal central nervous system response to hormonal fluctuations, cellular vulnerability to the effect of sex hormones, and heritability. Additionally, environmental factors contribute to the disorder, including stress, history of interpersonal trauma, seasonal changes, and cultural influences.[6,8]

Depressive symptoms may be caused by other factors, such as substances, medications, medical conditions, or other causes. In these cases, an individual may be diagnosed with substance/medication-induced depressive disorder, depressive disorder due to another medical condition, other specified depressive disorder, and unspecified depressive disorder.[6]

Disruptive Mood Disorders

Disruptive mood dysregulation disorder (DMDD) may be diagnosed in children demonstrating chronic, severe, and persistent irritability with frequent temper outbursts for 12 months or longer. The symptoms must be inconsistent with the child's developmental level and grossly disproportionate to the situation.[6] Multiple factors may contribute to the development of disruptive mood dysregulation disorder. Physiological risk factors include a family history of depression and information-processing deficits. Environmental risk factors include abuse, neglect, parental mental illness, limited parental education, single-parent household, early trauma, parental death, divorce, and malnutrition. Children with disruptive mood dysregulation disorder are at a higher risk of developing depressive or anxiety disorders in adulthood.[6,7]

Bipolar and Related Disorders

The diagnostic criteria for bipolar and related disorders are based on mood episodes. A mood episode is a distinct period when mood is notably disturbed. Mood episodes are categorized as manic, hypomanic, or major depressive (Table 23.1).[6]

TABLE 23.1 Mood Episodes

Episode Type	Symptoms Affecting Occupational Performance	Duration	Functional Impact
Manic[6,9]	Abnormally and persistently elevated, expansive, or irritable mood and abnormally and persistently increased activity or energy, including three or more of the following symptoms: • Inflated self-esteem • Decreased need for sleep • More talkative than usual • Flight of ideas or racing thoughts • Distractibility • Increase in goal-directed activity or psychomotor agitation • Excessive involvement in risky activities	Symptoms last at least 1 week.	Marked impairment in social or occupational function, hospitalization is required, or psychotic features are present.
Hypomanic[6,9]	Abnormally and persistently elevated, expansive, or irritable mood and abnormally and persistently increased activity or energy, including three or more of the following symptoms: • Inflated self-esteem • Decreased need for sleep • More talkative than usual • Flight of ideas or racing thoughts • Distractibility • Increase in goal-directed activity or psychomotor agitation • Excessive involvement in risky activities	Symptoms last at least 4 consecutive days.	A change in functioning that is uncharacteristic of the individual and observable by others, typically not severe enough to cause marked impairment in social or occupational function nor include psychotic features that require hospitalization.
Major depressive[6,9]	Five or more of the following symptoms: • Depressed mood • Diminished interest or pleasure in activities • Increase or decrease in weight or appetite • Insomnia or hypersomnia • Psychomotor agitation or retardation • Fatigue • Feelings of worthlessness or guilt • Diminished ability to think, concentrate, or make decisions • Thoughts of death or suicide	Symptoms last at least 2 weeks.	Clinically significant distress or impairment in social or occupational function.

Bipolar I Disorder

Bipolar I disorder is characterized by recurring mood episodes, which may be manic, hypomanic, or major depressive. The diagnosis requires the occurrence of at least one manic episode.[6,9]

Bipolar II Disorder

Bipolar II disorder is also characterized by recurring mood episodes. The diagnosis requires the occurrence of at least one hypomanic episode and at least one major depressive episode.[6,9]

Cyclothymic Disorder

Cyclothymic disorder may be diagnosed in adults who experience at least 2 years of both hypomanic and depressive symptoms that do not meet the criteria for manic, hypomanic, or major depressive episodes.[6,9]

Bipolar I disorder, bipolar II disorder, and cyclothymic disorder are associated with various risk factors. Genetic heredity is a significant predisposing factor. In twin studies of bipolar disorder, heritability is estimated to be approximately 90%. Environmental factors, such as childhood adversity, life stress, and substance use, are also risk factors.[6,9]

Manic-like symptoms resembling bipolar disorder may be caused by other factors, such as substances, medications, medical conditions, or other causes. In these cases, an individual may be diagnosed with substance/medication-induced bipolar and related disorder, bipolar and related disorder due to another medical condition, other specified bipolar and related disorder, or unspecified bipolar and related disorder.[6,9]

The OT Scope of Practice

The occupational therapy (OT) scope of practice for individuals with mood disorders is similar to the OT scope of practice for any population: evaluate occupational performance and provide interventions to improve occupational performance.[10–12] Occupational therapy practitioners (OTPs) support clients in applying individualized strategies to increase participation in occupations, including activities of daily living, instrumental activities of daily living, rest and sleep, education, work, play, leisure, social participation, and health management. OTPs can educate clients on evidence-based self-management strategies and support clients in integrating these strategies into their occupational habits and routines. Interventions are client-centered and depend on individual occupations, needs, interests, and symptoms[10] (Table 23.2).

TABLE 23.2 Mood Disorders Sometimes Seen by Occupational Therapy Practitioners

Condition	Symptoms Affecting Occupational Performance	OT Intervention
Bipolar disorders	*Manic or hypomanic symptoms:* • Inflated self-esteem • Decreased need for sleep • More talkative than usual • Flight of ideas or racing thoughts • Distractibility • Increase in goal-directed activity or psychomotor agitation • Excessive involvement in risky activities *Depressive symptoms:* • Depressed mood • Diminished interest or pleasure in activities • Increase or decrease in weight or appetite • Insomnia or hypersomnia • Psychomotor agitation or retardation • Fatigue • Feelings of worthlessness or guilt • Diminished ability to think, concentrate, or make decisions • Thoughts of death or suicide	Increase engagement in healthy occupations such as social activities, exercise, leisure, or spirituality[13,14] Supported education and employment[13,14] Living skills training[13] Self-management interventions[13,15–18] Problem-solving interventions for improved occupational engagement[1,19,20] Wellness planning[17,19] Peer support[13,15,21,22] Family psychoeducation[14,23,24]
Major depressive disorder	Depressed mood Diminished interest or pleasure in activities Increase or decrease in weight or appetite Insomnia or hypersomnia Psychomotor agitation or retardation Fatigue Feelings of worthlessness or guilt Diminished ability to think, concentrate, or make decisions Thoughts of death or suicide	Increase engagement in healthy occupations such as social activities, exercise, leisure, or spirituality[13,14] Supported education and employment[13,14] Living skills training[13] Self-management interventions[13,19,25,26] Problem-solving interventions for improved occupational engagement[19,20] Wellness planning[19] Peer support[13,21,22] Family psychoeducation[9,14,23,24]

Application—Case Study

CASE EXAMPLE 23.1

A 34-year-old male presented to an OT outpatient clinic for his weekly OT session addressing functional deficits related to bipolar I disorder.

1. **Screen:** When the client presented for his weekly OT appointment, the certified occupational therapy assistant (COTA) noticed the client uncharacteristically demonstrated an irritable mood, hopelessness, and dark humor.
2. **Take a Closer Look:** The COTA informed the occupational therapist (OTR) who screened for suicidal ideation, asking, "Have you had any thoughts of killing yourself?" The client responded, "Yes." Next, the OTR screened for a suicidal plan, asking, "Have you been thinking about how you might do this?" The client responded, "I would swallow my bottle of pills." Next, the therapist screened for suicidal intent, asking, "Do you intend to carry out this plan?" The client responded, "I'm planning to do it on Friday after I see my brother."
3. **Determine Flag Status:** The client screened positive for suicidal ideation, plan, and intent, indicating a high risk of danger. The OTR and COTA both determined this to be a red flag.
4. **Take Action if Needed:** With the client present, the OTR and COTA called the client's psychiatrist on speakerphone and described the client's situation to the psychiatrist. The psychiatrist recommended immediate assessment in the psychiatric hospital, which was attached to the OT outpatient clinic. The OTPs walked the client to the psychiatric hospital admissions room.
5. **Document the Findings:** The COTA documented the client's initial presentation, the OTR's suicide screening results, the subsequent phone call with the psychiatrist, and the transition to the psychiatric hospital admissions room.
6. **Take a Second Look:** Upon admission to the psychiatric hospital, the admissions nurse determined the client to be at high risk of harm to himself, requiring hospitalization.
7. **Determine the Flag Status:** This remained a red flag situation.
8. **Take Action if Needed:** The client was admitted to the secure inpatient psychiatric hospital for treatment of his depressive episode. The client received treatment in this safe environment for 2 weeks until his symptoms subsided. After hospitalization, he returned to living independently, taking a different medication that better managed his symptoms and continued with outpatient OT and psychotherapy.

This is a true case. The COTA perceptively noticed mood and behaviors which were unusual for this client. The occupational therapist asked questions to screen for suicide risk, determined the client was indeed at risk for suicide, and ensured he received treatment. The COTA's perceptive observations, the occupational therapist's focused screening, and the collaborative critical thinking of both the COTA and OTR were what likely saved this man's life.

References

1. APA. *Mood.* APA Dictionary of Psychology; 2018. https://dictionary.apa.org/mood.
2. Sekhon S, Gupta V. Mood disorder. In: *StatPearls.* National Institutes of Health; 2023. https://www.ncbi.nlm.nih.gov/books/NBK558911/.
3. Longe JL, ed. Mood. In: *The Gale Encyclopedia of Psychology.* 4th ed. vol. 2. Gale; n.d.:821. https://link.gale.com/apps/doc/CX8273700543/GVRL?u=tel_a_belmont&sid=bookmark-GVRL&xid=7022aadb.
4. Longe JL, ed. Emotion. In: *The Gale Encyclopedia of Psychology.* 4th ed. vol. 1. Gale; 2022:381–384. https://link-gale-com.bunchproxy.idm.oclc.org/apps/doc/CX8273700263/GVRL?u=tel_a_belmont&sid=bookmark-GVRL&xid=9da97fd8.
5. Harvard. *What Causes Depression?* Harvard Medical School; 2022. https://www.health.harvard.edu/mind-and-mood/what-causes-depression.
6. American Psychiatric Association. *Diagnostic and Statistical Manual of Mental Disorders.* 5th ed. American Psychiatric Association; 2022. Text Revision. https://doi.org/10.1176/appi.books.9780890425787.
7. Mayo Clinic. *Mood Disorders.* The Mayo Clinic; 2021. https://www.mayoclinic.org/diseases-conditions/mood-disorders/symptoms-causes/syc-20365057.
8. Hantsoo L, Payne JL. Towards understanding the biology of premenstrual dysphoric disorder: from genes to GABA. *Neurosci Biobehav Rev.* 2023;149:105168–105168. https://doi.org/10.1016/j.neubiorev.2023.105168.
9. Mayo Clinic. *Bipolar Disorder.* Mayo Clinic; 2022. https://www.mayoclinic.org/diseases-conditions/bipolar-disorder/symptoms-causes/syc-20355955.
10. Bonder B. *Psychopathology and Function.* 6th ed. Slack Incorporated; 2022.
11. Wagman P, Håkansson C, Gunnarsson AB. Occupational performance issues in a longitudinal perspective in people with depression and/or anxiety on sick leave, returning to work or working. *Scand J Occup Ther.* 2023;30(2):159–169. https://doi.org/10.1080/11038128.2022.2046847.
12. Krpalek D, Achondo N, Daher N, Javaherian H. Reducing veterans' symptoms of depression, anxiety, stress, and posttraumatic stress, and enhancing engagement in occupations with SCUBA diving and OT. *J Veterans Stud.* 2020;6(1):98–106. https://doi.org/10.21061/jvs.v6i1.158.
13. Noyes S, Lannigan EG. *Occupational Therapy Practice Guidelines for Adults Living With Serious Mental Illness.* AOTA Press; 2019.
14. Brown C, Stoffel V, Muñoz J. *Occupational Therapy in Mental Health: A Vision for Participation.* 2nd ed. F.A. Davis Company; 2019.
15. Cai S, Zhou L, Yang X, Ma C, Xu L, Qian R. Investigation on the status quo of self-health management of patients with bipolar disorder and analysis of influencing factors. *J Nanomaterials.* 2021;2021:1–6. https://doi.org/10.1155/2021/9993172.
16. Geerling B, Kelders SM, Stevens AWM, Kupka RW, Bohlmeijer ET. A web-based positive psychology app for patients with bipolar disorder: development study. *JMIR Formative Res.* 2022;6(9):e39476–e39476. https://doi.org/10.2196/39476.
17. Johansen KK, Marcussen J, Hansen JP, Hounsgaard L, Fluttert F. Early recognition method for patients with schizophrenia or bipolar disorder in community mental health care: illness insight, self-management and control. *J Clin Nurs.* 2022;31(23–24):3535–3549. https://doi.org/10.1111/jocn.16181.

18. Ngooi BX, Wong SR, Chen JD, Yin Koh VS. Exploring the use of activity-based group therapy in increasing self-efficacy and subjective well-being in acute mental health. *Hong Kong J Occup Ther*. 2022;35(1):52–61. https://doi.org/10.1177/15691861221075798.
19. Petros R, Solomon P. Examining factors associated with perceived recovery among users of wellness recovery action plan. *Psychiatr Rehabil J*. 2020;43(2):132–139. https://doi.org/10.1037/prj0000389.
20. Nielsen TL, Holst-Stensborg HW, Nielsen LM. Strengthening problem-solving skills through OT to improve older adults' occupational performance – a systematic review. *Scand J Occup Ther*. 2023;30(1):1–13. https://doi.org/10.1080/11038128.2022.2112281.
21. Kelly JF, Hoffman L, Vilsaint C, Weiss R, Nierenberg A, Hoeppner B. Peer support for mood disorder: characteristics and benefits from attending the Depression and Bipolar Support Alliance mutual-help organization. *J Affect Disord*. 2019;255:127–135. https://doi.org/10.1016/j.jad.2019.05.039.
22. Bjørkedal STB, Bejerholm U, Hjorthøj C, Møller T, Eplov LF. Meaningful Activities and Recovery (MA&R): a co-led peer OT intervention for people with psychiatric disabilities. Results from a randomized controlled trial. *BMC Psychiatry*. 2023;23(1):406–406. https://doi.org/10.1186/s12888-023-04875-w.
23. Sari A, Duman ZÇ. Effects of the family support and psychoeducation program based on the Calgary Family Intervention Model on the coping, psychological distress and psychological resilience levels of the family caregivers of chronic psychiatric patients. *Arch Psychiatr Nurs*. 2022;41:1–10. https://doi.org/10.1016/j.apnu.2022.07.014.
24. Knaifel E. Cultural competence in multi-family psychoeducation groups: the experiences of Russian-speaking immigrant mothers of adults with severe mental illness. *Transcult Psychiatry*. 2023;60(1):156–166. https://doi.org/10.1177/13634615211058351.
25. Grieken RA, Tricht MJ, Koeter MW, Brink W, Schene A. The use and helpfulness of self-management strategies for depression: the experiences of patients. *PLoS One*. 2018;13(10):e0206262–e0206262. https://doi.org/10.1371/journal.pone.0206262.
26. Murphy J, Oanh PT, Goldsmith CH, Jones W, Nguyen VC. Introducing supported self-management for depression to primary care in Vietnam: a feasibility study in preparation for a randomized controlled trial. *Families Syst Health*. 2018;36(2):210–215. https://doi.org/10.1037/fsh0000337.

24
Anxiety Disorders

KATY SCHMIDT

OBJECTIVES

By the end of this chapter, the reader should be able to:

- Define the word *anxiety*.
- Demonstrate a basic understanding of the physiology involved in the fight-or-flight response.
- Compare and contrast fear versus anxiety.
- Differentiate between the symptoms of fear versus phobia.
- Explain and/or predict the possible symptoms resulting from the pathophysiology of various anxiety disorders.
- Assess and justify how a specific symptom resulting from an anxiety disorder could constitute a yellow or red flag.

Anxiety

Anxiety is an emotion typically experienced by healthy individuals.[1] Occasional anxiety is a part of life, resulting from adaptive responses developed to protect oneself from danger.[2] These feelings of anxiety are linked to the fight-or-flight response, keeping an individual alert and wary of potentially dangerous situations.

Fight-or-Flight Response

The fight-or-flight response is an adaptation that originally evolved to protect humans from predators, such as wild animals, in an effort to promote survival. In response to danger, the fight-or-flight response prepares the body to defend itself.[2] In today's society, most people are not threatened by wild animals, but the fight-or-flight response can still be triggered by modern life stressors such as academic exams, work pressures, or relationship conflicts.[3] The fight-or-flight response is a physiological response of both the parasympathetic and sympathetic divisions of the autonomic nervous system (Fig. 24.1).[3]

First, the sensory organs, such as the eyes or ears, sense the signs of danger. The amygdala then processes this sensory information (Fig. 24.2).

If the amygdala perceives a threat of danger, it activates the hypothalamus.[3] The hypothalamus signals the pituitary and adrenal glands, resulting in the release of three stress hormones: adrenaline, norepinephrine, and cortisol.[2] The release of stress hormones causes many changes throughout the body.[2–4] Energy is directed away from the parasympathetic nervous system, resulting in decreased activity in the digestive systems and the cerebral cortex (which controls conscious thought). The sympathetic nervous system is activated, which can cause muscle tension, increased heart rate, increased breathing rate, sweating, dry mouth, increased blood pressure, dilated pupils, and reduced pain sensitivity[2–4] (Fig. 24.3).

In healthy individuals, the fight-or-flight response eventually ceases, and the body returns to homeostasis after the threat of danger subsides. The physiological changes caused by the stress hormones are reversed. The parasympathetic nervous system is reactivated, and rest-and-digest functions return. The return to equilibrium typically takes 20 to 30 minutes after the danger passes.[4]

Fear

Fear is a strong emotional response to a real, immediate threat.[5] Fear is the internal emotional experience associated with the fight-or-flight response. People first experience fear as infants at approximately 7 months.[6] Some fears seem to be instinctive, such as the fear of loud noises, pain, injury, and animals such as snakes. Other fears are learned through experience and association. For example, an individual who experienced a motor vehicle accident may feel fear while driving.[6]

Anxiety

While fear is an emotional response to an immediate threat, anxiety is an emotional response to a future threat.[7] Anxiety may be experienced when entering a possibly threatening situation or when anticipating future dangers.[6] It can be caused by either real or imagined threats. Anxiety can be experienced by healthy

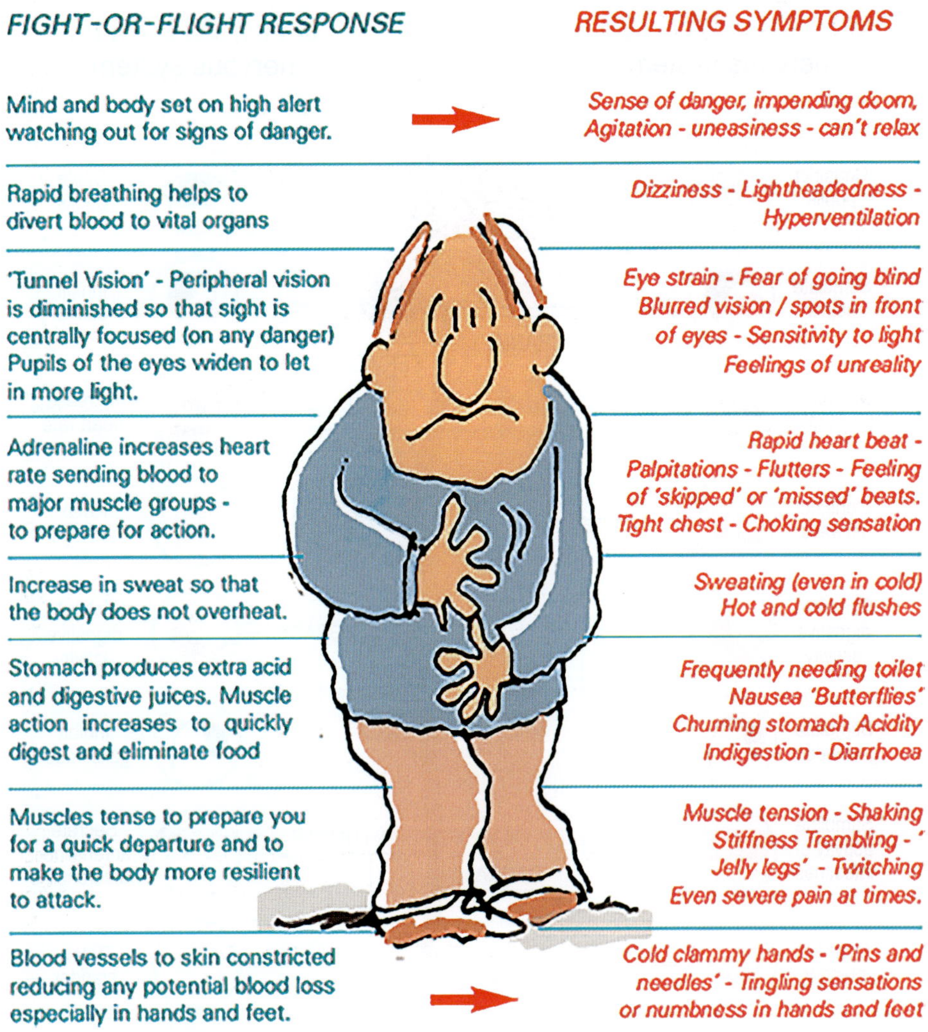

• **Fig. 24.1** Fight-or-flight response. (Copyright Robin Hall, CBT4Panic.org.)

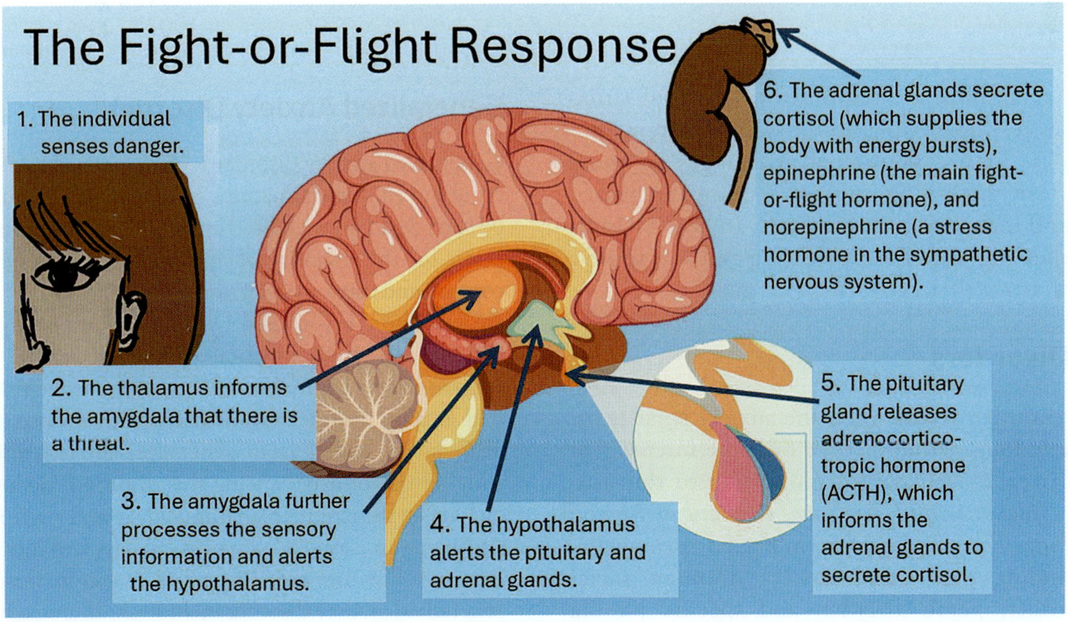

• **Fig. 24.2** The body's response to danger in the fight-or-flight response. (Image modified from iStock/blueringmedia, Brain Illustration: ID 2162347428; Data from Longe JL, eds. Fight/flight reaction. In: *The Gale Encyclopedia of Psychology*. 3rd ed., vol. 1. Gale eBooks; 2016:419–422. https://gale.com/apps/doc/CX3631000290/GVRL?u=tel_a_belmont&sid=bookmark-GVRL&xid=f4d20402.)

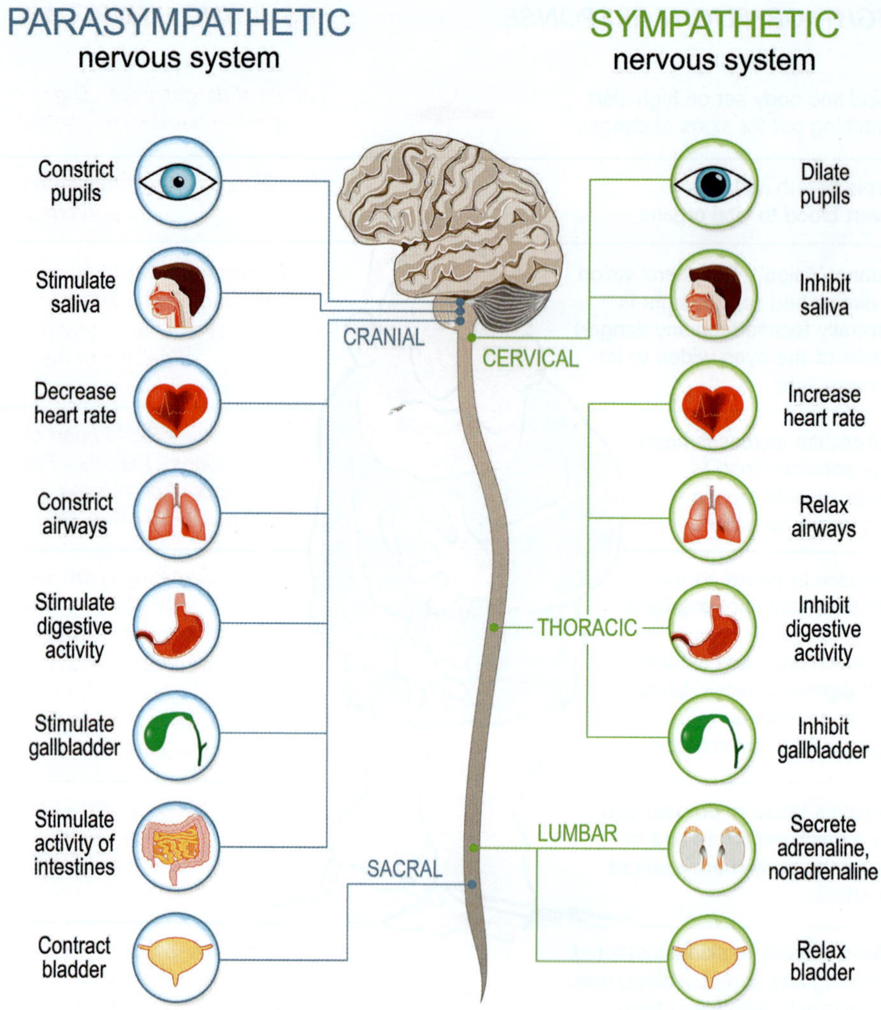

• **Fig. 24.3** The sympathetic nervous system. (From https://www.iStock.com/ttsz.)

individuals as appropriate responses to stressful situations, such as feeling anxious about starting a new job,[8] and results in similar physiological changes to those related to fear, including muscle tension, increased heart rate, and increased breathing rate. In healthy individuals, the feeling of anxiety is fleeting and will resolve with time.[8]

Anxiety Disorders

An anxiety disorder occurs when the anxiety persists for an abnormally long period of time or if the intensity of the anxiety is excessively out of proportion to the situation. The *Diagnostic and Statistical Manual of Mental Disorders, Fifth Edition* describes multiple anxiety disorders, including generalized anxiety disorder, social anxiety disorder, panic disorder, and specific phobia (Fig. 24.4).[9]

Generalized Anxiety Disorder

Generalized anxiety disorder is characterized by extreme anxiety about multiple situations, activities, or responsibilities. To be considered a generalized anxiety disorder, the anxiety must occur for the majority of at least 6 months, be difficult to control, and cause dysfunction in daily activities.[9] Generalized anxiety disorder is caused by a combination of genetic, biological, and environmental factors.[10] Genetic factors are responsible for approximately one-third of the risk of generalized anxiety disorder.[9] Individuals with a close (first-degree) relative who suffers from generalized anxiety disorder are at a higher risk of experiencing this disorder.[9] Biological factors include dysfunction in the amygdala and prefrontal cortex, leading to an elevated state of awareness and increased risk of anxiety.[11] Environmental factors that can increase the risk of generalized anxiety disorder include childhood adversity, traumatic events, stressful environments, and chronic illnesses.[10]

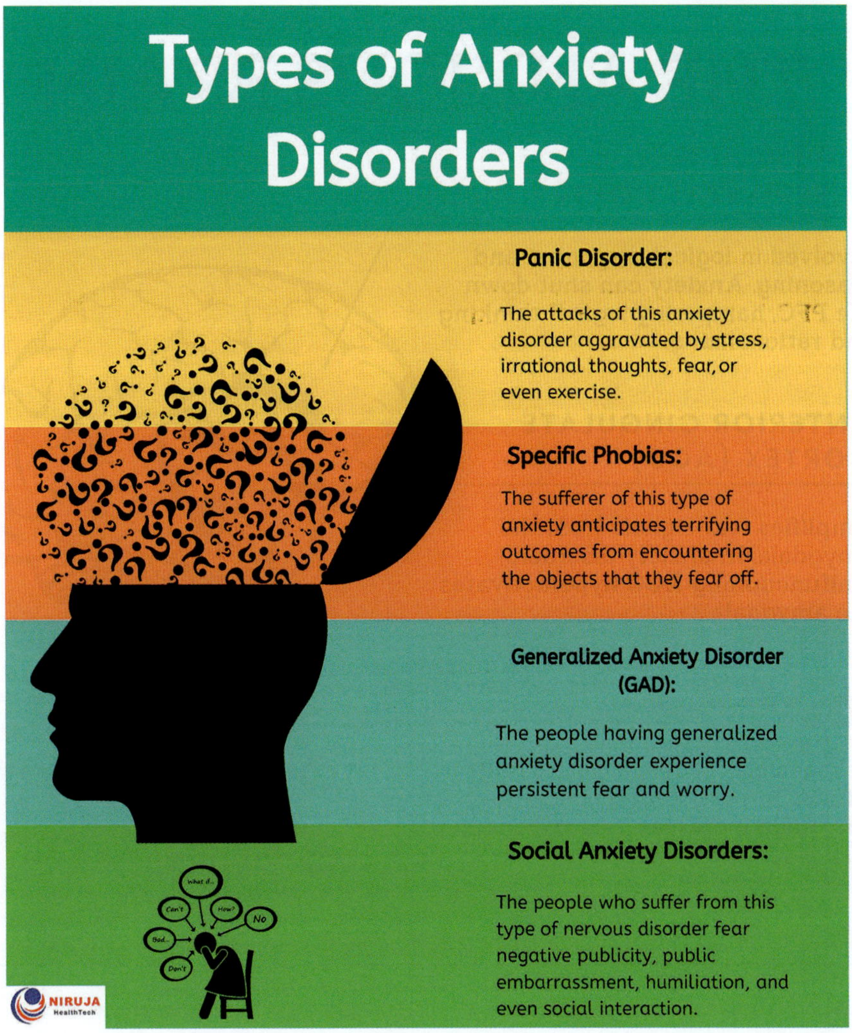

• **Fig. 24.4** Types of anxiety disorders. (From https://www.nirujahealthtech.com/types-of-anxiety-disorders/.)

Social Anxiety Disorder

Social anxiety disorder is defined by fear of social interactions, such as meeting new people, eating or drinking in front of others, or performing for others. The fear is out of proportion to the situation, may lead the individual to avoid social situations, and can cause problems with daily functions.[9] Social anxiety disorder is influenced by both genetic and environmental factors. Individuals with a close (first-degree) relative with social anxiety disorder are two to six times more likely to experience the same.[9] Genetic factors seem to impact the transmission of chemicals in the brain, including norepinephrine, dopamine, and serotonin. Individuals with social anxiety disorder have been found to experience dysfunction in the fronto-amygdala circuit as well as the fronto-parietal and temporal regions of the brain (Fig. 24.5).[11,12] Environmental risk factors include history of negative social situations, parents who demonstrate social anxiety, childhood adversity, and racism.[9,13]

Panic Disorder

Panic disorder is characterized by recurrent panic attacks or a sudden feeling of intense fear that typically peaks and subsides over the course of minutes.[14] Common symptoms of panic attacks include increased heart rate, heart palpitations, sweating, shaking, shortness of breath, chest discomfort, nausea, abdominal distress, dizziness, lightheadedness, altered sensations of temperature, tingling, numbness, feelings of unreality, feelings of detachment, fear of losing control, and fear of dying.[9,14] Individuals with panic disorder often experience fear of having additional panic attacks. They may, therefore, try to avoid anxiety-inducing situations to prevent panic attacks.[9,14]

Panic disorder is caused by genetic, biological, and environmental factors. Having parents with anxiety, depressive, or bipolar disorders increases one's risk of panic disorder.[9] Individuals with panic disorder have been found to have

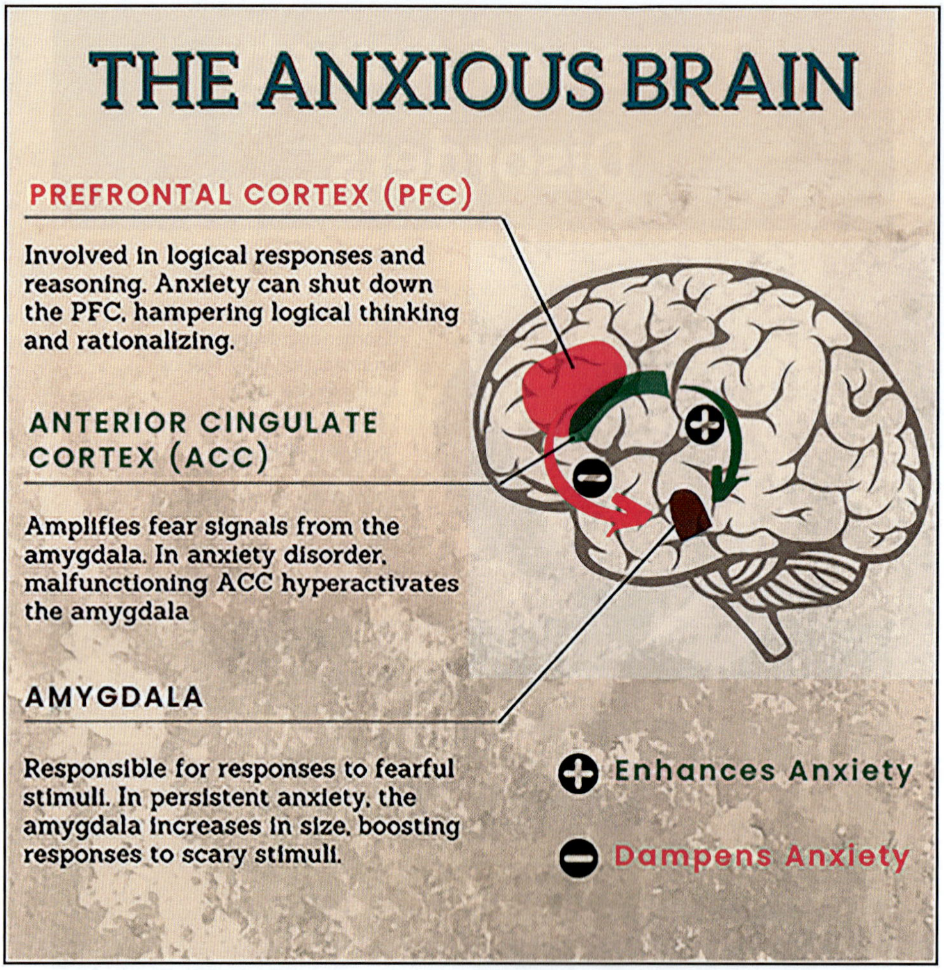

• **Fig. 24.5** The brain and anxiety. (From https://www.xcode.in/genes-and-health/how-anxiety-affects-brain/.)

differences in the gray matter of their frontal and temporal lobes, sensitized fear circuitry in the amygdala and insula, and respiratory sensitivities.[9,11] Environmental factors include life stressors, childhood adversity, history of trauma, overprotective parents, limited economic resources, and smoking.[9]

Specific Phobia

Specific phobia is the intense fear of a specific object or situation. Common sources of specific phobias include flying, heights, enclosed spaces, animals, insects, blood, and injections. The phobia causes avoidance of the feared object or situation and is out of proportion to the actual threat, causing dysfunction in daily activities.[9,15] Specific phobia can be caused by past experiences, genetic factors, or neurological functions. Phobias sometimes arise after a negative experience with the feared object or situation.[15] Genetic factors may contribute to the development of a phobia. Twin studies suggest that specific phobias have heritability rates between 25% and 33%.[9] Specific phobia is associated with altered brain activation patterns in the angular gyrus and occipital cortex of the brain.[13]

Obsessive-Compulsive Disorder

Obsessive-compulsive disorder (OCD) is an anxiety disorder in which an individual has upsetting, recurrent thoughts that are attempted to be controlled by repetitious behaviors.[16] These thoughts are unwarranted and intrusive, and because people with OCD realize that these thoughts are unreasonable, they experience extreme anxiety. Although individuals with OCD may realize that their symptoms are interfering with everyday life, they still feel compelled to perform the compulsions that go along with it.[16]

Occupational Therapy Approaches to Addressing Anxiety Disorders

Occupational therapy practitioners (OTPs) can support individuals with anxiety disorders by evaluating occupational

TABLE 24.1 Anxiety Disorders Sometimes Seen by Occupational Therapy Practitioners

Condition	Symptoms Affecting Occupational Performance	Occupational Therapy Intervention
Generalized anxiety disorder	Excessive anxiety about various events or activities	• Increase engagement in healthy occupations such as physical activity[18,19] • Problem-solving interventions for improved occupational engagement[20,21] • Self-management interventions[22] • Virtual reality exposure therapy[17] • Mindfulness-based interventions[23,24] • Sensory interventions[25] • Psychoeducational groups[26]
Social anxiety disorder	Excessive anxiety about social situations	
Panic disorder	Recurrent panic attacks	
Specific phobia	Excessive fear of a specific object or situation	

performance and providing interventions to improve occupational performance.[11] Anxiety disorders often result in avoidance of the feared objects, situations, or activities, leading to impairment in daily function.[9] OTPs can provide interventions to decrease the intensity of anxiety, such as through exposure to the feared environment or activity. OTPs may also improve self-management, adaptation, and healthy routines to improve the participation of individuals with anxiety disorders[17] (Table 24.1).

Application—Case Study

CASE EXAMPLE 24.1

A 68-year-old female presented to an occupational therapy assistant (COTA) in a skilled nursing facility for functional deficits related to a pelvic fracture.

1. **Screen:** The COTA started a session addressing functional mobility. As the COTA prepared the client for a transfer into the shower, the client began to sweat, breathe rapidly, clutch her chest, and yell "I'm having a heart attack!"
2. **Take a Closer Look:** The COTA took the client's vital signs and found her blood pressure was higher than usual for her, but still within the normal range.
3. **Determine Flag Status:** The client's behavior was concerning, but her vital signs did not indicate an emergency, so the COTA, along with guidance from the supervising occupational therapist, determined this to be a yellow flag situation.
4. **Take Action if Needed:** The OTPs provided immediate support to the client using therapeutic use of self and mindfulness exercises. Within minutes, the client calmed and reported her symptoms subsided. The COTA concluded the session and reported the events to nursing staff.
5. **Document the Findings:** The COTA documented the events of the session, including the client's presentation, interventions provided, and communication with the nursing staff.
6. **Take a Second Look:** After multiple professionals reported similar incidents with this client, the psychiatrist evaluated the client and diagnosed her with panic disorder.
7. **Determine the Flag Status:** This remained a yellow flag situation.
8. **Take Action if Needed:** The client received psychiatric treatment for panic disorder, including medication and psychotherapy. The client continued to engage in occupational therapy services to address functional deficits related to the pelvic fracture as well as panic disorder.

This is a true case. The occupational therapist and the COTA worked together as a team to support the client as she experienced a panic attack and then communicated with her team to ensure the client received appropriate treatment.

References

1. NIH. *Anxiety Disorders*. NIH: National Institute of Mental Health; 2023. https://www.nimh.nih.gov/health/topics/anxiety-disorders.
2. Encyclopedia Gale. Fight/flight reaction. In: Longe JL, ed. *The Gale Encyclopedia of Psychology*. 4th ed. Gale; 2022:821. https://link.gale.com/apps/doc/CX8273700543/GVRL?u=tel_a_belmont&sid=bookmark-GVRL&xid=7022aadb.
3. Harvard Health. *Understanding the Stress Response*. Harvard Health; 2020. https://www.health.harvard.edu/staying-healthy/understanding-the-stress-response.
4. Cleveland Clinic. *What Happens to Your Body During the Fight-or-Flight Response?* Cleveland Clinic; 2019. https://health.clevelandclinic.org/what-happens-to-your-body-during-the-fight-or-flight-response/.
5. American Psychological Association. *Fear*. American Psychological Association; 2025. https://dictionary.apa.org/fear.
6. Fear. In: Longe JL, ed. *The Gale Encyclopedia of Psychology*. 4th ed. Gale; 2022:821. https://link.gale.com/apps/doc/CX8273700543/GVRL?u=tel_a_belmont&sid=bookmark-GVRL&xid=7022aadb.
7. American Psychological Association. *Anxiety*. American Psychological Association Dictionary of Psychology. https://dictionary.apa.org/anxiety.
8. Encyclopedia Gale. Anxiety and anxiety disorders. In: Longe JL, ed. *The Gale Encyclopedia of Psychology*. 4th ed. Gale; 2022:821. https://link.gale.com/apps/doc/CX8273700543/GVRL?u=tel_a_belmont&sid=bookmark-GVRL&xid=7022aadb.
9. American Psychiatric Association. *Diagnostic and Statistical Manual of Mental Disorders*. 5th ed. American Psychiatric Association; 2022.
10. Cleveland Clinic. *Generalized Anxiety Disorder*. Cleveland Clinic; 2022. https://my.clevelandclinic.org/health/diseases/23940-generalized-anxiety-disorder-gad.

11. Bonder B. *Psychopathology and Function*. 6th ed. Slack Incorporated; 2022.
12. Mizzi S, Pedersen M, Lorenzetti V, et al. Resting-state neuroimaging in social anxiety disorder: a systematic review. *Mol Psychiatry*. 2022;27:164–179. https://doi.org/10.1038/s41380-021-01154-6.
13. Mayo Clinic. *Social Anxiety Disorder (Social Phobia)*. Mayo Clinic; 2021. https://www.mayoclinic.org/diseases-conditions/social-anxiety-disorder/symptoms-causes/syc-20353561.
14. National Institute of Mental Health. *Panic Disorder: When Fear Overwhelms*. https://www.nimh.nih.gov/health/publications/panic-disorder-when-fear-overwhelms#part_6101.
15. Mayo Clinic. *Specific Phobias*. 2023. https://www.mayoclinic.org/diseases-conditions/specific-phobias/symptoms-causes/syc-20355156.
16. Black R. OCD versus OCPD: symptoms and treatments. *Psycom*. 2018. https://www.psycom.net/ocd-vs-ocpd.
17. Donnelly MR, Reinberg R, Ito KL, et al. Virtual reality for the treatment of anxiety disorders: a scoping review. *Am J Occup Ther*. 2021;75(6):7506205040. https://doi.org/10.5014/ajot.2021.046169.
18. Noyes S, Lannigan EG. *Occupational Therapy Practice Guidelines for Adults Living With Serious Mental Illness*. AOTA Press; 2019.
19. Byrne GJ. Interventions for generalized anxiety disorder. *Curr Opin Psychiatry*. 2023;36(2):134–139. https://doi.org/10.1097/YCO.0000000000000840.
20. Petros R, Solomon P. Examining factors associated with perceived recovery among users of wellness recovery action plan. *Psychiatr Rehabil J*. 2020;43(2):132–139. https://doi.org/10.1037/prj0000389.
21. Nielsen TL, Holst-Stensborg HW, Nielsen LM. Strengthening problem-solving skills through occupational therapy to improve older adults' occupational performance – a systematic review. *Scan J Occup Ther*. 2023;30(1):1–13. https://doi.org/10.1080/11038128.2022.2112281.
22. Cao X, Feng M, Ge R, Wen Y, Yang J, Li X. Relationship between self-management of patients with anxiety disorders and their anxiety level and quality of life: a cross-sectional study. *PLoS One*. 2023;18(5):e0284121. https://doi.org/10.1371/journal.pone.0284121.
23. Yamamoto A, Tsukuda B, Minami S, et al. Effectiveness and changes in brain functions by an occupational therapy program incorporating mindfulness in outpatients with anxiety and depression: a randomized controlled trial. *Neuropsychobiology*. 2023;82(5):306–318. https://doi.org/10.1159/000531487.
24. Amanat Y, Morikawa S, Newman R. Systematic review brief—interventions for anxiety and depression for adults living with and beyond cancer (2018–2022). *Am J Occup Ther*. 2023;777710393280. https://doi.org/10.5014/ajot.2023.77S10028.
25. Ohene R, Logan C, Loresto F, et al. Assessing the impact of weighted blankets on anxiety among patients with anorexia nervosa and avoidant–restrictive food intake disorder: a randomized controlled trial. *Am J Occup Ther*. 2022;767606205100. https://doi.org/10.5014/ajot.2022.049295.
26. Holmes LG, Goebel RJ, Hollingue C, et al. Reductions in depression and anxiety among autistic adults participating in an intervention to promote healthy relationships. *Am J Occup Ther*. 2023;777702185070. https://doi.org/10.5014/ajot.2023.050108.

25

Personality Disorders

KATY SCHMIDT

OBJECTIVES

By the end of this chapter, the reader should be able to:

- Demonstrate a basic understanding of personality theory.
- Demonstrate a basic understanding of the various personality disorders.
- Differentiate between the symptoms of paranoid personality disorder versus schizoid personality disorder.
- Compare and contrast obsessive-compulsive personality disorder versus obsessive-compulsive disorder.
- Explain and/or predict the possible symptoms resulting from the pathophysiology of various personality disorders.
- Assess and justify how a specific symptom resulting from a personality disorder could constitute a yellow or red flag.

Personality Theory

Personality is defined as the pattern of characteristics, making each individual unique and influencing one's thoughts, emotions, and behavior.[1] There are many theories of personality. This chapter will briefly cover trait theory, humanistic theory, and social cognitive theory.

Trait Theory

The trait theory of personality defines personality as a combination of multiple qualities and characteristics. For instance, the Big Five personality model has identified five major dimensions of personality: extraversion, neuroticism, agreeableness, conscientiousness, and openness to experience (Fig. 25.1).[2]

Certain personality traits are associated with regions of the brain. For example, extraversion is associated with the medial orbitofrontal cortex, and conscientiousness is associated with the lateral prefrontal cortex (Fig. 25.2).[3]

Humanistic Theory

The humanistic approach to understanding personality focuses on the idea that personality relies heavily on how an individual feels about themselves and who they think they are.[4] Carl Rogers supported this idea with his writings about self-actualization, and Abraham Maslow also supported this idea with his hierarchy of needs.[4]

Social Cognitive Theory

Social cognitive theories encompass a combination of ideas from social learning theory, behaviorism, and expectancy-value theory.[4] The idea is that our behavior is often dictated by rewards and punishments, by observing others who act as models and then thinking things through before acting, and by believing that control over an outcome is possible through knowledge of past events and expectations of future rewards.[4]

Nature Versus Nurture

Personality is shaped by multiple factors, including genetic factors (nature). It is estimated that around half of the characteristics that make up personality are influenced by genetic factors.

Personality is also influenced by environmental factors, including early childhood experiences, primary relationships, and group belonging (nurture).[1] Culture also impacts personality. For example, Americans demonstrate greater independence (value of unique individualism) and East Asians demonstrate greater interdependence (value of relational harmony).[5]

Personality Over Time

Most theorists believe that personality stays relatively stable over time. Some personality traits, such as temperament, introversion, and extraversion, can be measured in

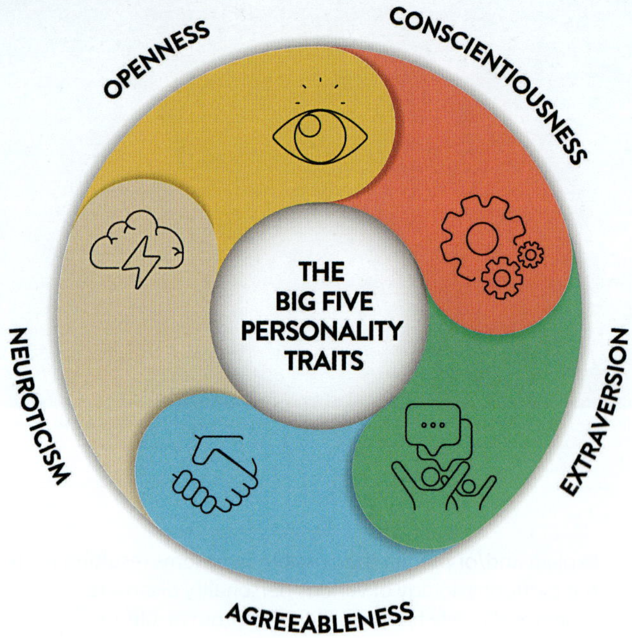

• **Fig. 25.1** The Big Five personality model. (From https://www.iStock.com/WhaleDesign).

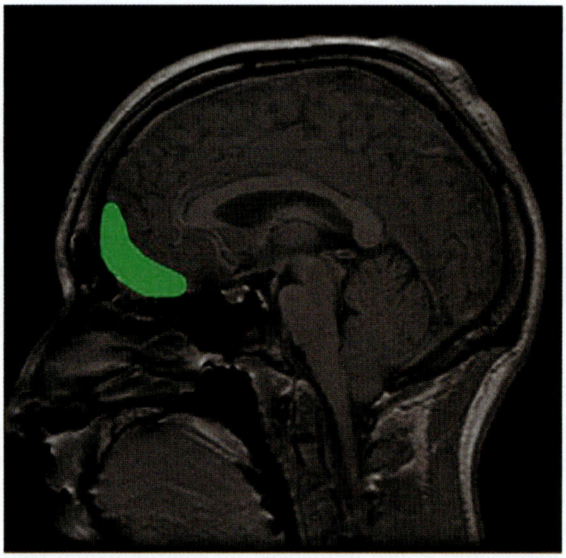

• **Fig. 25.2** The brain shows the orbitofrontal cortex and the prefrontal cortex. (From https://commons.wikimedia.org/wiki/File:MRI_of_orbitofrontal_cortex.jpg.)

infants and mostly remain stable for decades into adulthood.[3] Most individuals are capable of adapting their personality traits and behavior to various environments and demands. Typically, personality has a degree of flexibility to maintain healthy relationships and effective coping with life stressors.[6]

Personality Disorders

Individuals whose personality is inflexible with characteristics that lead to problems in daily life could be diagnosed with a personality disorder, as described by the *Diagnostic and Statistical Manual of Mental Disorders, Fifth Edition, (DSM-5)*.[7] Personality disorders are characterized by impairments in cognitive beliefs, emotional regulation, social skills, and impulse control. Individuals with personality disorders demonstrate behavior that is inflexible, consistent in many situations, and stable over time. These behavioral patterns are typically apparent from adolescence or young adulthood. The impairments can cause dysfunction in daily activities, with relationship problems listed as one of the more common difficulties.[7] The *DSM-5* identifies 10 specific personality disorders (Fig. 25.3).[7]

Paranoid Personality Disorder

Paranoid personality disorder is characterized by suspicion of others and concern that others will harm oneself. Individuals with the disorder often isolate themselves socially because of their distrust of others.[8] The prevalence of this disorder is estimated to be around 3.2%, and it is believed to be more common in men, with some increased prevalence in families.[9]

Schizoid Personality Disorder

Schizoid personality disorder is defined by feelings of indifference toward other people. Individuals with this disorder may appear detached or distant. They often avoid social situations due to a lack of interest in social activities or relationships.[10]

Schizotypal Personality Disorder

Schizotypal personality disorder is represented by unusual beliefs, speech, behaviors, and appearance. They may experience discomfort in social situations and have difficulty developing and maintaining relationships.[11] They are often described by others as eccentric or odd, which can cause anxiety and a tendency to avoid situations that require social interaction.[12]

Antisocial Personality Disorder

Antisocial personality disorder is characterized by recurrent violations of the rights of others without feelings of guilt or remorse. Common behaviors include lying, committing illegal acts, destroying property, and harming animals or people. These behaviors can cause relationship problems and possibly legal issues.[13]

Borderline Personality Disorder

Borderline personality disorder is defined by turbulent emotions and relationships. Individuals with borderline personality disorder are often highly sensitive to how others

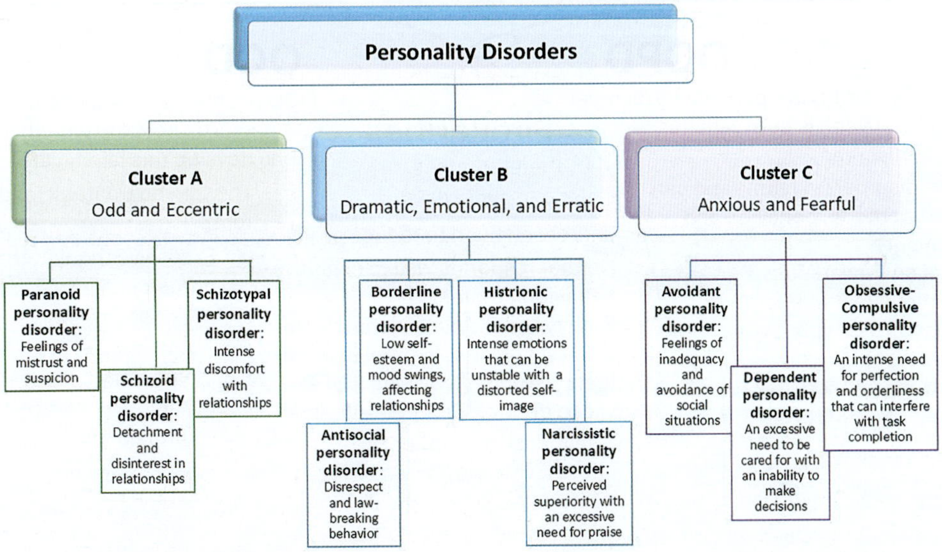

• **Fig. 25.3** The 10 personality disorders. (From: Cleveland Clinic. Personality disorders. 2022. https://my.clevelandclinic.org/health/diseases/9636-personality-disorders-overview.)

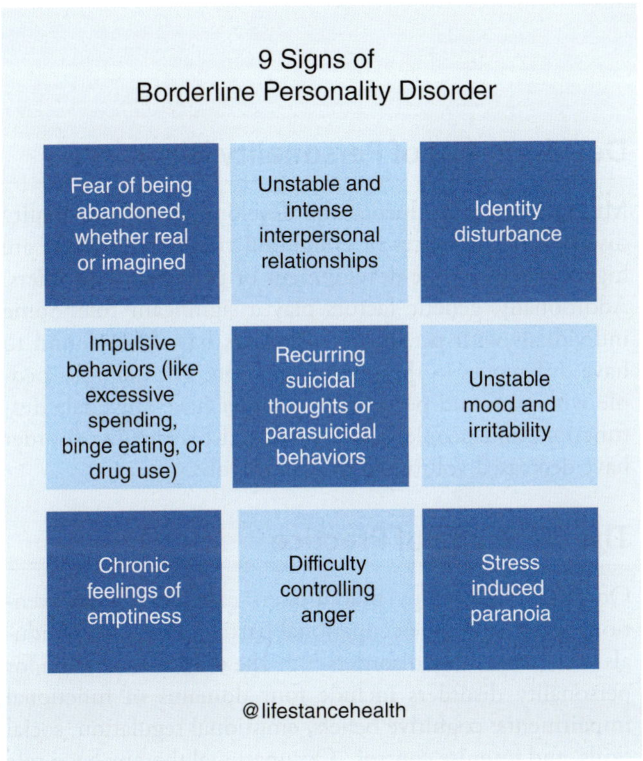

• **Fig. 25.4** Nine signs of borderline personality disorder. (From *Unveiling Borderline Personality Disorder: 9 Common Signs You Should Know*. LifeStance, https://lifestance.com/blog/signs-of-borderline-personality-disorder/.)

perceive them and experience severe fear of abandonment. They are at risk of impulsivity, self-injury, and suicide.[14]

Some of the signs of borderline personality disorder can be found in Fig. 25.4.

Histrionic Personality Disorder

Histrionic personality disorder is represented by a strong need for approval and attention from others. Individuals with this disorder may appear highly emotional, sensitive, flirtatious, or self-centered.[15] Individuals with this condition often demonstrate unstable emotions, with a distorted self-image, often behaving dramatically and erratically, and not realizing that their behavior is problematic.[16]

Narcissistic Personality Disorder

Narcissistic personality disorder appears as an inflated sense of self-worth, preoccupation with oneself, and minimal empathy for others. Individuals may be highly sensitive to criticism, often because their self-worth is insecure.[17]

Avoidant Personality Disorder

Avoidant personality disorder is defined by feelings of low self-esteem, shyness, and fear of rejection. These fearful

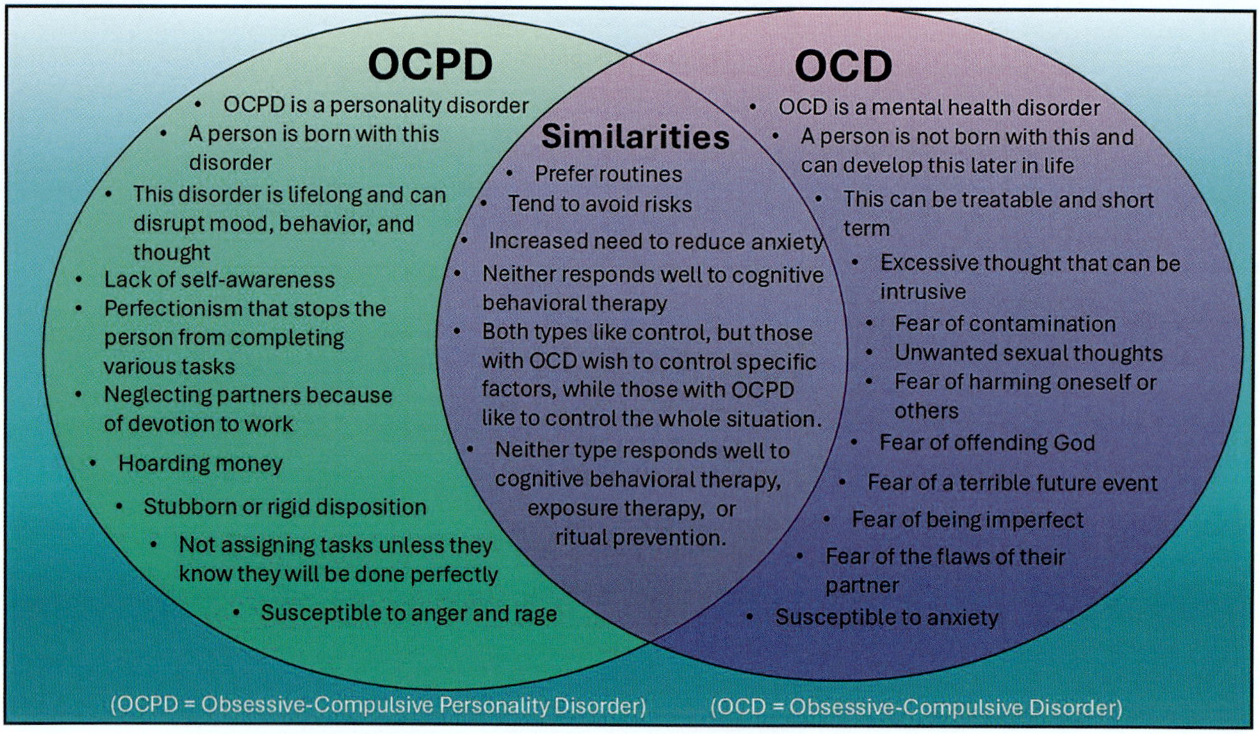

• **Fig. 25.5** Comparison of obsessive-compulsive personality disorder (OCPD) to obsessive-compulsive disorder (OCD). (Data from Felton A. (Reviewed by Bhandari S) *OCD vs. OCPD: What's the Difference?* WebMD; 2024. https://www.webmd.com/mental-health/ocd-vs-ocpd-whats-the-difference.)

feelings typically cause an individual to avoid social activities and relationships.[18]

Dependent Personality Disorder

Dependent personality disorder is represented by a high degree of reliance on others to meet one's emotional and physical needs. Individuals with this disorder often feel distrust toward themselves, helplessness, indecision, and passivity.[19]

Obsessive-Compulsive Personality Disorder

Obsessive-compulsive personality disorder (OCPD) is characterized by preoccupation with rules, orderliness, and control. This personality disorder has some similarities with obsessive-compulsive disorder (OCD). However, individuals with OCPD believe their thoughts are correct, and their behavior is appropriate. They may appear high-achieving and inflexible.[20] OCPD is a personality disorder, unlike OCD which is an anxiety disorder, discussed in Chapter 24. See Fig. 25.5 for a comparison of the two.

Development of Personality Disorders

Multiple factors influence the development of personality disorders. Experiences of childhood trauma and abuse are highly related to the development of personality disorders. Additionally, genetic factors play a significant role. Some individuals with personality disorders have been found to have differences in their brain function. For example, people with paranoid personality disorder have amygdala dysfunction, and people with schizotypal personality disorder have decreased volume in the frontal lobe.[21]

The OT Scope of Practice

Occupational therapy practitioners can provide interventions addressing the occupational participation of individuals with personality disorders.[22–24] The diagnostic criteria for personality disorders include four domains of functional impairments: cognitive beliefs, emotional regulation, social skills, and impulse control.[7] Occupational therapy has a role to address these functional impairments through improving skills, adapting activities, and modifying the environment (Table 25.1).[24]

TABLE 25.1 Personality Disorders Sometimes Seen by Occupational Therapy Practitioners

Condition	Symptoms	Occupational Therapy Intervention
Paranoid personality disorder	Suspicion of others	Increase engagement in healthy occupations[22–24] Problem-solving interventions for improved occupational engagement[24,25] Dialectical behavior therapy[26,27] Wellness planning[22,25] Skills training[26] Sensory interventions[28] Peer support[29] Psychoeducational groups[30] Family therapy and education[31,32]
Schizoid personality disorder	Indifference toward others	
Schizotypal personality disorder	Unusual beliefs and behaviors	
Antisocial personality disorder	Violations of the rights of others without remorse	
Borderline personality disorder	Turbulent emotions and relationships	
Histrionic personality disorder	Strong need for approval and attention from others	
Narcissistic personality disorder	Inflated self-worth	
Avoidant personality disorder	Low self-esteem and fear of rejection	
Dependent personality disorder	High degree of reliance on others to meet one's needs	
Obsessive-compulsive personality disorder	Preoccupation with rules, orderliness, and control	

Application—Case Study

CASE EXAMPLE 25.1

A 22-year-old female presented to an inpatient psychiatric hospital after a suicide attempt. The client was referred to occupational therapy to address functional deficits.

1. **Screen:** The occupational therapist (OTR) reviewed the client's medical chart and found that the client had diagnoses of bipolar disorder and borderline personality disorder. The client had a history of three suicide attempts and related psychiatric hospitalizations over the last 2 years.
2. **Take a Closer Look:** The OTR conducted an OT evaluation. During the conversations, the client excessively complemented the OTR's appearance and made a joke with a sexual innuendo.
3. **Determine Flag Status:** The client was in a safe environment in the inpatient psychiatric hospital, so risk of self-harm was minimal. The OTR felt concerned about the client's perception of their therapeutic relationship and decided that this needed to be addressed, so the OTR determined this to be a yellow flag situation.
4. **Take Action if Needed:** The OTR concisely explained the nature of the therapeutic relationship to the client. The OTR stated professional boundaries, including that personal appearance and sexual activities cannot be discussed with the members of the medical team. Knowing that individuals with borderline personality disorder are often highly sensitive to judgment or rejection, the OTR also briefly expressed concern for the client's well-being and reassured the client that OT intervention will continue as scheduled. The client apologized, expressing, "I'm so embarrassed, I'm just nervous."
5. **Document the Findings:** When documenting the evaluation, the OTR included the observations of the client's behavior, their communication, and the client's response.
6. **Take a Second Look:** The following day, the OTR saw the client for an OT group intervention. When the OTR entered the room, the client winked at the therapist. The client immediately apologized, expressing, "It was a friendly wink, not a flirty wink. It won't happen again."
7. **Determine the Flag Status:** The client demonstrated understanding of the therapeutic relationship and professional boundaries that the OTR had previously described. The client-therapist relationship improved dramatically over the days that followed. As no additional actions were required to address the nature of the relationship at this time, the therapist determined this to be a green flag situation.
8. **Take Action if Needed:** The OTR provided interventions as usual while remaining aware of any potential boundary violations from this client.

This is a true case. The client maintained a professional and therapeutic relationship with the OTR until she was discharged 2 weeks later. This story illustrates the importance of clear communication and intervening early to prevent problems in the therapeutic relationship.

References

1. American Psychological Association. *Personality.* American Psychological Association Dictionary of Psychology. https://dictionary.apa.org/personality.
2. American Psychological Association. *Big Five Personality Model.* American Psychological Association Dictionary of Psychology. https://dictionary.apa.org/big-five-personality-model.
3. Encyclopedia Gale. Personality. In: Longe JL, ed. *The Gale Encyclopedia of Psychology.* 4th ed. Gale; 2022:821. https://link.gale.com/apps/doc/CX3631000580/GVRL?u=tel_a_belmont&sid=bookmark-GVRL&xid=50c49837.

4. Gilette H. Theories of personality: these are the 6 main frameworks. *Psych Central*. 2022. https://psychcentral.com/health/personality-theories-in-psychology.
5. Na J, Grossmann I, Varnum MEW, et al. Culture and personality revisited: behavioral profiles and within-person stability in interdependent (vs. independent) social orientation and holistic (vs. analytic) cognitive style. *J Pers*. 2020;88(5):908–924. https://doi.org/10.1111/jopy.12536.
6. Mayo Clinic. *Personality Disorders*. 2023. https://www.mayoclinic.org/diseases-conditions/personality-disorders/symptoms-causes/syc-20354463.
7. American Psychiatric Association. *Diagnostic and Statistical Manual of Mental Disorders. 5th Ed. Text Revision*. American Psychiatric Association; 2022.
8. National Library of Medicine. Paranoid personality disorder. *MedlinePlus*. 2022. https://medlineplus.gov/ency/article/000938.htm.
9. Zimmerman M. Paranoid personality disorder (PPD). In: *MSD Manual: Professional Version*. 2023. https://www.msdmanuals.com/professional/psychiatric-disorders/personality-disorders/paranoid-personality-disorder-ppd.
10. National Library of Medicine. *Schizoid Personality Disorder*. MedlinePlus; 2022. https://medlineplus.gov/ency/article/000920.htm.
11. National Library of Medicine. *Schizotypal Personality Disorder*. MedlinePlus; 2022. https://medlineplus.gov/ency/article/001525.htm.
12. Mayo Clinic. *Schizotypal Personality Disorder*. Mayo Clinic; 2022. https://www.mayoclinic.org/diseases-conditions/schizotypal-personality-disorder/symptoms-causes/syc-20353919.
13. National Library of Medicine. *Antisocial Personality Disorder*. MedlinePlus; 2022. https://medlineplus.gov/ency/article/000921.htm.
14. National Library of Medicine. *Borderline Personality Disorder*. MedlinePlus; 2022. https://medlineplus.gov/ency/article/000935.htm.
15. National Library of Medicine. *Histrionic Personality Disorder*. MedlinePlus; 2022. https://medlineplus.gov/ency/article/001531.htm.
16. Cleveland *Clinic. Histrionic Personality Disorder*. Cleveland Clinic; 2022. https://my.clevelandclinic.org/health/diseases/9743-histrionic-personality-disorder.
17. National Library of Medicine. *Narcissistic Personality Disorder*. MedlinePlus; 2022. https://medlineplus.gov/ency/article/000934.htm.
18. National Library of Medicine. *Avoidant Personality Disorder*. MedlinePlus; 2022. https://medlineplus.gov/ency/article/000940.htm.
19. National Library of Medicine. *Dependent Personality Disorder*. MedlinePlus; 2022. https://medlineplus.gov/ency/article/000941.htm.
20. National Library of Medicine. *Obsessive-Compulsive Personality Disorder*. MedlinePlus; 2022. https://medlineplus.gov/ency/article/000942.htm.
21. Cleveland Clinic. *Personality Disorders*. 2022. https://my.clevelandclinic.org/health/diseases/9636-personality-disorders-overview.
22. Harding K. Enhancing the occupational therapy role around "personality disorder" and self-harm. *Br J Occup Ther*. 2020;83(9):547–548. https://doi.org/10.1177/0308022620947642.
23. Wasmuth S, Mokol E, Szymaszek K, Gaerke KJ, Manspeaker T, Lysaker P. Intersections of occupational participation and borderline personality disorder: a grounded theory approach. *Cogent Psychol*. 2020;7(1):1803580. https://doi.org/10.1080/23311908.2020.1803580.
24. Connell C, Furtado V, McKay EA, Singh SP. Developing an intervention to improve occupational participation for justice-involved people with a personality disorder: defining and describing intervention components. *Int J Offender Ther Comp Criminol*. 2022;66(6–7):774–788. https://doi.org/10.1177/0306624X211013520.
25. Petros R, Solomon P. Examining factors associated with perceived recovery among users of wellness recovery action plan. *Psychiatr Rehabil J*. 2020;43(2):132–139. https://doi.org/10.1037/prj0000389.
26. Machnik K, Ghneim H, Leep A, et al. Potential OT interventions for people with borderline personality disorder: a scoping review. *Am J Occup Ther*. 2023;77(Supplement_2):7711505186–7711505186p1. https://doi.org/10.5014/ajot.2023.77S2-PO186.
27. Wetterborg D, Dehlbom P, Långström N, Andersson G, Fruzzetti AE, Enebrink P. Dialectical behavior therapy for men with borderline personality disorder and antisocial behavior: a clinical trial. *J Pers Disord*. 2020;34(1):22–39. https://doi.org/10.1521/pedi_2018_32_379.
28. Matson R, Kriakous S, Stinson M. The experiences of women with a diagnosis of borderline personality disorder (BPD) using sensory modulation approaches in an inpatient mental health rehabilitation setting. *Occup Ther Ment Health*. 2021;37(4):311–331. https://doi.org/10.1080/0164212X.2021.1933674sss.
29. Barr KR, Townsend ML, Grenyer BFS. Using peer workers with lived experience to support the treatment of borderline personality disorder: a qualitative study of consumer, carer and clinician perspectives. *Borderline Personal Disord Emot Dysregul*. 2020;7:20. https://doi.org/10.1186/s40479-020-00135-5.
30. Kallis AC, Saeed SA. Borderline personality disorder: 6 studies of psychosocial interventions: evidence suggests benefits from several forms of psychoeducation and psychotherapy. *Curr Psychiatr*. 2022;21(2):18–26. https://doi.org/10.12788/cp.0218.
31. Nuntavisit L, Porter M. Mediating effects of discipline approaches on the relationship between parental mental health and adolescent antisocial behaviours: retrospective study of a multisystemic therapy intervention. *Int J Environ Res Public Health*. 2022;19(20):13418. https://doi.org/10.3390/ijerph192013418.
32. Martin K, Holz T, Woodward G, Cameron M. Exploring the impact of a peer-led education group for loved ones of individuals with borderline personality disorder: a pilot study. *Contemp Fam Ther*. 2020;42(3):240–249. https://doi.org/10.1007/s10591-020-09543-9.

26

Psychotic Disorders

KATY SCHMIDT

OBJECTIVES

By the end of this chapter, the reader should be able to:

- Demonstrate a basic understanding of the physiology involved when thinking.
- Compare and contrast delusions and hallucinations.
- Differentiate between the symptoms of schizophrenia and schizoaffective disorder.
- Explain and/or predict the possible symptoms resulting from the pathophysiology of various psychotic disorders.
- Assess and justify how a specific symptom resulting from a psychotic disorder could constitute a yellow or red flag.

The Physiology of "Thinking"

The term "thinking" refers to the cognitive functions that help an individual to perceive, process, and use information. These mental functions include attention, perception, memory, decision-making, problem-solving, and language.[1] The brain receives electrical and chemical signals from the body through a complex integration of neurons. Many of these signals are processed and interpreted in the cerebrum, the largest part of the brain. The cortex is the outer layer of the cerebrum, and it is highly involved in thinking. The cerebrum is divided into four lobes, which are responsible for these unique functions[2] (Fig. 26.1).

Each of the four lobes plays a part in enabling an individual to tell what is real in the world and what is not. The frontal lobe is responsible for executive functions, which are complex mental actions that control other simpler mental functions. Executive functions include the formation of ideas, the organization of thoughts, the ability to make decisions and solve problems, the capacity to plan actions, adaptability to change, and the regulation of impulses.[3] The parietal lobe integrates sensory information for the perception and recognition of tastes, sounds, sights, smells, and textures. It is also involved in spatial relationships, navigation, and body awareness.[4]

The temporal lobe is important for understanding information and communication. It contributes to memory, language processing, and emotional experience. The temporal lobe also processes sensory information, especially auditory and visual input.[5] The occipital lobe is primarily responsible for vision.[2] This lobe also plays an important role in reading, storing memories, and recognizing faces and places.[6]

Psychotic Disorders

Psychosis refers to a collection of symptoms that involve altered thinking and disconnection from reality.[7] Individuals with psychotic disorders often struggle to distinguish what aspects of their life are real and not. They might see things that are not really there or believe things to be true that are impossible.[8] The *Diagnostic and Statistical Manual of Mental Disorders, Fifth Edition*, identifies five key symptoms of psychotic disorders.[7]

Psychotic Symptoms

Delusions

Delusions are firmly held beliefs that contradict reality. Even if presented with opposing evidence, someone experiencing a delusion will not be swayed. Some beliefs are commonly held within a culture, and even if they seem unparalleled in reality, these beliefs cannot be considered delusions.[9] The most common types of delusions are as follows: persecutory, referential, and grandiose.[10] A persecutory delusion is the belief that an individual is being conspired against, for example, believing they are being followed by investigators. A referential delusion is the belief that ordinary events and behaviors have significant meaning for the individual, such as believing a newscaster on television is sending them a message. A grandiose delusion inflates a person's perception of their worth, identity, and abilities, for instance, a person believing they are a famous, talented singer.[10]

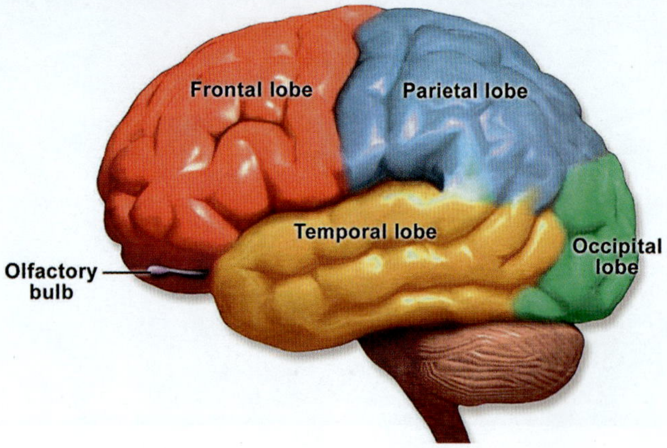

• **Fig. 26.1** Brain anatomy. (From https://en.wikipedia.org/wiki/Lobes_of_the_brain.)

"Positive" symptoms	"Negative" symptoms
• Delusions • Hallucinations • Disorganized speech • Disorganized behavior • Agitation	• Lack of interest • Difficulties organizing • Concentration difficulties • Social isolation • Lack of emotions • Lack of energy

• **Fig. 26.2** The positive and negative symptoms of psychosis. (From https://www.e-hospital.co.uk/resources/psychosis-in-children/.)

Hallucinations

A hallucination is a sensory experience of something that is not real. The person experiencing the hallucination perceives the sensation as if it is truly real, but it is only occurring in their mind. Auditory hallucinations are the most common type of hallucinations. Examples of auditory hallucinations are hearing voices, footsteps, banging, music, or other sounds that are not occurring in reality.[11] Visual hallucinations are also common, such as seeing lights, objects, beings, or patterns that are not there. Tactile hallucinations are false sensations of touch, such as feeling something crawling on the skin or the movement of internal organs. Olfactory hallucinations (smelling unreal odors) and gustatory hallucinations (tasting false flavors) are possible but less common.[11]

Disorganized Thought

Disorganized thinking is defined by illogical thoughts and loosely associated with one another. These ideas may even be completely unrelated and unfocused. A person experiencing disorganized thinking is unable to sequence steps logically or complete goal-oriented actions. Because a person's thoughts cannot be directly observed, disorganized thinking is typically made apparent through an individual's speech patterns.[12] Disorganized speech may be circumstantial (including irrelevant details), tangential (digressing from the main point without returning), perseverating (repeating words or statements), or incoherent (using an assortment of unrelated words).[12]

Disorganized Behavior

Disorganized behavior is characterized by actions that are purposeless, illogical, or unusual. Individuals with disorganized behavior have difficulty completing goal-directed actions or performing daily activities.[13] Disorganized behavior can include unexpected expressions of emotion, such as suddenly laughing or yelling without apparent cause. Movements may be excessive or purposeless, like repeatedly gesturing without meaning. Actions may be inappropriate for the situation, such as wearing winter clothing on a hot summer day or engaging in sexual activities in public.[13]

Negative Symptoms

Negative symptoms refer to a variety of behaviors typically seen in the average person but decreased or absent in an individual with a psychotic disorder. Flat affect is a lack of emotional expression. Alogia is a reduction in the quantity of words spoken. Avolition is a lack of motivation to complete tasks.[14] Asociality is a reduction in social interactions. Anhedonia is a decreased experience of pleasure. Out of all the key symptoms of psychosis, negative symptoms have the greatest association with long-term disability and poor quality of life (Fig. 26.2).[14]

The vast majority of individuals experiencing psychosis are not aggressive. In fact, they are more likely to be victims of violence than the general population.[15]

Schizophrenia

Schizophrenia is the most common psychotic disorder. The symptoms of schizophrenia are the five key symptoms of psychosis: delusions, hallucinations, disorganized thinking, disorganized behavior, and negative symptoms. What makes schizophrenia different from other psychotic conditions is the degree of severity and the combination of all five conditions of psychosis, plus other symptoms that interfere with normal daily life. The symptoms lead to decreased function in daily activities and must persist for a minimum of 6 months.[16]

The development of schizophrenia is highly associated with genetic and physiological factors. Schizophrenia has a heritability between 70% and 80%.[17] Pregnancy and birth complications are risk factors for developing schizophrenia.[15] In individuals with schizophrenia and schizoaffective disorder (see later), the frontal, parietal, and temporal cortices have been found to be thinner than those without psychotic disorders. The thinner the cortex, the more severe the psychotic symptoms.[18] For those with a genetic predisposition to schizophrenia, the risk and severity of symptoms are increased by environmental factors, such as adverse child experiences, low socioeconomic status, discrimination, and racism (Fig. 26.3).[7]

Other Psychotic Disorders

Schizoaffective disorder includes symptoms of both psychotic disorders and mood disorders. In addition to the five key symptoms of psychosis, individuals with schizoaffective disorder also experience mood symptoms such as mania

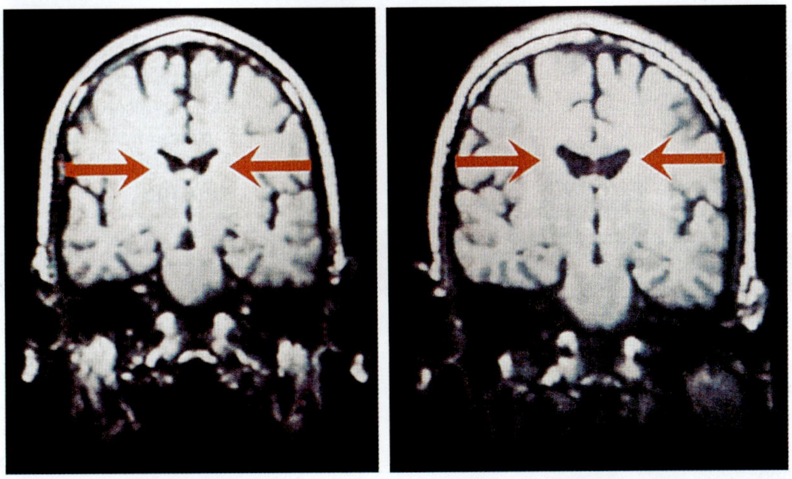

• **Fig. 26.3** The healthy brain compared to the brain of their twin with schizophrenia. (Courtesy Daniel R. Weinberger, MD, Director and CEO, Lieber Institute for Brain Development Maltz Research Laboratories. Professor of Psychiatry, Neurology, Neuroscience and Genetic Medicine Johns Hopkins University School of Medicine Baltimore, Maryland.)

TABLE 26.1 Psychotic Disorders Sometimes Seen by Occupational Therapy Practitioners

Condition	Symptoms That Could Affect Occupational Performance	Occupational Therapy Intervention
Schizophrenia	Psychotic symptoms Delusions Hallucinations Disorganized thinking Disorganized behavior Negative symptoms	Individualized interventions for ADLs, IADLs, and sleep performance[22,23] Supported education and employment[22] Increase engagement in healthy occupations such as exercise, art, or leisure[20–22] Self-monitoring and wellness planning[20] Skills training[21,22] Sensory interventions[24] Peer support[21] Psychoeducational groups[20]
Schizoaffective disorder	Psychotic symptoms Delusions Hallucinations Disorganized thinking Disorganized behavior Negative symptoms Mood symptoms Mania Depression	

ADL, Activities of daily living; *IADL*, instrumental activities of daily living.

and/or depression. The causes of schizoaffective disorder are similar to those of schizophrenia.[19]

Other psychotic disorders may be diagnosed depending on the presentation and cause. Psychotic symptoms can be caused by substances, medications, medical conditions, or other mental disorders.[7]

OT Approaches to Addressing Psychotic Disorders

Occupational therapy practitioners evaluate and provide interventions addressing the occupational performance of individuals with psychotic disorders. Because the presentation and functional impact of psychotic symptoms can vary drastically, individualized interventions are particularly effective.[20] Cognitive impairments are common in psychotic disorders; therefore, occupational therapy practitioners should carefully assess how cognition impacts occupational performance and consider providing interventions such as cognitive skill training, compensatory strategies, or environmental modifications[21] (Table 26.1).

Application—Case Study

CASE EXAMPLE 26.1

A 13-year-old boy presented to the school-based occupational therapist (OTR) to address his poor academic performance and disruptive behaviors in the classroom. The student was diagnosed with attention-deficit/hyperactivity disorder (ADHD).

1. **Screen:** During the OT evaluation, the student showed flat affect and reluctance to share information about himself.
2. **Take a Closer Look:** The OTR was concerned about the student's unusual behavior. After learning more about his situation, she administered the two-item screen for early psychosis, first asking the student, "Do you see things that others can't or don't see?" The student denied this experience. Second, the OTR asked the student, "Have you ever felt that someone was playing with your mind?" The student responded "Yes," and described feelings that the teachers and staff were playing tricks on him and plotting to suspend him.
3. **Determine Flag Status:** The student screened positively for early psychosis, so the OTR determined this to be a yellow flag situation, recognizing the need for additional assessment.
4. **Take Action if Needed:** The OTR notified the school psychologist of the situation.
5. **Document the Findings:** The OTR documented her observations of the student, the results of the early psychosis screening, and her communication with the school psychologist.
6. **Take a Second Look:** The school psychologist referred the student to a pediatric psychiatrist. After months of monitoring and assessing, the student was eventually diagnosed with schizophrenia.
7. **Determine the Flag Status:** This remained a yellow flag situation, as the student required immediate intervention.
8. **Take Action if Needed:** The student received mental health services. He transitioned from middle school to high school, and high school staff were informed of the situation as appropriate.

This is a true case. The student demonstrated unusual behaviors, which can be potential signs of early psychosis. The OTR's referral led to the student receiving interventions for schizophrenia. Early interventions for psychosis are vital for preventing exacerbation of symptoms and functional decline, which should have long-term benefits over the course of the student's life.

References

1. Cognition. In: Longe JL, ed. *The Gale Encyclopedia of Psychology*. 4th ed. Gale; 2022:821. https://link.gale.com/apps/doc/CX8273700543/GVRL?u=tel_a_belmont&sid=bookmark-GVRL&xid=7022aadb.
2. Johns Hopkins Medicine. *Brain Anatomy and How It Works*. 2024. https://www.hopkinsmedicine.org/health/conditions-and-diseases/anatomy-of-the-brain.
3. American Psychological Association. *Executive Functions*. American Psychological Association Dictionary of Psychology. 2023. https://dictionary.apa.org/executive-functions.
4. Cleveland Clinic. *Parietal Lobe*. 2023. https://my.clevelandclinic.org/health/body/24628-parietal-lobe.
5. Cleveland Clinic. *Temporal Lobe*. 2023. https://my.clevelandclinic.org/health/body/16799-temporal-lobe.
6. Cleveland Clinic. *Occipital Lobe*. Cleveland Clinic; 2022. https://my.clevelandclinic.org/health/body/24498-occipital-lobe
7. American Psychiatric Association. *Diagnostic and Statistical Manual of Mental Disorders*. 5th ed. Text Revision. American Psychiatric Association; 2022. https://www.khanacademy.org/science/health-and-medicine/executive-systems-of-the-brain/psychotic-disorders/a/what-are-psychotic-disorders.
8. Khan Academy. *What Are Psychotic Disorders?* Khan Academy; 2024. https://www.khanacademy.org/science/health-and-medicine/executive-systems-of-the-brain/psychotic-disorders/a/what-are-psychotic-disorders.
9. Joseph SM, Siddiqui W. Delusional disorder. In: *StatPearls [Internet]*. StatPearls Publishing; 2024. https://www.ncbi.nlm.nih.gov/books/NBK539855/.
10. Collin S, Rowse G, Martinez AP, Bentall RP. Delusions and the dilemmas of life: a systematic review and meta-analyses of the global literature on the prevalence of delusional themes in clinical groups. *Clin Psychol Rev*. 2023;104:102303. https://doi.org/10.1016/j.cpr.2023.102303.
11. National Library of Medicine. *Hallucinations*. MedlinePlus; 2022. https://medlineplus.gov/ency/article/003258.htm.
12. Calabrese J, Khalili YA. Psychosis. In: *StatPearls [Internet]*. StatPearls Publishing; 2024. https://www.ncbi.nlm.nih.gov/books/NBK546579/.
13. American Psychological Association. *Disorganized Behavior*. American Psychological Association Dictionary of Psychology. https://dictionary.apa.org/disorganized-behavior.
14. Correll CU, Schooler NR. Negative symptoms in schizophrenia: a review and clinical guide for recognition, assessment, and treatment. *Neuropsychiatr Dis Treat*. 2020;16:519–534. https://doi.org/10.2147/NDT.S225643.
15. NIH. *Schizophrenia*. National Institute of Mental Health; 2023. https://www.nimh.nih.gov/health/topics/schizophrenia.
16. Mayo Clinic. *Schizophrenia*. Mayo Clinic; 2020. https://www.mayoclinic.org/diseases-conditions/schizophrenia/symptoms-causes/syc-20354443.
17. St Clair D, Lang B. Schizophrenia: a classic battle ground of nature versus nurture debate. *Sci Bull*. 2021;66(10):1037–1046. https://doi.org/10.1016/j.scib.2021.01.032.
18. Stan AD, Tamminga CA, Han K, et al. Associating psychotic symptoms with altered brain anatomy in psychotic disorders using multidimensional item response theory models. *Cereb Cortex*. 2020;30(5):2939–2947. https://doi.org/10.1093/cercor/bhz285.
19. Cleveland Clinic. *Schizoaffective Disorder*. 2023. https://my.clevelandclinic.org/health/diseases/21544-schizoaffective-disorder.
20. Shimida T, Kobayashi M, Ohori M, Inagaki Y, Shimooka Y, Ishihara I. Cost-effectiveness of individualized occupational therapy for schizophrenia: results from a two-year randomized controlled trial. *Asian J Occup Ther*. 2020;16:29–35. https://doi.org/10.11596/asiajot.16.29.
21. Anggraini Y, Wahyudi A, Larasati DI, Yusuf A. The effectiveness of occupational therapy on patients with schizophrenia or another mental illness: a systematic review. *J Ners (Surabaya)*. 2020;15(1):538–547. https://doi.org/10.20473/jn.v15i1Sp.20523.
22. Noyes S, Lannigan EG. *Occupational Therapy Practice Guidelines for Adults Living With Serious Mental Illness*. AOTA Press; 2019.
23. Faulkner SM, Drake RJ, Ogden M, Gardani M, Bee PE. A mixed methods expert opinion study on the optimal content and format for an occupational therapy intervention to improve sleep in schizophrenia spectrum disorders. *PLoS One*. 2022;17(6):e0269453. https://doi.org/10.1371/journal.pone.0269453.
24. Zengin G, Yazici MR, Huri M. Sensory integration based program developed according to the model of creative ability in an individual with schizophrenia: an occupational therapy case report. *Int J Disabil Sports Health Sci*. 2022;5(1):66–74. https://doi.org/10.33438/ijdshs.1099222.

27

Eating Disorders

KATY SCHMIDT

OBJECTIVES

By the end of this chapter, the reader should be able to:

- Demonstrate a basic understanding of the behaviors involved in healthy eating.
- Discuss statistics related to eating disorders among various populations.
- Differentiate between the symptoms of anorexia nervosa and bulimia nervosa.
- Explain and/or predict the possible symptoms resulting from avoidant/restrictive food intake disorder.
- Assess and justify how a specific symptom resulting from an eating disorder could constitute a yellow or red flag.

Eating

Eating is not just a response behavior to hunger, but it is a function that produces nutrients, energy, and growth necessary for survival. Eating behaviors are controlled by multiple parts of the brain. The brain is divided into three structures: the forebrain, midbrain, and hindbrain (Fig. 27.1).[1]

The forebrain is the largest part of the brain and is highly developed.[1] Deep within the forebrain is the hypothalamus, which is responsible for maintaining stability and homeostasis. Among other functions, the hypothalamus creates the senses of hunger and fullness.[2] The hypothalamus helps maintain a consistent body weight, by estimating how much food a person needs to consume in order to compensate for the energy the person expends.[3] The hypothalamus will then generate signals to start or stop eating as needed by the body.

The hindbrain, which includes the upper part of the spinal cord, part of the brainstem, the pons, medulla oblongata, and cerebellum (see Fig. 27.1), is responsible for vital functions of survival, such as heart rate and breathing.[1] The hindbrain also contains circuits that lead to the termination of eating. If a person has eaten enough or is ill, the hindbrain can create sensations of satiety or nausea. These functions also contribute to the maintenance of a stable body weight.[3]

Definitions of the term *healthy eating* can vary greatly depending on an individual's situation and needs, but there are some consistent key features. A person is considered to have healthy eating when they consume food while hungry and stop consuming food once they have satiety (or when they feel full).[4] Healthy eating requires regularity, with routine meals and snacks throughout the day. For most people, eating three meals and a few snacks each day is typical. Healthy eating also requires variety, with numerous foods from all food groups (Fig. 27.2), and flexibility, adapting to changes in routine, context, or situation. Finally, healthy eating can provide pleasure by enjoying what is eaten as well as the social contexts and special occasions that may be celebrated through food.[5]

Typically, there are occasions when eating may not seem particularly healthy, such as eating the same meal repeatedly, skipping meals, avoiding certain food groups, or eating because the individual is feeling bored, sad, or stressed. A person might feel concerned about their health, weight, or appearance, causing them to follow a strict diet. These behaviors are fairly common. If these behaviors are not impacting the individual's function or health, they can be considered aspects of typical eating.[4,6]

Eating Disorders

Whenever function or health are impacted, these maladaptive behaviors may be classified as eating disorders.[4,6] *The Diagnostic and Statistical Manual of Mental Disorders, Fifth Edition* identifies several unique eating disorders.[7] Some statistics related to these disorders are depicted in Fig. 27.3.

Disordered eating behaviors, weight gain, or weight loss can cause changes in the hypothalamus and brain circuitry responsible for experiencing reward and regulating food consumption. These changes in the brain may reinforce disordered eating behaviors or contribute to the development of an eating disorder.[8,9]

Anorexia Nervosa

Anorexia nervosa is defined by restricted eating, severe fear of gaining weight, and distorted body image, resulting in

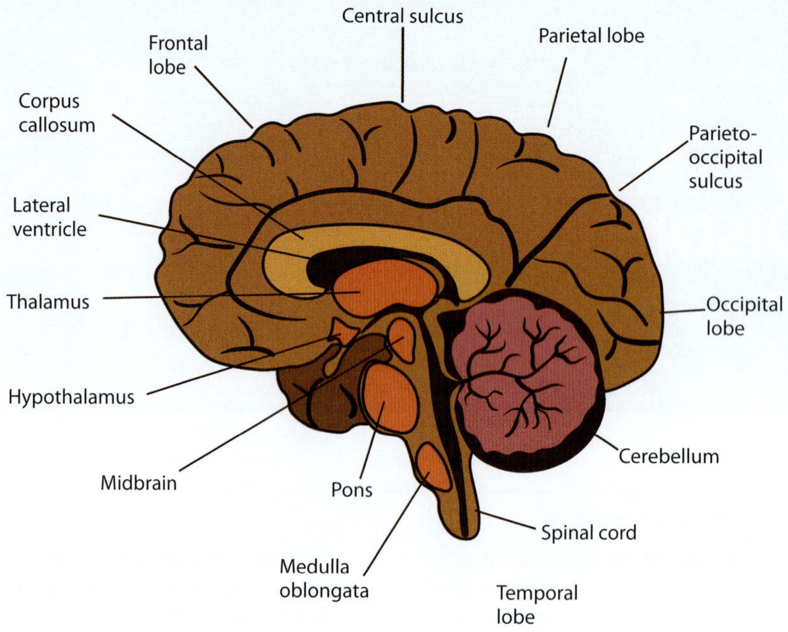

• **Fig. 27.1** Brain anatomy. (From www.istockphoto.com/be_moll.)

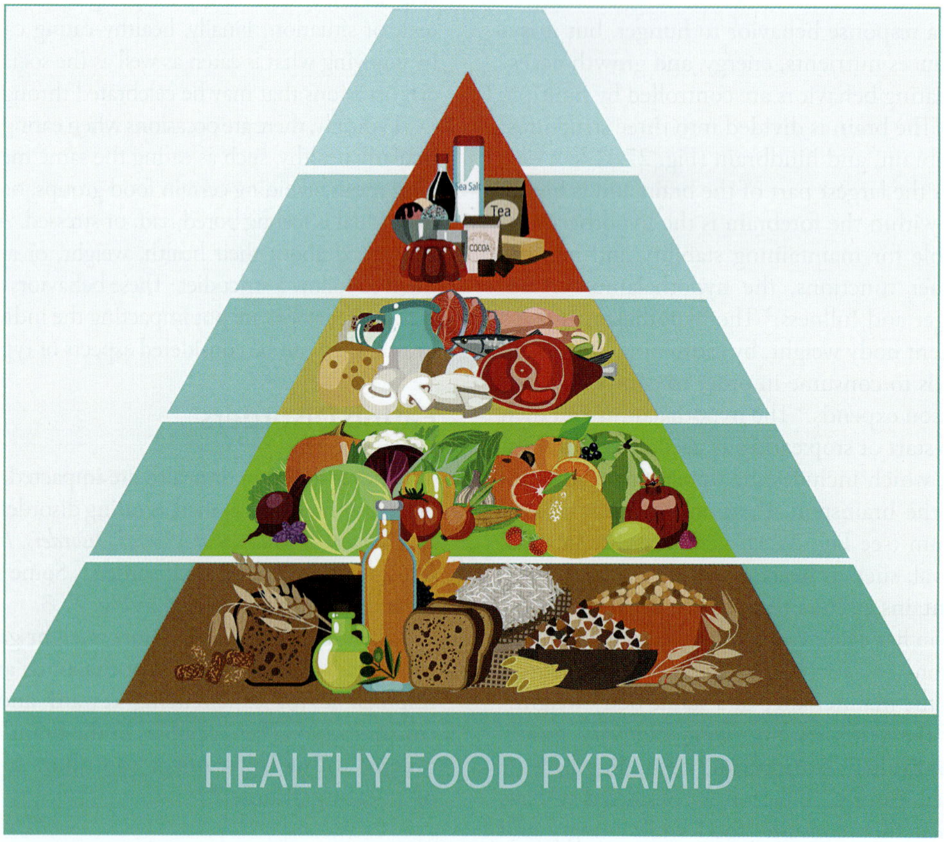

• **Fig. 27.2** The food pyramid. (From https://sustainable.harvard.edu/tools-resources/how/healthy-eating-plate.)

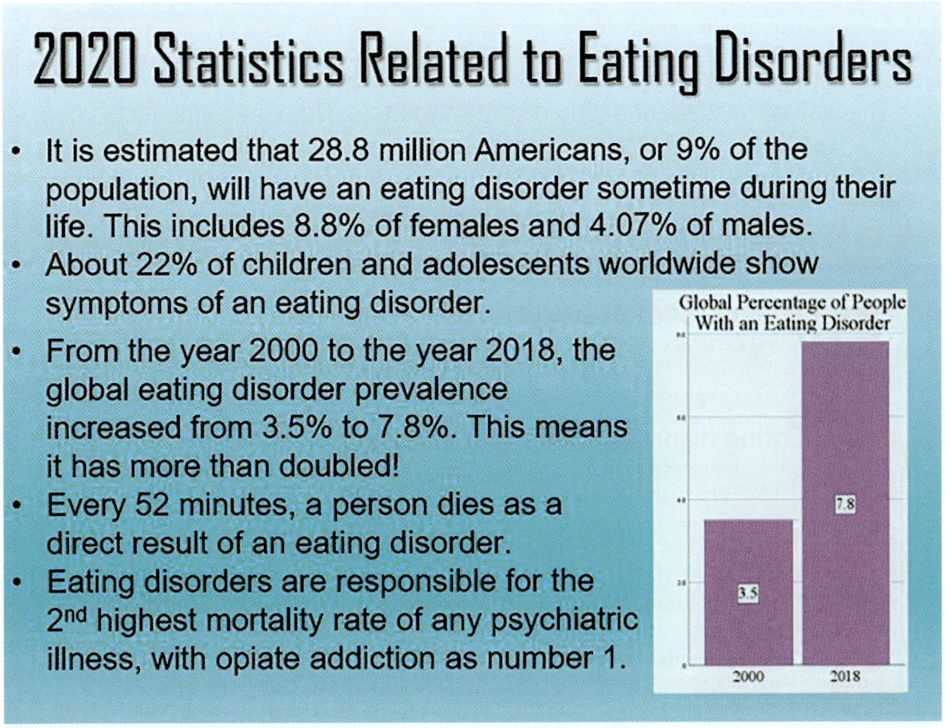

• **Fig. 27.3** Eating disorder statistics. (Adapted from Bunnell D. *Eating Disorder Statistics*. National Eating Disorders Association; 2025. https://staging.nationaleatingdisorders.org/statistics/.)

significantly low weight.[10] There are two types of anorexia nervosa. Restricting type is characterized by weight loss through dieting, fasting, or excessive physical activity. Binge-eating/purging type includes episodes of binge eating (overeating in a short period while feeling out of control) and/or purging (behaviors to prevent weight gain such as self-induced vomiting or misusing laxatives).[10]

The behaviors associated with anorexia nervosa can cause serious, potentially fatal medical conditions such as malnutrition or organ failure.[10] Depressive symptoms and obsessive-compulsive features commonly occur with anorexia nervosa, and the risk of suicide is high in individuals with this disorder.[10]

Multiple factors contribute to the development of anorexia nervosa. Genetic factors are involved, as biological relatives of individuals with anorexia nervosa are at a higher risk of developing the disorder.[11] People who show anxiety or obsessive qualities in childhood are at a higher risk of developing this disorder. Exposure to cultures or environments where thinness is valued, such as certain athletic or modeling industries, also increases an individual's risk of developing anorexia nervosa.[11]

Bulimia Nervosa

Bulimia nervosa is characterized by repeated episodes of binge eating and purging, which happen at least weekly for 3 months. Individuals with bulimia nervosa also place high importance on body weight, which significantly impacts their self-esteem.[12] They typically have a normal weight or are overweight. Behaviors related to bulimia nervosa may cause serious medical conditions, such as gastrointestinal problems, esophageal tears, or cardiac dysfunction.[12]

Various factors influence the development of bulimia nervosa. Genetic vulnerabilities to the disorder are possible. Physiological factors, such as childhood obesity and early puberty, increase one's risk of developing the disorder. Certain temperaments, including anxiety, depressive symptoms, poor self-esteem, or weight concerns, are associated with bulimia nervosa. Individuals who have experienced child abuse are at a greater risk of the disorder.[7]

Binge-Eating Disorder

Binge-eating disorder is defined by repeated episodes of binge eating, which happen at least weekly for 3 months. Binge eating may involve eating very quickly, eating when not hungry, eating past feelings of satiety, eating alone, and experiencing subsequent feelings of shame, guilt, or disgust. Binge eating causes feelings of distress about eating behaviors. This disorder does not include restrictive or purging behaviors.[13]

Individuals with binge-eating disorders are at an increased risk of health problems and healthcare utilization. Individuals with binge-eating disorder can be within the range of

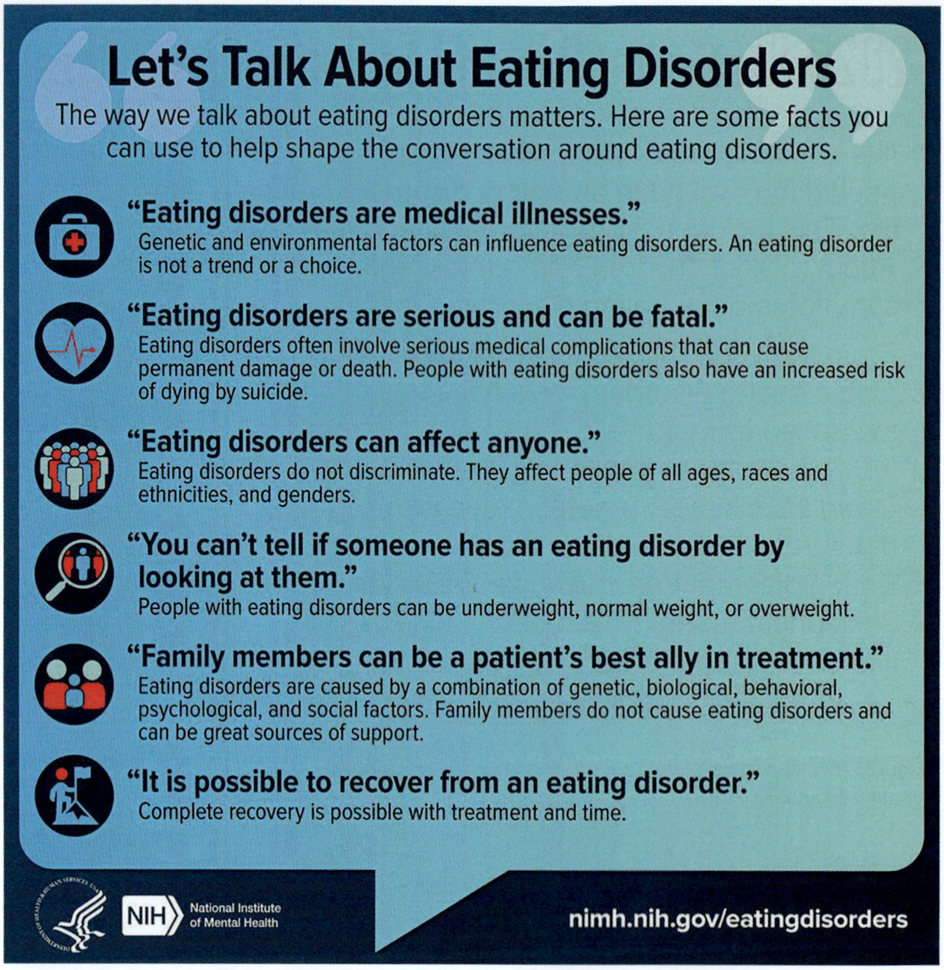
Let's Talk About Eating Disorders
The way we talk about eating disorders matters. Here are some facts you can use to help shape the conversation around eating disorders.
"Eating disorders are medical illnesses."
Genetic and environmental factors can influence eating disorders. An eating disorder is not a trend or a choice.
"Eating disorders are serious and can be fatal."
Eating disorders often involve serious medical complications that can cause permanent damage or death. People with eating disorders also have an increased risk of dying by suicide.
"Eating disorders can affect anyone."
Eating disorders do not discriminate. They affect people of all ages, races and ethnicities, and genders.
"You can't tell if someone has an eating disorder by looking at them."
People with eating disorders can be underweight, normal weight, or overweight.
"Family members can be a patient's best ally in treatment."
Eating disorders are caused by a combination of genetic, biological, behavioral, psychological, and social factors. Family members do not cause eating disorders and can be great sources of support.
"It is possible to recover from an eating disorder."
Complete recovery is possible with treatment and time.
NIH National Institute of Mental Health
nimh.nih.gov/eatingdisorders

• **Fig. 27.4** Eating disorder facts. (From https://www.nimh.nih.gov/health/publications/lets-talk-about-eating-disorders.)

normal BMI, overweight, or obese. It is important to distinguish obesity from binge-eating disorder, as most obese individuals do not binge eat.[14] The development of binge-eating disorder is affected by multiple factors. A family history of the disorder, along with a history of dieting, poor body image, or stress, can increase a person's risk of developing binge-eating disorder.[14]

Avoidant/Restrictive Food Intake Disorder

When an individual has avoidant/restrictive food intake disorder (ARFID), they severely limit eating or completely refuse to eat certain foods.[15] This is not because they want to lose weight, but rather due to various other reasons, such as the color, texture, or smell of the food. Some of these individuals have a fear of choking or a fear of stomach problems. This disorder can happen at any age but is more common among children. This limitation can lead to problems with growth or cause illness.[15] More information about eating disorders can be found in Fig. 27.4.

Occupational Therapy Approaches to Addressing Individuals with Eating Disorders

Eating disorders clearly impact an individual's engagement in any occupation that relates to food, including eating, meal preparation, shopping, and social participation. In addition, the psychological, emotional, cognitive, physical, and medical factors associated with eating disorders further complicate engagement in all occupations. Occupational therapy practitioners can provide evaluations and interventions to improve the occupational performance of individuals with eating disorders[15] (Table 27.1).

A case example of an OT client with an eating disorder is provided below.

TABLE 27.1 Eating Disorders Sometimes Seen by Occupational Therapy Practitioners

Condition	Symptoms	Occupational Therapy Intervention
Anorexia nervosa	Restricted eating Significantly low weight Severe fear of gaining weight Distorted body image	Increase engagement in occupations that provide identity, purpose, and meaning[16] Occupation-based groups (e.g., meal preparation or grocery shopping)[17,18] Community reintegration (e.g., swimming or eating in restaurants)[18] Coping skills training to manage distress during occupational performance[16] Goal-setting and problem-solving interventions[16] Environmental adaptations[16] Relapse prevention planning[16] Peer support[19]
Bulimia nervosa	Binge eating Purging Overvaluation of body weight	
Binge-eating disorder	Binge eating Distress about binge eating	

Application—Case Study

CASE EXAMPLE 27.1

A 20-year-old female presented to an occupational therapist (OTR) in an inpatient eating disorder unit of a psychiatric hospital for occupational performance deficits related to anorexia nervosa.

1. **Screen:** The OTR completed an occupational profile during the evaluation and then assigned the client's case to the certified occupational therapy assistant (COTA) for interventions. The client described disordered behaviors related to eating and exercise. It was apparent that these behaviors gave the client a sense of routine, identity, and purpose.
2. **Take a Closer Look:** Besides the disordered eating and exercise, the client was unable to identify any other occupations that felt meaningful to her. With prompts from the COTA, the client explained that, before the exacerbation of her symptoms, her college classes and pursuit of a nursing career felt meaningful.
3. **Determine Flag Status:** The COTA determined this to be a yellow flag situation and recommended continuing OT services throughout the client's length of stay on the inpatient unit.
4. **Take Action if Needed:** The OTR and COTA collaborated to develop a treatment plan to reengage the client in school and career-related occupations, which were previously meaningful, in order to give the client a sense of routine, identity, and purpose unrelated to the disordered behaviors.
5. **Document the Findings:** The OTR documented the occupational profile and treatment plan.
6. **Take a Second Look:** Through OT intervention, the client made a plan to return to school. The client experienced distress at the thought of returning to school and self-imposed pressure to achieve high academic success.
7. **Determine the Flag Status:** The COTA observed that the client's distress was a barrier to occupational performance and determined this to be a yellow flag situation requiring additional OT intervention.
8. **Take Action if Needed:** Through OT intervention, the client learned to implement functional coping strategies to prevent or manage distress while engaging in occupations. For example, the client learned to reframe negative thoughts that appeared while completing school-related activities.

This is a true case. The client regained routine, identity, and meaning from functional occupations. As the client engaged in treatment and no longer engaged in disordered behaviors related to eating and exercise, she no longer required the sense of purpose they once provided her. The client discharged from the hospital and returned to nursing classes, armed with the coping strategies developed in OT.

References

1. *Brain Basics: Know Your Brain*. National Institute of Neurological Disorders and Stroke; 2023. https://www.ninds.nih.gov/health-information/public-education/brain-basics/brain-basics-know-your-brain.
2. *Hypothalamus*. Cleveland Clinic; 2022. https://my.clevelandclinic.org/health/body/22566-hypothalamus.
3. Cheng W, Gordian D, Ludwig MQ, et al. Hindbrain circuits in the control of eating behaviour and energy balance. *Nat Metab*. 2022;4:826–835. https://doi.org/10.1038/s42255-022-00606-9.
4. Zucker T. *Eating Disorders vs. Disordered Eating: What's the Difference?* National Eating Disorders Association; n.d. https://www.nationaleatingdisorders.org/blog/eating-disorders-versus-disordered-eating.
5. Walsh J. *Disordered Eating vs. Eating Disorders*. Change Creates Change Eating Disorder Care; 2020. https://changecreateschange.com/disordered-eating-vs-eating-disorders-whats-the-difference/.
6. Green A. *Eating Disorders vs. Disordered Eating, What's the Difference?* University of Arizona; 2022. https://nutrition.arizona.edu/news/2022/02/eating-disorders-vs-disordered-eating-whats-difference.
7. American Psychiatric Association. *Diagnostic and Statistical Manual of Mental Disorders, Text Revision*. 5th ed. American Psychiatric Association; 2022.
8. Florent V, Baroncini M, Jissendi-Tchofo P, et al. Hypothalamic structural and functional imbalances in anorexia nervosa. *Neuroendocrinology*. 2020;110(6):552–562. https://doi.org/10.1159/000503147.
9. *Eating Disorder Behaviors Alter Reward Response in the Brain*. National Institute of Mental Health; 2021. https://www.nih.gov/news-events/news-releases/eating-disorder-behaviors-alter-reward-response-brain.

10. *Anorexia Nervosa*. Johns Hopkins Medicine; n.d. https://www.hopkinsmedicine.org/health/conditions-and-diseases/eating-disorders/anorexia-nervosa.
11. Moore CA, Bokor BR. *Anorexia Nervosa*. National Library of Medicine; 2023. https://www.ncbi.nlm.nih.gov/books/NBK459148/.
12. *Bulimia Nervosa*. Cleveland Clinic; 2022. https://my.clevelandclinic.org/health/diseases/9795-bulimia-nervosa.
13. *Binge Eating Disorder*. Cleveland Clinic; 2023. https://my.clevelandclinic.org/health/diseases/17652-binge-eating-disorder.
14. *Definitions and Facts for Binge Eating Disorder*. National Institute of Diabetes and Digestive and Kidney Diseases; 2021. https://www.niddk.nih.gov/health-information/weight-management/binge-eating-disorder/definition-facts.
15. Mayo Clinic. *Eating Disorders*. Mayo Clinic; 2023. https://www.mayoclinic.org/diseases-conditions/eating-disorders/symptoms-causes/syc-20353603.
16. Mack RA, Stanton CE, Carney MR. The importance of including occupational therapists as part of the multidisciplinary team in the management of eating disorders: a narrative review incorporating lived experience. *J Eat Disord*. 2023;11(37). https://doi.org/10.1186/s40337-023-00763-6.
17. Mack RA, Kelleher K, Bhattarai J, Spence T. Individuals with eating disorders' perspectives on a meal preparation intervention. *Occup Ther Ment Health*. 2023:1–20. https://doi.org/10.1080/0164212X.2023.2262761.
18. Coelho JS, Fernandes A, Suen J, Keidar A, Cairnes J. Perceived occupational performance in youth with eating disorders: treatment-related changes. *Can J Occup Ther*. 2020;87(5):423–430. https://doi-org.bunchproxy.idm.oclc.org/10.1177/0008417420953229.
19. Bray B, Rodríguez-Martín BC, Wiss DA, Bray CE, Zwickey H. Overeaters anonymous: an overlooked intervention for binge eating disorder. *Int J Environ Res Public Health*. 2021;18(7303). https://doi.org/10.3390/ijerph18147303.

28
Posttraumatic Stress Disorder

KATY SCHMIDT

OBJECTIVES

By the end of this chapter, the reader should be able to:

- Define the word *trauma.*
- Demonstrate a basic understanding of the physiological response to threat.
- Demonstrate a basic understanding of the possible neurological changes in the amygdala and hippocampus resulting from posttraumatic stress disorder.
- Assess and justify how a specific symptom resulting from posttraumatic stress disorder could constitute a yellow or red flag.

Trauma

Trauma is defined as an emotional response to a disturbing event that causes intense fear or other negative feelings. Trauma can have a significant impact on an individual's behavior, function, and health.[1]

Traumatic Events

Definitions of the term *traumatic events* vary greatly, depending upon the person and situation, but these events typically include some sort of exposure to serious injury, violence, or death. Both actual violence and threats of violence can be considered traumatic.[2] Traumatic events include personally experiencing the event, witnessing others experience the event, learning that close family or friends have experienced the event, or experiencing repeated exposure to details of the event. Examples of traumatic events include military combat, natural disasters, abuse, sexual violence, and severe accidents.[2]

Physiological Response to Threats

During a traumatic event, the fight-or-flight response is triggered[2] (see Chapter 24 for more information on the fight-or-flight response). Memories of the traumatic event are stored in the hippocampus (Fig. 28.1).[3]

Responses to threat are primarily controlled by a circuit between the amygdala, hippocampus, and parts of the prefrontal cortex.[3,4] The amygdala receives sensory input, and if a threat is detected, it signals the hippocampus and prefrontal cortex.[5] The hippocampus processes these threat signals and analyzes them while referring to stored memories of fear.[3,4] The medial prefrontal cortex inhibits responses to threats, if action is unnecessary.[3,4] If this circuit functions correctly, an individual can respond to threats appropriately. If danger is truly present, they will take action to ensure their safety. If no danger is present, they should return to a calmer state.[3] Fig. 28.2 highlights key brain regions involved in processing trauma.

The majority of individuals who face a traumatic event will experience dysfunction in the threat response circuit for a few moments, hours, days, or weeks.[4] Approximately 75% of individuals who have experienced severe trauma will not have a long-term impact. These individuals may be described as possessing resilience, the ability to recover from some form of hardship. The disposition for resilience is influenced by genetics, coping styles, and brain activity patterns.[3]

Posttraumatic Stress Disorder

Posttraumatic stress disorder (PTSD) may be diagnosed if the dysfunctional symptoms that follow a traumatic event persist for longer than 1 month and cause functional impairments in daily activities.[6]

Posttraumatic Stress Disorder Pathophysiology

PTSD can be considered a disorder of the responses to threat and fear.[3] Individuals with PTSD often have notable differences in the structure and function of the amygdala,

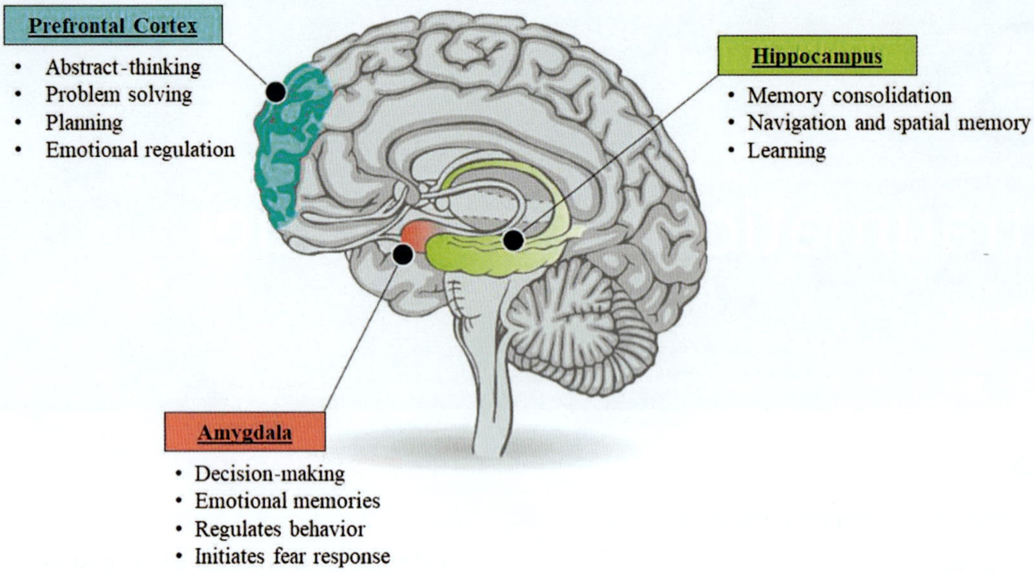

• **Fig. 28.1** Centers of the brain responsible for fear response and emotional regulation. (Courtesy Center for Whole-Child Education, Mary Lou Fulton Teachers College at Arizona State University.)

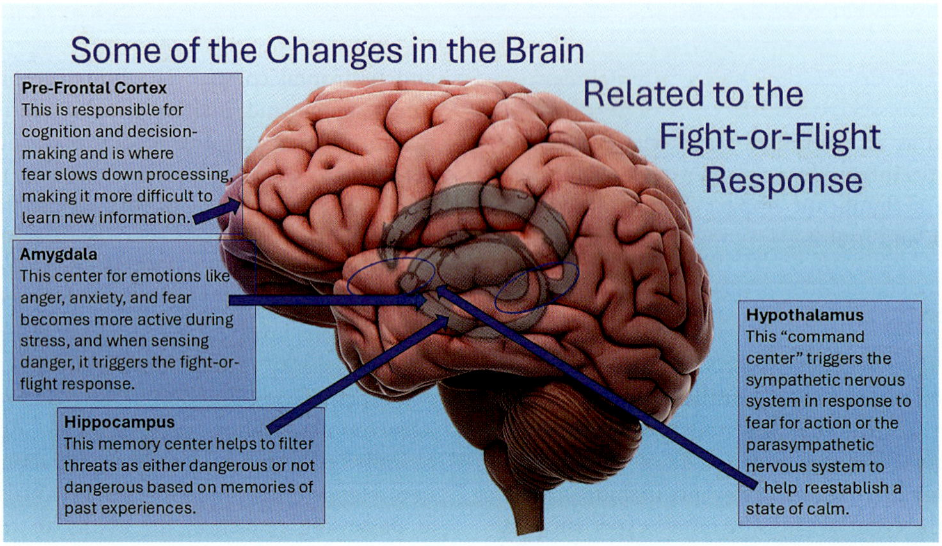

• **Fig. 28.2** Changes in the brain related to the fight-or-flight response. (Image from iStock.com/3dMediaSphere, Brain Illustration: ID 484757150; Data from Neurolaunch. *Brain's Fight or Flight Response: Understanding the Neural Control Center*. 2024. https://neurolaunch.com/what-part-of-the-brain-controls-fight-or-flight/.)

hippocampus, and parts of the prefrontal cortex, which control responses to threats.[3,4]

In individuals with PTSD, the amygdala is sometimes hyperactivated, causing the individual to excessively judge benign sensory information as a potential threat.[4,7] Additionally, the hippocampus often has a smaller volume and decreased activity in individuals with PTSD, resulting in dysfunctional processing of threat signals and increased stress response.[3,4] Furthermore, the prefrontal cortex often has decreased volume and reduced activation, causing poor inhibition of behaviors responding to threat.[4,7] Overall, the changes in the threat response circuit associated with PTSD lead to excessive fear responses to benign stimuli.[3,4,7] Some of these possible brain changes can be seen in Fig. 28.3.

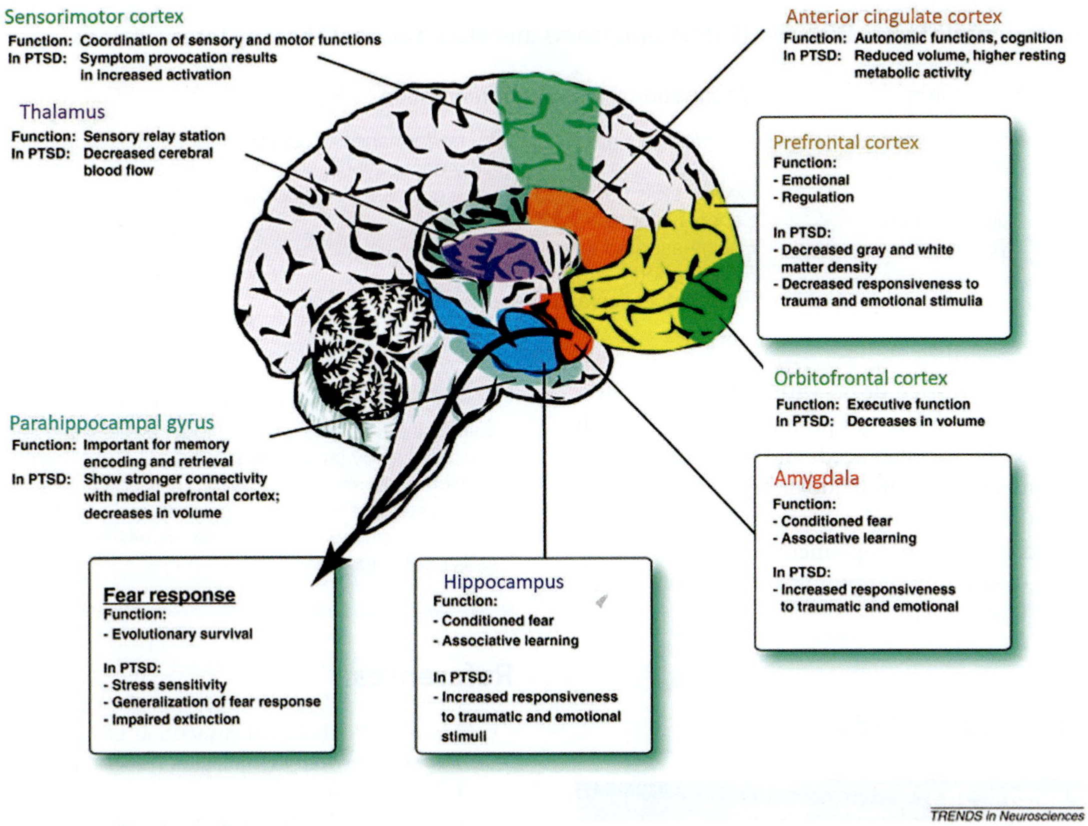

• **Fig. 28.3** Changes in the brain during posttraumatic stress disorder. (From Mahan AL, et al. Fear conditioning, synaptic plasticity and the amygdala: implications for posttraumatic stress disorder. *Trends Neurosci*. 2012;35(1):24–35.)

Posttraumatic Stress Disorder Symptoms

The symptoms of PTSD can vary from case to case.[6] Memories of the traumatic event may be intrusive, disrupting daily life. An individual may dissociate or experience a flashback, feeling as if the traumatic event is happening again. Dreams may be distressing and relate to the traumatic event. Ordinary occurrences may remind an individual of the traumatic event and cause significant distress.[8]

To prevent distress, an individual may avoid stimuli related to the traumatic event. A person may avoid internal stimulation, such as averting difficult memories, thoughts, or feelings. The individual might also avoid external stimuli, like people, places, items, or activities, that remind them of the traumatic event.[9]

Cognitive and emotional problems are common in PTSD, including memory loss related to the traumatic event, negative beliefs about oneself or the world, decreased interest in activities, negative emotions, and diminished ability to feel positive emotions.[10] A person with PTSD may experience hyperarousal and increased reactivity, such as heightened startle response, poor attention, sleep problems, irritability, anger, recklessness, and aggression. Hypervigilance might also occur. This is a state of high alertness for threats and an elevated fear of danger.[11]

Contributing Factors

Multiple factors contribute to the development of PTSD. The genetic heritability of PTSD is 30%–40%.[3] Preexisting differences in the amygdala and hippocampus may also contribute to the risk of developing this disorder.[4] Early adverse experiences during the prenatal period and childhood (such as domestic violence) can significantly impact a child's neurobiological development and heighten stress reactivity, which can increase risk of later developing PTSD.[3,4] If an individual has a mental illness prior to the traumatic event, this also increases the likelihood of developing PTSD. Additionally, the more severe, threatening, and personal a traumatic event is, the greater the risk of developing this disorder.[6] If a physical injury occurs during the traumatic event, this doubles the risk of PTSD.[4]

Occupational Therapy Approaches to Addressing PTSD

The symptoms of PTSD can cause impairments in all occupations. The core symptom of avoidance may particularly limit occupational engagement and community integration. Occupational therapy practitioners (OTPs) are trained to evaluate and provide interventions to improve occupational

TABLE 28.1 Posttraumatic Stress Disorder (PTSD) Symptoms and Occupational Therapy Interventions

Condition	Symptoms	Occupational Therapy Intervention
PTSD	Intrusive memories Avoidance Cognitive deficits Negative mood Hyperarousal	Individualized interventions for performance of occupations, such as work or sleep[12] Increase engagement in healthy occupations, such as leisure, art, or exercise[13] Coping skills training to manage distress during occupational performance[12] Sensory interventions[14] Equine-assisted therapy[15] Peer support[16] Family education and support[17]

performance, and they often do so with individuals suffering from PTSD. Due to the unique presentation of each case of PTSD and the personal needs and wants of each client, interventions should be individualized. OTPs can support individuals while they initiate or return to meaningful occupations and help them implement functional coping skills to manage distressing symptoms during occupational performance[12] (Table 28.1).

Application—Case Study

CASE EXAMPLE 28.1

A 46-year-old female presented to community-based OT for functional deficits related to PTSD symptoms and significant life transitions. The client had a history of domestic violence perpetrated by her ex-boyfriend. In the previous year, the client separated from her ex-boyfriend, moved across the country alone into supported housing, and began working two jobs to establish financial independence.

1. **Screen:** While completing an occupational profile during the evaluation, the occupational therapist (OTR) discovered the client worked an average of 70 hours each week. She also regularly helped her neighbor with household tasks for additional income. When not working, the client engaged in home management, social activities, and exercise.
2. **Take a Closer Look:** The OTR asked the client about her sleep. The client described an average total of 3 hours of sleep each day, obtained during multiple naps during the day and night. The client explained how her PTSD symptoms, including hypervigilance and nightmares, made it difficult for her to rest and sleep.
3. **Determine Flag Status:** The OTR determined this to be a yellow flag situation requiring OT services.
4. **Take Action if Needed:** The OTR wrote a treatment plan, including goals to improve occupational performance in rest/sleep and health management.
5. **Document the Findings:** The OTR documented the evaluation and treatment plan.
6. **Take a Second Look:** The OTR provided weekly interventions to the client for 3 months, training the client to implement coping skills into her occupational routines for improved rest/sleep and health management.
7. **Determine the Flag Status:** The OTR determined this was now a green flag situation.
8. **Take Action if Needed:** The client achieved her goals, and the OTR discharged her from OT services.

This is a true case. Before OT, the client avoided distressing thoughts and memories of her traumatic experiences by constantly staying busy, but this negatively impacted her sleep and health. Through OT interventions, she learned the value of life balance and how to manage symptoms during restful time alone, which brought her much satisfaction and peace.

References

1. American Psychological Association Dictionary of Psychology. *Trauma.* American Psychological Association. https://dictionary.apa.org/trauma.
2. MedlinePlus. *Post-traumatic Stress Disorder.* https://medlineplus.gov/posttraumaticstressdisorder.html.
3. Ressler KJ, Berretta S, Bolshakov VY, et al. Post-traumatic stress disorder: clinical and translational neuroscience from cells to circuits. *Nat Rev Neurol.* 2022;18(5):273–288. https://doi.org/10.1038/s41582-022-00635-8.
4. Sherin JE, Nemeroff CB. Post-traumatic stress disorder: the neurobiological impact of psychological trauma. *Dialogues Clin Neurosci.* 2022;13(3):263–278. https://doi.org/10.31887/DCNS.2011.13.2/jsherin.
5. Vogt KM, Pryor KO. Anesthesia and the neurobiology of fear and post-traumatic stress disorder. *Curr Opin Anaesthesiol.* 2022;35(5):593–599. https://doi.org/10.1097/ACO.0000000000001176.
6. American Psychiatric Association. Text Revision *Diagnostic and Statistical Manual of Mental Disorders.* 5th ed. American Psychiatric Association; 2022.
7. Carletto S, Panero M, Cavallo M, Pagani M. Neurobiology of posttraumatic stress disorder. In: Dierckx RA, Otte A, de Vries EFJ, van Waarde A, Sommer IE, eds. *PET and SPECT in Psychiatry.* Springer; 2021. https://doi.org/10.1007/978-3-030-57231-0_11.
8. Mayo Clinic. *Post-traumatic Stress Disorder (PTSD).* https://www.mayoclinic.org/diseases-conditions/post-traumatic-stress-disorder/symptoms-causes/syc-20355967.
9. Substance Abuse and Mental Health Services Administration. *Post-traumatic Stress Disorder (PTSD).* https://www.samhsa.gov/mental-health/post-traumatic-stress-disorder.
10. American Psychiatric Association. *What Is Posttraumatic Stress Disorder (PTSD)?* https://www.psychiatry.org/patients-families/ptsd/what-is-ptsd.
11. National Institute of Mental Health. *Traumatic Events and Post-Traumatic Stress Disorder (PTSD).* https://www.nimh.nih.gov/health/topics/post-traumatic-stress-disorder-ptsd.

12. Kerr NC, Ashby S, Gerardi SM, Lane SJ. Occupational therapy for military personnel and military veterans experiencing post-traumatic stress disorder: a scoping review. *Aust Occup Ther J*. 2020;67:479–497. https://doi.org/10.1111/1440-1630.12684.
13. King L, Campbell D, Finkbeiner M, et al. The mySELF group: recreation- and art-based group therapy as adjunct treatment for posttraumatic stress disorder. *J Mil Veteran Fam Health*. 2023;9(3):97–105. https://doi.org/10.3138/jmvfh-2022-0062.
14. Kimball JG. Sensory modulation challenges: one missing piece in the diagnosis and treatment of veterans with PTSD. *Occup Ther Ment Health*. 2023;39(3):314–331. https://doi.org/10.1080/0164212X.2022.2131695.
15. Punski-Hoogervorst JL, Avital A, Engel-Yeger B. Challenges in basic and instrumental activities of daily living among adults with posttraumatic stress disorder: a scoping review. *Occup Ther Ment Health*. 2023;39(2):184–210. https://doi.org/10.1080/0164212X.2022.2094523.
16. Goetter EM, Hoeppner SS, Khan AJ, et al. Combat-related posttraumatic stress disorder and comorbid major depression in U.S. veterans: the role of deployment cycle adversity and social support. *J Trauma Stress*. 2020;33:276–284. https://doi.org/10.1002/jts.22496.
17. Campbell SB, Caska Wallace CM. Development of a brief support and education intervention for loved ones of veterans with posttraumatic stress disorder. *J Trauma Stress*. 2023;36:557–566. https://doi.org/10.1002/jts.22914.

29

Substance Use Disorders

KATY SCHMIDT

OBJECTIVES

By the end of this chapter, the reader should be able to:

- Define the word *reward*.
- Demonstrate a basic understanding of the reward system physiology.
- Demonstrate a basic understanding of the possible neurological changes in the ventral tegmental area in the midbrain and hippocampus resulting from a rewarding stimulus.
- Compare and contrast physical withdrawal versus psychological withdrawal.
- Assess and justify how a specific symptom resulting from substance use disorder could constitute a yellow or red flag.

Substance Use and Reward System Physiology

The mesolimbic system of the brain controls the responses and experiences of reward. Reward is an adaptive process that associates pleasurable feelings with positive stimuli and also increases a person's engagement in activities necessary for survival, such as eating, drinking, and mating.[1] When an individual interacts with a positive stimulus, it activates the mesolimbic system.

Neurons of the ventral tegmental area in the midbrain release the neurohormone dopamine throughout the brain. The hippocampus forms memories of the rewarding stimulus. The amygdala associates positive emotions with the rewarding stimulus, and the nucleus accumbens creates feelings of pleasure, satisfaction, and motivation. The prefrontal cortex (PFC) analyzes the entire experience to make future plans and decisions regarding engagement with the rewarding stimulus again (Fig. 29.1).[2]

Stressful events also impact the mesolimbic system. Severe, chronic stressors decrease the quantity of dopamine released when experiencing reward. This response may result in behaviors that avoid stressful stimuli and may also produce depressive symptoms.[3]

Substance Use Disorders

When use of a substance affects the PFC in a positive way, the individual will be more likely to repeat the behavior.[2] After a while, more of the substance might be required to produce the same effect.[4] This can lead to a substance use disorder (SUD). SUDs are chronic, treatable disorders characterized by a pattern of overuse of a substance (typically drugs or alcohol), leading to physiological, cognitive, and/or behavioral problems.[5] In the year 2022, more than 1 out of every 6 Americans over the age of 12 reported having had a SUD.[5]

SUDs consist of a cluster of physiological, cognitive, and behavioral symptoms related to the use of addictive substances.[5] The presentation and treatment of SUD vary depending on the type of substance involved. The *Diagnostic and Statistical Manual of Mental Disorders, Fifth Edition* categorizes SUD by 10 classes of drugs: alcohol, caffeine, cannabis, hallucinogens, inhalants, opioids, sedatives, stimulants, tobacco, and other substances.[6]

Substance Use Disorder Pathophysiology

As an SUD forms, the mesolimbic system changes. Many substances cause an enormous release of dopamine, significantly higher than any natural reward could create. The brain learns to associate the substance with dopamine.[7] Over time as tolerance to the substance builds, the brain becomes less sensitive to dopamine and greater levels of a substance are required to obtain the same effects. The physiological changes associated with SUD also cause cognitive problems, such as deficits in attention, memory, learning, and judgment.[7]

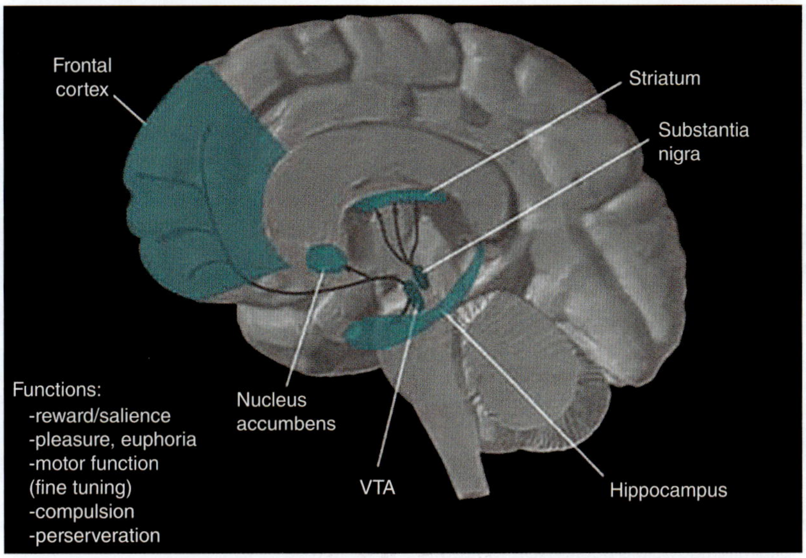

• **Fig. 29.1** The mesolimbic system. *VTA*, Ventral tegmental area. (From National Institutes of Health. https://cs.wikipedia.org/wiki/Ventr%C3%A1ln%C3%AD_tegment%C3%A1ln%C3%AD_oblast.)

Substance Use Disorder Symptoms

Impaired control is a key symptom of SUD. A person may consume increasingly large quantities of the substance over time, despite original intentions or desire to decrease substance use. The substance use may feel out of control.[8] Cravings, intense urges to use the substance, are common. A person may spend much of their time in activities related to substance use, including gaining access to the substance, using the substance, and recovering from the substance use.[8]

People with SUD often experience social impairments, including difficulties keeping up with their roles and responsibilities. For example, a person with SUD may experience problems as a spouse, parent, family member, friend, employee, homemaker, or hobbyist.[9] Risk-taking behavior is another key symptom of SUD. Despite the obvious health consequences, a person with SUD is likely to continue using the substance, and a person with SUD may also use substances in dangerous situations, such as using substances while driving.

The pharmacological criteria associated with SUD are tolerance and withdrawal. Tolerance is the decreased sensitivity to substances over time, requiring increasingly higher doses of the substance to obtain the effect.[10] Withdrawal refers to the cluster of symptoms experienced when substance levels decline after significant use. Withdrawal symptoms vary depending on the type of substance but often include anxiety, depression, agitation, confusion, insomnia, fatigue, aches, and gastrointestinal distress (Fig. 29.2).[10]

Contributing Factors

Multiple factors contribute to the development of SUD. Genetic factors account for 30% to 80% of risk, depending on substance type.[6] Specifically, genetic factors related to stress response are associated with SUD risk, which is not surprising considering the negative impact chronic stress has on the reward system, which is highly involved in SUD. Adverse childhood experiences are directly related to an increased risk of future SUD; the greater the trauma exposure, the higher the risk (Fig. 29.2).[11]

Individuals with mental illness are at a higher risk of SUD than the general population.[11] Co-occurring mental disorders can include anxiety disorders, personality disorders, attention-deficit/hyperactivity disorder, depression, bipolar disorder, schizophrenia, or posttraumatic stress disorder (Fig. 29.3).[12]

While SUD and another mental disorder can occur together, this does not imply cause and effect. Although one can lead to the other, there can be other variables, including common risk factors, that cause both in an individual.[12]

OT Approaches to Addressing Substance Use Disorders

The time-consuming nature of SUD typically impacts all occupations.[13] A key feature of the disorder is impaired control, which may require a person to spend the majority of their time in the substance use cycle of obtaining, using, and recovering from substances. This cycle can provide

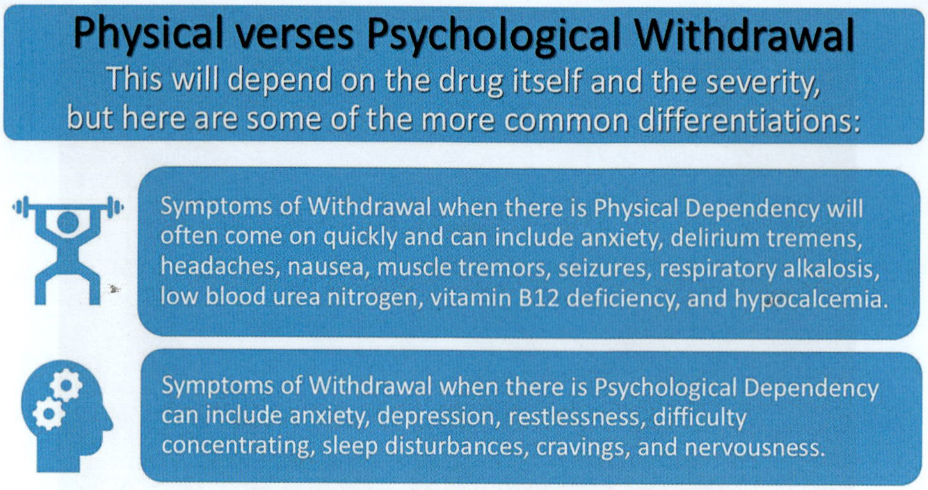

• **Fig. 29.2** Common physical and psychological symptoms of substance withdrawal. (Data from https://www.ncbi.nlm.nih.gov/sites/books/NBK459239.)

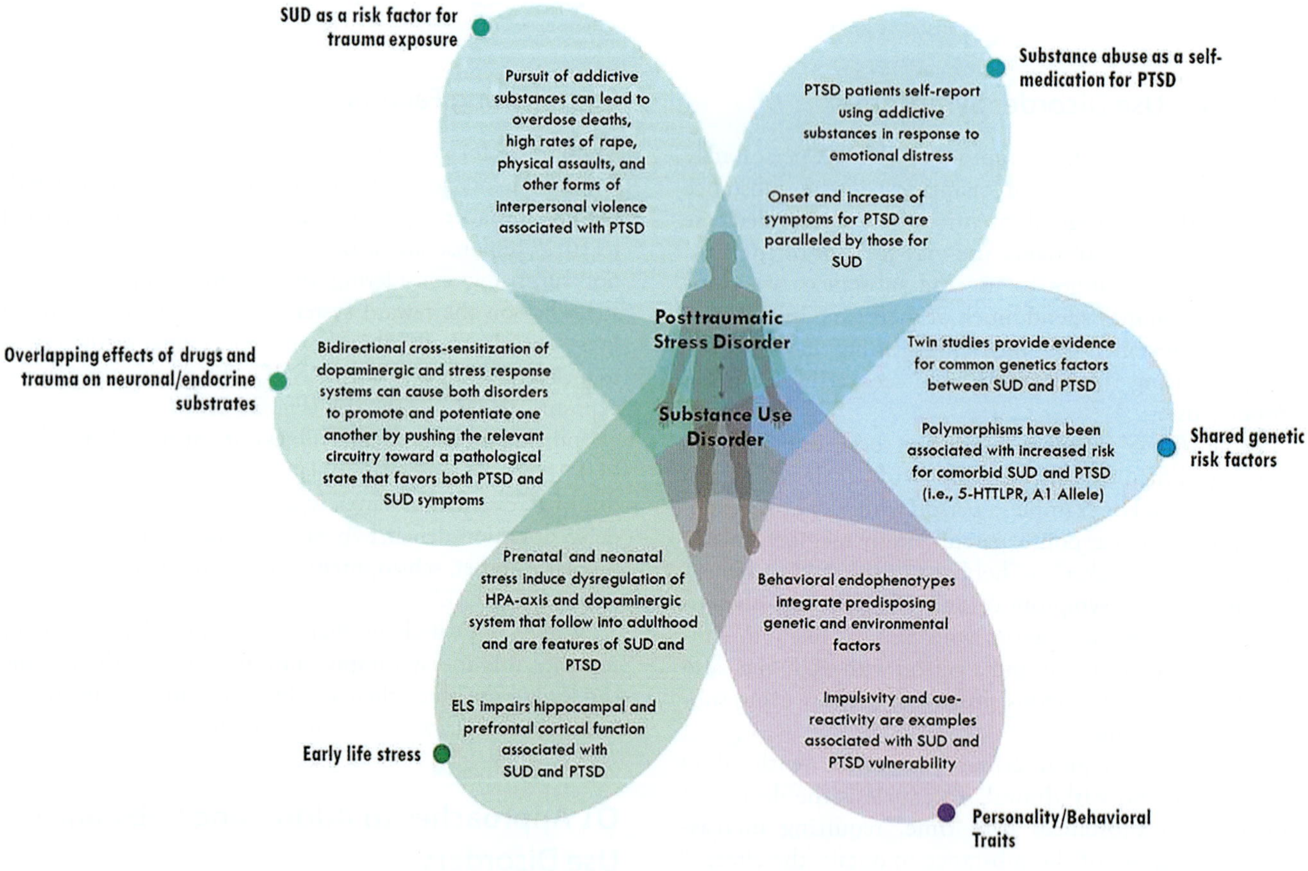

• **Fig. 29.3** Connection between posttraumatic stress disorder (PTSD) and substance use disorder (SUD). (From https://www.frontiersin.org/articles/10.3389/fnbeh.2020.00006/full.)

TABLE 29.1 Substance Use Disorder (SUD) Symptoms and Occupational Therapy Interventions

Condition	Symptoms Affecting Occupational Performance	Occupational Therapy Intervention
SUD	Impaired control Social impairments Risky substance use Tolerance Withdrawal	Individualized interventions for performance of occupations such as work, parenting, or sleep[13–15] Increase engagement in healthy occupations such as leisure, art, or exercise[13] Skills training[13] Community reintegration[13] Establish routines for healthy time use and identity[13] Metacognitive-focused occupational therapy[16] Relapse prevention planning[17] Screening, brief intervention, and referral to treatment[18] Occupation-based groups[18] Peer support[19] Family education and support[20]

a maladaptive sense of routine, purpose, and identity. Occupational therapy practitioners (OTPs) evaluate occupational performance and provide interventions to improve the participation of individuals with SUD. A person recovering from SUD must typically discover or reconnect with meaningful occupations to spend their newfound free time. Occupations also give individuals with SUD a healthy experience of routine, purpose, and identity (Table 29.1).[13]

Application—Case Study

CASE EXAMPLE 29.1

A 24-year-old male presented to occupational therapy (OT) in an inpatient psychiatric hospital for functional deficits related to hallucinogen use disorder.

1. **Screen:** While developing an occupational profile during the evaluation, the occupational therapist (OTR) learned about the client's history of methylenedioxymethamphetamine (MDMA) abuse. Before admission, the client was entrenched in the substance use cycle, selling his plasma weekly in order to purchase MDMA, using the MDMA, then repeating the process.
2. **Take a Closer Look:** The client's substance use negatively impacted all occupations. The client was unhoused and rarely completed ADLs. The client reported he would not get any sleep for weeks. All his time was spent obtaining and using MDMA.
3. **Determine Flag Status:** The client was in a safe and secure setting in the hospital but required OT intervention before discharge, so the OTR determined this to be a yellow flag situation.
4. **Take Action if Needed:** The OTR developed a treatment plan including individual and group OT services to reengage the client in meaningful occupations. This plan was shared with the occupational therapy assistant, and both occupational therapy practitioners (OTPs) worked together on the client's treatment plan.
5. **Document the Findings:** The OTR documented the evaluation and treatment plan.
6. **Take a Second Look:** The client explored leisure activities in OT groups and rekindled his passion for art and making comics. In individual OT sessions, the client identified motivation to work with animals, set goals, learned strategies, and accessed resources in order to find a job related to animals after discharge. After 2 weeks, the client prepared for discharge to a residential program.
7. **Determine the Flag Status:** The client was transitioning to a setting with adequate support, so this was a green flag situation.
8. **Take Action if Needed:** Before the client was discharged, he and the OTPs developed a relapse prevention plan, including triggers, warning signs, coping strategies, safe places, and professional supports for him to utilize in the residential program and to share with staff.

This is a true case. Initially, the client was involuntarily admitted to the hospital for his own safety, and he explicitly planned to return to his former lifestyle after discharge. In OT, he rediscovered occupations which made sober life worth living, which significantly contributed to his willingness to enter a residential program and pursue recovery.

References

1. Cleveland Clinic. *Dopamine*. Cleveland Clinic; 2022. https://my.clevelandclinic.org/health/articles/22581-dopamine.
2. Lewis RG, Florio E, Punzo D, Borrelli E. The brain's reward system in health and disease. *Adv Exp Med Biol*. 2021;1344:57–69. https://doi.org/10.1007/978-3-030-81147-1_4.
3. Baik JH. Stress and the dopaminergic reward system. *Exp Mol Med*. 2020;52:1879–1890. https://doi.org/10.1038/s12276-020-00532-4.
4. Mayo Clinic. *Drug Addiction (Substance Use Disorder)*. 2022. https://www.mayoclinic.org/diseases-conditions/drug-addiction/symptoms-causes/syc-20365112.
5. CDC. *Treatment of Substance Use Disorders (SUDs)*. Centers for Disease Control and Prevention; 2024. https://www.cdc.gov/overdose-prevention/treatment/index.html.

6. American Psychiatric Association. *Text Revision Diagnostic and Statistical Manual of Mental Disorders*. 5th ed. American Psychiatric Association; 2022.
7. Yale Medicine. *How an Addicted Brain Works*. Yale Medicine; 2022. https://www.yalemedicine.org/news/how-an-addicted-brain-works.
8. Cleveland Clinic. *Substance Use Disorder (SUD)*. Cleveland Clinic; 2022. https://my.clevelandclinic.org/health/diseases/16652-drug-addiction-substance-use-disorder-sud.
9. APA. *What Is a Substance Use Disorder?* American Psychiatric Association; 2020. https://www.psychiatry.org/patients-families/addiction-substance-use-disorders/what-is-a-substance-use-disorder.
10. Sharp A. *Drug Withdrawal Symptoms, Timelines, & Treatment*. American Addiction Centers; 2023. https://americanaddictioncenters.org/withdrawal-timelines-treatment.
11. Jahan AR, Burgess DM. Substance use disorder. *Natl Library Med*. 2023. https://www.ncbi.nlm.nih.gov/books/NBK570642/.
12. NIH. *Substance Use and Co-occurring Mental Disorders*. National Institute of Mental Health; 2024. https://www.nimh.nih.gov/health/topics/substance-use-and-mental-health.
13. Ryan DA, Boland P. A scoping review of occupational therapy interventions in the treatment of people with substance use disorders. *Ir J Occup Ther*. 2021;49(2):104–114. https://doi.org/10.1108/IJOT-11-2020-0017.
14. Gardner J, Swarbrick M, Dennis S, Franklin M, Pricken M, Palmer K. Sleep habits and routines of individuals diagnosed with mental and/or substance-use disorders. *Occup Ther Ment Health*. 2021;37(2):158–177. https://doi.org/10.1080/0164212X.2021.1877592.
15. Jirikowic T, Graham JC, Grant T. A trauma-informed parenting intervention model for mothers parenting young children during residential treatment for substance use disorder. *Occup Ther Ment Health*. 2023;39(2):156–183. https://doi.org/10.1080/0164212X.2022.2089315.
16. Lam KCK, Fung EML, Chan HF, Louie FTM, Chan F. Metacognitive-focused occupational therapy for substance abuse in medical–social service collaboration: a case report. *East Asian Arch Psychiatry*. 2021;31(1):19–20. https://doi.org/10.12809/eaap2008.
17. Carter T, Heaton K, Merlo LJ, Roche BT, Puga F. Relapse prevention and prediction strategies in substance use disorder: a scoping review. *J Addict Nurs*. 2023;34(2):146–157. https://doi.org/10.1097/JAN.0000000000000527.
18. Matilla AM, Santacecilia G, LaCroix R. Perceptions and knowledge around substance use disorders and the role of occupational therapy: a survey of clinicians. *Subst Abuse*. 2022;16:1–6. https://doi.org/10.1177/11782218221130921.
19. Hutchison SL, MacDonald-Wilson KL, Karpov I, Herschell AD, Carney T. Peer support to reduce readmission in Medicaid-enrolled adults with substance use disorder. *J Subst Abuse Treat*. 2023;144:108901. https://doi.org/10.1016/j.jsat.2022.108901.
20. Kane EM, Snethen JA, Gwon SH, Oh HK. Affected family members social support experiences when assisting an individual with substance use disorder. *J Nurs Scholarsh*. 2022;55:590–598. https://doi.org/10.1111/jnu.12893.

SECTION V

Pathophysiology and the Occupational Therapy Practitioner

Introduction to Section V

This section contains the final chapter of the book: Chapter 30.

This chapter brings together the content of this textbook with a focus on its application to occupational therapy practice. Why does an occupational therapy practitioner (OTP) need to be knowledgeable about the symptoms associated with various pathophysiological conditions? First, the most obvious reason: understanding a client's diagnosis helps all healthcare professionals provide appropriate care tailored to the individual's specific needs.

It is also important to address those symptoms that fall outside the cluster typically expected with a client's diagnostic condition. This is another reason why an OTP's knowledge of pathophysiology is so valuable. It is an area where OTPs can truly excel. Unlike physicians and many other healthcare professionals, OTPs often work with clients one-on-one several times a week, or even multiple times during a day. This frequent interaction provides OTPs with extended opportunities to observe signs and symptoms that others might miss. Additionally, the consistent presence of the OTP fosters trust and rapport, often encouraging clients to share concerns or symptoms they might not disclose to their physician.

Chapter 30 comes full circle from Chapter 1, revisiting the International Classification of Functioning, Disability, and Health (ICF) and applying it to the field of pathophysiology and the OTP's role. The authors hope that the reader will gain new insights into the importance of recognizing client signs and symptoms through the unique observational skills that OTPs bring to health care.

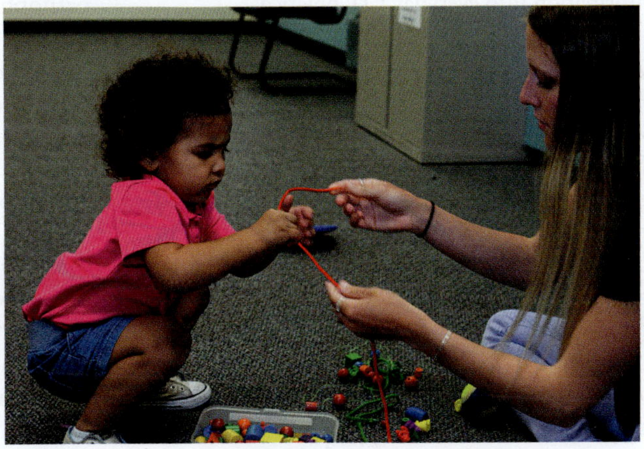

(From O'Brien JC, Conners BL. (2024). Introductory questions. In: *Introduction to Occupational Therapy*. 6th ed. Elsevier; 2024.)

30

Pathophysiology and the Role of the Occupational Therapy Practitioner

OBJECTIVES

By the end of this chapter, the reader should be able to:

- Demonstrate an understanding of how a strong working knowledge of pathophysiology ties into the occupational therapy scope of practice.
- Compare and contrast the basic components of the International Classification of Functioning, Disability, and Health with the American Occupational Therapy Association's Occupational Therapy Scope of Practice.
- Justify how having foundational knowledge of pathophysiology enables the occupational therapy practitioner to better evaluate, communicate, and advocate for their clients and for the profession.

This book has summarized the following topics: the client interview, pathophysiology with respect to the various stages of human development, pathophysiology as it relates to bodily systems, and disorders related to cognition and mental health. According to Bloom's taxonomy, as discussed in Chapter 21, the bridge between knowledge and application is understanding.[1] Chapter 30 will attempt to tie this information together and demonstrate how occupational therapy (OT) fits into the bigger picture. The authors hope that this will provide the reader with a better understanding of pathophysiology and the ability to apply this information into everyday OT practice.

The OT Scope of Practice Revisited

The scope of OT practice was previously covered in Chapter 1. This information is interconnected in practice, so it is revisited in this chapter to bring the ideas offered throughout this text full circle. As previously discussed in Chapter 1, both occupational therapists (OTRs) and certified occupational therapy assistants (COTAs) are responsible for identifying red and yellow flags, making appropriate clinical decisions related to pathophysiological conditions or changes, and collaborating with the interprofessional team. COTAs are responsible for communicating and coordinating with their supervising occupational therapist regarding each client's therapeutic plan of care. According to the American Occupational Therapy Association (AOTA), the scope of practice for both OTRs and COTAs (collectively referred to as occupational therapy practitioners [OTPs]) depends on the laws of the state in which the practitioner is working. The scope will depict both the domain and the services the OTP is able to perform under the guidelines of state law.[2] OTPs are strongly encouraged to consult with the Occupational Therapy Regulatory Authority in their particular state for the OT scope of practice in that region.[3]

The AOTA defines OT as the therapeutic use of life's daily occupations in an effort to enhance or support participation for individuals, groups, or communities.[2] Occupations act as the foundation for OT intervention, and understanding pathophysiology across different body systems helps bridge the gap to clinical application. This understanding enables the OTP to more effectively screen and evaluate their clients, find symptoms that may fall outside what is expected for their specific condition(s), communicate relevant findings to the physician, and develop more appropriate occupation-based interventions, when applicable.

The *Occupational Therapy Practice Framework: Domain and Process, 4th edition (OTPF-4)* acts as a guide for the OT profession, serving as the AOTA's official document to describe OT practice.[4] In the *OTPF-4*, the scope of OT practice consists of two components: the *Domain*, or focus of OT, and the *Process*, or delivery of OT.[4] The diagram below depicts an adaptation of the interaction between domain and process, including the five corresponding aspects of domain and the three corresponding aspects of process (Fig. 30.1).[4] While this is one way to illustrate the scope of OT practice, and will be further explored later in the chapter, there is another framework that encompasses and aligns with many attributes of the OT scope of practice.

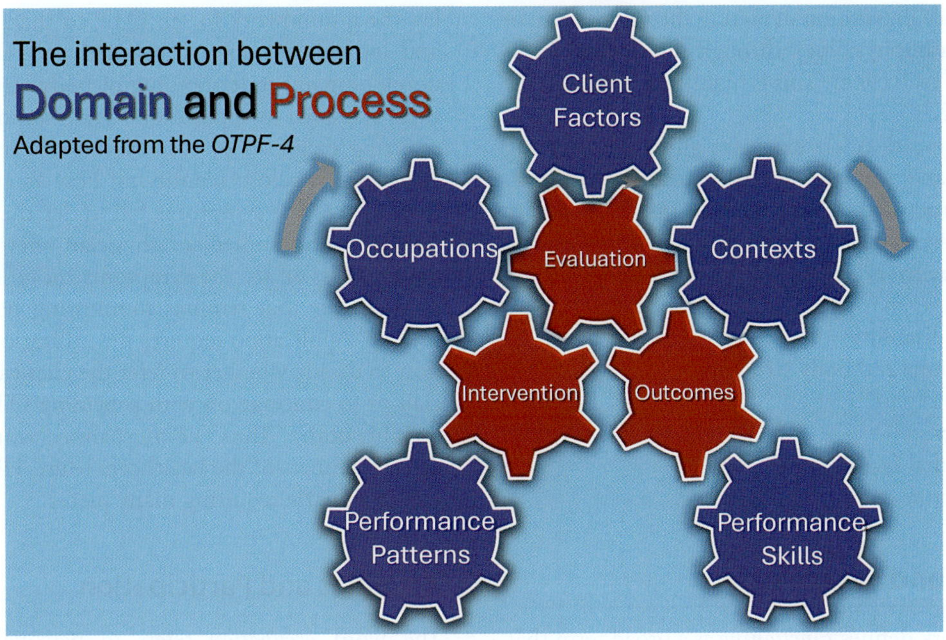

• **Fig. 30.1** The OT scope of practice: domain and process. (Adapted from American Occupational Therapy Association. Occupational therapy practice framework: domain and process (4th ed.). *Am J Occup Ther*. 2020; 74(suppl 2):7412410010p1–7412410010p87.)

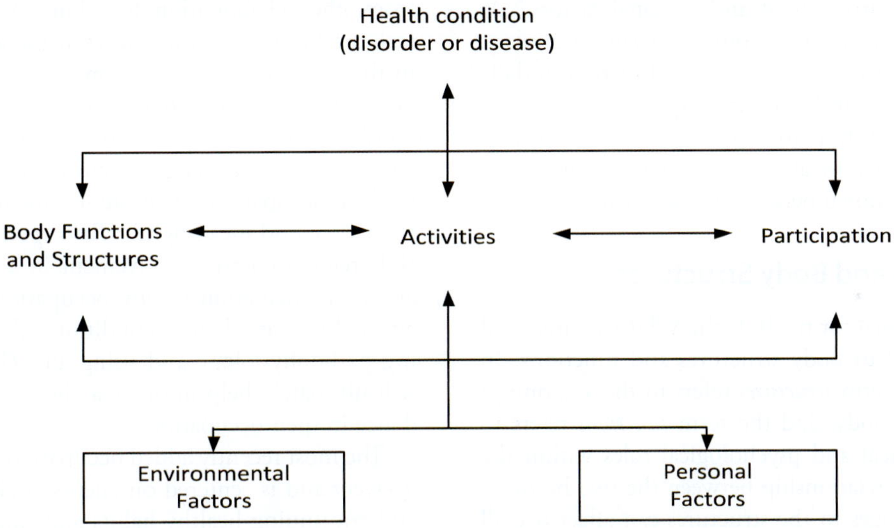

• **Fig. 30.2** The International Classification of Functioning, Disability, and Health framework. (From https://cdn.who.int/media/docs/default-source/classification/icf/drafticfpracticalmanual2.pdf?sfvrsn=8a214b01_4&download=true.)

The International Classification of Functioning, Disability, and Health

The World Health Organization (WHO) created a framework called the International Classification of Functioning, Disability, and Health (ICF) to provide healthcare practitioners with a common language for measuring health and disability.[5] This was introduced in Chapter 1. As a profession, OT is holistic and client-centered; therefore, a physical or mental disability is considered within the context of each client's participation in daily life activities or occupations.[6] The ICF model utilizes that same holistic principle by considering the interaction between a person's bodily functions, activities, participation, and other environmental circumstances as it relates to overall health, well-being, and functional status (Fig. 30.2).[5]

The ICF framework demonstrates how an individual's ability to participate in activities can be influenced by multifaceted factors, including pathological conditions that affect body functions and structures.[5] One of the main objectives of OT is to improve meaningful participation, which varies from client to client. A 2018 study by Abarghuei et al. found that the ICF model complements OT clinical practice, as both focus on a comprehensive or holistic view of the client, the personalized functional components of recovery, the therapeutic plan of care, the goal of increasing participation, and the influence of social and environmental factors on overall health.[7] In sum, the ICF model is an interdisciplinary illustration depicting the importance of understanding pathophysiology through the unique, individualized lens of each client. This is highly applicable to the foundation of OT.

The ICF framework offers extensive guidance, utilizing building blocks and statistics to help measure function. This chapter is structured to align with Section 2 of *How to Use the ICF: A Practical Manual for Using the International Classification of Functioning, Disability and Health (ICF)*[5] by organizing the material into the following sections:

Functioning and disability:
- Body functions and body structures
- Activities and participation

Contextual factors:
- Environmental factors
- Personal factors

Functioning and Disability

The ICF framework defines *functioning* as a broad term that encompasses body functions and structures, as well as activities and participation, focusing on the positive elements of the interaction between an individual with a medical condition and their environmental and personal factors.[5] As OTPs, the word *function* is in our everyday vocabulary. While it is important to analyze a client's function in daily activities, occupations, and roles, it is equally important to understand the bodily function within the client's current health condition and how all of these functions interconnect to affect occupational performance and participation.

Body Functions and Body Structures

In the practical manual for the ICF, the WHO summarized the domains related to body structures and functions. In this document, the term *structures* refers to the anatomical components of the body, and the term *functions* refers to both the physiological and psychological roles within the bodily systems. The relationship between the two becomes evident in how changes to the structures can affect overall health and function. Chapters 3 through 9 of this book specifically outline human development. Chapters 10 through 20 outline each bodily system (neuromuscular, cardiovascular, pulmonary, etc.) and its related structures and functions, and Chapters 21 through 29 outline cognition and mental health. The ICF framework depicts domains for both body functions and structures.[6,8] Chapters from this book that align with ICF domains on body functions and structures can be found in Table 30.1.

As seen in Table 30.1, OTPs, along with other members of the healthcare team, are responsible for understanding the basics of pathophysiology within cognitive, sensory, neuromuscular, and body system functions in association with occupational performance.[4,5] The disease process provides insight into how signs, symptoms, and etiologies may affect a person. Learning about a disease, disorder, or health condition from a physiological perspective is one of the first steps in developing clinical reasoning skills. This will lay the groundwork for an OTP to then view each disease and individual from a functional perspective. Specifically, developing an understanding of body structures and functions is crucial to application. Understanding how a client's referring diagnosis or comorbidity affects them physically is necessary before identifying how it affects them functionally. Do the symptoms fall under the category of a *red flag*, requiring immediate physician referral or a call to the paramedics, or are the symptoms more in the category of a *yellow flag* that requires monitoring but not immediate action?[9] Application requires the utilization of this information to decide whether to refer the client back to the physician or to continue on with providing OT intervention (or possibly both).[9] The OTP must always work closely with the other members of the healthcare team. High-quality health care is a puzzle requiring many pieces.

Activities and Participation

The word *occupation* refers to personal engagement in meaningful, everyday life activities, and there are nine types of occupations.[4] The work to help improve a client's participation in meaningful occupations is what differentiates OT from other rehabilitation disciplines. As expected, pathological conditions can interfere with the ability to participate in these occupations. The term *activity* is similar to that of occupation, as it signifies a type of action or execution of a task.[4] Activities are typically more objective and less specific to meaningful engagement or to a particular context, whereas occupations are more specific to the individual and what they find meaningful.[4] *Participation*, according to the ICF, refers to active involvement in a life activity or situation.[5] Participation in any occupation or activity can be affected by pathological conditions; therefore, understanding pathophysiology and using an OTP's unique skill set will ultimately help improve a client's functional independence in their occupations.

The most recently added occupation is called *health management* and is centered on clients establishing, overseeing, and continuing healthy habits and routines to improve or maintain their health.[4] Epley et al. suggested that occupational therapists have a unique role in assisting clients with chronic diseases. These researchers embedded healthy habits into the daily routines of their clients by modifying the environment to reinforce these habits, with the overall purpose of promoting health and wellness.[10] OTPs can educate clients and assist with developing new lifestyle routines or habits. Examples include creating a grocery list together to follow a "heart-healthy" diet, designing a home exercise program to increase daily physical activity as a weight management strategy, brainstorming ways to manage stress, educating individuals on the importance of self-monitoring blood pressure or other vitals, and keeping a daily log of pain levels, fatigue, or joint stiffness. In essence, OTPs can work alongside their clients to consider the pathophysiological effects of a disease or condition, collaborate on ways to manage symptoms and medications, and adopt healthier lifestyle alternatives to support their participation.

TABLE 30.1 Some Body Functions Adapted (In-Part) From the ICF Framework and Biopsychosocial Model, Along With Book Chapters Containing Analogous Information

Body Functions-Physiological Functions That Include Both Physical and Psychological[6,8]	
Category	Applied Pathophysiology Chapters
Mental Functions	
The human brain and cognition, neurocognitive disorders, other systems affecting cognition	Chapters 21 and 22
Mood disorders, anxiety disorders, personality disorders, psychotic disorders, eating disorders, posttraumatic stress disorder, substance use disorders	Chapters 23–29
Sensory Functions and Pain	
The perception of sensation, proprioception, interoception, touch and pain; the systemic connection to neuromuscular pain	Chapter 20
Neuromuscular and Musculoskeletal-Related Functions	
The head, neck, back, spine, sacrum, chest, shoulder, upper extremity, ribs, abdomen, gluteal region, and lower extremity	Chapter 20 and Development Chapters 3 through 9
Cardiovascular, Hematological, Immunological, and Pulmonary/Respiratory Functions	
Cardiovascular system functions	Chapter 13
Hematological and immune system functions	Chapter 11
Respiratory system functions	Chapter 14
Digestive, Metabolic, and Endocrine System Functions	
Digestive, metabolic, and endocrine system functions	Chapters 15, 16, and 18
Genitourinary and Reproductive Functions	
Genitourinary and reproductive functions	Chapter 17
Skin and Related Structures	
Skin and related structure functions	Chapters 10 and 12
External Factors Affecting Health	
Environmental pathogens	Chapter 19

Contextual Factors

The ICF framework includes two contextual elements: environmental factors and personal factors.[5] *Context* is how each person views the world, and both environmental and personal factors can influence their overall health, function, and participation.[11]

Environmental Factors

Environmental factors refer to external surroundings or influences, either positive or negative, that affect a person's physical health or engagement in occupations.[4,5] An example of considering environmental factors to facilitate participation in toileting and bathing occupations would be a remodeled bathroom with proper lighting and ventilation, grab bars installed near the toilet, a shower chair for safety, a long-handled sponge to help a client wash their legs independently, and a supportive family member living in the client's house for the first few days after being released from the hospital. Examples of environmental factors that could act as a barrier to participation in occupations include instances like exposure to secondhand smoke due to living in a house with a cigarette smoker, limited opportunities to go to a support group secondary to living in a rural town, asbestos found in a client's place of employment that might predispose them to future illness, not having access to a ramp as a wheelchair user in a movie theater, or exposure to other pathogens that could eventually lead to the development of a long-term neurological condition. Chapter 19 of this book covers some of these environmental pathogens. Knowing and understanding a person's environmental factors is crucial in recognizing how their physical and social surroundings can influence their occupational performance or function, through the ICF perspective, in a positive or negative way.[5]

Personal Factors

Personal factors refer to the unique characteristics and background of a person, their demographics (i.e., social determinants of health), and how they interpret and participate in societal and cultural norms.[4,5] Personal factors can influence how the OTP may relate to the client, tailor interventions specific to the client, or address occupational performance in general. The Ecology of Human Performance is a framework used in OT theory and practice that highlights the relationship between occupational performance and context.[11] A person, with unique skills and abilities, must first embrace their context and then view the task at hand through the context to find meaning and maximize their performance of the task.[11]

Within the realm of personal factors, it is important to consider how a person's habits, rituals, routines, and individualized roles can support or hinder engagement in occupations.[4] *Habits* are automatic, nearly instinctive behaviors.[4] While there are healthy habits that positively influence performance (i.e., appropriate daily water intake, routine exercise, getting the recommended amount of sleep, meditating, or taking supplements as part of a morning routine), there are unhealthy habits that may be detrimental to health and limit participation in meaningful occupations and eventually lead to pathological conditions (i.e., smoking, drinking alcohol excessively, or eating fast food for breakfast every day). *Roles* are identities a person adopts, typically with behavioral or social expectations.[12] While being a member of a religious organization, a community volunteer, or a parent may be fulfilling some roles, such as being a full-time caregiver to a disabled family member, can negatively influence health outcomes and opportunities for occupational balance. Roles can change dramatically in the face of injury, disability, or chronic disease.[13] OTPs are the professionals charged with analyzing a client's personal factors to see how they invest their time and why. This allows OTPs to identify beneficial and harmful habits, help establish new or revamp existing routines, foster meaningful spiritual rituals, or discover how a role may facilitate or limit occupational performance. These factors can be affected by pathological conditions, life experiences, or stages of development (see Chapters 3–9 of this book).

Delivery of OT Services

For the purposes of this section, delivery of OT services is divided into four parts: screening, evaluation, intervention, and results or outcomes. It is imperative that OTPs work within their scope of care from the initial evaluation to the therapeutic intervention phase until the client's discharge from OT services. Although OTPs do not make a medical diagnosis, they do diagnose the occupational implications of their client's condition and how it may impact everyday life. Evaluation, intervention, and outcomes will be discussed below along with a review of the importance of the screening process found in Chapter 1.

Screening

Screening can serve as a less formal precursor to evaluation for these reasons: (1) screening acts as a means of consultation to ensure that a client is appropriate for and would benefit from OT services prior to an initial evaluation, and (2) screening the client throughout their plan of care acts to ensure that they are still an appropriate candidate for OT services. The AOTA provides evaluation checklists and quality measures in their AOTA Toolkit that can assist when deciding whether a person is a suitable candidate for OT services.[14]

According to Catherine C. Goodman, MBA, PT, an important part of the screening process is the ability to identify yellow flags (those signifying caution) and red flags (those signifying warning).[9] Signs and symptoms are typically found within identifiable clusters that could signify a possible disorder. Although the medical diagnosis is not made by the OTP, but rather a physician, OTPs do use activity analysis and clinical reasoning skills to determine the occupational implications of their condition that impact everyday life. Therefore, OTPs need to be able to identify signs and symptoms that fall outside the cluster of symptoms expected with a given diagnosis. It is also important to know how to communicate this to the physician so the appropriate tests can be ordered, especially if potential findings could make OT services contraindicated.

A real-life example of this follows: An OTP was working in a hospital-based inpatient therapy department when a family member entered the therapy gym in panic. They said their mother was in the room across the hall and suddenly became unresponsive with her left side "just hanging there." They were afraid that their mother was having a stroke and could not find the nurse. The OTP ran to the woman's room and found that she was flaccid on her left side and unable to sit upright in her wheelchair. Her face was also drooping, and it did appear that she was having a stroke. Although the OTP was aware of what was happening and recognized the definitive red flag, she did not state this to the family, as it was outside her scope to do so. The son asked, "Is my mother having a stroke?" and the OTP replied, "I can't say, but we do need to get help right away." Since the client was already in the hospital, the OTP alerted nursing, who called a "stroke alert" after performing a quick neurological assessment. The "stroke alert" team of physicians and nurses took immediate action to get new brain imaging and to place her on Heparin to thin the blood, along with other interventions. Although she was experiencing symptoms of a stroke, all symptoms subsided, and the diagnosis was changed to a transient ischemic attack. The doctors stated that this was because they were able to treat the client quickly and thanked the OTP for her quick action. The OTP's quick thinking may have saved this woman's life.

Here is another example of the importance of distinguishing between what to expect versus not expect and what can be seen as yellow or red flags. For many cardiac conditions, it is important for an OTP to monitor vitals before, during, and after therapeutic activities. Knowing a client's cardiac comorbidities is essential for acknowledging what each client's average heart rate may look like during an evaluation or treatment session. For a client without cardiac comorbidities, the expectation is a resting heart rate between 60 and 100. If an OTP enters a room knowing the client has diagnosed bradycardia with an average heart rate of 45–55 beats per minute, the client's heart rate of 50 while sitting edge of bed might not be alarming or an immediate red flag. Although this is more of a yellow flag, it still requires close monitoring, detailed documentation of the heart rate, and clear communication with the physician.

Evaluation

After a client receives a referral for OT services from a physician, there is typically an informal screening (see above) followed by the initial OT evaluation. The evaluation can take place in a variety of practice settings: a hospital, rehab facility, outpatient clinic, school, or client's home. When reviewing a client's chart, the OTR typically first takes note of the referring diagnosis and what physiological implications may affect their current level of function, potential recovery, and whether they are appropriate or contraindicated for an OT evaluation. In addition, the therapist will also need to review a client's past medical history and contemplate how comorbidities may impact the same factors as above or, furthermore, how they may interact with the referring diagnosis. An example of an OT evaluation form can be found below (Fig. 30.3).

Although medical questionnaires completed in the waiting room of an outpatient clinic, or information provided in a client's electronic medical chart, can provide adequate information about the reason for the visit and past medical history, nothing compares to the conversation the OTR has with the client. This interview not only provides answers to important questions but also enables the therapist to observe nonverbal cues that may signify pain or discomfort from the client.

Although completed by the OTR, the initial interview will help both the evaluating OTR as well as the treating OTR or COTA learn about a client's prior level of function and engagement in occupations before needing OT services. This interview helps to clarify current strengths, barriers, or limitations; their living situation, support system, and personal interests; and any additional information related to environmental factors.[4,5] The interview also enables the OTR to observe body language and vocal inflections to gain some insight regarding level of pain or client distress. Understanding the limitations associated with the client's diagnosed pathology, while listening and looking for other symptoms that may fall outside the expected cluster, will enable the OTR and the client to have a more effective interaction. After the OTR synthesizes all the information learned about the client through the questionnaire/chart, interview, observations, and standardized or nonstandardized assessments, the therapist will create an occupational profile as well as a therapeutic plan of care and can begin interventions if the client is appropriate for OT services.

Intervention

There are various types of approaches to intervention.[4] Since OTPs are focused on facilitating engagement in meaningful occupations, many interventions are occupation-based or otherwise support occupations in some way. Through skilled interventions, OTPs can increase a client's participation in meaningful occupations using creative problem-solving in environmental modifications, teaching adaptive equipment and strategies, or even educating on health management. The OTP must determine how to approach meeting a client's occupational needs, especially with respect to symptoms related to their diagnostic condition.

An example follows: A client is admitted to the hospital for a chronic obstructive pulmonary disease (COPD) exacerbation as the referring diagnosis. One of the primary symptoms is shortness of breath or dyspnea on exertion. The OTP must problem solve how this may affect the client's ability to perform her favorite occupations. How will difficulty breathing limit her? What barriers will she need to overcome? Whether the COPD is an acute or chronic condition of hers, one major role OTPs have is education and training on energy conservation techniques to maximize participation in meaningful occupations, from as early as the acute care stage all the way through clients in an outpatient clinic. The general public may not initially consider an OTP as part of the healthcare team when thinking about COPD, but a recent scoping study by Snyder et al. demonstrated an improvement in client care outcomes when OT was added to pulmonary rehabilitation.[15]

Results/Outcomes

Outcomes are the achievable goals or measurable results of OT services.[4] The *OTPF-4* outlines eight categories of therapeutic outcomes.[4] Some of these categories will be briefly summarized below as they relate to pathophysiology.

Prevention

Prevention refers to educational and health initiatives aimed at identifying risk factors or educating individuals to help avoid or reduce the incidence of physiological disorders or injuries.[4] An OTP's role within the health management occupation, as discussed in the "Activities and Participation" section, demonstrates how symptom and condition management, medication management, and lifestyle management can prevent certain diagnoses from occurring or reoccurring.[4] Muntefering et al. found that an OTP's professional values, clinical skill set, and proactive mindset are optimal in preventing the onset of obesity in vulnerable adults through therapeutic interventions in health management.[16] Another factor to consider within prevention is readmission rates. A study by Rogers et al. showed that increased spending

Occupational Therapy Evaluation

Patient Last Name, First Name, M.I.	Patient #	HIC #

Reason for Referral:

Precautions:

Level of Assistance: Independent=I; Modified Independent=M; Stand By Assist=SBA; Supervision=S; Contact Guard Assis=CGA; Minimum=Min; Moderate=Mod; Maximum=Max; Dependent=D

Activities of Daily Living (MDS G-1g,h,j,2)	**Level of Assist.**	**Comments**
Feeding		
Grooming		
UB Bath		
LB Bath		
UB Dressing		
LB Dressing		
Toileting/Hygiene		
Homemaking Skills		
Functional Mobility (MDS G-1g,b, I)	**Level of Assist.**	
Rolling		
Supine to Sit		
Sit to Supine		
Bed to W/C		
Toilet		
Tub/Shower		

Adaptive Equipment/Positioning:

Current Seating	Yes	No
W/C		
Geri Chair		
Other		
Appropriate?		
Further assessment		

Other:

Balance (MDS G-3)	**Static**	**Dynamic**
Sitting		
Standing		

Activity Tolerance:

ROM and Strength/Voluntary Movement (MDS G-4: A/B)

Left					**Body Part**	**Right**				
Coordination	Tone	Strength	AROM	PROM	**Upper**	Coordination	Tone	Strength	AROM	PROM
					Shoulder					
					Elbow					
					Wrist					
					Hand					

Left Upper Extremity Comments:

Right Upper Extremity Comments:

Sensory Integration

Key: I=Intact; Imp=Impaired; A=Absent; NT=Not Tested

Sensation	L	R	Perception	L	R
Stereognosis			Visual Field		
Proprioception			Figure-Ground		
Sharp/Dull			Body Scheme		
Light Touch			R/L Discrimination		
Temperature			R/L Neglect		
Pain:					

Cognitive Function

Orientation:	Person	Place	Time
Follows Commands:	One-Step	Multi-Step	Unable
Communication:	Verbal	Non-verbal	None
Attention Span:			
Judgment:			
Memory:			
Safety Awareness:			
Comments:			

Assessment:

Therapist Signature/Credentials/Date: ______________________

Physician's Name: ______________________ **Patient's Room #** ____________

• **Fig. 30.3** Example of an occupational therapy evaluation form. (From Occupational Therapy Evaluation-Fill and Sign Printable Template Online. https://www.uslegalforms.com/form-library/493846-20occupational-therapy-evaluation.)

for OT services within an acute care setting had a statistically significant association with decreased readmission rates for clients with myocardial infarction, pneumonia, or heart failure, stating the OT lens into social and functional needs may be related to the lower readmission rates.[17] OTPs can be changemakers for health promotion and disease prevention within their scope of practice, working inside the box while thinking outside the box.

Health and Wellness, Well-Being, Quality of Life, and Participation

One of the main goals of OT is to empower individuals to achieve a healthy life, a sense of well-being, and active participation in meaningful occupations.[4] OTPs emphasize the idea of meaningful participation over mere performance with a focus on enhancing an individual's quality of life, well-being, physical health, and mental health.[18] It is the performance of meaningful occupations that drives an individual to achieve, especially in the face of pathological conditions. The balance of occupations not only helps the health of the clients but also addresses the needs of their families and ultimately their communities.[19] OTPs assist clients to perform meaningful activities in the face of pathology but also work with the community to help prevent various pathologies from occurring in the first place.[19]

As illustrated in this text, pathophysiology has not only physical implications but also psychological and social implications. This biopsychosocial approach to health care is in line with the outcomes of the OT process.[4,18] The biopsychosocial model uses a multisystem lens to look at physical and mental health.[18] Developed by Engel and Romano, this approach recognizes the interplay among the biological, psychological, and social systems as well as an individual's self-awareness, relationships, and life context (Fig. 30.4).[20]

The model has been applied to OT practice due to its focus on the social, biological, and psychological aspects of an individual.[21,22] Application of this model with reference to pain can be found in Fig. 30.5.

The Pursuit of Occupation

The field of OT is based on the core belief in the positive relationship between the health of an individual and the perception of an individual as an occupational being. These daily activities that bring us meaning are at the core of OT. The field emphasizes the importance of occupational identity for a more productive, healthy, and satisfying life.[23] This puts OTPs in a unique role when helping clients address health management issues related to chronic conditions in an effort to improve or maintain their ability to perform meaningful occupations.[23]

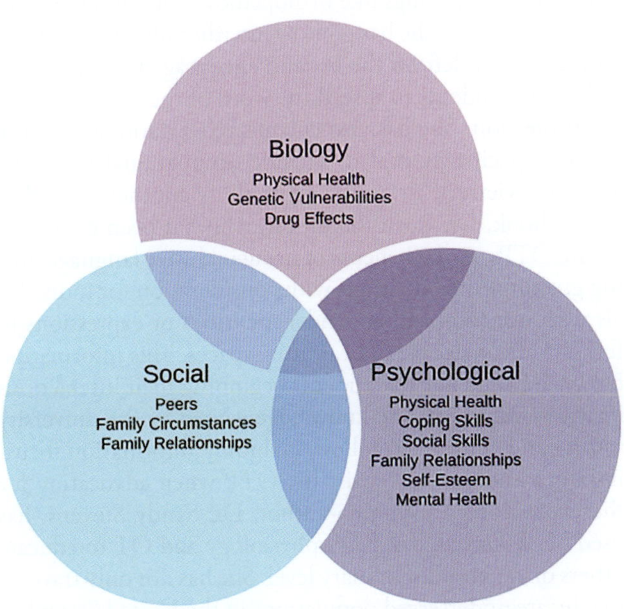

• **Fig. 30.4** Biopsychosocial approach to health care. (From https://commons.wikimedia.org/wiki/File:Biopsychosocial_Model_of_Health_1.svg.)

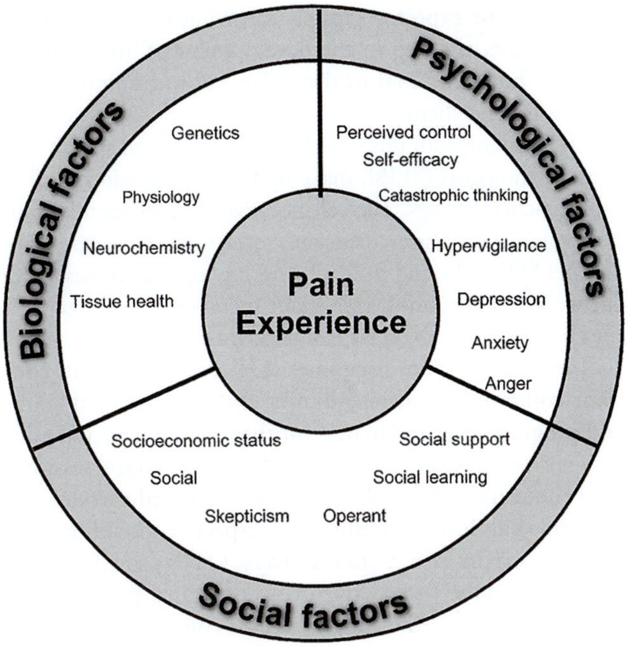

• **Fig. 30.5** The biopsychosocial approach to pain. (From Adams LM, Turk DC. Central sensitization and the biopsychosocial approach to understanding pain. *J Appl Biobehav Res*. 2018;23(2):e12125.)

Occupational Science

Occupational science is the study of individuals as occupational beings and the human ability throughout the lifespan to pursue meaningful occupations.[24] It looks at how occupations influence an individual's well-being and the relationship between occupations and health.[4] This scientific study explores the complex interplay of community, social, behavioral, sociocultural, developmental, and environmental factors.[25] Additionally, occupational science justifies the need for OTPs in the field as client advocates, therapists, innovators, and researchers.[24]

OTPs as Important Members of the Medical Team

A thorough understanding of the symptoms involved in various pathological conditions will aid the OTP dramatically as a member of the healthcare team in the provision of quality health care. Recognizing specific symptoms related to a client's diagnosis helps ensure the client's symptoms fall within the expected cluster. Knowing this information could be the first step in the development of interventions that will hopefully lead to the pursuit of meaningful occupations for the client.

OTPs, along with physical therapists (PTs) and speech-language pathologists (SLPs), make up the rehabilitation team in most practice settings. The collaborative medical team is composed of doctors, nurses, dieticians, social workers (or case managers), OTPs, PTs, and SLPs all working together to best serve clients' needs. The most important member of both teams is the client, followed by their family, advocates, and caregivers.[26]

The rehabilitation disciplines (OT, PT, SLP) are in constant communication regarding a client's functional status and progress, appropriateness for therapy services, and education on successful strategies used during therapy sessions. This communication will lead to an improved carryover of care and skills learned within each respective discipline's sessions. To maximize a client's recovery, OTPs provide insight from the unique perspective of occupational participation and performance. Another important component of interprofessional collaboration is an OTP's clinical reasoning related to safe discharge recommendations.

In medical model settings, such as acute care or inpatient rehab, there is often extensive collaboration regarding a client's medical as well as functional status and eventual discharge plan. OTPs treat clients in these settings to determine what would be the safest option for discharge: returning home with or without the need for family/caregiving support or transferring to a rehabilitation floor or facility. An OTP's perspective and understanding of pathophysiological conditions are essential in discharge planning to advocate for the client's safety, functional needs, and specific goals and desired outcomes.

OT, Client Advocacy, and Advocacy for the Profession

Advocacy within the field of OT is defined as initiatives that focus on advancing occupational justice and enabling clients to access and secure resources that support their health, promote well-being, and facilitate participation in occupations.[4] Advocacy can be provided to individuals, groups, or even systems.[5] OTPs are responsible for advocating for the profession by educating and promoting awareness of OT, the value of the profession as part of the healthcare team, how OT services can benefit various populations, and how an OTP's unique lens is beneficial for social policy reform or health care in general. Understanding pathophysiology, therefore, becomes imperative when advocating not only for the care of individual clients but also for groups of people with a given diagnostic condition in the community.[26] The case study examples provided at the end of most chapters in this text exemplified how an OTP's pathophysiology knowledge, rapport building with clients, and advocacy skills to other members of the medical team could prevent, detect, or decrease medical emergencies. By reading this text, you, the reader, have already taken the first crucial step in becoming an advocate for your future clients and the profession of OT as a whole. Moreover, the various roles assumed when advocating for individuals with rare diseases can be found in Fig. 30.6.

At the individual level, OTPs not only advocate for their clients but also teach clients how to be their own self-advocate.[4] An example of both points is the communication an OTP has with the physician when a client's diagnostic condition falls outside the typical presentation for their stated diagnosis. It can also be seen in a hypothetical "family training" session on the inpatient rehab floor with an overprotective spouse. The spouse insists on fully dressing the client when she goes home. The OTP can discuss the benefits of the client performing these Activities of Daily Living (ADLs) to improve occupational performance and recovery outcomes, or the client, with encouragement from her OTP, can show the spouse the adaptive equipment she learned to use during rehab to improve independence and safety when getting dressed. OTPs have the power to advocate for clients' needs to other medical professionals or insurance companies as well. An example is an OTP sending a letter of medical necessity to a client's pediatrician for a splint to prevent deformity and subsequent consequences to their fine motor skill development. Another example is an OTP writing a note to an insurance company requesting a bedside commode be financially covered because this client would not otherwise have a safe toileting option upon discharge home from their current rehabilitation facility.

Next, OTPs can advocate to groups of people to reinforce the knowledge and/or values of the profession.[4] An example is an OTP providing an in-service at a local YMCA educating the public (older adults mostly in attendance) on fall prevention. One of the co-authors of this book, Dr. Natalie Norman Michaels, has been teaching for years in an OT curriculum as a PT. She has been able to attend healthcare functions to educate individuals on the need to increase OT in various settings like orthopedics or aquatic intervention. In addition, she has gone to interdisciplinary functions where OT was left off the list and encouraged the inclusion of her OT students to spread the word of the importance of the profession. She has also encouraged a national physical therapy-specific journal to include occupational therapists as peer reviewers. A second example is another co-author of this book, Dr. Roya Rezadoost, who has been educating future OTPs on the benefits of using inclusive language during greetings/introductions with consideration for individuals with nonconforming gender identities or expressions to feel safe and welcome in healthcare spaces. This information has been invaluable for students beginning their interactions in the community. The knowledge gained in the university setting and clinics that follow, including information focusing on pathology, will assist the OTP when advocating for the profession. Another co-author, Dr. Sandy Stevens, has used her knowledge of pathophysiology and OT to educate others on an interdisciplinary level. She has not only traveled to educate underserved populations in the United States but has also educated people in Honduras, Guatemala, Ecuador, Hungary, Romania, Cameroon, and Kenya.

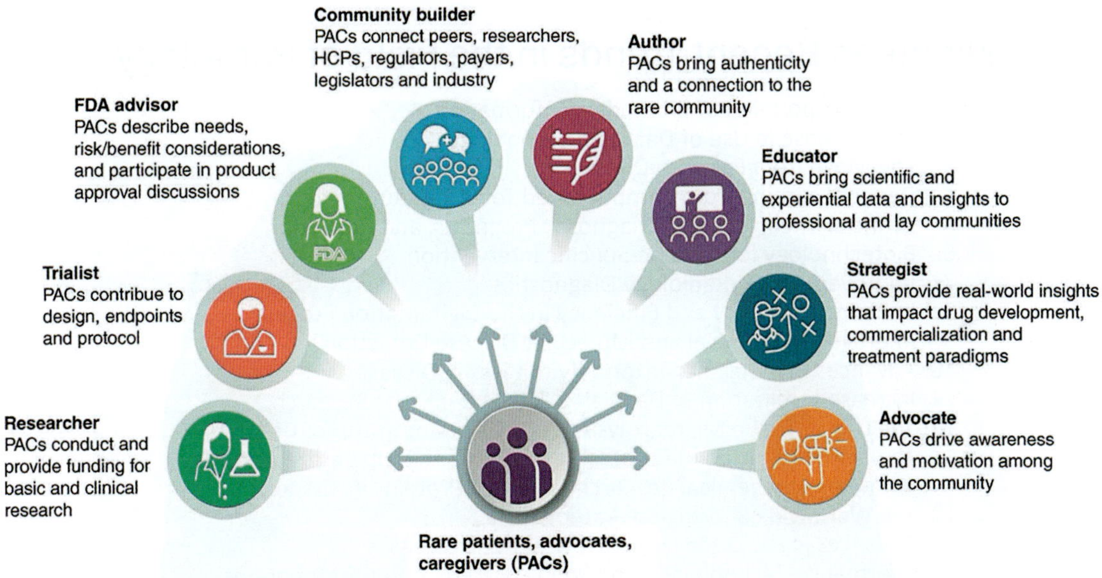
Community builder
PACs connect peers, researchers, HCPs, regulators, payers, legislators and industry
Author
PACs bring authenticity and a connection to the rare community
FDA advisor
PACs describe needs, risk/benefit considerations, and participate in product approval discussions
FDA
Educator
PACs bring scientific and experiential data and insights to professional and lay communities
Trialist
PACs contribute to design, endpoints and protocol
Strategist
PACs provide real-world insights that impact drug development, commercialization and treatment paradigms
Researcher
PACs conduct and provide funding for basic and clinical research
Advocate
PACs drive awareness and motivation among the community
Rare patients, advocates, caregivers (PACs)

• **Fig. 30.6** Possible roles assumed by clients, advocates, and caregivers. (Reproduced with permission ©rareLife solutions.)

Furthermore, an OTP has the power to advocate for the advancement of inclusive legislation to expand rights for disabled or vulnerable populations on a systemic level. OTPs can be policy changemakers and influence the contexts that impact a person's ability to participate in occupations. Another author of this book, Dr. Ashley Rabuck, was able to meet with a state-level politician to advocate passing a bill for adult-sized changing tables in public spaces for disabled teenagers and adults who require assistance with toileting, with the ultimate benefit of community reintegration to maximize occupational opportunities for these individuals and their caregivers. This demonstrates the importance of having knowledge of human development, pathophysiology, and the human condition. Good news: the bill was passed because of these advocacy efforts!

No matter how big or small, advocacy is an important role of OTPs. The AOTA has created an "Everyday Advocacy Decision Guide" with a list of tips to encourage OTPs to take action.[27] The more we advocate for the profession, the better we can advocate for our clients.

The Endless Pursuit of Knowledge

This textbook's focus was to cover pathophysiology for the OT student in a way that would be applicable in the clinical setting. OT students are encouraged to look into both of the important resources used within this chapter to expand their understanding and appreciation of health care and OT practice: the ICF framework[5] and the *OTPF-4*.[4] With each passing day, more is learned about the human body and pathophysiological conditions. OTPs work with other members of the healthcare team to provide the highest quality care possible. The advancement of technology has made medical diagnostics more sensitive and specific than ever before.[28] The use of artificial intelligence in the form of digital pathology has risen in both cytology (the examination of cells from body fluids) and histology (the study of anatomy at a microscopic level).[26] The recent utilization of computational pathology algorithms is now being used to analyze histopathological images. This advancement has led to the discovery of predictive biomarkers for various disorders.[29] Over the past 10 years, there have been many more trends in medicine that have greatly impacted the field of pathology and the future of diagnostics.[30] The editorial team of *Medical Trends Now* listed 19 trends in medicine that directly affect pathology.[30] These trends can be found in Fig. 30.7.

Advancement in the field of pathophysiology is why it is important for all OTRs and COTAs to continue to read the latest journals and stay on top of changes that could affect the field of OT and the provision of care. OTPs should strive to be autonomous, lifelong learners, independently using reflective, higher order, critical thinking skills.[31] The field of OT is ever-changing, as is the field of pathology. These are not static systems. Like trying to get your bearings on a rocking boat at sea, OTPs are in a fluid, dynamic system and need to go with the flow and learn as they go. This transformative learning might even change one's thinking as the world changes around them.[32] Lifelong learning for OTPs is a major key to the continued growth of the profession.

OTPs are in a very unique work situation, as they are surrounded by knowledgeable individuals. Working within an interprofessional team not only supports learning about various diagnostic conditions but also deepens understanding of the roles of each member of the healthcare team.[33,34] Much can be learned from these professionals; yet, it is possible these professionals will learn the most from the OTPs.[33,34] There is so much to tell them about this important, life-changing profession (Fig. 30.8).

Nineteen Recent Trends in the Field of Pathology

1. The Incorporation of Biomedical Information
2. The Increase in Use of Data and Technology
3. The Move from Paper to Digital
4. Deeper Learning from Computerized Tools and Automation
5. Artificial Intelligence for Diagnosis, Prognosis, and Prediction
6. Biotechnology for Genetic-Specific Intervention
7. Improvements in Radiology Diagnostics
8. Improved Accuracy and Efficiency in the Digitalization Process
9. Improved Anatomical and Molecular Disease Detection
10. Advances in Molecular Taxonomy to Classify Diseases
11. Increased Utilization of Dedicated Tissue Banks for Research
12. The Use of Tissue Microarrays to Study Proteins in Tumor Cells
13. The Standardization of Processing Protocols to Help Ensure Accuracy
14. Immunohistochemical Research to Detect Proteins in Tissues
15. The Worldwide Shortage of Pathologists
16. Advances in the Discovery of New Genetic Diseases
17. Information Technology Using Sophisticated Computer Programs
18. Digital Imaging Techniques to Create Images of Organs and Tissues
19. Advances Histopathology to Better Understand Cellular Pathophysiology

• **Fig. 30.7** Nineteen trends in the field of pathology. (Adapted from https://medicaltrendsnow.com/pathology/trends-in-pathology/#Advances_in_Molecular_Taxonomy.)

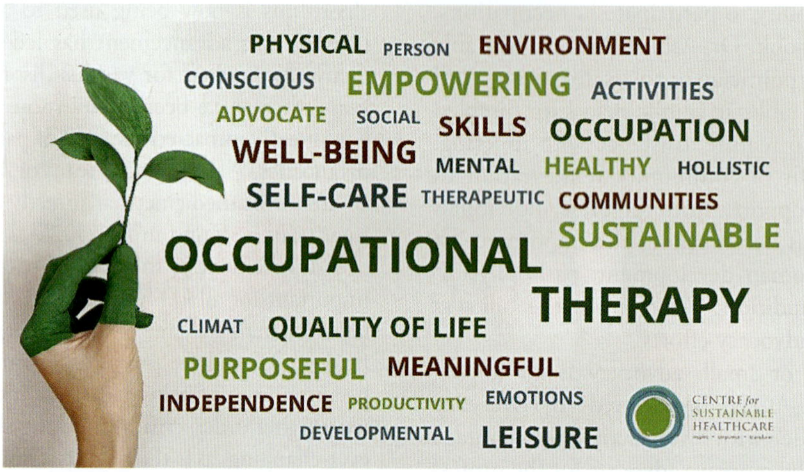

• **Fig. 30.8** Word cloud of some of the many perspectives of OT. (From Sustainable Occupational Therapy | Centre for Sustainable Healthcare.)

Conclusion

The purpose of this book was to provide the soon-to-be OTP with an introduction to the ever-changing field of pathophysiology. One book cannot cover the endless array of diagnostic conditions an OTP may encounter in the field. This book was written to provide the reader with a systematic way of thinking, with the ability to take a client's case and determine whether the symptoms of that client fell within the range typically seen with their given disorder. If symptoms appear outside what is expected, we hope the reader will then cluster those unusual symptoms together and communicate these findings to the referring physician for further exploration or testing.[9] As stated earlier in this text, OTPs do not diagnose. They must work within their scope of service. Although they must work within the box, OTPs need to be thinking outside the box with the appropriate knowledge to know which symptoms justify possible caution (*yellow flags*) or which could signify potential danger (*red flags*).

According to the AOTA, the OT evaluation process focuses on what the client wants to do and identifies supports as well as barriers to their participation, well-being, and health.[35] Although the organization of the client evaluation will often depend on the practice setting, each evaluation needs to focus on the unique needs of the specific client, which can be complicated and multifaceted. The most important components of the OT evaluation include the occupational profile (or summary of client's values, needs, and past and present occupational experience) and the OTR's occupational performance analysis.[35] Although the evaluation is seen as the initial step in the OT intervention process, the OTP is always listening, observing, and watching for new or changed signs and symptoms until the client has been discharged from services. This requires the organization of a great deal of information as well as clinical reasoning strategies and decision-making skills that become easier with each year of OT practice.

Case scenarios were introduced in Chapters 4 through 20 and again in Chapters 22 through 29 to provide examples of OT application. Each scenario used the same format for organization of information collected during the initial screening or evaluation process. This is just one way to organize client information so that higher order, reflective, critical thinking strategies can be utilized when making client care decisions and justifying these decisions to other members of the healthcare team. This system is reviewed in Fig. 30.9.

The authors of this book hope that the information in these pages will help the reader to use critical thinking and thorough, clinical reasoning skills when making decisions that can greatly impact their clients. The hope is that through reading this text, one will have the tools to better organize the multidimensional and complex information gained through active listening and close observation. Most importantly, the authors hope that the reader will prioritize treating each individual as just that, an individual, honoring each person's unique complexity of dreams, wishes, and goals for meaningful participation in occupations.

Systematic Process for OT Critical Thinking and Decision-Making in Client Care with Respect to Pathophysiology

1. Screen
2. Take a Closer Look
3. Determine Flag Status
4. Take Action if Needed
5. Document the Findings
6. Take a Second Look
7. Determine the Flag Status
8. Take Action if Needed

• **Fig. 30.9** The systematic process used in this book. (Adapted from Heick J, Lazaro RT. *Goodman and Snyder's Differential Diagnosis for Physical Therapists: Screening for Referral*. 7th ed. Elsevier; 2023.)

References

1. New World. *Benjamin Bloom*. New World Encyclopedia; 2023. https://www.newworldencyclopedia.org/entry/Benjamin_Bloom
2. AOTA. Occupational therapy scope of practice. *Am J Occup Ther*. 2021;75(suppl 3): 7513410020. https://doi.org/10.5014/ajot.2021.75S3005.
3. AOTA. *State Occupational Therapy Regulatory Authority Contact Information*. AOTA; 2024. myaota.aota.org/regulatorycontacts.aspx?
4. AOTA. The Occupational Therapy Practice framework: domain and practice: 4th ed. *Am J Occup Ther*. 2020;74(Suppl. 2). https://doi.org/10.5014/ajot.2020.74S2001.
5. WHO. *How to Use the ICF: A Practical Manual for Using the International Classification of Functioning, Disability and Health (ICF)*. World Health Organization; 2013. https://www.who.int/publications/m/item/how-to-use-the-icf---a-practical-manual-for-using-the-international-classification-of-functioning-disability-and-health.
6. CDC. *ICF*. National Center for Health Statistics; 2024. https://www.cdc.gov/nchs/icd/icf/
7. Abarghuei AF, Mehraban AH, Lajevardi L, Yousefi M. The clinical application of ICF model for occupational therapy in a patient with stroke: a case report. *Med J Islamic Repub Iran*. 2018;32:65. https://pmc.ncbi.nlm.nih.gov/articles/PMC6325290/.
8. CDC. *The ICF: An Overview*. Centers for Disease Control and Prevention; 2024. https://www.cdc.gov/nchs/data/icd/icfoverview_finalforwho10sept.pdf
9. Heick J, Lazaro RT. *Goodman and Snyder's Differential Diagnosis for Physical Therapists: Screening for Referral*. 7th ed. Elsevier; 2023.
10. Epley E, Wolske J, Lee J, Mirza M, Fisher G. Habits and health promotion in occupational therapy: a scoping review. *Ann Int Occup Ther*. 2021;4(4):e269–e277. https://doi.org/10.3928/24761222-20210921-04.
11. Dunn W, Brown C, McGuigan A. The ecology of human performance: a framework for considering the effect of context. *Am J Occup Ther*. 1994;48:595–607. https://ottheory.com/index.php/therapy-model/ecology-human-performance-framework-ehp.
12. Mcleod S. Social roles and social norms in psychology. *Simply Psychology*; 2023. https://www.simplypsychology.org/social-roles.html.
13. John Hopkins. The effects of rehabilitation on the family. In: *Health*. John Hopkins; 2024. https://www.hopkinsmedicine.org/health/treatment-tests-and-therapies/effects-of-rehabilitation-on-the-family.
14. AOTA. *Quality Toolkit*. American Occupational Therapy Association; 2024. https://www.aota.org/practice/practice-essentials/quality/quality-toolkit
15. Snyder N, Wilson R, Finch L, et al. The role of occupational therapy in pulmonary rehabilitation programs: protocol for a scoping review. *J Med Internet Res: Res Protoc*. 2021;10(7):e30244. https://doi.org/10.2196/30244.
16. Muntefering C, Fields B, Christensen JR. Going beyond management and maintenance: occupational therapy's role in primary prevention for adults at risk of obesity. *Am J Occup Ther*. 2023;77(5). https://doi.org/10.5014/ajot.2023.050154.

17. Rogers AT, Bai G, Lavin RA, Anderson GF. Higher hospital spending on occupational therapy is associated with lower readmission rates. *Med Care Res Rev*. 2017;74(6):668–686. https://doi.org/10.1177/1077558716666981.
18. Pizzi MA, Richards LG. Promoting health, well-being, and quality of life in occupational therapy: a paradigm shift for the next 100 years. *Am J Occup Ther*. 2017;71(4): 7104170010p1–7104170010p5. https://doi.org/10.5014/ajot.2017.028456.
19. Reitz SM, Scaffa ME. Occupational therapy in the promotion of health and well-being. *Am J Occup Ther*. 2020;74(3): 7403420010p1-7403420010p14. https://doi.org/10.5014/ajot.2020.743003.
20. Marschall A. Understanding the biopsychosocial model of health and wellness: a holistic approach to well-being. *Very Well Mind*; 2023. https://www.verywellmind.com/understanding-the-biopsychosocial-model-7549226.
21. Gentry K, Snyder K, Barstow B, Hamson-Utley J. The biopsychosocial model: application to occupational therapy practice. *Open J Occup Ther*. 2018;6(4): Article 12. https://doi.org/10.15453/2168-6408.1412.
22. Chamberlain M. *The Biopsychosocial Model and Occupational Therapy.* OT Flourish; 2024. https://otflourish.com/biopsychosocial-model-occupational-therapy/
23. AOTA. *Domain and Process: Occupations and Everyday Activities*. American Occupational Therapy Association; 2024. https://www.aota.org/practice/domain-and-process/occupations-everyday-activities
24. Clark FA, Parham D, Carlson ME, et al. Occupational science: academic innovation in the service of occupational therapy's future. *Am J Occup Ther*. 1991;45(5):300–301. https://doi.org/10.5014/ajot.45.4.300.
25. USC. *Occupational Science*. USC Chan/Division of Occupational Science and Occupational Therapy; 2019. https://chan.usc.edu/about-us/occupational-science
26. Mukund N, Fisher-Vance D, Wuerth L, et al. The global role of patients, advocates and caregivers in rare diseases. *Future Rare Dis*. 2022;2(2). https://doi.org/10.2217/frd-2022-0003.
27. AOTA. *Everyday Advocacy Decision Guide*. American Occupational Therapy Association; 2024. https://www.aota.org/advocacy/everyday-advocacy/everyday-advocacy-decision-guide
28. HCBT Editorial Team. The future of diagnosis: 2023 trends in pathology. *Health Care Business Today*; 2023 https://www.healthcarebusinesstoday.com/the-future-of-diagnosis-2023-trends-in-pathology/
29. Giovagnoli MR, Giansanto D. Artificial intelligence in digital pathology: what is the future! Part 1: From the digital slide onwards. *Healthcare*. 2021;9(7):858. https://doi.org/10.3390/healthcare9070858.
30. Verghese G, Lennerz JK, Ruta D, et al. Computational pathology in cancer diagnosis, prognosis, and prediction—present day and prospects. *J Pathol*. 2023;260(5):551–563. https://doi.org/10.1002/path.6163.
31. MTN Editorial Team. 19 trends in pathology: the future of diagnosis. *Medical Trends Now*. 2022. https://medicaltrendsnow.com/pathology/trends-in-pathology/
32. Lee HC-Y, Flavell H, Parsons D, et al. Developing agentic learners for 21st century practice: a pedagogical approach in occupational therapy. *J Appl Health*. 2016;45(1):8–13. https://pubmed.ncbi.nlm.nih.gov/26937876/.
33. Taylor L. Doing, being and becoming—the synergistic relationship of occupational therapy practice and employability. *Br J Occup Ther*. 2021;85(1):3–4. https://doi.org/10.1177/03080226211062489.
34. Leveille W, Brandes J, Boos K, et al. The positive impact of occupational therapy involvement in interprofessional education. *J Occup Ther*. 2020;4(4). https://doi.org/10.26681/jote.2020.040405.
35. AOTA. *Domain and Process. Evaluation and Assessment*. American Occupational Therapy Association; 2024. https://www.aota.org/practice/domain-and-process/evaluation-and-assessment.

Glossary of Pathophysiological Conditions

Introduction to the Glossary

Welcome to the glossary of diagnostic conditions for this textbook. This glossary can serve as a reference tool for occupational therapy (OT) students, providing quick access to information related to various conditions, the underlying pathophysiology of those conditions, and their most typical symptoms. It can also support occupational therapy practitioners (OTPs) who have reviewed a client's chart and are familiar with their conditions and comorbidities but seek a deeper understanding of potential complications and associated symptoms. Additionally, this glossary can help practicing OTPs discern whether a client's symptoms fall within the expected cluster for a given diagnosis or if further collaboration the referring physician is warranted. While comprehensive, this glossary is not all-inclusive.

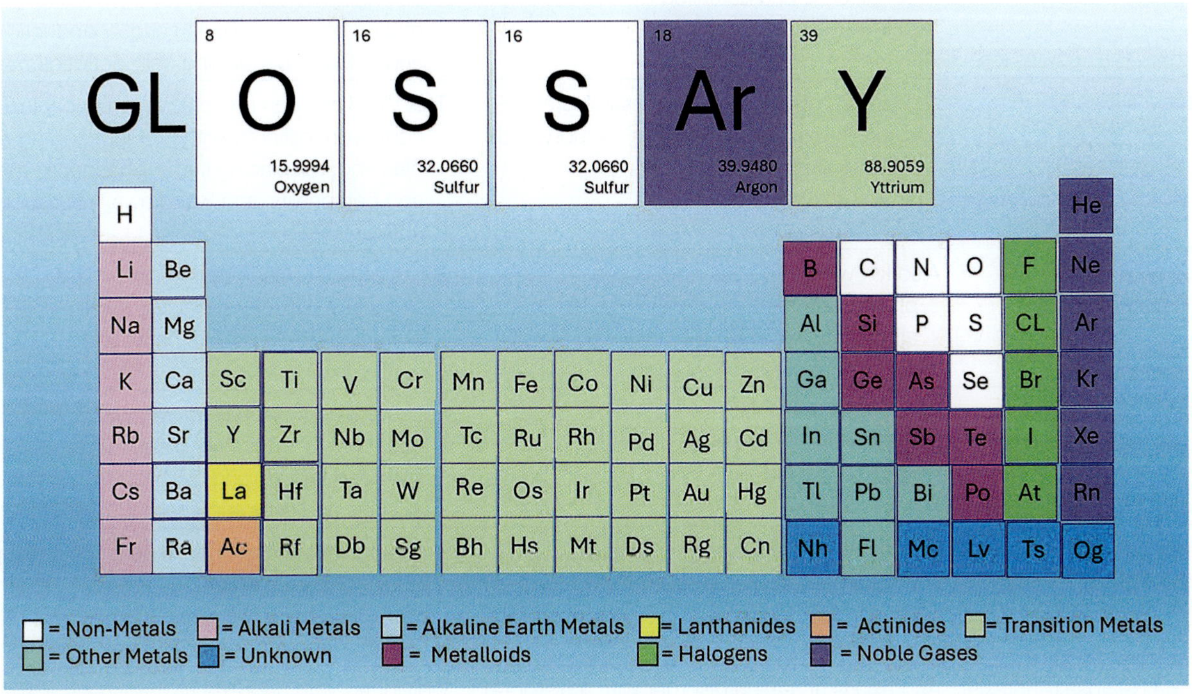

(Courtesy Natalie Norman Michaels.)

Glossary of Medical Conditions and Comorbidities

Most Often Seen by Occupational Therapy Practitioners

Condition	Pathophysiology	Most Common Signs and Symptoms
Abdominal Aortic Aneurysm (AAA)	AAA is a bulge or swelling in the aorta, the main blood vessel that runs from the heart down through the chest and abdomen.[1]	While AAA is often asymptomatic, common signs and symptoms may be deep, constant pain in the abdomen or side, back pain, pulsating sensation in the abdomen, and other symptoms if the aneurysm expands or ruptures.[1]
Abscess—Liver	A liver abscess is a fluid-filled sac in the liver, typically with infection.[2]	Signs and symptoms include fever, chills, pain in the upper-right abdomen, jaundice, nausea, vomiting, and weight loss.[2]
Abscess—Obturator Internus or Psoas Major	This condition includes fluid-filled sacs (typically infected) located in the obturator internus or psoas muscles.[3]	Fever, localized pain in the pelvic or lower back region, difficulty moving the affected limb, and other signs of infection are all potential signs and symptoms.[3]
Adhesive Capsulitis of the Shoulder	Commonly known as frozen shoulder, this condition is characterized by stiffness and pain in the shoulder joint.[4]	Common signs and symptoms include pain and stiffness in the shoulder joint, limited range of motion of forward flexion and/or abduction, and difficulty performing daily activities.[4]
Alzheimer's Disease	Alzheimer's disease is a progressive brain disorder that slowly destroys memory and thinking skills.[5,6]	This condition can present with memory loss, confusion, difficulty with problem solving or planning, misplacing items, changes in mood and personality, and withdrawal from social activities.[5]
Amyotrophic Lateral Sclerosis (ALS)	Also known as Lou Gehrig disease, ALS is a progressive nervous system disease that affects nerve cells in the brain and spinal cord.[7,8]	Signs of ALS include muscle weakness; twitching; difficulty speaking, swallowing, or breathing; and eventual paralysis.[7,8]
Anemia	Anemia is lower-than-normal red blood cell count or hemoglobin level, which can lead to reduced oxygen flow to tissues and organs.[9]	Fatigue, weakness, pale or yellowish skin, irregular heartbeat, shortness of breath, dizziness or lightheadedness, and cold hands and feet are all signs and symptoms related to anemia.[9]
Angina Pectoris	Commonly known simply as "angina," angina pectoris is chest pain or discomfort caused by reduced blood flow to the heart muscle.[10,11]	A person with angina may experience chest pain or discomfort; pain or discomfort in the arms, neck, jaw, shoulder, or back; shortness of breath; nausea; fatigue; and anxiety.[12]
Anorexia Nervosa (Anorexia)	Anorexia is an eating disorder with a distorted perception of body weight.[13]	Individuals with anorexia typically have a low body weight and an intense fear of gaining weight. There may also be fatigue, abnormal blood counts, dizziness or fainting, hair breakage, insomnia, and/or absence of menstruation.[13]

Condition	Pathophysiology	Most Common Signs and Symptoms
Aortic Valve Stenosis	Aortic valve stenosis is characterized as a narrowing of the heart's aortic valve, which restricts blood flow from the heart to the rest of the body.[14]	Signs and symptoms are chest pain, shortness of breath, fatigue, heart palpitations, fainting, and heart murmur.[14]
Aphasia	Aphasia is a communication disorder that results from damage to parts of the brain that control language. There are two main types: *Receptive aphasia* (typically from damage to Wernicke's area of the brain in the temporal lobe) and *Expressive aphasia* (typically from damage to Broca's area of the brain in the frontal lobe).[15,16]	General signs and symptoms of aphasia are difficulty speaking, understanding speech, reading, and writing; using incorrect words; and difficulty with word recall. Understanding is the main concern with receptive aphasia, whereas speech production becomes the major concern with expressive aphasia.[15]
Appendicitis	Appendicitis is inflammation of the appendix, a small pouch attached to the large intestine.[17]	Sudden pain that starts near the navel and moves to the lower right abdomen, pain that worsens with movement, nausea, vomiting, loss of appetite, fever, and abdominal swelling may all be indicative of appendicitis.[17]
Arterial Septal Defect (ASD)	ASD is a hole in the wall between the heart's upper chambers (atria).[18]	An ASD is often asymptomatic; however, some signs and symptoms may include shortness of breath; fatigue; swelling in legs, feet, or abdomen; heart palpitations; and frequent respiratory infections.[18]
Arthritis—Osteoarthritis (OA)	OA is a degenerative joint disease that occurs when the protective cartilage that cushions the ends of bones wears down over time.[19]	Signs and symptoms of OA include joint pain, tenderness, stiffness, loss of flexibility, grating sensation, bone spurs, and swelling.[19]
Arthritis—Rheumatoid Arthritis (RA)	RA is an autoimmune disorder that causes chronic inflammation of the joints and other areas of the body. The joints most often affected are the smaller joints of the fingers and wrists.[20]	Signs and symptoms of RA include joint pain, swelling, stiffness, fatigue, fever, loss of appetite, and deformity.[20]
Arthroplasty—Hip or Knee	Hip or knee arthroplasty is a surgical procedure to replace a damaged hip or knee joint with an artificial joint.[21]	The aftermath may include pain relief, improved joint function, stiffness, swelling, and possible complications related to surgery.[21]
Arthroplasty—Shoulder	Shoulder arthroplasty is a surgical procedure to replace a damaged shoulder joint with an artificial joint.[22]	Following a shoulder arthroplasty, an individual may experience pain relief, improved shoulder function, stiffness, swelling, and possible complications related to surgery.[22]
Asthma	Asthma is a chronic respiratory condition characterized by inflammation and narrowing of the airways.[23]	Shortness of breath, wheezing, chest tightness, coughing (especially at night or early morning), and exacerbations triggered by allergens or irritants may result from asthma.[23]
Autism Spectrum Disorder (ASD)	This is a developmental condition that affects how a person interacts with others. ASD can affect communication, behavior, and social interaction.[24]	ASD may present as difficulty with communication (verbal and nonverbal), difficulty with social interactions, repetitive behaviors, limited interests, and sensory sensitivities.[24]

(Continued)

Condition	Pathophysiology	Most Common Signs and Symptoms
Bipolar Disorder, formerly known as Manic-Depressive Disorder	This is a mood disorder that causes shifts in energy levels, moods, and behaviors, which can last from hours to days or even weeks.[25]	Signs and symptoms can include manic episodes with elevated irritability or emotions, garrulous, or activity level that is noticed by others as unusual from typical behavior of that individual. There will also be depressive periods of fatigue, loss of appetite, or feelings of worthlessness.[25]
Borderline Personality Disorder (BPD)	This is a mental health condition in which the individual is emotionally unstable.[26]	Individuals with BPD have a hard time managing their emotions, with extreme anger, severe mood swings, and fear of abandonment and have trouble with daily tasks, life events, and obligations. They may also be prone to suicide and might also misuse food or alcohol to cope.[26]
Bulimia Nervosa (Bulimia)	This is a potentially life-threatening condition in which the individual will binge eat in one sitting and then try to rid themselves of the food by vomiting or misusing laxatives.[27]	Signs and symptoms include a negative body image, fear of gaining weight, extreme mood swings, repeatedly eating large quantities in one sitting with a loss of control while doing this (binge), induced vomiting (purge), damaged teeth and gums, calloused fingers, and overuse of laxatives and diuretics.[27]
Cardiac Arrest	Cardiac arrest presents as a sudden loss of heart function, breathing, and consciousness.[28,29]	Signs of cardiac arrest include sudden collapse, no pulse, no breathing, loss of consciousness, and death if not treated immediately.[28,29] This is a red flag situation, requiring immediate medical attention.
Carcinoma—Basal Cell	Basal cell carcinoma is a type of skin cancer that begins in the basal cells, which are responsible for producing new skin cells.[30]	Observable signs include a shiny, bumpy, pink growth; open sore; red patch; scar-like area; or a white, waxy area on the skin.[30]
Carcinoma—Merkel Cell	Merkel cell carcinoma is a rare and aggressive skin cancer that usually appears as a painless lump on the skin.[31,32]	This is typically a fast-growing, painless lump or nodule on the skin that is usually red, pink, or purple in color.[31,32]
Carcinoma—Squamous Cell	Squamous cell carcinoma is a common form of skin cancer that develops in the squamous cells, which are thin, flat cells that look like fish scales.[33,34]	The skin lesion will present as a firm, red nodule; a flat sore with a scaly crust; or a new growth on the skin that does not heal.[33,34]
Cerebral Palsy (CP)	CP is a group of disorders that affect movement, posture, and muscle coordination, caused by damage to the developing brain, usually before birth.[35] Subtypes of CP are based on the body part involved: • Diplegic—the lower extremities are affected more than the upper extremities[36] • Quadriplegic—affecting all four extremities • Hemiplegic—affecting one side of the body • Monoplegic—affecting one extremity • Paraplegic—affecting the lower extremities.[37]	General signs and symptoms of CP include the lack of muscle coordination when performing voluntary movements (ataxia), stiff or tight muscles and exaggerated reflexes (spasticity), walking with one foot or leg dragging, and difficulty walking.[35] There are three primary types of CP: • Spastic (the most common type) with stiff muscles and jerky movements • Dyskinetic with slow and uncontrollable movements • Ataxic with balance and depth perception deficits.[38]

Condition	Pathophysiology	Most Common Signs and Symptoms
Cerebrovascular Accident (CVA) (Stroke)	A stroke, or CVA, occurs when blood flow to the brain is disrupted, causing brain cells to die.[39]	The most common symptoms observed when someone is experiencing a stroke include sudden numbness or weakness in the face, arm, and/or leg (typically affecting only one side of the body); confusion; trouble speaking or understanding speech; sudden trouble seeing in one or both eyes; sudden trouble walking; dizziness; loss of balance or coordination; and severe headache with no known cause.[39] This is a red flag situation, requiring immediate medical attention.
Cholelithiasis (gallstones)	Cholelithiasis or gallstones are hardened deposits of digestive fluid that can form in the gallbladder.[40]	Signs and symptoms can include sudden and rapidly intensifying pain in the upper-right portion of the abdomen; pain in the center of the abdomen between your breastbone and belly button; back pain between the scapula; pain in the right shoulder, and nausea or vomiting.[40]
Chronic Obstructive Pulmonary Disease (COPD)	COPD is a group of lung diseases that block airflow and make breathing difficult, including emphysema and chronic bronchitis.[41]	Signs and symptoms of COPD include shortness of breath, especially during physical activities; wheezing; chest tightness; chronic cough; producing a lot of mucus (sputum); frequent respiratory infections; lack of energy; unintended weight loss (in later stages); and swelling in ankles, feet, or lower extremities.[41]
Cholangiocarcinoma (CCC)	CCC is a cancer that forms in the bile ducts, the tubes that carry bile from the liver to the small intestine.[42]	CCC may cause jaundice, abdominal pain, itching, fever, weight loss, and general malaise.[42]
Congestive Heart Failure	CHF is a chronic condition in which the heart muscle is unable to pump blood efficiently, leading to fluid buildup in various parts of the body.[43,44]	Various signs and symptoms for CHF include shortness of breath (especially during exertion or in supine); fatigue; weakness; edema in lower extremities, ankles, and feet; rapid or irregular heartbeat; reduced ability to exercise; persistent cough or wheezing with white or pink blood-tinged phlegm; and sudden weight gain due to fluid retention.[43,44]
COVID-19	COVID-19 is also called coronavirus disease and is caused by the SARS-CoV-2 virus.[45]	For most people, the symptoms resemble a mild to moderate respiratory illness, but some people, especially those with preexisting conditions, will become seriously ill.[45]
Crohn's Disease	Crohn's Disease is an inflammatory bowel disease, causing chronic inflammation of the digestive tract.[46]	Each individual experiences different patterns of flares and remission. Typical symptoms include persistent diarrhea, rectal bleeding, abdominal cramps and pain, urgent need to move bowels, sensation of incomplete bowel evacuation, and constipation that can lead to fecal impaction.[46]
Cystic Fibrosis	Cystic fibrosis is an inherited disorder, affecting the cells that produce mucus, digestive juices, and sweat. It causes severe damage to the lungs and to the gastrointestinal system.[47]	The symptoms vary depending on the severity of the disease. Those diagnosed earlier will have more severe symptoms. Signs include a persistent productive cough with thick mucus, wheezing, repeated lung infections, lack of endurance for exercise, and a recurrent runny or stuffy nose.[47]

(Continued)

Condition	Pathophysiology	Most Common Signs and Symptoms
Deep Vein Thrombosis (DVT)	A DVT is a blood clot in one of the deep veins of the arm or leg. This can lead to a pulmonary embolism if it dislodges.[48,49]	Symptoms include pain and swelling in the extremity, sometimes with red and hot skin, dilated veins, and tenderness on palpation.[48,49] This is a red flag situation, requiring immediate medical attention.
Dehydration	Dehydration is the absence of an adequate amount of water in the body to sustain normal bodily functions, caused by activity on a hot day, fever, diarrhea, or vomiting.[50]	Signs include dryness in the mouth or lips, absence of tears, decreased urination, dark discolored urine, dry and easily wrinkled skin, deep and rapid breathing, dizziness, headache, low blood pressure, loss of appetite, heat intolerance, or chills.[50]
Dementia	Dementia is a symptom and not a disease by itself. It is caused by other disorders, such as Alzheimer's or Parkinson's, involves an atypical decline in cognition, and includes a group of symptoms affecting memory and social ability.[51]	Signs of dementia vary depend on the cause but include memory loss, problems with reasoning and problem solving, trouble planning and organizing, confusion and disorientation, and problems communicating and word finding. There can also be psychological symptoms like depression and anxiety.[51]
Diabetes Insipidus	This is a rare disorder caused by a deficiency of or resistance to arginine vasopressin (antidiuretic hormone [ADH]), leading to an imbalance of fluids in the body. ADH is made in the hypothalamus and stored in the pituitary.[52-55]	Symptoms of diabetes insipidus include severe thirst, large amounts of pale urine, or feeling the need to drink water or urinate after bedtime. The individual may also have bed wetting, weight loss, fever, constipation, headache, vomiting, and problems sleeping.[52-55]
Diabetes Mellitus (DM)	Diabetes mellitus (DM), commonly called "diabetes," happens when the pancreas does not produce a sufficient amount of insulin to control the glucose in the blood. There are two types. Type I DM, also called insulin-dependent diabetes, occurs when antibodies attack the pancreas, so the pancreas cannot produce enough insulin. Type II, non–insulin-dependent, DM occurs when the pancreas produces some insulin but not enough, or the body does not respond to insulin like it should.[52-55]	Symptoms of diabetes mellitus are similar to the symptoms above for diabetes incipitus, but for different reasons. Individuals will still be thirsty with large amounts of urine, as well as fatigue and blurred vision.[52-55]
Down Syndrome	Down syndrome occurs when a person has an extra chromosome 21. It is a congenital condition.[56]	Signs and symptoms include distinct facial features like a flattened bridge of the nose, epicanthal folds in the eyes, a thickened tongue, and a short neck. They might also have hypotonicity, atlantoaxial instability, hearing loss, congenital heart anomalies, and sleep apnea.[56]
Ectopic Pregnancy	This is when a fertilized egg implants in an area of the body that is outside of the uterus.[57] It is more common if a female becomes pregnant while wearing an intrauterine device (IUD) or has a history of smoking, endometriosis, or tubal ligation. This can be life-threatening, requiring emergency intervention.[57]	At first, the symptoms might be the same as with a normal pregnancy, but as the egg grows, there will be vaginal bleeding, pain in the lower abdomen, dizziness, weakness, fainting, low blood pressure, and possible feelings of rectal pressure. This can be determined by using standard pregnancy tests and diagnostic ultrasound.[57]

Condition	Pathophysiology	Most Common Signs and Symptoms
Encephalitis	This is an inflammation of the encephalon of the brain.[14] This can be caused by a bacterial infection, a viral infection, or simply a mistaken autoimmune response with no infection present.[58]	Symptoms include fever, headache, and constitutional signs and symptoms such as malaise and fatigue.[58] There will be neck pain and possible confusion, seizures, trouble with speech, irregular movements, loss of consciousness, and even coma. This condition is a medical emergency requiring immediate intervention.[58]
Endocarditis	This is an inflammation of the lining of the heart, typically caused by injected bacteria.[59] Diagnosis typically requires an echocardiogram. Intervention includes antibiotics or possible surgery.[59]	When mild, the individual only has flu-like symptoms, but when severe, it can cause headaches, drowsiness, seizures, vomiting, confusion, and a fever with a sudden onset.[59]
Endometritis	This is an inflammation of the inner lining of the uterus. It can cause long-term effects if not treated. It is typically caused by an infection. If this spreads to the fallopian tubes and pelvic peritoneum, it is then called pelvic inflammatory disease. Subtypes include acute endometritis, chronic endometritis, and postpartum endometritis.[60]	Symptoms include pelvic pain, abdominal pain, fever, chills, vaginal bleeding or discharge, fatigue, and pain when going to the bathroom.[60]
Endometriosis	This is when the endometrium (the lining of the uterus) grows outside the uterus. This affects about 10% of all females between ages 15 and 44 years.[61] This tissue typically grows near the uterus or outside of the uterus, on the fallopian tubes or ovaries, but it can also grow on other organs like the bladder, cervix, rectum, or intestines.[61]	Symptoms include painful cramps during menstruation, pain after sex, diarrhea or constipation during periods, heavy or irregular periods, pain with urination or bowel movements, or bleeding between periods. There are both nonsurgical and surgical interventions for this diagnosis.[61]
Fatty Liver Disease (FLD), now known as Steatotic Liver Disease (SLD)	This is when there is excess fat in the liver, typically caused by excessive alcohol use (alcohol-related liver disease [ALD]) or by metabolic conditions (metabolic dysfunction-associated steatotic liver disease [MASLD], formerly called non–alcohol-related fatty liver disease [NASLD]).[62] Some fat in the liver is normal, but when this becomes over 5% of the organ's weight, it is considered to be steatotic or "fatty."[62]	Typically, there are no symptoms, but when present, they include abdominal pain, fatigue, nausea, loss of appetite, jaundice, ascites (swelling in the abdomen), and swelling in the hands and feet. If left untreated, the individual might experience hepatitis, cirrhosis, or other liver disease.[62]
Fetal Alcohol Spectrum Disorders (FASD)	This is a range of conditions in infancy caused by the mother drinking during pregnancy. Fetal alcohol syndrome is at the most severe end of the spectrum.[63]	This range of conditions includes the following: • Fetal alcohol syndrome (FAS) (see definition in the box below) • Alcohol-related neurodevelopmental disorder (ARND): mainly intellectual disabilities • Alcohol-related birth defects (ARBD): mainly physical disabilities[63] • Neurobehavioral disorder associated with prenatal alcohol exposure (ND-PAE): mainly problems with everyday life activities • Partial fetal alcohol syndrome (PFAS): some symptoms of FAS but not severe enough for the FAS diagnosis.[63]

(Continued)

Condition	Pathophysiology	Most Common Signs and Symptoms
Fetal Alcohol Syndrome (FAS)	This is a congenital condition caused by the mother drinking during pregnancy. It is at the most severe end of fetal alcohol spectrum disorders (FASD).[64] See above. The excessive consumption of alcohol can kill various parts of the developing fetus leading to behavioral and physical anomalies.[64]	Symptoms include problems with social interactions, behavior, and cognition[64] but also include physical anomalies like a smaller-than-average head circumference, smaller eye openings, a smooth philtrum (the area above the lip), and abnormal limb development. Symptoms can also include learning disabilities, hyperactivity, poor coordination, and poor reasoning and judgment skills.[64]
Folic Acid (Folate or Vitamin B-9) Deficiency Anemia	Folate is an important vitamin for the production of red blood cells. It is found in green leafy vegetables, beans, nuts, and fruits like bananas and strawberries.[65,66] Folic acid deficiency results when the body does not get enough in the diet, when the person consumes excessive alcohol, or when there is a stomach problem like celiac disease.[65]	Laboratory results will show a low red blood cell (RBC) count, and the mean corpuscular volume will be above 100, indicating enlargement of the red blood cells (macrocytic anemia).[65] Other possible symptoms include a decreased sensation in taste, diarrhea, muscle weakness, headaches, feeling of pins and needles in the feet and hands, shortness of breath, racing heart, decreased appetite, lack of energy, and depression.[67]
Gastroesophageal Reflux Disease (GERD)	This is when the stomach contents repetitively (more than twice per week) move backwards up into the esophagus. This is a common disorder affecting approximately 20% of the people in the United States. If left untreated, it can lead to serious problems.[68]	An individual with GERD will feel a burning feeling in the stomach that can rise up as high as the chest or throat.[68] There may be a chronic cough, a hoarse voice, a sour taste in the back of the throat, and bad breath. There is also a feeling of fullness or a lump feeling in the back of the throat (a globus sensation). Antacids help some individuals whereas others need diet changes or even surgery.[68]
Glenohumeral (Shoulder) Instability	Because the shoulder joint has a large range of motion, larger than any other joint in the human body, it is inherently more prone to instability. Shoulder instability is defined as a loss of comfort and function due to increased translation of the humeral head in the glenoid fossa.[69] If this translation is severe, the individual might have a subluxation or dislocation of the humeral head.[70]	Symptoms include pain in the shoulder joint, an inability to move the shoulder, a "popping" sensation when moving the shoulder, a feeling that the shoulder is stuck in a position or that there is increased mobility in the joint, and muscle weakness.[70]
Kidney Failure	This is the most severe stage of kidney disease that happens when one or both kidneys are no longer working on their own.[71] Risk factors include diabetes, high blood pressure, diabetes, over the age of 60 years, and a long history of nonsteroidal anti-inflammatory drug use.[71]	An individual with kidney failure might experience nausea, vomiting, fatigue, brain fog, cramps, dry or itchy skin, and changes in urination. Intervention includes possible dialysis or kidney transplant.[71] The individual will also have a decreased glomerular filtration rate (GFR) found on blood testing.[72] This is a measurement of how well your kidneys are filtering waste from the blood.

Condition	Pathophysiology	Most Common Signs and Symptoms
Hemophilia	This is a disorder involving the blood clotting proteins (clotting factors). There are different types that depend on the type of clotting factor that is missing.[73] Most cases of hemophilia are caused by a genetic mutation. The two most common types of hemophilia (hemophilia A and B) are carried on the X chromosome.[73] It is recessive, and this makes the symptoms more evident in males than in females (a female has an additional X chromosome that, if healthy, could help mask the symptoms).	Symptoms include multiple large bruises; joint pain and swelling; unusual bleeding after injections such as immunizations; nosebleeds without a cause; unexplained bleeding from cuts; and blood in the urine or stool. There might even be bleeding in the brain with prolonged headache, repeated vomiting, lethargy, double vision, convulsions, or seizures.[74]
Hepatic (Portosystemic) Encephalopathy	This is a disorder that occurs when the liver is not filtering blood effectively, leading to a buildup of blood toxins that begin to affect brain function.[75]	Some of the signs and symptoms are confusion, disorientation, and changes in memory, concentration, coordination, mood, impulse control, sleep patterns, behavior, and ability to care for oneself.[75]
Hepatitis	Hepatitis is inflammation of the liver. It can be due to a virus (viral hepatitis), or it can be due to other factors like alcoholism and certain medications (nonviral hepatitis).[76] There is also autoimmune hepatitis, caused by the body's antibodies attacking the liver.[76]	Symptoms of hepatitis include fatigue, dark urine, pale stool, decreased appetite, flu-like symptoms, abdominal pain, weight loss, and jaundice (yellowing of the skin and eyes).[76]
Hepatocellular Carcinoma (HCC)	This is the most common type of primary liver cancer. Risk factors include past or current hepatitis B or hepatitis C, fatty liver disease, or drinking alcohol in excess.[77]	Individuals with HCC might have abdominal pain, weight loss, and the feeling of a mass in the right upper abdominal quadrant. If not diagnosed early, this type of cancer can be fatal.[77]
Human Papillomavirus (HPV)	There are more than 100 strains of HPV, but 30 of these strains are considered to be sexually transmitted infections (STI) affecting the genitalia. HPV infection is the most common STI in the United States. Some of these strains, like those that cause genital warts, are harmless, but some can lead to cervical cancer.[78]	There are typically no symptoms except possible genital warts. The high-risk forms of HPV typically have no symptoms until after they have progressed to cancer. It is strongly advised that sexually active individuals get the HPV vaccine, use protection like condoms and dental dams during sex, get tested for STIs regularly, and inform their partner if they have an STI so their partner can get tested too.[78]
Human Immunodeficiency Virus (HIV)	HIV is a virus that attacks an individual's own immune system. This is also the virus that causes acquired immunodeficiency syndrome (AIDS). HIV is a sexually transmitted infection (STI), but it also can be spread through shared needles, via breast milk, or during pregnancy to the fetus.[79]	Symptoms vary depending on the phase of the infection. There may be no symptoms at all with HIV infection. Once symptoms begin, however, a person may have fever, headache, rash, muscle pain, cough, weight loss, night sweats, swollen lymph nodes, and diarrhea. Once the AIDS diagnosis is made (this happens when the CD4 T cell count falls below 200), the individual may have chills, sweats, recurrent fever, constant fatigue, weakness, rapid weight loss, skin rashes or bumps, swollen glands, ongoing diarrhea, and constant white spots or lesions in the mouth.[79]

(Continued)

Condition	Pathophysiology	Most Common Signs and Symptoms
Huntington Disease	Huntington disease (formerly Huntington chorea) is an inherited disease in which nerve cells in the brain, mainly those that control voluntary movement, break down and eventually die.[80]	Symptoms typically occur during middle age. They include clumsiness, problems with balance, problems with cognition, uncontrollable movements called chorea, and abnormal posturing of the body. There are also problems with behavior, thinking, emotion, and personality.[80]
Hypocalcemia	Hypocalcemia occurs when there is too little calcium in the blood, due to genetics, deficiencies in the diet, or other conditions, like parathyroid conditions or metabolic problems.[81]	Symptoms include numbness; tingling; twitching of the hands, face, or feet; depression; memory loss; rough texture of the hair; scaly skin; cramps; or seizures.[81]
Hypokalemia	Hypokalemia occurs when there is too little potassium in the blood, due to vomiting, diarrhea, laxative use, or deficiencies in the diet.[78] Potassium is an electrolyte and is needed for the nerves and muscles to function properly.[82]	Symptoms include constipation, extreme fatigue, heart palpitations, muscle weakness, numbness and tingling, muscle twitches, cramps, paralysis, polyuria (excessive urination), and polydipsia (excessive thirst).[82]
Hyponatremia	Hyponatremia is a condition resulting from low sodium concentration in the blood (<135 mEq/L) due to excess water in the body, thus diluting the sodium levels. Sodium is an important electrolyte, and it regulates water in and around the cells, helps control blood pressure, and supports muscles and nerves.[83]	Signs and symptoms of hyponatremia include nausea and vomiting; headache; confusion; loss of energy, drowsiness, or fatigue; restlessness and irritability; muscle weakness, spasms, or cramps; seizures; and/or coma.[83]
Hypoproteinemia	Hypoproteinemia results from low protein levels in the blood, which can have diet-related etiology (by not consuming enough protein daily, malnutrition, or undereating) or be caused by underlying conditions that affect the kidneys, liver, or digestive system.[84]	Symptoms of hypoproteinemia include weakness, hair thinning or breakage, brittle nails, mood changes, and stress fractures.[84]
Hyperlipidemia	Also known as high cholesterol (≥200 mg/dL) or dyslipidemia, hyperlipidemia is an umbrella term for a group of disorders characterized by extra fats or lipids in the blood, caused by diet, lifestyle habits, medications, and other health conditions.[85]	It is hard to identify symptoms as most individuals do not know they have hyperlipidemia without a blood test. It can affect blood pressure (due to the narrowing of arteries) and one's susceptibility to other problems such as coronary artery disease, MI, or stroke.[85]
Hypertension (HTN)	Also known as high blood pressure, hypertension is a consistent blood pressure of 130/80 mm Hg or higher, and it typically develops over time. Risk factors include family history, health conditions, and lifestyle choices.[86]	There are typically no symptoms, but it can increase an individual's risk for stroke, heart disease, heart attack, or kidney disease.[86]
Hyperthyroidism	Also known as overactive thyroid, hyperthyroidism occurs when the thyroid gland overproduces thyroid hormones (the two main hormones being triiodothyronine, T-3, and thyroxine, T-4), resulting in high metabolism.[87]	Some signs due to high metabolism include weight loss, hand tremors, and rapid or irregular heartbeat. Other symptoms include heart palpitations; increased hunger; sweating; nervousness, anxiety, and irritability; changes in menstrual cycles; heat sensitivity; changes in bowel patterns; enlarged thyroid; tiredness; muscle weakness; sleep problems; warm, moist or clammy skin often showing signs of thinning, and/or fine, brittle hair.[87]

Condition	Pathophysiology	Most Common Signs and Symptoms
Hypothyroidism	Also known as underactive thyroid, hypothyroidism occurs when the thyroid gland fails to make enough of the thyroid hormones.[88]	Initially, noticeable symptoms may be missed early on as they develop slowly. The earliest symptoms are typically fatigue and weight gain. As an individual's metabolism slows down, some additional symptoms may be cold sensitivity; constipation; dry skin; puffy face; hoarse voice; coarse hair and skin; muscle weakness; muscle aches, tenderness, and stiffness; heavier or irregular menstrual cycles; slowed heart rate (bradycardia); depression; and memory problems.[88] (Notice how many of the symptoms here are "opposite" of the hyperthyroidism symptoms above.)
Inflammatory Bowel Disease (IBD)	IBD is an autoimmune disorder. Its name is used to represent two different inflammatory conditions of the gastrointestinal (GI) tract: ulcerative colitis (UC) and Crohn's disease. UC typically affects the large intestine, whereas Crohn's disease can affect any part of the entire digestive tract (mouth to anus). Those with IBD are at an increased risk for colorectal cancer.[89]	The most common IBD symptoms are as follows: abdominal pain, (bloody) diarrhea, bowel urgency and sometimes fecal incontinence, rectal bleeding, weight loss, fever, anemia, anxiety and depression, and/or malnutrition and delayed growth (when diagnosed as a child).[89]
Irritable Bowel Syndrome (IBS)	IBS is a common disorder that is noted to cause discomfort in the abdomen and changes in bowel movements or habits. Research suggests symptoms related to IBS may be secondary to sensitivity to the nerves found within the walls of the GI tract. There are four subtypes of IBS that are characterized by the most prevalent symptom: IBS-D, IBS-C, IBS-Mixed, and IBS-U. Common triggers are specific foods, emotions, and stress.[90]	Abdominal pain/discomfort and altered bowel movement are the main symptoms, along with mucus in the stool, bowel urgency, and a feeling of incomplete bowel movement. Relevant symptoms not related to the intestine include migraines, sleep disturbances, anxiety, depression, fibromyalgia, and chronic pelvic pain.[90]
Iodine Deficiency	Iodine deficiency is due to a diet lacking the required amount of iodine for normal bodily functions. This deficiency leads to an inability of the thyroid gland to function properly with a resultant decline in thyroid hormones. Iodine deficiency can cause severe complications, especially during pregnancy.[91]	The main symptoms of iodine deficiency are an enlarged thyroid (goiter) and hypothyroidism. Other symptoms include infertility; puffy skin; hoarseness; confusion; scaly or dry skin; and coarse, thinning hair.[91]
Kaposi Sarcoma	Kaposi sarcoma is a term to describe cancer cells found within the skin or mucous membranes lining the GI tract. It is often triggered by a weak immune system after contracting a human herpesvirus 8 (KSHV) infection. It is typically found in HIV-positive individuals, those undergoing a transplant who take immunosuppressant drugs, or those living in specific areas of the world (Mediterranean, Middle Eastern, Eastern European, and Equatorial Africa).[92]	Symptoms of Kaposi sarcoma include lesions on the skin, on mucous membranes, or inside the body (in the lungs, can cause breathing difficulties, and in the GI tract, can cause bleeding and anemia). There may be involvement of the lymph nodes, especially in the groin area, which can cause swelling in the lower extremities.[92]

(Continued)

Condition	Pathophysiology	Most Common Signs and Symptoms
Kwashiorkor	Kwashiorkor is a severe protein deficiency with low antioxidant levels due to malnutrition. It is usually found in infants and children.[93]	The disease is characterized by pitting edema in bilateral extremities. Other clinical signs include marked muscle atrophy; abdominal distension; round "moon" face; thin, dry, peeling skin with scaly or hyperpigmented presentation; dry, full, hypopigmented hair that easily falls out; hepatomegaly; stunted growth; skin lesions/dermatitis; subcutaneous fat retention with loose inguinal skin folds; and psychic changes (anorexia, apathy).[93]
Leukemia	Leukemia is the name given to a group of malignant blood disorders that affect bone marrow and the lymphatic system. The bone marrow is responsible for the production of white blood cells (WBCs), so with this type of cancer, the bone marrow is producing a superabundant number of abnormal WBCs.[94]	Signs and symptoms of leukemia include fever; chills; fatigue; weakness; frequent or severe infections; swollen lymph nodes, liver, or spleen; recurrent nosebleeds; loss of appetite; weight loss; easy bruising or bleeding; night sweats; petechiae (small red dots on skin); and bone or joint pain.[94]
Leukocytosis	Leukocytosis is an abnormally high number of leukocytes (white blood cells) (>11,000 per μL) in the bloodstream which can represent the body's natural response to infection, inflammation, or injury or be an indication of an immune system disorder or other serious condition (such as leukemia or lymphoma).[95]	Warning signs of leukocytosis are fever, fatigue, pain, difficulty breathing, wheezing, night sweats, rash, and unexpected weight loss.[95]
Leukopenia	Leukopenia is an abnormally low number of leukocytes (white blood cells), especially neutrophils (<4000 per μL) in the bloodstream and can occur secondary to certain medical conditions, medications, or vitamin deficiencies.[96]	Leukopenia itself does not have symptoms, but it can make an individual more prone to infection, which would present with the following signs: fever and chills, swelling and redness, mouth sores, red or white patches found in the mouth, sore throat, severe cough or shortness of breath (SOB), painful urination, foul urine, diarrhea, pus-filled cuts or sores, and unusual vaginal discharge or itch.[96]
Liver Cirrhosis	Cirrhosis is a late stage of scarring (fibrosis) of the liver caused by many forms of liver diseases and conditions, such as hepatitis and chronic alcoholism.[97]	Fatigue, easy bruising, itchy skin, swelling in the abdomen (ascites) and lower extremities (edema), loss of appetite, nausea, spider-like blood vessels on the skin, weight loss, and yellowing of the skin and eyes (jaundice) are all typical signs and symptoms of cirrhosis.[97]
Liver Disease	Liver disease, whether inherited or caused by a virus or lifestyle choices, is an umbrella term for damage to the liver that can lead to cirrhosis (scarring) and liver failure.[98]	When liver disease produces symptoms, it can include jaundice of the eyes or skin, abdomen pain and swelling, bilateral lower extremity swelling, itchy skin, dark-colored urine, pale-appearing stool, constant state of tiredness, nausea or vomiting, loss of appetite, and easy bruising.[98]
Long COVID	Long COVID is a term used to describe a chronic condition encompassing a wide range of symptoms that continue for at least 3 months after the SARS-CoV-2 infection has passed. These symptoms can last up to several months or even years. When an individual has contracted the virus more than once, there is an increased likelihood of developing long COVID.[99]	Symptoms of long COVID include fatigue, brain fog, and postexertional malaise (PEM), which are the three most reported symptoms, but more than 200 symptoms, some unexplainable, have been identified.[16] Other more common symptoms include SOB, chronic cough, headaches, insomnia, loss of or altered sense of smell or taste, depression, anxiety, heart palpitations, chest pain, and diarrhea.[100]

Condition	Pathophysiology	Most Common Signs and Symptoms
Lung Cancer	Lung cancer begins as a growth in the lungs. Smoking is the greatest risk factor, and lung cancer accounts for the leading cause of all cancer deaths.[101] There are two main types of lung cancer: non–small cell lung cancer (NSCLC) and small cell lung cancer (SCLC). NSCLC makes up >80% of lung cancers, whereas SCLC tends to grow and metastasize quicker.[101,102]	Lung-related signs and symptoms include a new and persistent cough, coughing up blood, hoarseness, SOB, and wheezing. Signs and symptoms of lung cancer once metastasized are bone pain, headache, unexplainable weight loss, loss of appetite, and swelling in the face or neck.[101,102]
Major Depressive Disorder	This is a mood disorder that is characterized by persistent feelings of worthlessness, loss of interest, and sadness.[103]	Reported signs and symptoms include feelings of sadness, angry outbursts, decreased appetite, anxiety, agitation and restlessness, sleep disturbances, and loss of interest in activities that typically bring pleasure like leisure activities, sex, and hobbies or sports.[103]
Melanoma	Melanoma is a potentially fatal type of skin cancer that originates in the melanocytes (cells that produce melanin) that easily metastasizes throughout the body secondary to ultraviolet light exposure.[104]	The first signs and symptoms of melanoma are a changing mole or an atypical, new growth.[104]
Metabolic Acidosis	Metabolic acidosis is the buildup of acids in bodily fluids, either caused by the storage of too many acids (thus eliminating bicarbonate) or insufficient removal of acids (a dramatic loss in bicarbonate) secondary to an underlying kidney condition, such as kidney failure or chronic kidney disease.[105]	Characteristics of metabolic acidosis include tachycardia, fatigue, confusion, and an overall “unwell” feeling. Other clinical symptoms include dizziness; loss of appetite; sweet- or fruity-smelling breath; rapid or long, deep breathing patterns; nausea and vomiting; headache; and weakness.[105] This can be a red flag situation, requiring immediate medical attention.
Metabolic Alkalosis	Alkalosis is defined as the excess of alkali, or bases, in bodily fluids, thus affecting the acid-base balance and pH levels of the body. Metabolic alkalosis is an excess of bicarbonate in bodily fluids, which can be a result of digestive issues (decrease in stomach acid); heart, liver, or kidney conditions; or excessive consumption of specific medications or supplements (laxatives, diuretics, steroids, etc.). Those at higher risk include those who are dehydrated.[106]	Metabolic alkalosis symptoms include irritability, muscle twitching, muscle cramps, muscle spasms, fatigue, confusion, tremors, numbness and tingling, arrhythmia, seizures, or coma.[106] This is a red flag situation, requiring immediate medical attention.
Metabolic Syndrome	Metabolic syndrome represents a group of conditions (HTN, high blood sugar, excess body weight in the abdomen, and atypical cholesterol levels) taking place simultaneously which increases one's risk for heart disease, stroke, and type 2 diabetes. Up to one-third of American adults have metabolic syndrome.[107]	The most observable sign for metabolic syndrome is a greater waist circumference, with an “apple” or “pear” body shape. Other signs and symptoms are often related to the diagnoses/conditions the individual has.[107]
Mitral Valve Prolapse	The mitral valve is located between the left atrium and left ventricle, and its leaflets (flaps) open and close during a heartbeat. With mitral valve prolapse, due to a bulge in the valve's leaflets, blood can leak backwards into the atrium because the valve “parachutes” and does not close properly during contraction.[108]	Mitral valve prolapse is typically asymptomatic, but it depends on the amount of blood leaking backward. Symptoms could include arrhythmia, dizziness or lightheadedness, difficulty breathing or SOB (especially with exercise or in supine position), and fatigue.[108]

(Continued)

Condition	Pathophysiology	Most Common Signs and Symptoms
Multiple Myeloma	This is a cancer that develops in the plasma cells. While typical plasma cells fight infections and make antibodies, cancerous plasma cells congregate in the bone marrow, take up too much space, and produce faulty proteins that cause problems and cannot be used in the same way as functioning antibodies. It is most often seen in people over the age of 60 years, those who are male, and those who are Black.[109]	In the early stages, there are typically no symptoms. When they begin, the symptoms include bone pain (especially hip, chest, and spinal pain), nausea, constipation, loss of appetite, mental fogginess or confusion, tiredness, infections, weight loss, weakness, thirst, and urinary frequency.[109]
Multiple Sclerosis (MS)	MS is an autoimmune disorder that is characterized by the body attacking and damaging the myelin found on nerves housed in the brain and spinal cord. The demyelination interrupts signals being sent to the rest of the body. There are four main types of MS and three rare variants.[110]	Typical symptoms of MS include vision changes (sometimes double vision); muscle weakness, stiffness, or spasms (tremors); numbness, abnormal sensations, or pain; clumsiness; balance and coordination deficits; fatigue; difficulty with cognitive function; and mood changes. Progressive symptoms may also lead to additional complications: difficulty walking, bowel or bladder control, memory loss, sexual dysfunction, depression, and anxiety.[110]
Myocardial Infarction (MI)	Also known as a heart attack, MI is a lack of blood flow to the heart, which causes damage to the heart muscle. These partial or complete blockages are typically created from a buildup of fat, cholesterol, or plaque, which narrows the arteries.[111]	Common symptoms include chest pain (pressure, tightness, squeezing, and aching); pain or discomfort that radiates to the shoulder, arm, back, neck, jaw, teeth, or upper abdomen; cold sweat; fatigue; heartburn or ingestion; lightheadedness or sudden dizziness; SOB; and nausea. Symptoms are typically different for males and females.[111] This is a red flag situation, requiring immediate medical attention.
Nerve Impairment (Impingement)—Median Nerve	A median nerve impairment can result from trauma, a humeral fracture, entrapment, or neuropathy (nerve damage). One of the most common median nerve impairments is carpal tunnel syndrome.[112]	Signs of a median nerve impairment include pain, numbness/tingling, burning, or numbness in the hand, wrist, or forearm; tenderness or pain at the elbow; hand pain at night that affects sleep; and/or difficulties grasping items.[112]
Nerve Impairment (Impingement)—Radial Nerve	Pressure on the radial nerve can lead to a pinched nerve or neuropathic pain from entrapment, radial tunnel syndrome, radial nerve palsy, or Wartenberg syndrome.[113]	Impairment can lead to radial nerve neuropathy and pain as well as pain, burning, itching, tingling, and/or numbness in the arm, wrist, and hand. Other signs may include arm, wrist, or hand weakness or paralysis; difficulty with elbow, wrist, hand, or digit extension; problems with grasping and pinching objects; and wrist drop.[113]
Nerve Impairment (Impingement)—Ulnar Nerve	Pressure on the ulnar nerve can lead to various conditions such as ulnar nerve entrapment, which includes cubital tunnel syndrome and Guyon's canal syndrome, as well as ulnar nerve dislocation.[114]	Signs of ulnar entrapment are "claw" hand, elbow or wrist pain, hand weakness, muscle loss in hand and affected digits, and numbness or tingling in the fourth and fifth digits.[114]

Condition	Pathophysiology	Most Common Signs and Symptoms
Obsessive-Compulsive Disorder (OCD)	This is a mental condition with frequent unwanted thoughts (obsessions) that cause a person to perform repetitive behaviors (compulsions).[115]	Symptoms include obsessions and compulsions that can take up hours of a person's day making it hard for them to function normally. Some symptoms can include fear of contaminated substances, unwanted mental images related to sex, excessive concerns over morality, need for constant reassurance, feelings of doubt or disgust, and rituals related to checking items, people, chants, or numbers.[115]
Orthostatic Hypotension (OH)	OH is a drop in systolic blood pressure of more than 20 mm Hg when moving from a seated or recumbent position to a standing position.[116]	Symptoms of OH include lightheadedness, dizziness, blurry vision, fainting, syncope, confusion, unsteadiness upon standing, possible fainting, and recurrent falls.[116]
Osteopenia	The term osteopenia refers to loss of bone density, which naturally occurs during the aging process as bones break down quicker than they are restored. Some have an increased risk of osteopenia with certain comorbidities, lifestyle habits, or medications, especially females. With osteopenia, the bones do not have as many minerals, making them weaker and more susceptible to fractures or injury.[117]	Osteopenia is considered a "silent disease" because there are no noticeable symptoms. This individual might, however, experience frequent fractures.[108]
Osteoporosis	This disease occurs with age in both males and females and is due to a remodeling of the bones in the body, causing them to weaken and become more prone to fracture.[1] It is diagnosed using a bone density test (DEXA Scan).[118]	There may be no symptoms at all until a bone breaks. The most common fractures are in the hips, wrists, or spine.[1] Some possible symptoms include a loss in height of an inch or more, kyphotic posture, shortness of breath, and lower back pain.[118]
Pancreatic Carcinoma (Cancer)	This cancer develops in the cells of the pancreas and is rarely detected during its earliest stages, when a cure is most possible, because symptoms do not typically appear until later.[119]	Symptoms include stomach pain and swelling, loss of appetite, weight loss, jaundice, light-colored and/or floating stools, itching, dark-colored urine, fatigue, and pain or swelling in an arm or leg.[119]
Parkinson's Disease	This disorder occurs when the nerve cells in the substantia nigra of the basal ganglia become impaired or die. This leads to a drop in a neurotransmitter needed for smooth coordinated movements called dopamine. There may also be a drop in norepinephrine and the presence of Lewy bodies in the brain cells.[120]	Individuals with Parkinson's disease often experience tremor in the hands, arms, jaw, or head; muscle stiffness (rigidity, even in the facial muscles); slow movement; difficulty initiating steps when walking (festination); problems with balance and coordination; possible increase in falls; depression; difficulty chewing and swallowing; constipation and/or urinary problems; and eventual changes in cognitive function, leading to dementia.[120]
Patent Ductus Arteriosus (PDA)	In a fetus, the blood supply does not go through the fetal lungs because the fetus receives oxygenated blood directly from the mother. The ductus arteriosus is a hole in the heart that allows the blood to bypass the fetal lungs. This hole typically closes immediately after birth, but in some newborns, the ductus arteriosus does not close, remaining patent.[121]	If the PDA is small, there might be no symptoms except for a distinct type of heart murmur. If it is larger, the heart and lungs will have to work harder. The child might be breathing harder and faster, and it might be harder for them to eat. These symptoms will get worse over the weeks following birth. This can often be surgically repaired. There are sometimes additional heart anomalies that accompany PDA.[121]

(Continued)

Condition	Pathophysiology	Most Common Signs and Symptoms
Pelvic Inflammatory Disease (PID)	This is an infection affecting one or more of the reproductive organs.[122] This is a very common condition in individuals assigned female at birth and is typically caused by chlamydia or gonorrhea. These infections typically occur during sex (STI), but some bacteria that cause PID can be also spread during menstruation, insertion of an intrauterine device, childbirth, abortion, or uterine surgery.[122]	This can cause pain in the lower abdominal area, heavy vaginal discharge, increased bleeding during menstruation, bleeding between periods, fever and chills, pain during sex, and pain during urination.[5] Emergency medical care is needed if there is severe abdominal pain, high fever, vomiting, fainting, or shock.[122] If left untreated, PID can eventually lead to difficulty getting pregnant.[122]
Peptic Ulcers	Peptic ulcers are sores in the lining of the stomach (gastric ulcer) or the beginning of the small intestine (duodenal ulcer).[123] These sores are created by digestive juices and stomach acids. This can be exacerbated by *Helicobacter pylori* (*H. pylori*) bacteria or by nonsteroidal anti-inflammatory drugs (NSAIDs).[123]	Symptoms vary but can include nausea, feeling full after eating only a small amount of food (early satiety), burping, weight loss, nausea, vomiting, bloody stool, or vomiting blood.[123]
Pericarditis	The pericardium is a thin sac of tissue surrounding the heart. When this tissue becomes inflamed (swollen and irritated), it is called pericarditis. This condition, if mild, might resolve without treatment, but when severe, it could require medication or even surgery. Some viruses, like COVID-19, can cause inflammation of the heart muscle (myocarditis) along with pericarditis.[124]	Chest pain is the most common symptom. This pain is typically felt behind the sternum or in the chest on the left side, and it can spread to the left shoulder and neck, or even to both shoulders. The pain is worse when coughing, taking a deep breath, or lying down, and gets better when sitting up or leaning forward. Other symptoms can include a low-grade fever, swelling in the legs and feet, shortness of breath when lying down, and abdominal swelling.[124]
Peripheral Vascular Disease (PVD)	PVD is a disorder affecting either the arteries and veins in the arms or legs and includes peripheral artery disease (PAD) and venous disease. PAD affects the vessels carrying blood away from the heart to the extremities, and venous disease or venous stasis affects the blood leaving the extremities to return to the heart.[125] The primary cause of PVD is progressive atherosclerosis.	Symptoms of PAD include intermittent claudication, exercise-induced cramping, pain on elevation of the leg, pain relief when the leg is in a dependent position, paresthesia, leg weakness, and cool extremities. There may also be limb discoloration, especially in the toes; decreased sensation, with pain at rest; and nonhealing wounds.[125] Venous disease can consist of blood clots, deep vein thrombosis, venous ulcers, or chronic venous insufficiency.[126] When venous insufficiency is chronic, there may be swelling of the lower extremities with oozing of fluid from the skin, discoloration of the skin, and leg ulcers. Pain decreases with leg elevation.[126]
Pernicious Anemia	This is an autoimmune disorder that causes an inability to absorb vitamin B12, which is needed for erythrocyte formation. This can result in megaloblastic anemia.[127]	There will be fatigue, headache, confusion, emotional lability, dyspnea, diarrhea, and decreased appetite.[127]
Pneumonia	This is an inflammation of the lungs with fluid accumulation caused by bacteria, a type of virus, or fungi. Common causes include the flu and the COVID-19 virus. It can affect only one or both lungs (double pneumonia).[128]	The most common symptoms are difficulty breathing, congestion, chest pain, high fever, rapid heart rate, and productive cough with yellow, green, or bloody sputum.[128]

Condition	Pathophysiology	Most Common Signs and Symptoms
Poikilocytosis	This is a condition when more than 10% of the red blood cells in a sample are abnormally shaped, and this can limit their ability to carry oxygen, leading to anemia. Intervention will depend upon the cause which can either be inherited or acquired.[129]	Symptoms are similar to those with anemia and include weakness and fatigue, arrhythmia, dyspnea, an occasional whooshing sound in the ear (pulsatile tinnitus), headache, chest pain, pale skin, and dizziness.[129]
Polycythemia or Polycythemia Vera	This is a type of blood cancer in which the bone marrow makes too many red blood cells. Although rare, it is typically found when a person is blood tested for another condition.[130]	There may be no signs or symptoms, but when present, they can include itchiness, numbness or tingling, a bloated feeling after eating, pain in the upper left abdomen from an enlarged spleen, shortness of breath, unusual bleeding, and painful swelling in the big toe.[130]
Posttraumatic Stress Disorder (PTSD)	This is a mental health disorder that is triggered by a past terrifying event.[131]	There may be flashbacks, severe anxiety, nightmares, and uncontrollable thoughts about the event. The individual might also feel detached from family and friends, have feelings of hopelessness, and lose interest in activities previously seen as meaningful.[131]
Primary Biliary Cholangitis (previously called Primary Biliary Cirrhosis)	This is an autoimmune disease that occurs when the bile ducts are inflamed and slowly destroyed. It is most common in females.[132]	There may be no symptoms, but typical signs include fatigue itchy skin, jaundice, dry mouth, swelling in the upper-right abdomen, swollen feet and ankles, hyperpigmentation not due to a suntan, buildup of fluid in the abdomen, bone, muscle or joint pain, spleen swelling, osteoporosis, weight loss, and diarrhea.[132]
Psoriasis	This skin disorder causes skin cells to multiply up to 10 times faster than the normal rate, leading to raised bumpy patches, mainly on the scalp, elbows, knees, and the lower part of the back. It is not contagious.[133]	The raised patches can be on the lighter side with silver-colored scales. These are called plaques which can appear on the scalp. There also might be some issues with fingernails or toenails that might change color or develop small pits.[133]
Pulmonary Embolism (PE)	This is a blood clot in the lungs. It is the most serious of all the complications from deep vein thrombosis (DVT).[134] It occurs after a piece from the DVT breaks off and travels through the bloodstream lodging in the smaller vessels of the lung. This can be very serious and even deadly.[134]	The individual might have had prior symptoms of a DVT including pain, tenderness, swelling, and redness of the skin.[134] Symptoms of a PE include dyspnea, chest pain, tachycardia, coughing up blood, lightheadedness, fainting, and low blood pressure.[134]
Pulmonary Valve Stenosis	This is a narrowing of the pulmonary valve.[135] This valve connects the right ventricle to the pulmonary artery. This makes the right ventricle work harder to get the needed amount of blood through. This can be congenital or caused by other conditions in adulthood.[135]	Individuals might have a heart murmur, fatigue, chest pain, dyspnea especially when active, and possibly fainting.[135]
Respiratory Acidosis	When the lungs are unable to remove enough carbon dioxide from the body resulting in a lower-than-normal blood pH (acidic). This can lead to breathing problems and other conditions affecting the nerves or muscles in the chest. When this occurs suddenly, it can be fatal.[136]	A person suffering from respiratory acidosis might have anxiety, blurry vision, headache, confusion, cyanosis, dyspnea, and wheezing. If not treated promptly, the person might develop muscle twitches, seizures, or even coma.[136] This is often a red flag situation, requiring immediate medical attention.

(Continued)

Condition	Pathophysiology	Most Common Signs and Symptoms
Respiratory Alkalosis	This happens after hyperventilation, when too much carbon dioxide is removed, resulting in a higher-than-normal blood pH (alkalinity).[137] Hyperventilation can occur when in extreme pain, after strenuous exercise, with cancer, drug overdose, fever, or during labor.[137]	An individual suffering from respiratory alkalosis might have dyspnea, nausea, irritability, fatigue, muscle spasms, fainting (syncope), or chest discomfort. This is typically a yellow flag situation.[137]
Rhabdomyolysis	When skeletal muscle breaks down, the cells release myoglobin into the blood. This is a protein that stores oxygen in muscle cells.[138] When there is too much of this substance in the blood, it can lead to kidney damage. There will also be an increase in blood potassium levels, high enough enough to disrupt the electrical rhythm of the heart muscle. This can be caused by strenuous exercise, trauma, heat stroke, or as a medication side effect.[138]	Some of the possible symptoms include fatigue, low urine output, weakness, bruising, fever, nausea, confusion, dark tea-colored urine, and agitation. The individual might also have high creatine kinase levels on blood testing along with high myoglobin and potassium.[138]
Rickets	This is a softening and weakening of the bones, typically in children and often due to vitamin D deficiency.[139]	Symptoms included delayed growth; pain in the spine, legs, and pelvis; muscle weakness; and delayed motor skills.[139]
Rotator Cuff Tear	The tendons of four muscles (the supraspinatus, infraspinatus, teres minor, and subscapularis) make up the rotator cuff in the shoulder. When one or more of these muscles are injured, it constitutes a rotator cuff tear.[140]	The individual will typically complain of severe pain, especially on active movement with an inability to use the arm.[140] There might also be popping or crackling sounds on attempted movement, with pain that is worse at night or at rest.[140]
Sarcoidosis	This is an inflammatory disease that involves the lungs and the lymph glands, causing the formation of red, swollen lumps called granulomas to form in the organs of the chest.[141] Although it does involve immune activity and inflammation, it is not considered to be an autoimmune disease.[141]	Individuals with this disorder might have fever, achy muscles, fatigue, swollen or painful joints, kidney stones, weight loss, and night sweats. If the granulomas are in the lungs, the individual might also exhibit coughing, wheezing, dyspnea, or chest pain.[141]
Schizoaffective Disorder	This is a mental health condition with symptoms of both schizophrenia and mood disorder.[142]	Symptoms of schizophrenia include hallucinations, delusions, and disorganized thinking. If this is coupled with a depressive mood disorder, symptoms can be sadness, emptiness, or feelings of worthlessness.[142] If this is coupled with a manic mood disorder, symptoms can include euphoria, risky thoughts, agitation, or other mania symptoms.[142]
Schizophrenia	This is a serious mental condition that can affect an individual's thoughts and behavior.[143]	There can be hallucinations (seeing or hearing things that are not there), delusions (believing things that are not true), and disorganized thinking. These individuals sometimes lose touch with reality.[143]

Condition	Pathophysiology	Most Common Signs and Symptoms
Scurvy	This is caused by a severe vitamin C deficiency. Vitamin C is an antioxidant that can protect the body against free radicals. In the United States, scurvy tends to primarily affect babies, children, and older adults.[144]	Symptoms include anemia, swollen legs, rough and scaly skin, wounds that will not heal, bleeding gums, bleeding under the skin, anemia, irritability, failure to gain weight, and loose teeth.[144]
Shingles (Herpes Zoster)	Shingles is a viral infection caused by the same virus that causes chickenpox (*Varicella zoster*), which can remain dormant in the nervous system after chickenpox, only to emerge as shingles years later.[145]	The characteristic symptoms include a red, painful, burning skin rash that appears on one side of the body, typically along a dermatomal distribution; itchiness; fever; fatigue; chills; headache; muscle weakness; and fluid-filled blisters.[145]
Shoulder Impingement (Swimmer's Shoulder)	This occurs when the muscles of the rotator cuff rub against the upper border of the shoulder, decreasing the space between the humeral head and the acromion, creating friction and pressure that irritates the bursa, tendons, and muscles. This is typically caused by overuse.[146]	Symptoms include shoulder weakness and constant pain in the anterior and lateral shoulder, which is worse with movement and increases at night.[146]
Sickle Cell Anemia	This is just one of the inherited sickle cell diseases. In sickle cell anemia, the red blood cells are shaped like crescent moons (or sickles), which become rigid and sticky, restricting blood flow. They are also less able to carry the necessary oxygen through the body.[147]	Symptoms include anemia, pain, bilateral swelling in the hands and feet, visual difficulties, frequent infections, delayed growth, or delays during puberty. There is an increased chance of stroke (CVA), with one-sided weakness or paralysis, paresthesia, confusion, difficulty walking or talking, and severe headache.[147]
Social Anxiety Disorder (Social Phobia)	This is a condition that causes fear and anxiety when an individual is with other people in social situations.[148]	Symptoms include fear of meeting new people, performing in front of people, dating, using public restrooms, and other social situations. These individuals fear being judged or watched by others.[148]
Substance Use Disorder	This is a disorder affecting an individual's ability to control their use of legal or illegal drugs or medications.[149]	Symptoms include intense urges to use the drug, blocking out other thoughts; over time, needing more of the medication to get the same effect; continuing use of the drug even knowing the problems it is causing; and taking more of the medication over time than intended. There may be problems at school or work, neglected appearance, changes in behavior, and health issues.[149]
Syphilis	This is a sexually transmitted infection caused by a bacterium (*Treponema pallidum*), typically starting as a painless sore (chancre) on the mouth, genitals, or rectum and spreading via direct contact. It can also be spread during pregnancy, childbirth, or breastfeeding. It is treated with antibiotics.[150]	Syphilis can stay in the body for many years without symptoms, but if left untreated, it can cause damage to the brain, heart, or other organs, and it can be life-threatening. Symptoms include a painless chancre, a rough red or reddish-brown rash that is not itchy, wart-like sores in the mouth or genital area, fever, hair loss, muscle aches, sore throat, weight loss, and swollen lymph nodes.[27] Advanced problems include confusion, stroke, or paralysis.[150]

(Continued)

Condition	Pathophysiology	Most Common Signs and Symptoms
Systemic Lupus Erythematosus (SLE)	This is an inflammatory condition considered to be of autoimmune origin damaging the skin, joints, organs, and other body tissue. There are other types of lupus, but SLE is the most common.[151]	Symptoms typically come in waves or flare-ups, when the symptoms are severe enough to affect the person's daily routine. These symptoms include a facial rash, fever, hair loss, headaches, joint pain, muscle pain, fatigue, dyspnea, swollen glands, confusion, dry eyes, photosensitivity, osteoporosis, heart disease, and kidney disease. Blood tests to check for infections and inflammation, as well as tests for antinuclear antibodies, can help with the diagnosis.[151]
Tetralogy of Fallot (TOF)	TOF is a congenital heart defect that features four different problems: a ventricular septal defect, an overriding aorta, pulmonary valve stenosis, and right ventricular hypertrophy.[152] The cause is unknown, but it is most common in children with Down syndrome or DiGeorge syndrome.[152]	Children born with this are typically cyanotic with dyspnea. Further testing would be done immediately to determine the cause, and if it is Tetralogy of Fallot, then surgery using a series of shunts and patches would be indicated.[152] This is a red flag situation, requiring immediate medical attention.
Thoracic Outlet Syndrome (TOS)	There is a passageway for the brachial plexus in the shoulder near the anterior and middle scalene muscles, known as the thoracic outlet. When this area becomes injured or swollen, it can place pressure on the structures in the outlet.[153]	Symptoms include a feeling of numbness or tingling in the arm (possibly down to the fingers), arm fatigue with activity, aches in the neck or shoulder, and a weakened grip. If an artery is impinged, there will be discoloration in the skin of the wrist and hand, cold fingers, and a weak pulse, especially upon arm elevation.[153]
Thrombocytopenia	This is a reduction in the required number of thrombocytes (platelets) produced in the bone marrow (less than 140,000 per microliter of blood).[154] These are necessary for blood clotting, making it hard to control bleeding after an injury. This can happen with various autoimmune disorders or as a side effect of certain medications.[154]	Some of the possible symptoms include bleeding gums, blood in the urine or stool, petechiae (tiny red or purple dots on the lower legs), blood in the vomit, heavy menstrual periods, easy bruising, and rectal bleeding.[154]
Thrombocytosis	This is a condition in which the body is producing too many thrombocytes (platelets).[155]	Most individuals are asymptomatic, but when symptoms occur, it can be due to a blood clot. These symptoms include headache, confusion, weakness, chest pain, burning in the hands or feet, and shortness of breath.[155]
Traumatic brain injury (TBI)	Traumatic brain injury (TBI) is a disruption in the normal function of the brain caused by a bump, blow, or jolt to the head or penetrating head injury.[156]	Headache, confusion, memory loss, difficulty concentrating, mood swings, changes in sleep patterns, and nausea are all potential signs and symptoms of a TBI.[156]
Tuberculosis	This is an infection caused by a bacterium that typically attacks the lungs, known as *Mycobacterium tuberculosis*.[157]	There are several forms of the disease, and not all produce symptoms. When symptoms do occur, they include fever, night sweats, coughing up blood, chest pain, loss of appetite, and weight loss.[157]
Ulcerative Colitis	This is a type of inflammatory bowel disease that causes ulcers in the lining of the large intestine (colon) and rectum.[158]	Symptoms typically develop slowly over time and include diarrhea, rectal pain, weight loss, fatigue, fever, and rectal bleeding.[158]
Urinary Tract Infection (UTI)	This is an infection in the urinary system.[159]	Symptoms include a burning sensation during urination; cloudy or dark-colored urine; pain in the penis, vaginal area, or rectum; a frequent and intense urge to urinate even if there is very little urine; confusion; bed wetting; and possible fever.[159]

Condition	Pathophysiology	Most Common Signs and Symptoms
Ventricular Septal Defect (VSD)	This is a hole between the two ventricles of the heart, typically occurring right after birth.[160]	There are usually no symptoms in the newborn if the hole is small, and the defect typically closes on its own by age 6 years. Larger holes, however, might need to be repaired surgically. Symptoms of a larger opening include shortness of breath, failure to thrive, fatigue, and frequent respiratory infections.[160]
Wilson Disease	This is a rare condition that is inherited and causes copper to build up in the liver, brain, and eyes.[161]	There is often a loss of appetite, jaundice, fluid buildup in the legs and stomach, problems with speech and swallowing, poor coordination, uncontrolled movements, and golden rings around the irises of the eyes (Kayser-Fleischer rings).[161]

References

1. Johns Hopkins. *Abdominal Aortic Aneurysm*. John Hopkins Medicine; 2024.
2. Cleveland Clinic. (2021). Liver abscess. Cleveland Clinic. Retrieved July 1, 2024. https://my.clevelandclinic.org/health/diseases/16823-liver-abscess.
3. Sankaran A, Karande G. *Obturator internus and psoas abscess. In National Institutes of Health*. StatPearls; 2021. https://www.ncbi.nlm.nih.gov/books/NBK556055/.
4. Mayo Clinic. *Adhesive Capsulitis (frozen shoulder)*. Mayo Clinic; 2022. https://www.mayoclinic.org/diseases-conditions/frozen-shoulder/symptoms-causes/syc-20372684.
5. Alzheimer's Association. *Alzheimer's Disease Facts and Figures*. Alzheimer's Association; 2021. https://www.alz.org/alzheimers-dementia/facts-figures.
6. Mayo Clinic. *Alzheimer's Disease*. Mayo Clinic; 2022. https://www.mayoclinic.org/diseases-conditions/alzheimers-disease/symptoms-causes/syc-20350447.
7. NIH. Amyotrophic lateral sclerosis (ALS) fact sheet. *National Institute of Neurological Disorders and Stroke, 2020*. Retrieved July 1, 2024. https://www.ninds.nih.gov/health-information/patient-caregiver-education/fact-sheets/amyotrophic-lateral-sclerosis-als-fact-sheet.
8. Mayo Clinic. *Amyotrophic Lateral Sclerosis (ALS)*. Mayo Clinic; 2022. https://www.mayoclinic.org/diseases-conditions/amyotrophic-lateral-sclerosis/symptoms-causes/syc-20354022.
9. WHO. *Anaemia*. World Health Organization; 2021. https://www.who.int/health-topics/anaemia.
10. American Heart Association. *Angina Pectoris*. American Heart Association; 2022. https://www.heart.org/en/health-topics/angina.
11. Mayo Clinic. *Angina Pectoris*. Mayo Clinic; 2022. https://www.mayoclinic.org/diseases-conditions/angina/symptoms-causes/syc-20369373.
12. American Heart Association. *Aortic Valve Stenosis*. American Heart Association; 2022. https://www.heart.org/en/health-topics/aortic-valve-stenosis.
13. Mayo Clinic. Anorexia nervosa. *Mayo Clinic*, 2018. Retrieved July 2, 2024. Anorexia nervosa - Symptoms and causes - Mayo Clinic
14. Mayo Clinic. *Aortic Valve Stenosis*. Mayo Clinic; 2022. https://www.mayoclinic.org/diseases-conditions/aortic-valve-stenosis/symptoms-causes/syc-20353129.
15. NIDCD. Aphasia. *National Institute on Deafness and Other Communication Disorders, 2017*. Retrieved July 1, 2024. https://www.nidcd.nih.gov/health/aphasia.
16. Biomed. Broca's Area & Wernicke's Area: Speech and Language Comprehension. *Biomed Guide, 2024*. Retrieved July 1, 2024. Broca's Area & Wernicke's Area: Speech and Language - Biomed Guide.
17. Mayo Clinic. *Appendicitis*. Mayo Clinic; 2021. https://www.mayoclinic.org/diseases-conditions/appendicitis/symptoms-causes/syc-20369543.
18. American Heart Association. *Atrial Septal Defect (ASD)*. American Heart Association; 2021. https://www.heart.org/en/health-topics/congenital-heart-defects/about-congenital-heart-defects/atrial-septal-defect-asd.
19. Mayo Clinic. *Osteoarthritis*. Mayo Clinic; 2022. https://www.mayoclinic.org/diseases-conditions/osteoarthritis/symptoms-causes/syc-20351925.
20. Mayo Clinic. *Rheumatoid Arthritis*. Mayo Clinic; 2021. https://www.mayoclinic.org/diseases-conditions/rheumatoid-arthritis/symptoms-causes/syc-20353648.
21. AAOS. *Hip Replacement*. American Academy of Orthopaedic Surgeons; 2020. https://orthoinfo.aaos.org/en/treatment/hip-replacement/.
22. AAOS. *Shoulder Replacement Surgery*. American Academy of Orthopaedic Surgeons; 2021. https://orthoinfo.aaos.org/en/treatment/shoulder-replacement-surgery/.
23. NHLBI. *Asthma*. National Heart, Lung, and Blood Institute; 2022. https://www.nhlbi.nih.gov/health-topics/asthma.
24. CDC. *Autism Spectrum Disorder (ASD)*. Centers for Disease Control and Prevention; 2021. https://www.cdc.gov/ncbddd/autism/facts.html.
25. Cleveland Clinic. *Bipolar Disorder*. Cleveland Clinic; 2022. Bipolar Disorder (Manic Depression): Symptoms & Treatment (clevelandclinic.org).
26. Johns Hopkins. *Borderline Personality Disorder*. Johns Hopkins Medicine; 2024. Borderline Personality Disorder | Johns Hopkins Medicine.
27. Mayo Clinic. *Bulimia Nervosa*. Mayo Clinic; 2024. Bulimia nervosa - Symptoms and causes - Mayo Clinic.
28. AHA. *Cardiac Arrest*. American Heart Association; 2022. https://www.heart.org/en/health-topics/cardiac-arrest.

29. Mayo Clinic. *Cardiac Arrest.* Mayo Clinic; 2022. https://www.mayoclinic.org/diseases-conditions/sudden-cardiac-arrest/symptoms-causes/syc-20350634.
30. Skin Cancer Foundation. *Basal Cell Carcinoma.* Skin Cancer Foundation; 2021. https://www.skincancer.org/skin-cancer-information/basal-cell-carcinoma/.
31. Mayo Clinic. *Merkel Cell Carcinoma.* Mayo Clinic; 2022. Merkel cell carcinoma - Symptoms and causes - Mayo Clinic.
32. ACS. *Merkel Cell Carcinoma.* American Cancer Society; 2021. https://www.cancer.org/cancer/merkel-cell-skin-cancer.html.
33. Skin Cancer Foundation. *Squamous Cell Carcinoma.* Skin Cancer Foundation; 2021. https://www.skincancer.org/skin-cancer-information/squamous-cell-carcinoma/.
34. ACS. *Squamous Cell Carcinoma.* American Cancer Society; 2021. https://www.cancer.org/cancer/squamous-cell-skin-cancer.html.
35. CDC. *Cerebral Palsy (CP).* Centers for Disease Control and Prevention; 2020. https://www.cdc.gov/ncbddd/cp/facts.html.
36. Horne B. *Understanding Spastic Diplegia Cerebral Palsy.* Medical News Today; 2023. What is spastic diplegia cerebral palsy? (medicalnewstoday.com).
37. Cleveland Clinic. *Cerebral Palsy.* Cleveland Clinic; 2023. Cerebral Palsy: What It Is, Causes, Symptoms & Treatment (clevelandclinic.org).
38. NIH. What are the types of cerebral palsy? *Eunice Kennedy Shriver National Institute of Child Health and Human Development, 2021.* Retrieved July 2, 2024. What are the types of cerebral palsy? | NICHD - Eunice Kennedy Shriver National Institute of Child Health and Human Development (nih.gov)
39. ASA. Stroke. American Stroke Association, 2021. Retrieved July 2, 2024. https://www.stroke.org/en/about-stroke
40. NIDDKD. *Gallstones (Cholelithiasis).* National Institute of Diabetes and Digestive and Kidney Diseases; 2021. https://www.niddk.nih.gov/health-information/digestive-diseases/gallstones.
41. NHLBI. *COPD.* National Heart, Lung, and Blood Institute; 2022. https://www.nhlbi.nih.gov/health-topics/copd.
42. ACS. *Cholangiocarcinoma (Bile Duct Cancer).* American Cancer Society; 2021. https://www.cancer.org/cancer/bile-duct-cancer.html.
43. Mayo Clinic. *Congestive Heart Failure.* Mayo Clinic; 2022. https://www.mayoclinic.org/diseases-conditions/heart-failure/symptoms-causes/syc-20373142.
44. AHA. *Congestive Heart Failure.* American Heart Association; 2022. https://www.heart.org/en/health-topics/congestive-heart-failure.
45. WHO. *Coronavirus Disease (COVID-19).* World Health Organization; 2024. https://www.who.int/health-topics/coronavirus#tab=tab_1.
46. Crohn's & Colitis. *What is Crohn's Disease?.* The Crohn's and Colitis Foundation; 2024. https://www.crohnscolitisfoundation.org/patientsandcaregivers/what-is-crohns-disease.
47. Mayo Clinic. *Cystic Fibrosis.* Mayo Clinic; 2024. https://www.mayoclinic.org/diseases-conditions/cystic-fibrosis/symptoms-causes/syc-20353700.
48. Douketis, J.D. Deep venous thrombosis (DVT). *Merck Manual: Professional Version*, 2023. Retrieved June 10, 2024. https://www.merckmanuals.com/professional/cardiovascular-disorders/peripheral-venous-disorders/deep-venous-thrombosis-dvt.
49. Waheed SM, Kudaravalli P, Hotwagner DT. *Deep Vein Thrombosis.* Stats Pearls: National Library of Medicine, NIH; 2023. https://www.ncbi.nlm.nih.gov/books/NBK507708/.
50. Cleveland Clinic. *Dehydration.* Cleveland Clinic; 2023. https://my.clevelandclinic.org/health/diseases/9013-dehydration.
51. Mayo Clinic. *Dementia.* Mayo Clinic; 2024. Dementia - Symptoms and causes - Mayo Clinic.
52. Mayo Clinic. *Diabetes insipidus.* Mayo Clinic, 2023. Retrieved June 12, 2024. https://www.mayoclinic.org/diseases-conditions/diabetes-insipidus/symptoms-causes/syc-20351269 Diabetes insipidus - Symptoms and causes - Mayo Clinic.
53. Sapra, A., Bhandari, P. *Diabetes.* NIH: State Pearls, 2023. Retrieved June 12, 2024. https://www.ncbi.nlm.nih.gov/books/NBK551501/. Diabetes - StatPearls - NCBI Bookshelf (nih.gov).
54. Mayo Clinic. *Diabetes.* Mayo Clinic, 2024. Retrieved June 12, 2024. https://www.mayoclinic.org/diseases-conditions/diabetes/symptoms-causes/syc-20371444. Diabetes - Symptoms and causes - Mayo Clinic.
55. Basina, M. *Warning signs and treatment options for insulin shock.* Healthline, 2020. Retrieved June 13, 2024. https://www.healthline.com/health/diabetes/insulin-shock. Insulin Shock: Warning Signs and Treatment Options (healthline.com).
56. CDC. Down Syndrome. Centers for Disease Control: Birth Defects, 2024. Retrieved June 13, 2024. Down Syndrome | Birth Defects | CDC.
57. Cleveland Clinic. Ectopic Pregnancy. Cleveland Clinic; 2023. Ectopic Pregnancy: Causes, Symptoms & Treatments (clevelandclinic.org).
58. Mayo Clinic. Encephalitis. Mayo Clinic, 2024. Retrieved June 13, 2024. Encephalitis - Symptoms and causes - Mayo Clinic.
59. Johns Hopkins. *Endocarditis.* Johns Hopkins: Health; 2024. Endocarditis | Johns Hopkins Medicine.
60. Taylor M, Jenkins SM, Pillarisetty LS. *Endometritis.* NIH: Stats Pearls; 2023. Endometritis - StatPearls - NCBI Bookshelf (nih.gov).
61. Johns Hopkins. *Endometriosis.* Johns Hopkins: Health; 2024. Endometriosis | Johns Hopkins Medicine.
62. Cleveland Clinic. *Steatotic (Fatty) Liver Disease.* Cleveland Clinic; 2023. Steatotic (Fatty) Liver Disease: Symptoms & Treatment (clevelandclinic.org).
63. Mayo Clinic. *Fetal Alcohol Syndrome.* Mayo Clinic; 2024. Fetal alcohol syndrome - Diagnosis and treatment - Mayo Clinic.
64. Cleveland Clinic. *Fetal Alcohol Syndrome.* Cleveland Clinic; 2022. Fetal Alcohol Syndrome (FAS): Symptoms, Causes & Treatment (clevelandclinic.org.
65. Mayo Clinic. *Folate (Folic Acid).* Mayo Clinic; 2023. Folate (folic acid) - Mayo Clinic.
66. DerSarkissian C. *What is Folic Acid Deficiency Anemia?.* WebMD; 2022. Folic Acid Deficiency Anemia (Low Folate): Causes, Symptoms, Treatment (webmd.com).
67. Kahn KM, Jialal I. *Folic Acid Deficiency, NIH: National Center for Biotechnology Information.* StatPearls; 2023. Folic Acid Deficiency - StatPearls - NCBI Bookshelf (nih.gov).
68. Chavoustle CT. *Everything You Need to Know About Acid Reflux and GERD.* Health Line; 2024. GERD (Acid Reflux): Symptoms, Treatment, Causes and More (healthline.com).
69. Physiopedia, Shoulder instability, Physiopedia, 2024. Retrieved June 13, 2024. Shoulder Instability - Physiopedia (physio-pedia.com).
70. Mayo Clinic. *Shoulder Instability.* Mayo Clinic: Orthopedics and Sports Medicine; 2024. Shoulder instability - Overview - Mayo Clinic Orthopedics & Sports Medicine.
71. Cleveland Clinic. *Kidney Failure.* Cleveland Clinic; 2023. Kidney Failure: Causes, Symptoms & Treatment (clevelandclinic.org).
72. Smith M, Mitchell K. *Glomerular Filtration Rate (GFR): What to Know.* WebMD; 2024. Estimated Glomerular Filtration Rate (GFR) Test for Your Kidneys (webmd.com).

73. Wexler M. *Types of Hemophilia*. Hemophilia News Today; 2023. Types of hemophilia | Hemophilia News Today.
74. Mayo Clinic. *Hemophilia*. Mayo Clinic: Orthopedics and Sports Medicine; 2024. Hemophilia - Symptoms and causes - Mayo Clinic.
75. Cleveland Clinic. *Kidney Failure*. Cleveland Clinic; 2023. Hepatic Encephalopathy: Symptoms, Causes, Grading & Treatment (clevelandclinic.org).
76. Kahn A. *Hepatitis*. Health Line; 2023. Hepatitis: What Is It? Types, Symptoms, Causes, and More (healthline.com).
77. Tholey D. *Hepatocellular Carcinoma*. Merck Manual; 2023. Hepatocellular Carcinoma - Liver and Gallbladder Disorders - Merck Manual Consumer Version (merckmanuals.com).
78. Cleveland Clinic. *HPV (Human Papillomavirus)*. Cleveland Clinic; 2022. HPV (Human Papillomavirus): Causes, Symptoms & Treatment (clevelandclinic.org).
79. Mayo Clinic. HIV/AIDS. *Mayo Clinic: Diseases and Conditions*, 2024. Retrieved June 13, 2024 HIV/AIDS - Symptoms and causes - Mayo Clinic.
80. NIH. *Huntington's Disease*. NIH: National Institute of Neurological Disorders and Stroke; 2023. Huntington's Disease | National Institute of Neurological Disorders and Stroke (nih.gov).
81. Swiner CN. *What is Hypocalcemia?*. WebMD; 2023. Hypocalcemia: Symptoms, Causes, Treatments, and more (webmd.com).
82. Cleveland Clinic. *Hypokalemia*. Cleveland Clinic; 2022. Low Potassium Level Causes (Hypokalemia) (clevelandclinic.org).
83. Mayo Clinic Staff. *Hyponatremia*. Mayo Clinic; 2022. https://www.mayoclinic.org/diseases-conditions/hyponatremia/symptoms-causes/syc-20373711.
84. MedicalNewsToday. *What to Know About Hypoproteinemia*. MedicalNewsToday; 2024. https://www.medicalnewstoday.com/articles/320050.
85. Fowler P, Seed S. *What is Hyperlipidemia?*. WebMD; 2024. https://www.webmd.com/cholesterol-management/hyperlipidemia-overview.
86. CDC. *High Blood Pressure*. Centers for Disease Control and Prevention; 2024. https://www.cdc.gov/bloodpressure/index.htm.
87. Mayo Clinic Staff. *Hyperthyroidism (Overactive Thyroid)*. Mayo Clinic; 2022. https://www.mayoclinic.org/diseases-conditions/hyperthyroidism/symptoms-causes/syc-20373659.
88. Mayo Clinic Staff. *Hypothyroidism (Underactive Thyroid)*. Mayo Clinic; 2022. https://www.mayoclinic.org/diseases-conditions/hypothyroidism/symptoms-causes/syc-20350284.
89. John Hopkins. *Inflammatory Bowel Disease (IBD)*. John Hopkins Medicine: Health; 2024. https://www.hopkinsmedicine.org/health/conditions-and-diseases/inflammatory-bowel-disease.
90. John Hopkins. *Irritable Bowel Syndrome (IBS)*. John Hopkins Medicine: Health; 2024. https://www.hopkinsmedicine.org/health/conditions-and-diseases/irritable-bowel-syndrome-ibs.
91. Cleveland Clinic. *Iodine Deficiency*. Cleveland Clinic: Diseases & Conditions; 2022. https://my.clevelandclinic.org/health/diseases/23417-iodine-deficiency.
92. John Hopkins. *Kaposi Sarcoma*. John Hopkins Medicine: Health; 2024. https://www.hopkinsmedicine.org/health/conditions-and-diseases/sarcoma/kaposi-sarcoma.
93. Benjamin O, Lappin SL. *Kwashiorkor*. NIH: StatPearls; 2023. https://www.ncbi.nlm.nih.gov/books/NBK507876/.
94. Mayo Clinic Staff. *Leukemia*. Mayo Clinic; 2022. https://www.mayoclinic.org/diseases-conditions/leukemia/symptoms-causes/syc-20374373.
95. Cleveland Clinic. *High White Blood Cell Count*. Cleveland Clinic: Diseases & Conditions; 2022. https://my.clevelandclinic.org/health/diseases/17704-high-white-blood-cell-count.
96. Cleveland Clinic. *Low White Blood Cell Count (leukopenia)*. Cleveland Clinic: Diseases & Conditions; 2022. https://my.clevelandclinic.org/health/diseases/17706-low-white-blood-cell-count.
97. Mayo Clinic. *Cirrhosis*. Mayo Clinic; 2022. https://www.mayoclinic.org/diseases-conditions/cirrhosis/symptoms-causes/syc-20351487.
98. Mayo Clinic Staff. *Liver Disease*. Mayo Clinic: Diseases & Conditions; 2024. https://www.mayoclinic.org/diseases-conditions/liver-problems/symptoms-causes/syc-20374502.
99. CDC. Long COVID basics. *CDC: COVID-19*, 2024. Retrieved June 26, 2024. https://www.cdc.gov/coronavirus/2019-ncov/long-term-effects/index.html.
100. Cleveland Clinic. Long COVID. *Cleveland Clinic: Disease & Conditions*, 2023. Retrieved June 26, 2024. https://my.clevelandclinic.org/health/diseases/25111-long-covid.
101. Mayo Clinic. *Lung Cancer*. Mayo Clinic: Diseases & Conditions; 2024. https://www.mayoclinic.org/diseases-conditions/lung-cancer/symptoms-causes/syc-20374620.
102. American Cancer Society. *What is Lung Cancer*. American Cancer Society: About Lung Cancer; 2024. https://www.cancer.org/cancer/types/lung-cancer/about/what-is.html.
103. Mayo Clinic. *Depression (Major Depressive Disorder)*. Mayo Clinic; 2022. Depression (major depressive disorder) - Symptoms and causes - Mayo Clinic.
104. Mayo Clinic Staff. *Melanoma*. Mayo Clinic: Diseases & Conditions; 2023. https://www.mayoclinic.org/diseases-conditions/melanoma/symptoms-causes/syc-20374884.
105. Cleveland Clinic. *Metabolic Acidosis*. Cleveland Clinic: Disease & Conditions; 2022. https://my.clevelandclinic.org/health/diseases/24492-metabolic-acidosis.
106. Cleveland Clinic. *Metabolic Alkalosis*. Cleveland Clinic: Disease & Conditions; 2021. https://my.clevelandclinic.org/health/diseases/21529-metabolic-alkalosis.
107. Mayo Clinic Staff. *Metabolic Syndrome*. Mayo Clinic: Diseases & Conditions; 2021. https://www.mayoclinic.org/diseases-conditions/metabolic-syndrome/symptoms-causes/syc-20351916.
108. Mayo Clinic Staff. *Mitral Valve Prolapse*. Mayo Clinic: Diseases & Conditions; 2024. https://www.mayoclinic.org/diseases-conditions/mitral-valve-prolapse/symptoms-causes/syc-20355446.
109. Mayo Clinic Staff. *Multiple Myeloma*. Mayo Clinic: Diseases & Conditions; 2023. https://www.mayoclinic.org/diseases-conditions/multiple-myeloma/symptoms-causes/syc-20353378.
110. Cleveland Clinic. *Multiple Sclerosis (MS)*. Cleveland Clinic: Disease & Conditions; 2024. https://my.clevelandclinic.org/health/diseases/17248-multiple-sclerosis.
111. Mayo Clinic Staff. *Heart Attack*. Mayo Clinic: Diseases & Conditions; 2023. https://www.mayoclinic.org/diseases-conditions/heart-attack/symptoms-causes/syc-20373106.
112. Cleveland Clinic. *Median Nerve*. Cleveland Clinic: Disease & Conditions; 2021. https://my.clevelandclinic.org/health/body/21889-median-nerve.
113. Cleveland Clinic. *Radial Nerve*. Cleveland Clinic: Disease & Conditions; 2024. https://my.clevelandclinic.org/health/body/21617-radial-nerve.
114. Cleveland Clinic. *Ulnar Nerve*. Cleveland Clinic: Disease & Conditions; 2021. https://my.clevelandclinic.org/health/body/21664-ulnar-nerve.
115. Cleveland Clinic. *Obsessive-Compulsive Disorder (OCD)*. Cleveland Clinic; 2022. OCD (Obsessive-Compulsive Disorder): Symptoms & Treatment (clevelandclinic.org).
116. Mayo Clinic Staff. *Orthostatic Hypotension (Postural Hypotension)*. Mayo Clinic; 2022. https://www.mayoclinic.org/diseases-conditions/orthostatic-hypotension/symptoms-causes/syc-20352548.

117. Cleveland Clinic. *Osteopenia*. Cleveland Clinic: Disease & Conditions; 2024. https://my.clevelandclinic.org/health/diseases/21855-osteopenia.
118. Cleveland Clinic. *Osteoporosis*. Cleveland Clinic; 2023. Osteoporosis: Symptoms, Causes and Treatment (clevelandclinic.org).
119. Mayo Clinic. *Pancreatic Cancer*. Mayo Clinic: Diseases and Conditions; 2024. Pancreatic cancer - Symptoms and causes - Mayo Clinic.
120. NIH. *Parkinson's Disease: Causes, Symptoms, and Treatments*. NIH: National Institute on Aging; 2022. Parkinson's Disease: Causes, Symptoms, and Treatments | National Institute on Aging (nih.gov).
121. AHA. *Patent Ductus Arteriosus (PDA)*. American Heart Association; 2024. Patent Ductus Arteriosus (PDA) | American Heart Association.
122. Watson S. *Pelvic Inflammatory Disease (PID): What Is It?*. WebMD; 2024. Pelvic Inflammatory Disease (PID): Symptoms, Causes, & Treatment (webmd.com).
123. Johns Hopkins. *Stomach and Duodenal Ulcers (Peptic Ulcers)*. Johns Hopkins: Health; 2024. Stomach and Duodenal Ulcers (Peptic Ulcers) | Johns Hopkins Medicine.
124. Mayo Clinic. *Pericarditis*. Mayo Clinic: Diseases and Conditions; 2024. Pericarditis - Symptoms and causes - Mayo Clinic.
125. Gul F, Janzer SF. *Peripheral Vascular Disease*. NIH: National Center for Biotechnology Information, Stat Pearls; 2023. Peripheral Vascular Disease - StatPearls - NCBI Bookshelf (nih.gov).
126. Cleveland Clinic. *Venous Disease*. Cleveland Clinic; 2023. Venous Disease: Types, Symptoms & Treatment (clevelandclinic.org).
127. Vaqar S, Shackelford KB. *Pernicious Anemia*. NIH: National Center for Biotechnology Information, Stat Pearls; 2023. Pernicious Anemia - StatPearls - NCBI Bookshelf (nih.gov).
128. Cleveland Clinic. *Pneumonia*. Cleveland Clinic; 2022. Pneumonia: Causes, Symptoms, Diagnosis & Treatment (clevelandclinic.org).
129. Cleveland Clinic. *Poikilocytosis*. Cleveland Clinic; 2023. Poikilocytosis: Causes, Symptoms & Treatment (clevelandclinic.org).
130. Mayo Clinic. *Polycythemia Vera*. Mayo Clinic: Diseases and Conditions; 2024. Polycythemia vera - Symptoms & causes - Mayo Clinic.
131. Mayo Clinic. *Post-Traumatic Stress Disorder (PTSD)*. Mayo Clinic; 2022. Post-traumatic stress disorder (PTSD) - Symptoms and causes - Mayo Clinic.
132. Mayo Clinic. *Primary Biliary Cholangitis*. Mayo Clinic: Diseases and Conditions; 2023. Primary biliary cholangitis - Symptoms and causes - Mayo Clinic.
133. Shaban D. *Psoriasis: Symptoms Causes, and Treatment*. WebMD; 2024. Psoriasis: Types, Causes, Symptoms, & Treatment (webmd.com).
134. Bull, T. Hountras, P. Pulmonary embolism (PE). *MDS Manual, 2023*. Retrieved June 20, 2024. Pulmonary Embolism (PE) - Lung and Airway Disorders - MSD Manual Consumer Version (msdmanuals.com).
135. Mayo Clinic. *Pulmonary Valve Stenosis*. Mayo Clinic: Diseases and Conditions; 2022. Pulmonary valve stenosis - Symptoms & causes - Mayo Clinic.
136. Cleveland Clinic. *Respiratory Acidosis*. Cleveland Clinic; 2023. Respiratory Acidosis: Causes, Symptoms & Treatment (clevelandclinic.org).
137. Cleveland Clinic. *Respiratory Alkalosis*. Cleveland Clinic; 2023. Respiratory Alkalosis: What Is It, Treatment & Prevention (clevelandclinic.org).
138. Case-Lo C. *Everything You Need to Know About Rhabdomyolysis*. Healthline; 2023. Rhabdomyolysis: Symptoms, Causes, Treatment, and More (healthline.com).
139. Mayo Clinic. *Rickets*. Mayo Clinic: Diseases and Conditions; 2021. Rickets - Symptoms & causes - Mayo Clinic.
140. Cleveland Clinic. *Rotator Cuff Tear*. Cleveland Clinic; 2023. Rotator Cuff Tear: Symptoms & Treatment (clevelandclinic.org).
141. Painter K. *Sarcoidosis*. WebMD; 2024. Sarcoidosis: Symptoms, Stages, Causes, and Treatment (webmd.com).
142. NAMI. *Schizoaffective Disorder*. National Alliance on Mental Illness; 2024. Schizoaffective Disorder | NAMI.
143. Mayo Clinic. *Schizophrenia*. Mayo Clinic; 2024. Schizophrenia - Symptoms and causes - Mayo Clinic.
144. Cleveland Clinic. *Scurvy*. Cleveland Clinic; 2022. Scurvy: Symptoms, Causes & Treatment (clevelandclinic.org).
145. Gotter A, Goldman L, Yetman D. *Shingles: Everything You Should Know*. Health Line; 2023. Shingles: Symptoms, Treatment, and Prevention (healthline.com).
146. Hersh E. *Shoulder Impingement*. Health Line; 2023. Shoulder Impingement: Symptoms, Causes, Treatment, and Exercises (healthline.com).
147. Mayo Clinic. *Sickle Cell Anemia*. Mayo Clinic: Diseases and Conditions; 2023. Sickle cell anemia - Symptoms & causes - Mayo Clinic.
148. Cleveland Clinic. *Social Anxiety Disorder*. Cleveland Clinic; 2022. Social Anxiety Disorder: Symptoms, Tests, Causes & Treatments (clevelandclinic.org).
149. Mayo Clinic. *Drug Addiction (Substance Use Disorder)*. Mayo Clinic; 2022. Drug addiction (substance use disorder) - Symptoms and causes - Mayo Clinic.
150. Mayo Clinic. *Syphilis*. Mayo Clinic: Diseases and Conditions; 2023. Syphilis - Symptoms and causes - Mayo Clinic.
151. Cleveland Clinic. *Lupus (Systemic Lupus Erythematosus)*. Cleveland Clinic; 2023. Lupus: Symptoms & Treatment (clevelandclinic.org).
152. AHA. *Tetralogy of Fallot*. American Heart Association; 2024. Tetralogy of Fallot | American Heart Association.
153. Mayo Clinic. *Thoracic Outlet Syndrome*. Mayo Clinic: Diseases and Conditions; 2024. Thoracic outlet syndrome - Symptoms and causes - Mayo Clinic.
154. Cleveland Clinic. *Thrombocytopenia*. Cleveland Clinic; 2022. Thrombocytopenia: Symptoms, Stages & Treatment (clevelandclinic.org).
155. Mayo Clinic. *Thrombocytosis*. Mayo Clinic; 2022. Thrombocytosis - Symptoms and causes - Mayo Clinic.
156. CDC. *Traumatic Brain Injury (TBI)*. Centers for Disease Control and Prevention; 2020. https://www.cdc.gov/traumaticbraininjury/index.html.
157. Shaban D. *Tuberculosis (TB): Causes, Symptoms, Treatment*. WebMD; 2023. Understanding Tuberculosis: Causes, Symptoms, and Treatment Options (webmd.com).
158. Mayo Clinic. *Ulcerative Colitis*. Mayo Clinic; 2022. Ulcerative colitis - Symptoms and causes - Mayo Clinic.
159. Kovacs JS, Whitbourne K. *Urinary Tract Infections (UTIs)*. WebMD; 2024. Urinary Tract Infection (UTI): Symptoms, Causes, Treatment (webmd.com).
160. Cleveland Clinic. *Ventricular Septal Defects (VSD)*. Cleveland Clinic; 2021. Ventricular Septal Defect (VSD): What Is It, Types, Causes & Symptoms (clevelandclinic.org).
161. Mayo Clinic. *Wilson's Disease*. Mayo Clinic; 2023. Wilson's disease - Symptoms and causes - Mayo Clinic.

Index

Note: Page numbers followed by *b* indicate boxes, *f* indicate figures, and *t* indicate tables.

R

S